Comprehensive
Review of Pathology

Second Edition

Dr. Sonam K. Pruthi
MD Pathology
Specialist Pathologist
Hindu Rao Hospital and NDMC Medical College
New Delhi-110007

PEEPEE PUBLISHERS AND DISTRIBUTORS (P) LTD.®

Comprehensive Review of Pathology

Published by
Pawaninder P. Vij and Anupam Vij

Peepee Publishers and Distributors (P) Ltd.
Head Office: 160, Shakti Vihar, Pitam Pura
Delhi-110 034 (India)

Correspondence Address:

7/31, First Floor, Ansari Road, Daryaganj
New Delhi-110002 (India)

Ph: 41512412, 23246245, 9811156083

e-mail: peepee160@yahoo.co.in

e-mail: peepee160@gmail.com

www.peepeepub.com

First Edition: **2016**
Second Edition: 2019

ISBN: 978-81-8445-263-1

This book is dedicated

to

my Loved ones

FOREWORD

Dr. Sonam Kumar Pruthi was my most sincere and hardworking postgraduate student during his MD Pathology training in Kasturba Medical College, Mangalore, Manipal University. It's my esteemed pleasure to write this foreword of his first book ***'Comprehensive Review of Pathology'***. This book is a well-structured and organized collection of skillfully drafted MCQs by the author, presented in a chapter-wise manner and based on 'Robbins and Cotran Pathologic Basis of Disease, 8th and 9th Edition'. The pathology MCQs of last 5 years AIIMS – New Delhi PG entrance exam, AIPGMEE and NEET have been amalgamated craftily in each chapter. Answers to the questions are justified with references from Robbins, Ackerman, WHO Classification of Tumors and Journals, as well as additionally supported by easy to remember tables and diagrams. Important topics in each chapter have been highlighted in the beginning of each chapter for the candidate to essentially focus on. Among an ocean of preparatory books and manuals for PG entrance exams, this books is unique in its mammoth collection of approximately 2000 MCQs of good standard, chapter-wise approach, along with simple and lucid explanations. This worthy compendium is definitely going to fill the longstanding void of a good preparatory book in pathology and the candidates will be truly benefited.

My heartfelt best wishes to Dr. Sonam Kumar Pruthi in his endeavor and God bless him with a roaring success.

Dr. Shrijeet Chakraborti
MD, DNB, PDF–Neuropath, DipRCPath, PGDEA, MNAMS
Specialty Doctor–Histopathology, Leighton Hospital, Crewe
Mid Cheshire Hospitals NHS Foundation Trust, Cheshire, United Kingdom
Ex-Associate Professor and In-Charge Blood Bank Department of Pathology
Kasturba Medical College, Mangalore
Manipal University, India

PREFACE TO THE FIRST EDITION

Why did I write this book?

During my MBBS days, and while preparing for postgraduate entrance exams, I always used to think and search for Pathology MCQ book, which would have been based on Robbins. During, end of my post-graduation course, I started writing it and slowly but steadily, I completed it after three years.

Brief description of the book:

Book is completely based on Robbins (8 ed. and 9th ed.) and the questions are made after going through each and every page, and the explanations are simple and up to the point, with references and diagrams (wherever must).

Explanations are kept short and point-wise, so that students can reproduce them easily during exams.

Why should you read this book?

Reading Robbins and recalling it is not an easy job, so I have given you to read MCQ based book on Robbins, which will reduce your time for preparing Pathology, so that you can concentrate on other remaining subjects.

In MD/DNB/FGMEE/DM/Fellowship/MBBS exams, MCQs are framed from individual lines of Robbins (refer past year MCQs).

Numerous books available in market, gives you pages of information, even for a single question, but as an MBBS graduate, one doesn't realize, what is important from exam point of view. In this book, I have provided you only important points to remember, and after being a post-graduate in same specialty, I know how the questions can be twisted and turned, to confuse students, so the same has been taken care of in making explanations.

MCQ books available in the market, will give you explanations paper-wise, here I provide you fresh bunch of MCQs (which will make your theory very strong) and also repeat MCQs of last five years (All India and AIIMS), and all this chapter-wise (because according to me, chapter-wise reading makes your concepts clear rather than reading different topics of different chapters at the same time).

How to read this book?

For MBBS students (2nd Prof.):

Simultaneously read each topic from Robbins (Pathologic Basis of Disease) and from this book and try to understand each MCQ (by ruling out each option), before coming to the final answer. This is the best possible way to gain maximum out of this book.

For Entrance exam preparation:

Revise this book thoroughly. Refer Robbins (Pathologic Basis of Disease) for figures and tables, given in references of the answers of this book. By doing this, you will save lots of your time, and you can gain maximum knowledge in less time.

How much time it took for me to complete this book?

It took me three years to write and finish this book, as I have to go through each page to frame new MCQs, to benefit you the most.

I started writing, referring 8th ed. Robbins, and after reaching mid-way; 9th ed. Robbins came into the market, so I have to go through for the first half again from the new edition and remaining half from both 8th and 9th ed.

So, it was not an easy journey, but the day, I decided to help students, I also decided, not to look back and so I stood firm with the decision of mine and finally, by God's grace, this book is in your hands to learn.

What I learned in writing this book?

I have learned a lot as an author. By referring multiple books for few questions and also reading the same topic from two different editions has improved my knowledge vastly about the subject.

Also, I am 100% confident and have firm belief that this book of mine will clear all your doubts regarding Pathology.

Have self-belief and you can do wonders in life!!

Your valuable suggestions to improve the book are always and most welcome.

PREFACE TO THE SECOND EDITION

After over-whelming response of first edition, I am happy to introduce the second edition of **"Comprehensive Review of Pathology"**. The book is more lucid in descriptions and includes recent postgraduate entrance exam questions and answers. The following points will help you to learn important things about the second edition of the book.

Why did I write this book?

During my MBBS days, and while preparing for postgraduate entrance exams, I always used to think and search for Pathology MCQ book, which would have been based on Robbins.

During, the near-end of my postgraduation course, I started writing it and slowly but steadily over the period of three years (2013-2016) the book was finally completed.

Brief description of the book

Book is based on Robbins (8th and 9th edition) and the questions are being made by me after going through each and every page of the textbook, and the explanations are simple and up to the point, with references, flowcharts and diagrams.

Explanations are kept short and point-wise, so that students can reproduce them easily during exams.

Why should you read this book?

Reading Robbins and recalling is a tough job, so I have given you one comprehensive MCQ based book based on Robbins, which will reduce your time for preparing Pathology.

In MD/DNB/FGMEE/DM/Fellowship entrance exams and in MBBS exams, each and every line of Robbins can be asked as MCQs.

In this book, I have provided you only important points to remember, and after being a postgraduate in same specialty, I know how the questions can be twisted and turned, to confuse students, and the same has been taken care of making explanations.

MCQ books available in the market, will give you explanations paper-wise, here I provide you fresh bunch of MCQ's (which will make your theory very strong) and also repeat MCQ's of last few years (NEET-PG and AIIMS), and all this is written chapter-wise.

How to read this book?

For MBBS students (2nd Prof.):

Simultaneously read each topic from Robbins (Pathologic basis of disease) and from this book and try to understand each MCQ (by ruling out each option), before coming to the final answer. This is the best possible way to gain maximum from this book.

For Postgraduate entrance exam preparation:

Revise this book thoroughly. Refer Robbins (Pathologic basis of disease) for figures and tables, given in references of the answers of this book. By doing this, you will save lots of your time, and you can gain maximum knowledge in less time.

For DM and fellowship entrance exam preparation:

Thorough knowledge of the book will be highly useful for DM Histopathology, DM Oncopathology, DM Hematooncology, DM Hematopathology entrance exams and also for various post-degree fellowship (PDF) entrance exams throughout India.

I am 100% confident and have firm belief that this book of mine will clear all your doubts regarding Pathology.

Have self-belief and you can do wonders in life!!

Your valuable suggestions to improve the book are always welcome.

Dr. Sonam Kumar Pruthi

Email: sonam_manipal@yahoo.com

ACKNOWLEDGEMENTS

I would like to express my gratitude to my teachers who saw me through this book.

I also want to thank my family for their unconditional love and immense support, which cannot be exemplified with words.

Last, but not the least I also want to thank, Mr. Pawaninder P. Vij and Mr. Anupam Vij, Directors, Peepee Publishers and Distributors (P) Ltd. for their hard work and efforts, which made publication of this book possible.

CONTENTS

ERRATA

1. **In chapter 1, page number 5, in explanation of answer 9, correct reference should be "refer to explanation of answer 8"**
2. **In chapter 5, correct answer of Q 58 on page 79 should be A: Prader-Willi syndrome**
3. **In chapter 8, correct answer of Q7 on page 126 should be A: CD8+T-cells**
4. **In chapter 13, correct answer of Q 71 on page 199 should be D. Mental retardation**
5. **In chapter 27, Q27 on page 380 should be read as: "All of the following features differentiate lymphoblasts from myeloblasts except"**
6. **In chapter 27, option A of Q 62 on page 382 should be read as A. t (11;14)**
7. **In chapter 29, correct answer to Q11 on page 452 should be B: Alcohol**

AIIMS November 2018

1. **Marker to differentiate mediastinal mass being a thymoma or ALL:**
(a) Cytokeratin (b) Tdt
(c) CD-3 (d) CD1a

2. **Which of the following vacutainer contain anti-metabolite sodium fluoride?**
(a) Blue (b) Gray
(c) Red (d) Black

3. **Identify the inheritance pattern in the pedigree chart given below:**

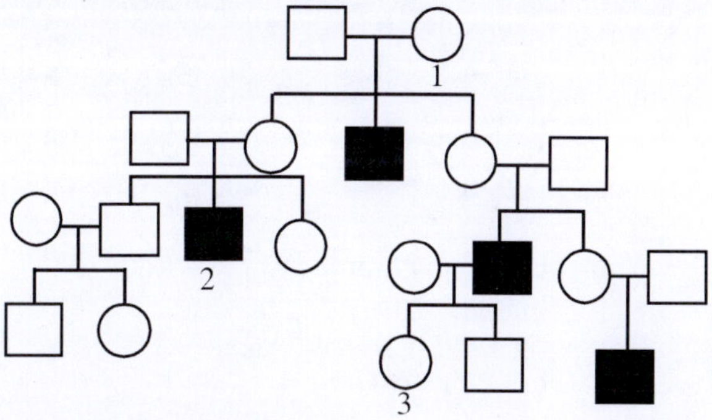

(a) X-linked recessive
(b) X-linked dominant
(c) Autosomal recessive
(d) Autosomal dominant

4. **Naïve T-cell gets activated by:**
(a) NK-cells (b) B-cells
(c) Macrophages (d) Dendritic cells

5. **A-50-year-old male presented with fever and retroperitoneal lymphadenopathy. Lymph node biopsy was done and the morphology of the lymph node is shown below. What does this histopathological image suggest?**
(a) Non-Hodgkin lymphoma
(b) Angiolymphoid hyperplasia with eosinophilia
(c) Castleman disease
(d) IgG4 related disease

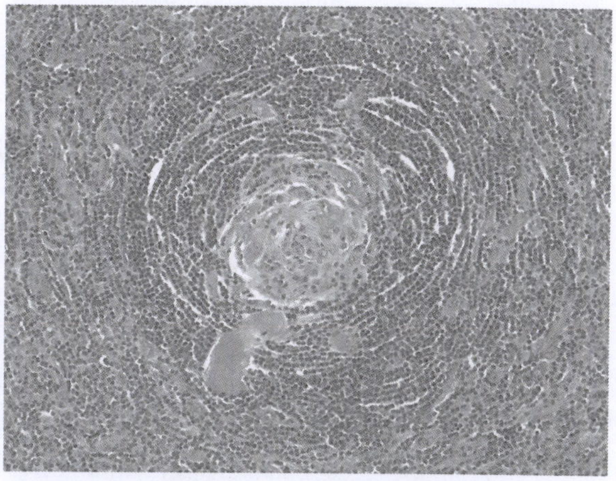

6. **Figure below demonstrates the following:**
(a) Phagocytosis (b) Killing
(c) Emperipolesis (d) Megakaryocyte

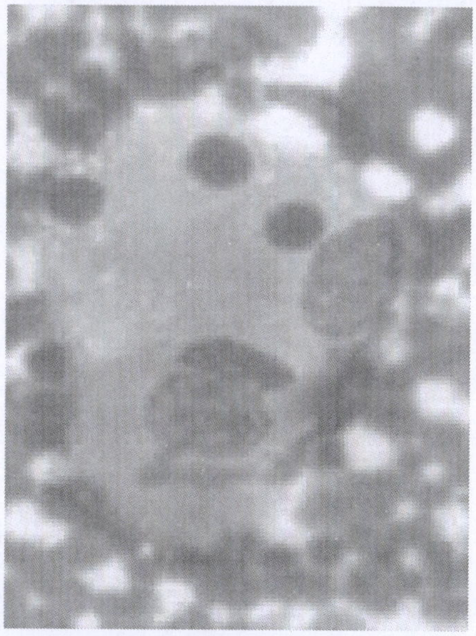

7. **False about apoptosis:**
(a) No inflammation
(b) Intact plasma membrane
(c) Affected by regulatory genes
(d) Cell swelling

8. **Fresh frozen plasma (FFP) of the following group can be given to the trauma patient, in emergency department when there is no time for cross matching?**
(a) O Rh-D+ (b) O Rh-D-
(c) AB Rh-D+ (d) AB Rh-D-

9. **Antibody dependent killing is mediated by:**
(a) NK-cells
(b) Neutrophils
(c) Macrophage
(d) NK-cell, neutrophils, macrophage

10. **Which of the following can recognize product of dead cells?**
(a) Inflammasome
(b) C-type lectin receptors
(c) Toll-like receptors
(d) Complement receptors

11. **Immune privileged site is:**
(a) Optic nerve (b) Seminiferous tubule
(c) Spinal cord (d) Area postrema

12. **Full house staining pattern on immuno-fluorescence is seen in:**
(a) Focal segmental glomerulosclerosis
(b) Post streptococcal glomerulonephritis
(c) SLE
(d) Good Pasteur's syndrome

13. **Diagnosis of which of the following cannot be made without the presence of antinuclear antibodies?**
(a) Scleroderma
(b) Sjogren's syndrome
(c) Drug induced lupus
(d) SLE

14. **Specific marker for alcoholic hepatitis is:**
(a) GGT (b) AST
(c) ALT (d) LDH

15. **An intern while collecting blood, split it over floor. What should be done next?**
(a) Mop the floor
(b) Put some absorbable material over it
(c) 1% sodium hypochlorite solution
(d) Inform hospital control board of hospital

16. **Identify the marked structure below:**

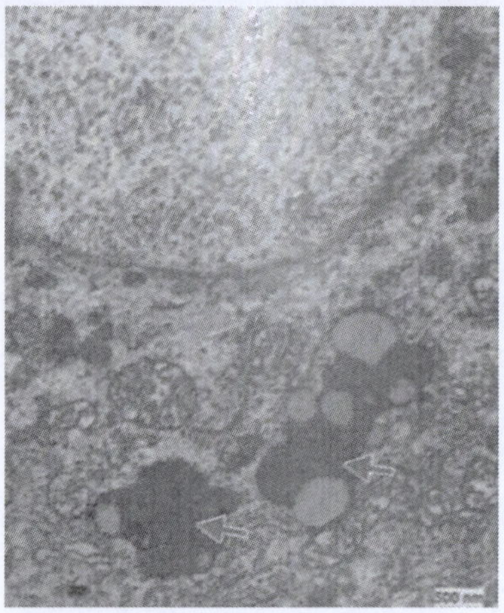

(a) Lipofuscin granules
(b) Lysosomes
(c) Secondary lysosomes
(d) Phagolysosome

AIIMS November 2018 – Answers

Ans: 1. **A. Cytokeratin**

- Cytokeratin is an epithelial marker and will be positive in thymoma and absent in lymphoma
- CD-1a is a marker of Langerhans cell
- CD-3 is T-cell marker

Note: To learn other markers, kindly refer to Q21-Q24 of chapter 27 of this book

Ans: 2. **B. Gray**

Different types of Vacutainer with their uses:

- Blue vacutainer has 3.2% tri-sodium citrate and is used for coagulation studies
- Red vacutainer is without anticoagulant and is used for serum studies
- Green vacutainer contains lithium heparin and is used for osmotic fragility tests, G-6PD deficiency tests, Arterial blood gas analysis, Pyruvate kinase deficiency tests
- Lavender vacutainer contains di-potassium EDTA and is used for routine hematological investigations
- Gray vacutainer contains di-potassium EDTA for blood glucose and has NaF as anti-metabolite
- Black vacutainer has 3.8% tri-sodium citrate and is used for ESR estimation studies

Ans: 3. **A. X-linked recessive**

Note: For details, kindly refer to chapter 5, Mendelian disorders section of this book

Ans: 4. **D. Dendritic cells**

Dendritic cells are the most potent stimulators of Naïve T-cells
Note: Also, refer to Q83 and Q101 of chapter 6 (Immunity) of this book

Ans: 5. **C. Castleman disease. Ref: Ackerman 11th edition, chapter 37, page 1554**

Two types of Castleman disease

(a) Hyaline vascular type:
- Lymphoid follicular hyperplasia with hyalinization of germinal centers
- Follicles at the periphery are surrounded by lymphocytes (onion-skin appearance)

(b) Plasma cell type:
- Follicular lymphoid hyperplasia without hyaline vascular changes
- In-between the follicles there is marked plasma cell infiltration

Clinical types:

1. **Solitary form**
   - Can present as mass in mediastinum, neck, mesentery, axilla, lung, retroperitoneum, soft tissues of extremities
2. **Multi-centric or systemic form**
   - Presents as generalized lymphadenopathy and involvement of spleen is common
   - Association with HHV-8 is seen

Ans: 6. **C. Emperipolesis**

- Figure shows one intact cell i.e. macrophage, ingesting another intact cell i.e. lymphocytes
- In phagocytosis the ingested cell is destroyed, which is not seen in emperipolesis

Ans: 7. **D. Cell swelling**

Note: For details, kindly refer to chapter 2, question number 7 of this book

Ans: 8. **C. AB Rh-D+**

- Universal Red cell donor – O negative (because type O blood has neither A nor B surface antigens and can donate blood cells to any other type)

- Universal red cell acceptor – AB positive
- Universal FFP donor – AB positive (because AB type FFP contains neither anti-A nor anti-B antibodies)
- Universal FFP acceptor – O-negative

Ans: 9. D. NK-cell, neutrophils, macrophage

Antibody dependent cell killing:

- Antibody mediated destruction of cells
- Cells that are coated with IgG antibody are killed by variety of cells which includes NK cells, macrophages, monocytes, neutrophils, dendritic cells

Ans: 10. A. Inflammasome

- Microbial products are recognized by Toll-like receptors
- C-type lectin receptors recognize fungal glycans
- RIG-like receptors recognize nucleic acid of viruses
- Inflammasome recognize products of dead cells and microbes and leads to secretion of IL-1
- Inflammasome is made up of a sensor protein (called NLRP3), an adapter, and enzyme caspase-1

Note: Also see Q2 of chapter 6 of this book

Ans: 11. B. Seminiferous tubule

Note: Refer Q23, chapter 6 of the book for details

Ans: 12. C. SLE

- Full house Immunofluorescence pattern is seen in patients of lupus nephritis
- Full house effect indicates that staining pattern for all five major Immunofluorescence stains i.e. IgG, IgM, IgA, C1q and C3 are positive
  Note: Refer Q29, Q30 of chapter 6 and portion of glomerular diseases of chapter 18 to learn about various disease entities including their Immunofluorescence and electron microscopic features

Ans: 13. D. SLE

- ANAs, are found in 100% of SLE patients, even though these are not specific for SLE
- Scleroderma patients show Anti-DNA topoisomerase-1 and Anti-centromeric proteins antibody positivity
- Sjögren syndrome patients show anti-Ro/SS-A and anti-La/SS-B antibody positivity
- Drug induced lupus: 80% of patients receiving Procainamide can show ANA positivity. Also, anti-histone antibody positivity is common in these patients

Ans: 14. A. GGT

- Alanine amino transferase (ALT): markedly elevated levels are seen in viral hepatitis, ischemic liver injury and toxin-induced liver damage
- Aspartate amino transferase (AST): elevated levels are seen in patients with cirrhosis
- AST/ALT ratio, greater than 2 is characteristically present in alcoholic hepatitis
- Gamma Glutamyl Transferase (GGT): elevated levels are seen in alcoholism and is the best indicator of excessive alcohol consumption

Ans: 15. B. Put some absorbable material over it

WHO guidelines for blood spillage

1. Wear a pair of gloves
2. Remove broken glass or container, if any, and discard it in sharps container
3. Use disposable paper towel to absorb spilled blood or body fluid
4. Wipe the area with water and detergent
5. Saturate the area with 0.5% sodium hypochlorite
6. Remove gloves and discard them
7. Wash hands with soap and water
8. Record the incident in the incident book if a specimen was lost, or if anyone was exposed to blood and body fluids

Ans: 16. A. Lipofuscin granules

- Lipofuscin is a brown perinuclear pigment

Note: Also refer to Q 23 of chapter 2 of this book for details

NEET PG December 2018

1. **Vitamin A is stored in:**
(a) Cells of ito (b) Hepatocyte
(c) Endothelial cell (d) Kupffer cell

2. **Glanzmann thrombasthenia is due to:**
(a) Decreased GpIb
(b) Decreased GpIIb/IIIa
(c) Anti-GpIIb/IIIa antibodies
(d) ADAMTS 13 deficiency

3. **Anti-apoptotic gene is:**
(a) Bax (b) Bcl-2
(c) Bcl-x (d) Mcl

4. **Alpha-1-antitrypsin works by:**
(a) Inhibition of trypsin
(b) Inhibition of trypsinogen
(c) Inhibition of elastase
(d) Inhibition of chymotrypsin

5. **Autosomal recessive disorder is:**
(a) Albinism
(b) Huntington's syndrome
(c) Marfan's syndrome
(d) Neurofibromatosis-1

6. **Fish mouth appearance of mitral valve in rheumatic heart disease is due to:**
(a) Rupture of valve
(b) Calcification and fibrosis
(c) Ventricular hypertrophy
(d) Any of the above

7. **Follicular lymphoma shows positivity of:**
(a) Bcl-1 (b) Bcl-6
(c) Bcl-2 (d) Bcl-x

8. **Best morphological difference's between ulcerative colitis and Crohn disease is:**
(a) Diffuse pseudo polyps
(b) Crypt abscess
(c) Mucosal edema
(d) Lymphoid aggregates

9. **Following is a cause of intravascular hemolysis:**
(a) PNH
(b) Sickle cell anemia
(c) Thalassemia
(d) Hereditary Spherocytosis

10. **Following type of necrosis is seen in blood vessels:**
(a) Fibrinoid (b) Caseous
(c) Coagulative (d) Ischemic

11. **In a patient with lipoprotein lipase deficiency, which of the following is increased following a fatty meal?**
(a) Chylomicron (b) LDL
(c) HDL (d) Apo-A

12. **Function of IL-1:**
(a) Increases hematopoiesis
(b) Mast cell stimulator
(c) Antibacterial properties
(d) Endogenous pyrogen

13. **IL-1 is activated by:**
(a) Caspase-1 (b) Caspase-3
(c) Caspase-8 (d) Caspase-5

14. **Benign mixed tumor of parotid is:**
(a) Pleomorphic adenoma
(b) Sebaceous adenoma
(c) Trichilemmal tumor
(d) Warthin's tumor

15. **Krabbe disease is due to deficiency of:**
(a) Beta-galactosylceramidase
(b) Aryl-sulphatase
(c) Alpha-galactosidase
(d) Acid lipase

16. **Treatment of Idiopathic thrombocytopenic purpura:**
(a) Blood transfusion
(b) Spontaneous recovery
(c) I.V. Fluids
(d) Splenectomy

NEET PG December 2018 – Answers

Ans: 1. **A.** Cells of ito
- Cells of Ito are also called as hepatic stellate cells
- Hepatic stellate cell in quiescent stage stores vitamin A

Note: Refer Q1, 6 and 7 of chapter 16 of this book, to learn more about stellate cells

Ans: 2. **B.** Decreased GpIIb/IIIa

Note: Refer Q 111 of chapter 28 of this book for details

Ans: 3. B. Bcl-2

Note: Refer Q16 of chapter 2 of this book

Ans: 4. **C.** Inhibition of elastase
- Function of alpha-1- antitrypsin is inhibition of neutrophilic elastase, cathepsin-G and proteinase 3

Note: Refer Q54 of chapter 16 of this book for details

Ans: 5. **A.** Albinism

Note: Refer Q6 of chapter 5 of this book

Ans: 6. **B.** Calcification and fibrosis

Note: refer Q27 of chapter 12 of this book

Ans: 7. **C.** Bcl-2

Note: Refer Q37 to Q39 of chapter 27 of this book

Ans: 8. **A.** Diffuse pseudopolyps
- In ulcerative colitis, there are no skip lesions thus there will be diffuse pseudopolyps whereas in Crohn's disease due to presence of skip lesions, pseudopdyps number is limited

Note: Refer Q 83-85 of chapter 15 of this book

Ans: 9. **A.** PNH

Note: Refer Q3-5 of chapter 28 of this book

Ans: 10. **A.** Fibrinoid

Note: Refer Q 9 of chapter 2 of this book for details

Ans: 11. **A.** Chylomicron
- LPLD (lipoprotein lipase deficiency) is caused by mutations in the LPL gene and is inherited in an autosomal recessive manner
- Deficiency of lipoprotein lipase results in accumulation of triglycerides in the plasma
- The clearance of chylomicrons is impaired and they appear in the bloodstream after ingestion of dietary fat
- Lipoprotein lipase recognizes a protein in chylomicrons called apo-lipoprotein C2
- Deficiency or lack of lipoprotein lipase results in the accumulation of chylomicrons and triglycerides

Ans: 12. **D.** Endogenous pyrogen

Note: Refer Q19 of chapter 3 of this book

Ans: 13. **A.** Caspase-1
- Nod-like receptors (NLRs) signal via inflammasome complex
- Inflammasome complex activate caspase-1
- Caspase-1 cleaves precursor form of IL-1 to active form of IL-1

Ans: 14. **A.** Pleomorphic adenoma

Note: refer Q 17 of chapter 14 of this book

Ans: 15. **A.** Beta-galactosylceramidase
- Krabbe disease is an autosomal recessive leukodystrophy
- Occurs due to the deficiency of beta-galactosidase (galactosylceramidase)
- Beta-galactosidase leads to catabolism of galactocerebroside to ceramide and galactose

Note: Refer Q 9 of chapter 26 of this book

Ans: 16. **D.** Splenectomy

Note: Refer Q 104, chapter 28 of this book

IMAGE BASED QUESTIONS

CHAPTER 2

1. **Following pathology of the lining epithelium is depicted in the figure:**

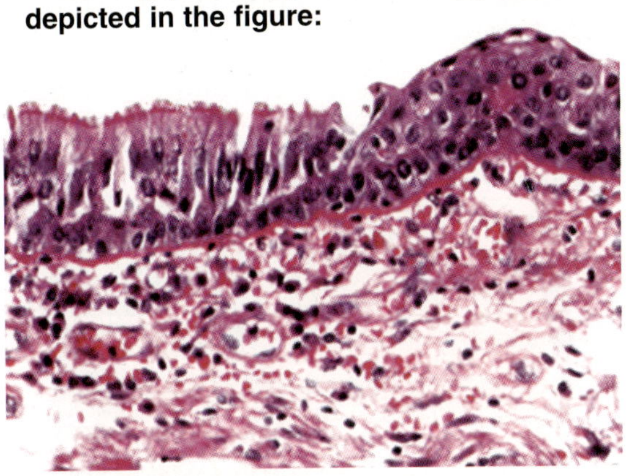

a) Metaplasia
b) Dysplasia
c) Carcinoma in situ
d) Tran-differentiation

2. **Infarct of the kidney due to obstruction of the vessel leads to following type of necrosis?**

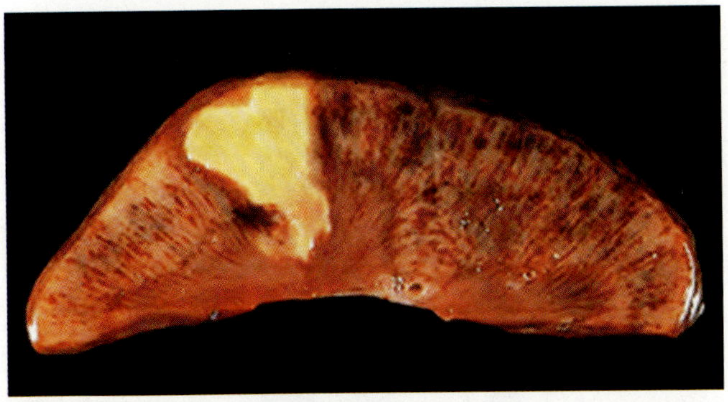

a) Coagulative necrosis
b) Caseous necrosis
c) Fibrinoid necrosis
d) Liquefactive necrosis

3. **Tuberculous infection of the lung parenchyma results in following necrosis:**

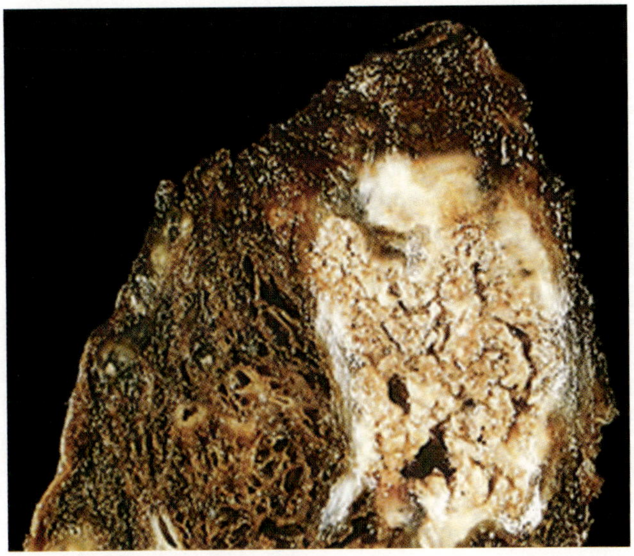

a) Caseous necrosis
b) Coagulative necrosis
c) Fibrinoid necrosis
d) Liquefactive necrosis

4. **Vasculitis of the vessel wall results in following pathology?**

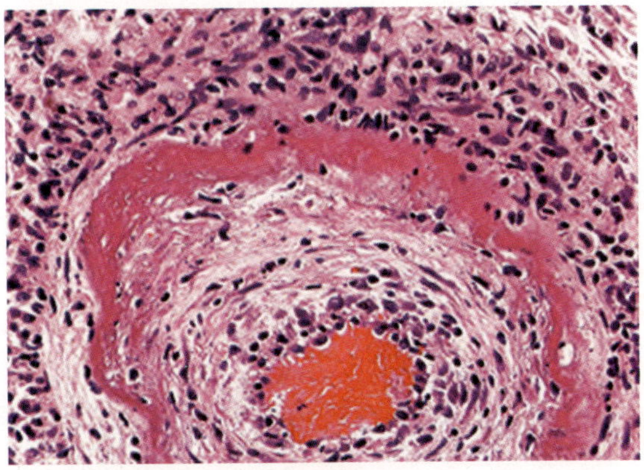

a) Fibrinoid necrosis
b) Caseous necrosis
c) Monckeberg's glomerulosclerosis
d) Hyaline arteriosclerosis

5. **Following pathology affects the pancreas:**

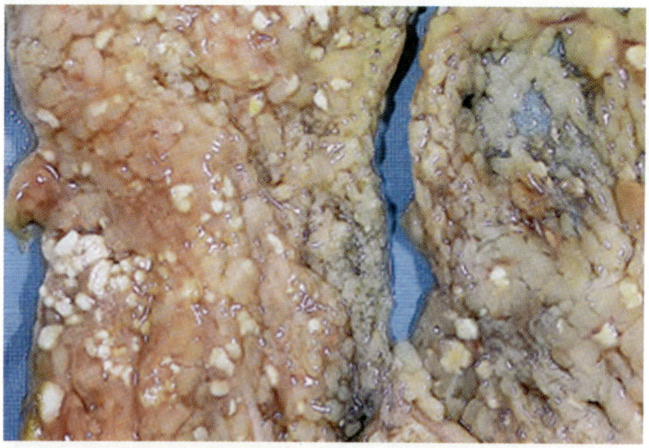

a) Fat saponification b) Tubercles
c) Bacterial abscesses d) Metastasis

6. **Figure below depicts:**

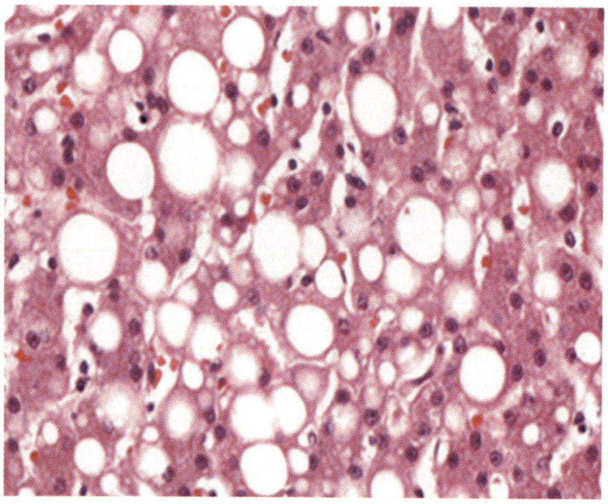

a) Steatosis b) Cirrhosis
c) Pancreatitis d) Signet ring cell carcinoma

CHAPTER 3

7. **Following figure gives a clue towards:**

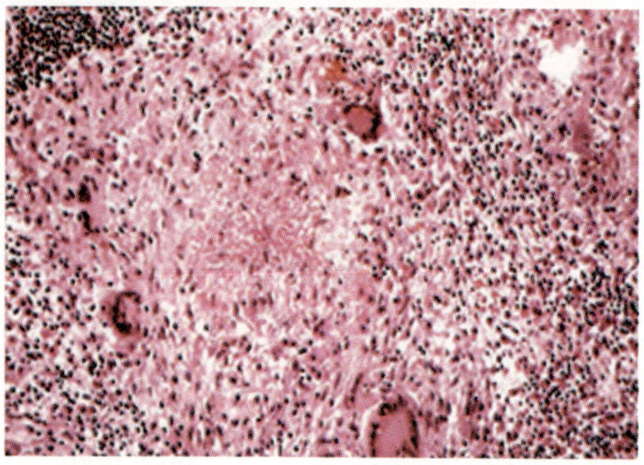

a) Tuberculosis b) Cat-Scratch disease
c) Berylliosis d) Sarcoidosis

CHAPTER 4

8. **Following is the appropriate term used for liver pathology as depicted in the figure.**

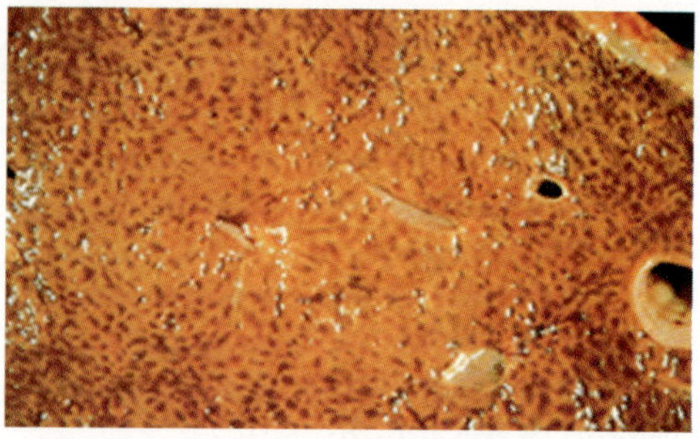

a) Hepatic necrosis b) Cirrhosis
c) Hepatitis d) Nutmeg liver

9. **Following consequence of Myocardial Infarction is seen grossly in heart?**

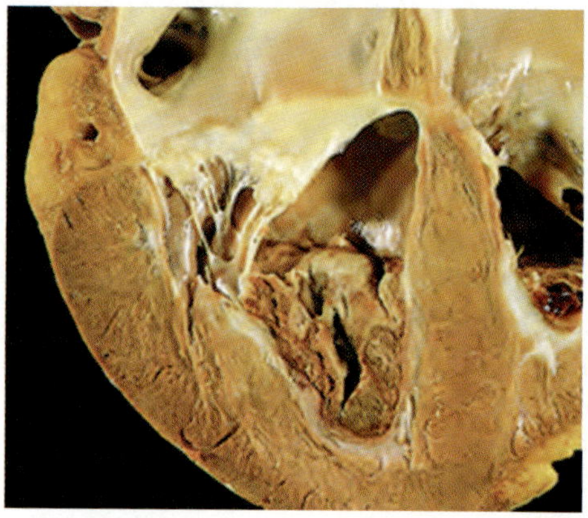

a) Mural thrombi b) Myocardial rupture
c) Papillary muscle tears d) Tendon rupture

10. **Following pathology is seen in the spleen below:**

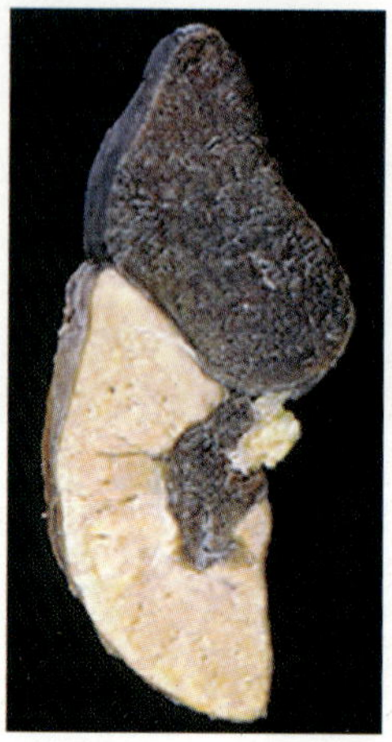

a) Red infarct b) White infarct
c) Caseous necrosis d) Septic infarct

CHAPTER 5

11. Following cell in the bone marrow suggests:

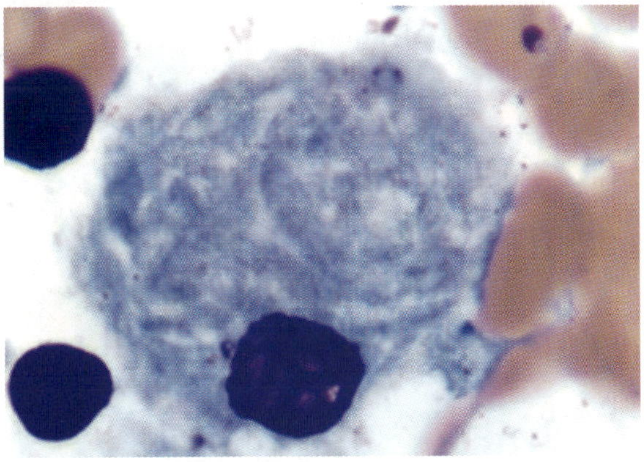

a) Gaucher's disease
b) Niemann-Pick disease
c) Tay-Sachs disease
d) Mucopolysaccharidoses

CHAPTER 6

12. Indirect immunofluorescence (shown in the figure) suggests the following anti-nuclear antibody:

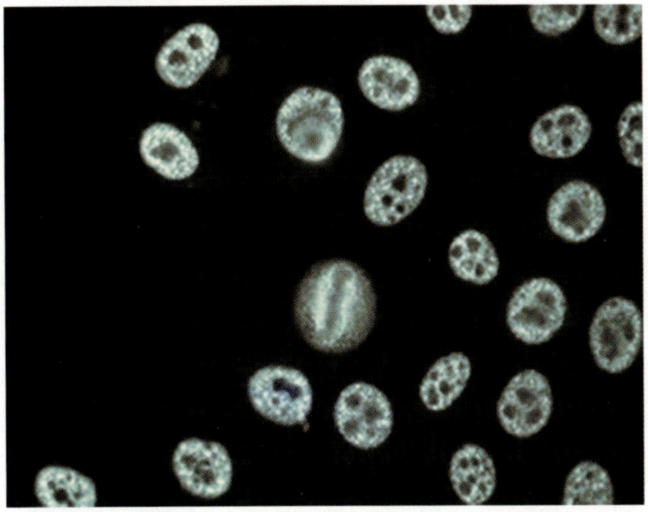

a) ds-DNA
b) Antibody to Sm antigen
c) Antibody to RNA
d) Ani-centromeric antibodies

13. Following figure depicts which type of Lupus nephritis?

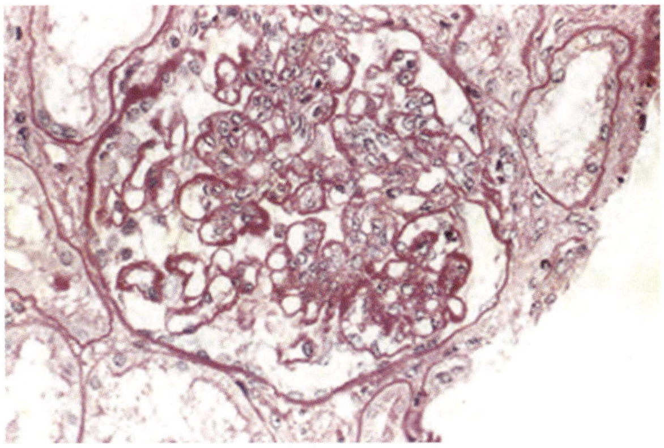

a) Class I
b) Class II
c) Class III
d) Class IV

14. Vegetations seen on the valves of heart are seen characteristically in:

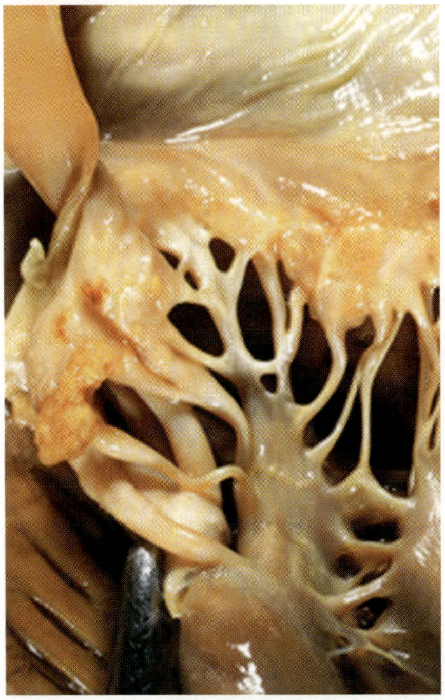

a) Infective endocarditis
b) Libman-Sack's endocarditis
c) Rheumatic heart disease
d) Non-Bacterial endocarditis

15. **Which stain shows green birefringence in liver biopsy:**

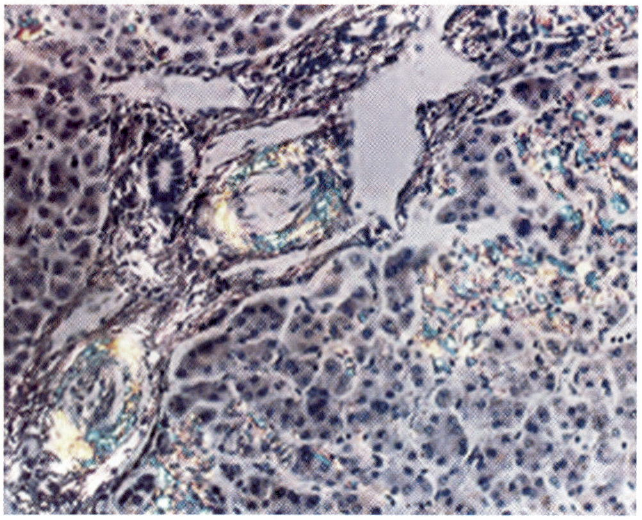

a) Congo-Red b) Hematoxylin & Eosin
c) Geimsa d) Pap stain

CHAPTER 7

16. **Following figure depicts:**

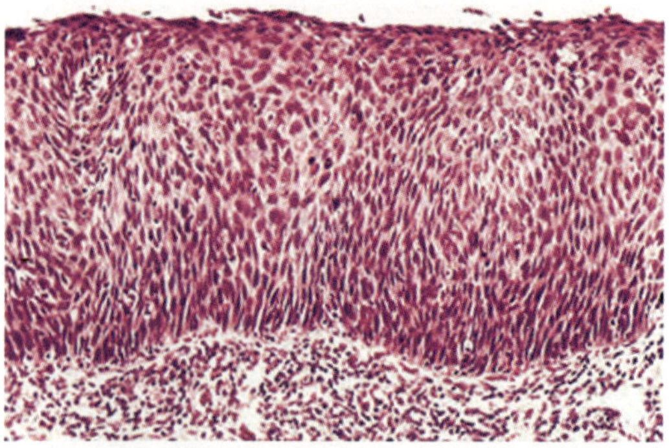

a) Carcinoma in-situ
b) Microinvasive cancer
c) Squamous cell carcinoma
d) Adenocarcinoma

17. **Figure depicts following pathology in liver:**

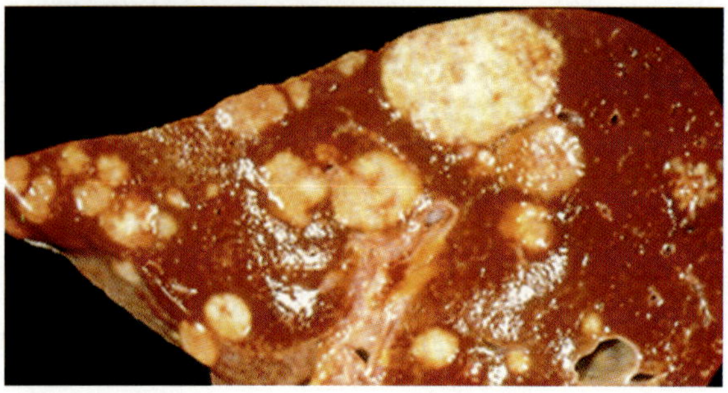

a) Metastasis b) Tubercles
c) Abscess d) Parasitic cyst

CHAPTER 9

18. **Multinucleate cells in lung biopsy with glassy eosinophilic intra-nuclear inclusions suggest the following infection:**

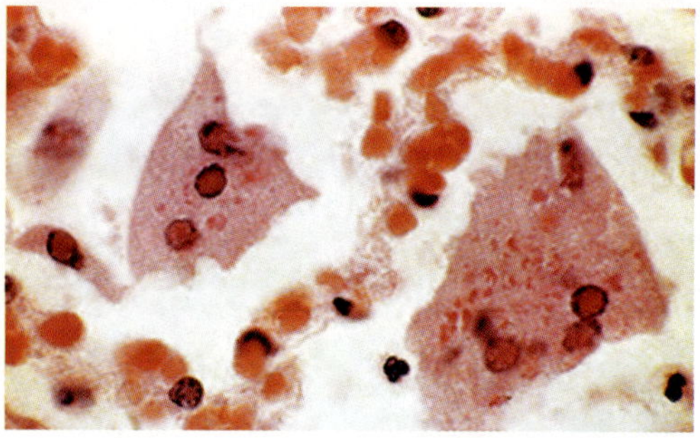

a) Measles b) Herpes
c) Polyoma virus d) CMV

19. **In lung biopsy, figure gives a clue towards:**

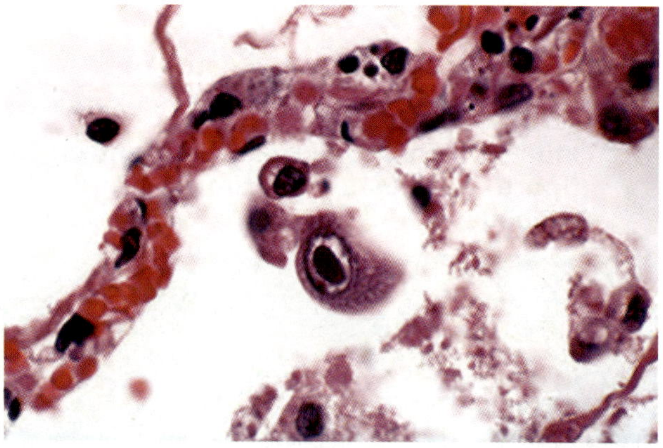

a) CMV b) Measles
c) Herpes d) Polyoma virus

20. **Abnormal lymphocytic population in peripheral smear indicates:**

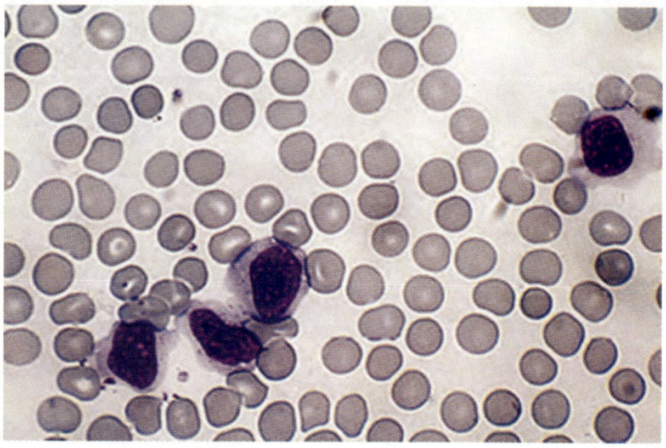

a) EBV infection b) CMV infection
c) Burkitt lymphoma d) Hodgkin disease

21. **Figure below indicates the following infection:**

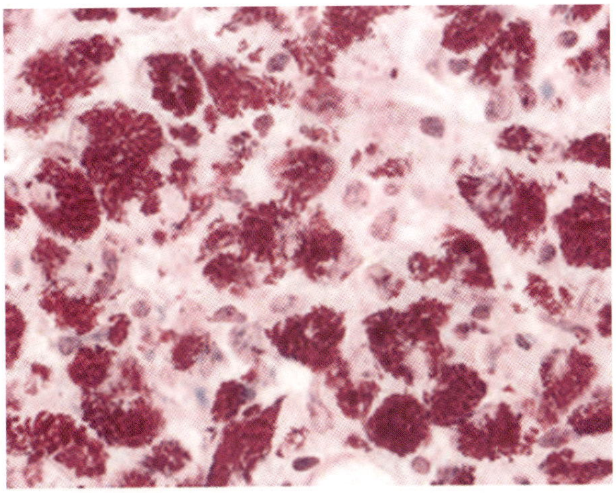

a) Tuberculosis b) Leprosy
c) Syphilis d) Lyme disease

22. **Figure depicts splenic involvement by the following pathology:**

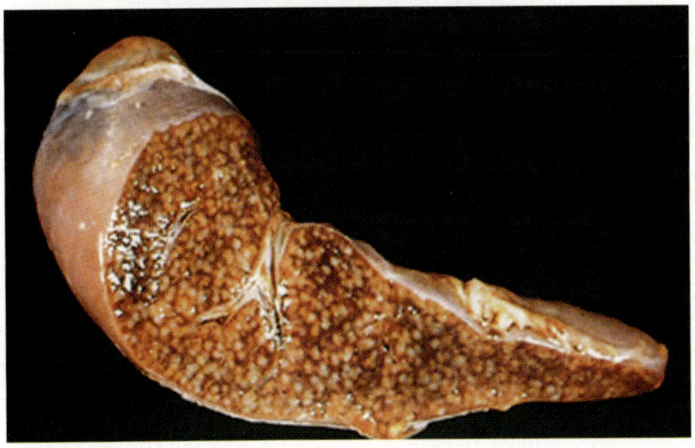

a) Miliary tuberculosis b) Metastasis
c) Infarction d) Abscess

23. **Grossly esophagus suggests following infection:**

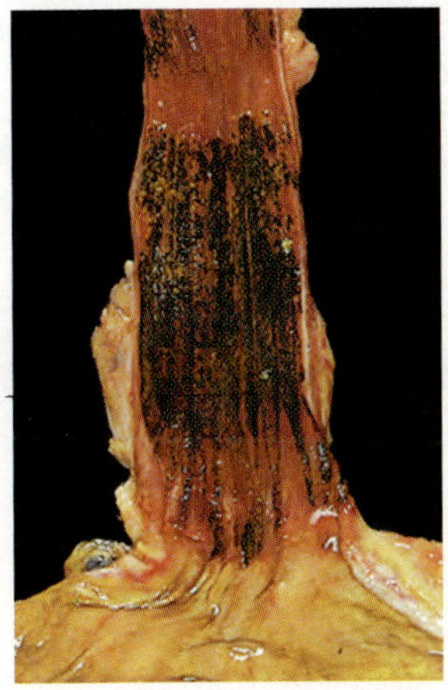

a) Candidiasis b) CMV
c) Cryptococcal infection d) Aspergillus infection

24. **Figure depicts:**

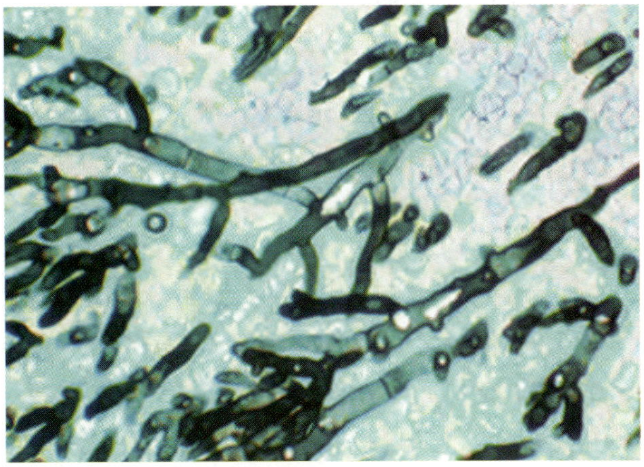

a) Aspergillus b) Candidiasis
c) Mucor d) Cryptococcus

25. **Following organism is visualized within macrophage using Giemsa stain:**

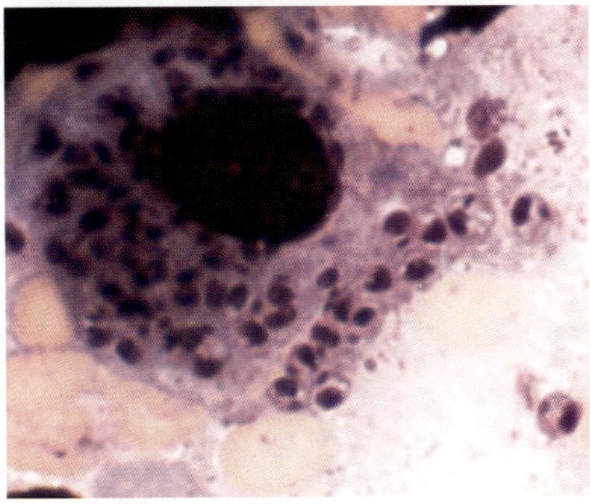

a) Leishmania Donovani
b) Trypanosoma
c) Plasmodium vivax
d) Plasmodium falciparum

26. **Following organism is visualized in the peripheral smear:**

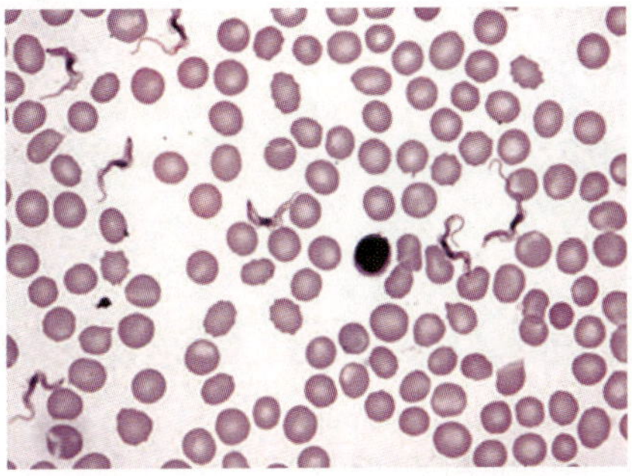

a) Trypanosoma b) Leishmania Donovani
c) Plasmodium vivax d) Plasmodium falciparum

27. Erythrocytes show infection with which of the following parasite?

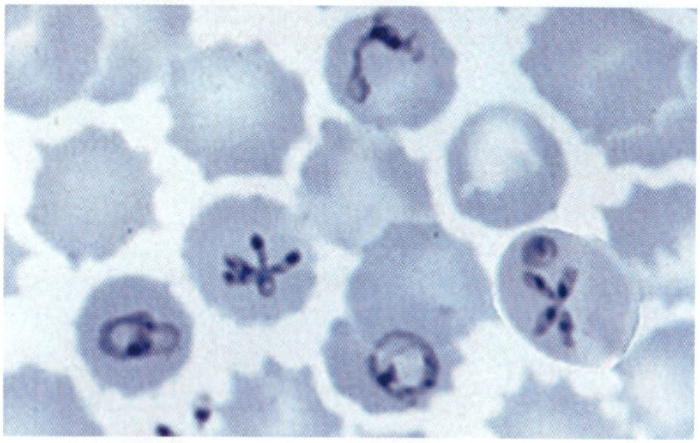

a) Babesiosis b) Trypanosoma
c) Plasmodium vivax d) Plasmodium falciparum

28. Erythrocyte shows infection with the following parasite:

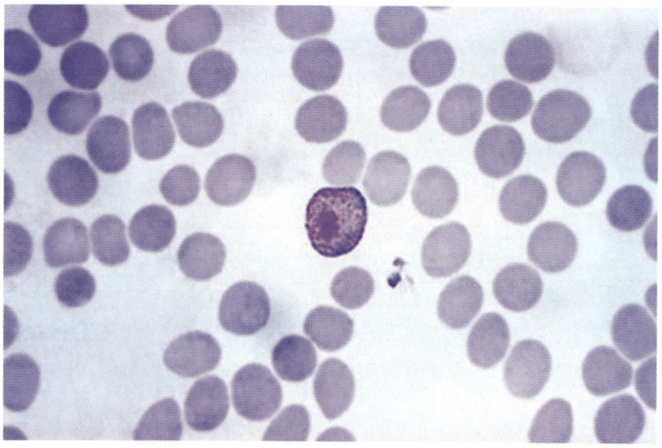

a) Plasmodium vivax
b) Plasmodium malaria
c) Plasmodium falciparum
d) Babesiosis

29. Gametocytes in peripheral smear suggests following infection:

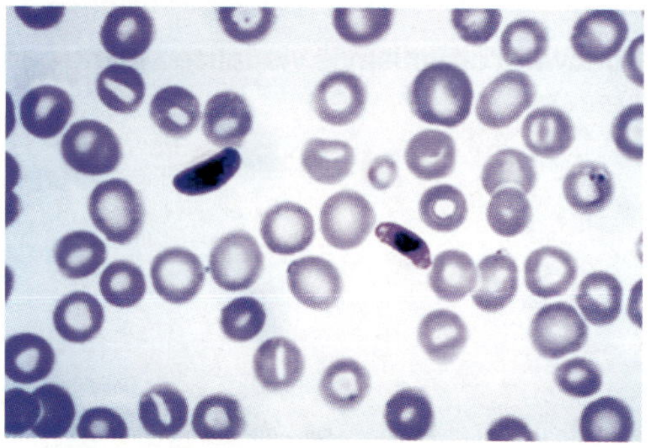

a) Plasmodium falciparum
b) Plasmodium malaria
c) Plasmodium vivax
d) Babesiosis

CHAPTER 10

29. 5-year-old male presents with abdominal mass. After surgery, grossly, adrenal gland was involved by the tumor as shown in the figure below, which also shows tumor characteristic histopathology. Gross and histopathology indicates the diagnosis of:

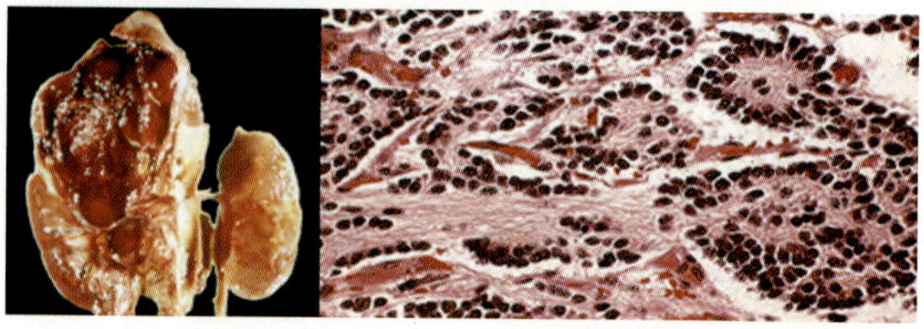

a) Neuroblastoma b) Renal cell carcinoma
c) Ganglioglioma d) Ganglioneuroblastoma

31. Following gross photograph indicate towards:

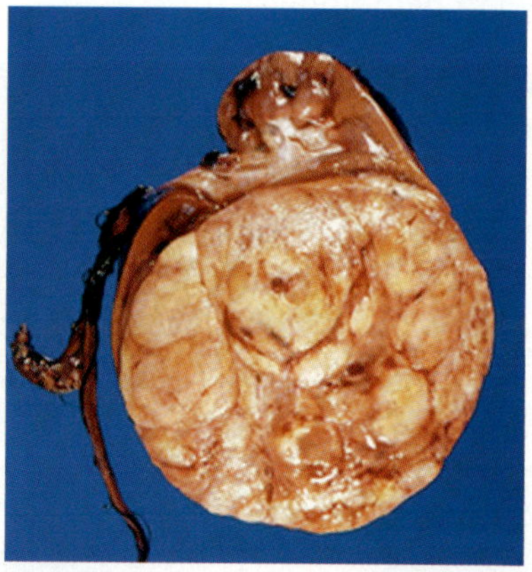

a) Wilms tumor b) Embryonal carcinoma
c) Renal cell cancer d) Sarcoma

CHAPTER 11

32. Arterial wall thickening due to increased protein deposition is seen in:

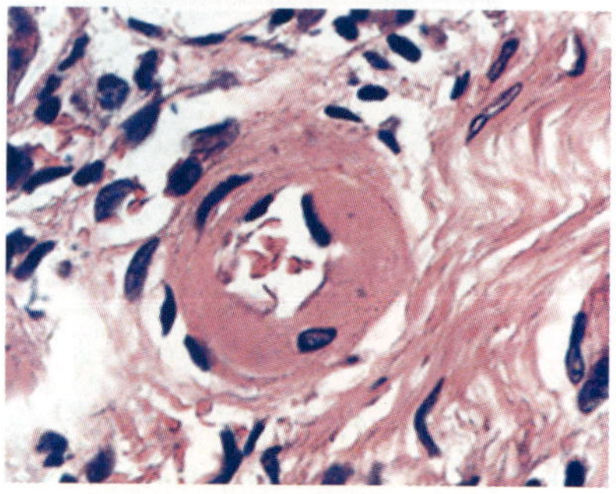

a) Hyaline arteriosclerosis
b) Hyperplastic arteriosclerosis
c) Atherosclerosis
d) Mönckeberg medial sclerosis

33. **Figure below suggests the following pathology in the vessel wall:**

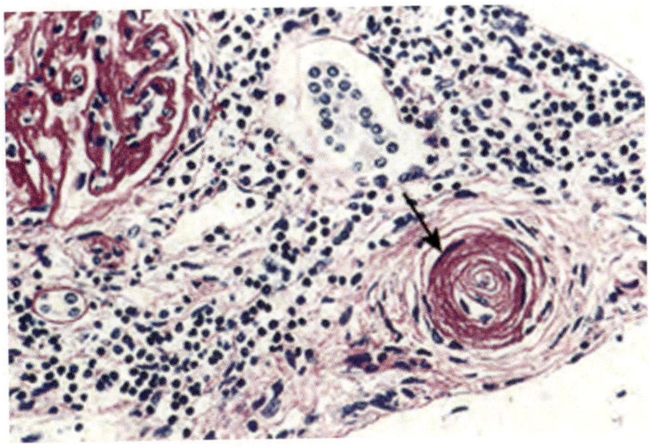

a) Hyperplastic arteriosclerosis
b) Hyaline arteriolosclerosis
c) Atherosclerosis
d) Mönckeberg medial sclerosis

34. **Figure below depicts:**

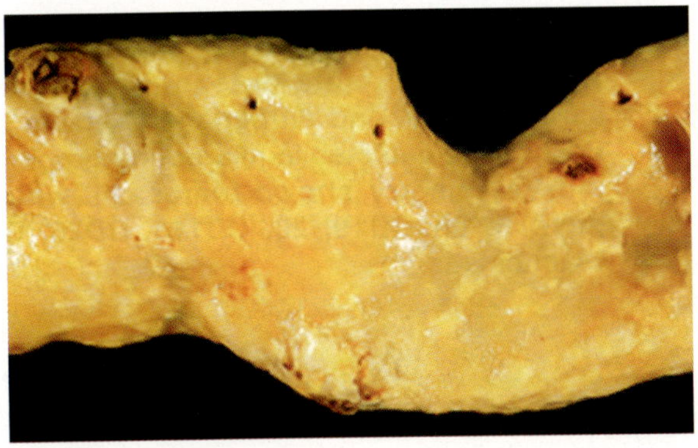

a) Atherosclerotic plaque
b) Aortic rupture
c) Aortic aneurysm
d) Atheroembolism

35. **Figure below depicts the following pathology in blood vessel:**

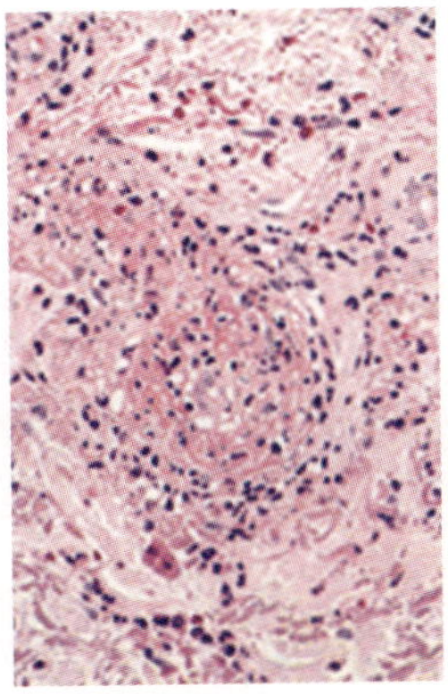

a) Leukocytoclastic vasculitis
b) Kawasaki disease
c) Takayasu disease
d) Wegener granulomatosis

36. **Figure depicts following vascular tumor:**

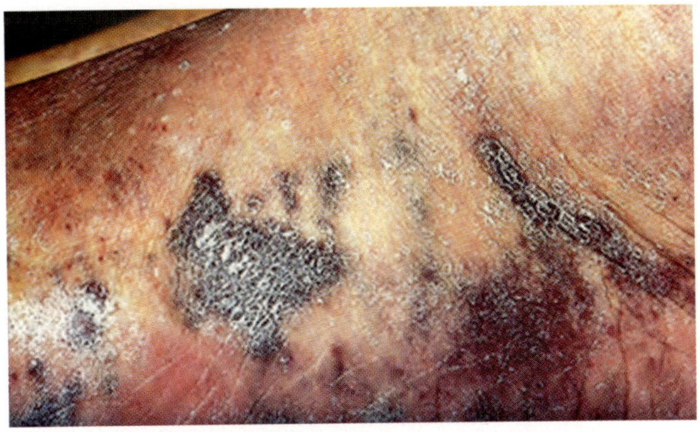

a) Kaposi sarcoma
b) Angisarcoma
c) Hemangioendothelioma
d) Glomus tumor

CHAPTER 12

37. **Following figure depicts:**

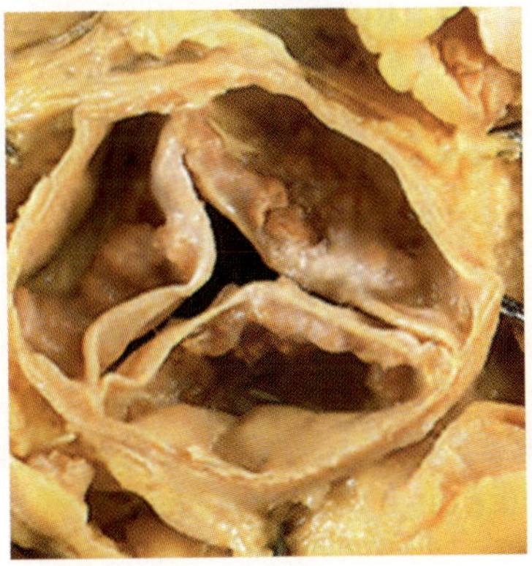

a) Calcific aortic stenosis
b) Calcified Bicuspid aortic valve
c) Mitral annular calcification
d) Pulmonary valvular stenosis

38. **Following pathology is seen in the atrium:**

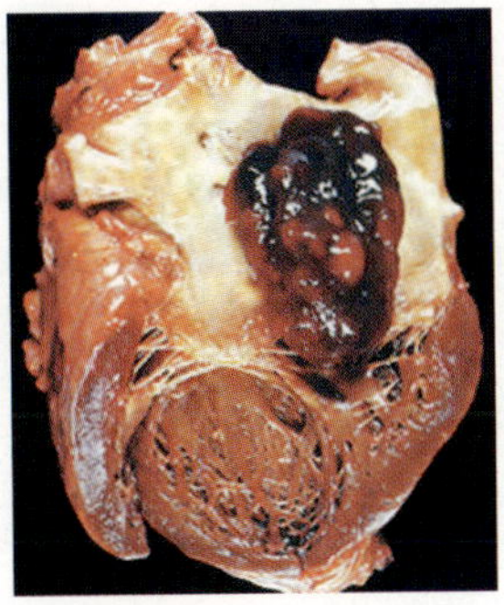

a) Atrial myxoma
b) Mural thrombus
c) Embolism
d) Myxomatous degeneration of atrial wall

CHAPTER 13

39. A 5-years-old male, presented with weakness and fever since 15 days with generalized lymphadenopathy. On Peripheral Smear – Cells shown in figure were seen, and flow-cytometry showed CD 19, CD22 and TdT positivity. The diagnosis will be:

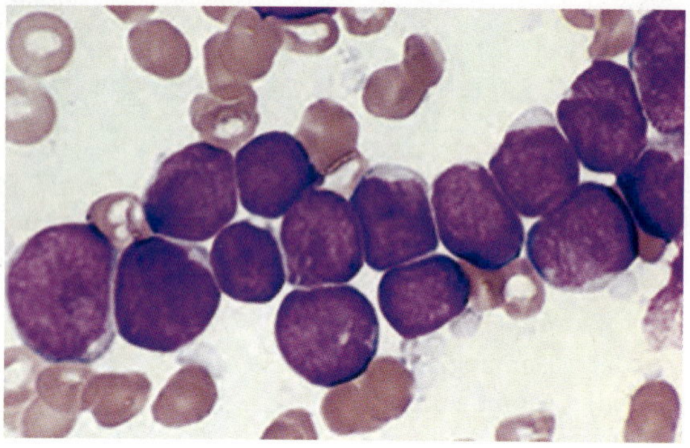

a) B-ALL b) T-ALL
c) AML d) CML

40. Large destructive mass of the spleen (as shown in the figure) signifies?

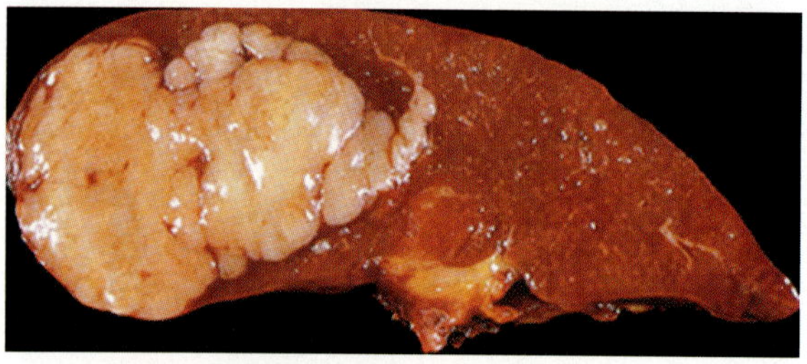

a) Diffuse Large B-cell Lymphoma
b) Mantle cell lymphoma
c) Marginal zone lymphoma
d) Hodgkin disease

41. Histopathology of the tumor shown in figure, shows cytogenetic abnormality of t(8;14). Diagnosis is:

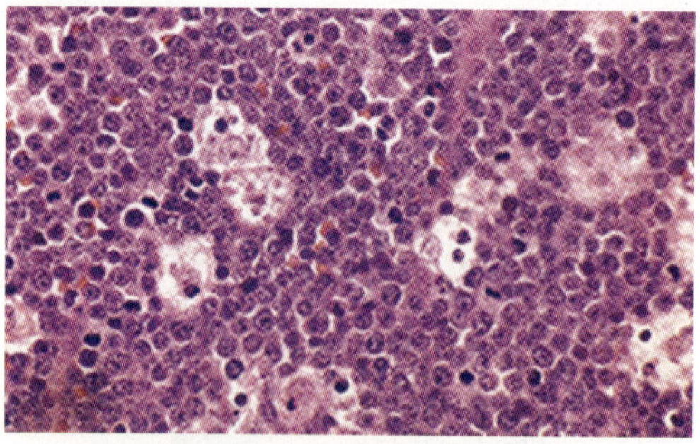

a) Burkitt lymphoma
b) MALToma
c) Diffuse large B-cell lymphoma
d) Mantle cell lymphoma

42. 60-year-old male, presents with lytic lesions on the skull and bone marrow aspirate shows the particular cells as shown in the microphotograph shown below. Diagnosis is:

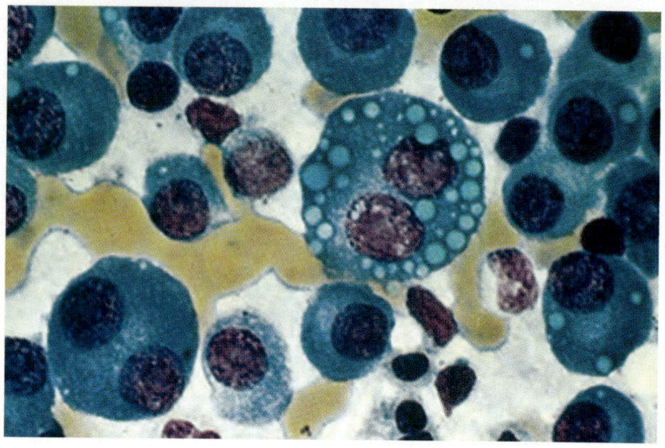

a) Multiple myeloma
b) Lymphoplasmacytic lymphoma
c) Osteoma
d) Osteoblastoma

43. A 70-year-old male presents with massive splenomegaly, and on peripheral smear shows the cells as depicted in microphotograph below. Flow-cytometry shows tumor cell which are positive for CD19, 20, CD11c, CD25, CD103. Diagnosis is:

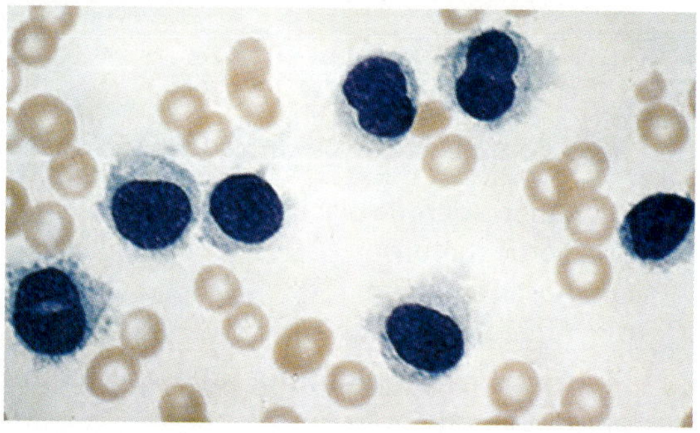

a) Hairy cell leukemia b) Marginal zone lymphoma
c) Mantle cell lymphoma d) Multiple myeloma

44. Characteristic cell shown in the figure below, gives a clue towards following diagnosis:

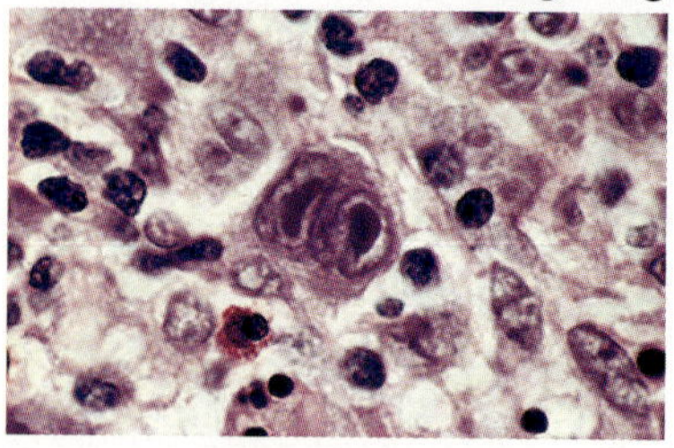

a) Hodgkin disease
b) Diffuse large B-cell lymphoma
c) Anaplastic large cell lymphoma
d) Poorly differentiated carcinoma

45. **18-year-old female, presents with bleeding diathesis. Peripheral smear (in microphotograph) favors towards the following diagnosis:**

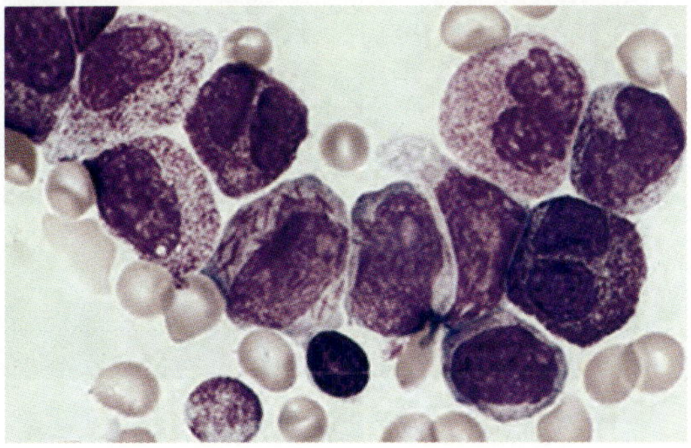

a) Acute-myeloid leukemia (AML)-M3
b) AML-M4
c) AML-M5
d) AML-M6

46. **Histopathological microphotograph showing tumor cells with grooved nuclei. Electron microscopy shows rod like Bireback granules. Diagnosis is:**

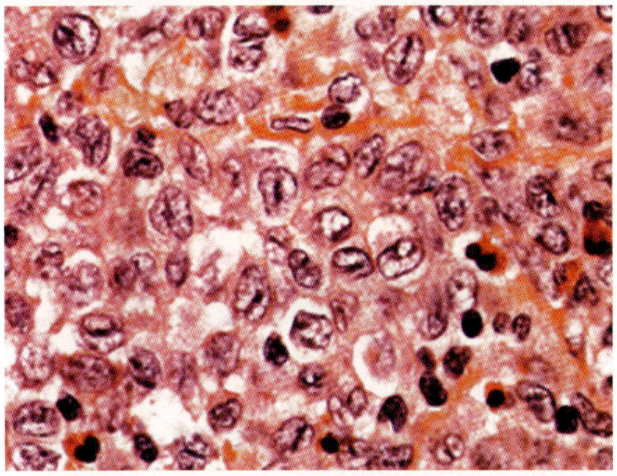

a) Langerhans cell histiocytosis (LCH)
b) Acute myeloid leukemia
c) Acute lymphoblastic lymphoma
d) Chronic lymphocytic lymphoma

CHAPTER 14

47. **Erythrocytes shown in microphotograph are:**

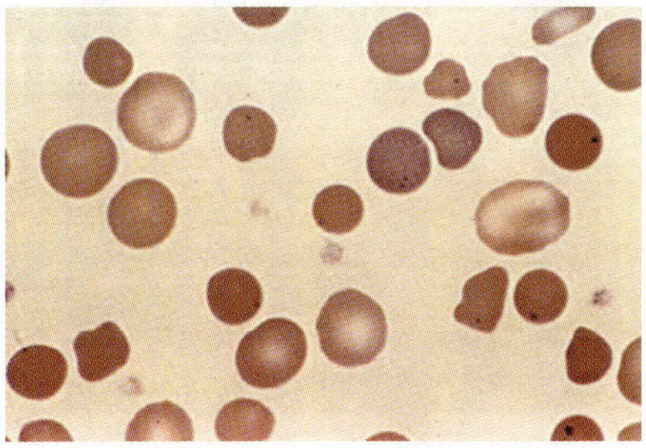

a) Spherocytes b) Bite cell
c) Microcytes d) Normocyte

48. **Characteristic cells shown in microphotograph:**

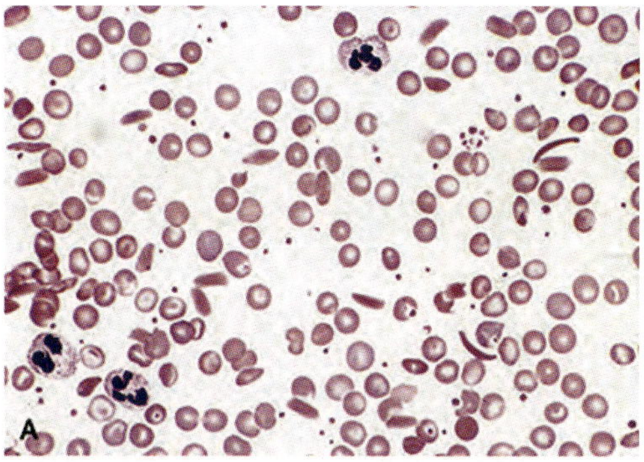

a) Sickle cells b) Spherocytes
c) Microcytes d) Bite cell

49. **Crew-cut appearance of the skull is seen in:**

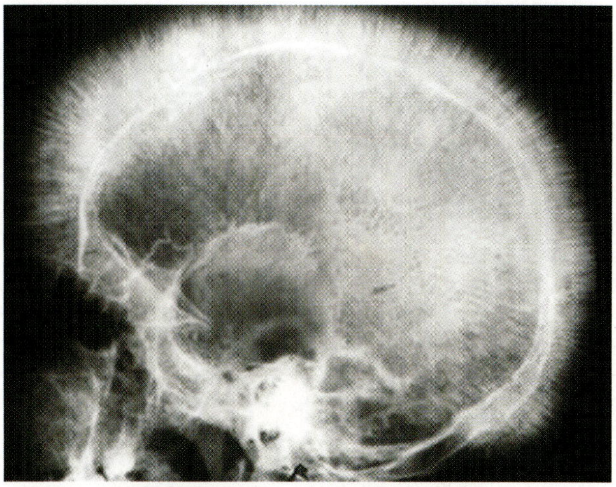

a) Thalassemia
b) Sickle cell anemia
c) Multiple myeloma
d) Hemolytic uremic syndrome

50. **Following figure shows features of:**

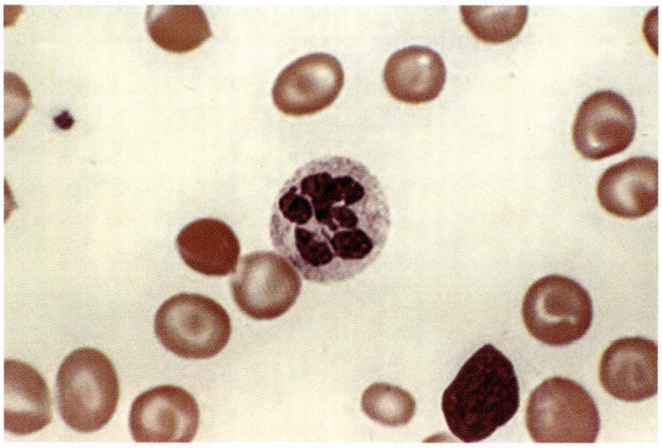

a) Megaloblastic anemia
b) Iron deficiency anemia
c) Hemolytic anemia
d) Aplastic anemia

CHAPTER 15

51. Figure below depicts:

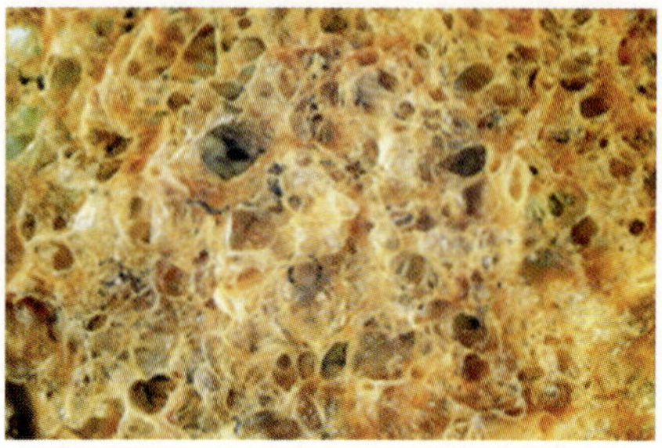

a) Emphysema b) Bronchiectasis
c) Asthma d) Interstitial pneumonia

52. Figure below depicts following underlying pathology?

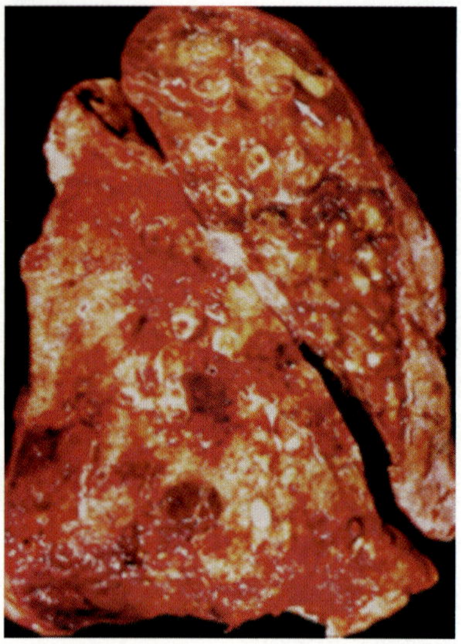

a) Bronchiectasis b) Emphysema
c) Asthma d) Pneumonia

53. Golden brown beaded rods, seen in the lung biopsy indicate:

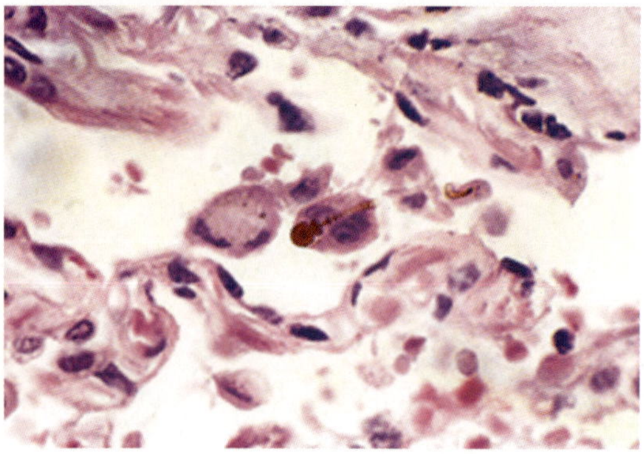

a) Asbestosis b) Silicosis
c) Asthma d) Pneumoconiosis

54. Plaques on the pleural surface are seen in:

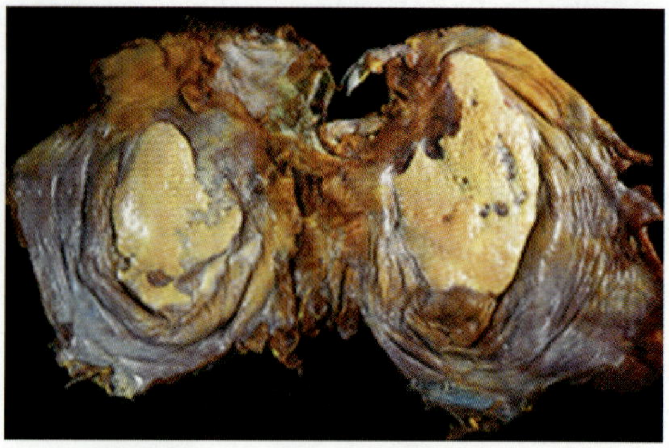

a) Asbestosis b) Silicosis
c) Asthma d) Pneumoconiosis

55. Figure below shows the following lung pathology:

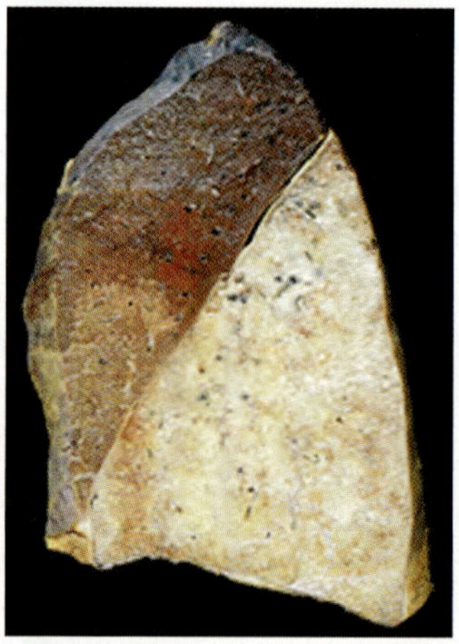

a) Lobar pneumonia b) Bronchopneumonia
c) Lung abscess d) Histoplasmosis

56. Figure below depicts the following pathology in lung parenchyma:

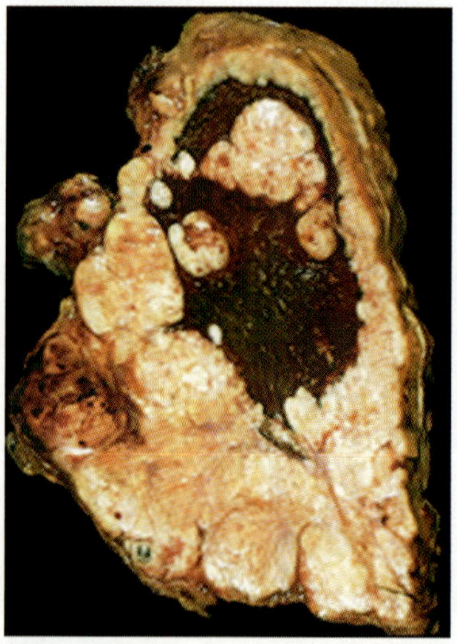

a) Mesothelioma b) Bronchiogenic carcinoma
c) Lung metastasis d) Histoplasmosis

CHAPTER 17

57. Following gross and microscopy gives a clue towards the following diagnosis?

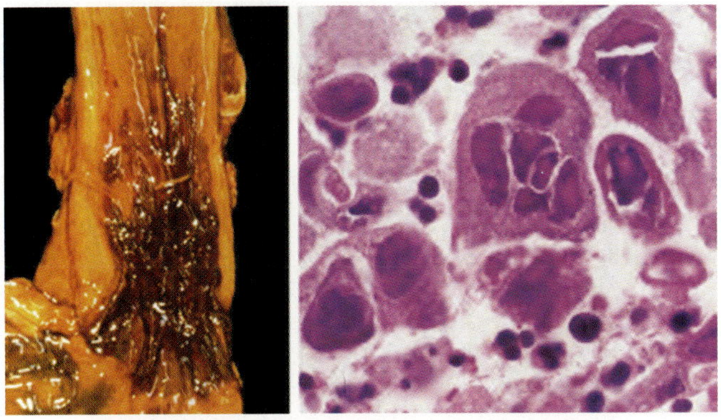

a) Viral esophagitis b) Tubercular esophagitis
c) Crohn disease d) Squamous cell carcinoma

58. Following figure depicts:

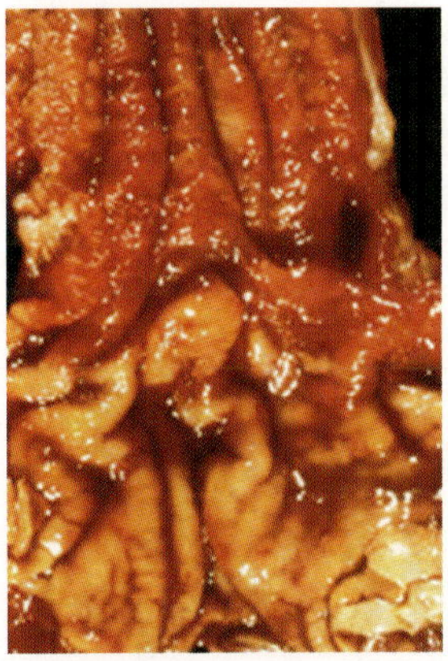

a) Barrett esophagus b) Herpetic esophagitis
c) Peptic ulcer disease d) Caustic injury

59. Gross and microscopic photographs confirm the diagnosis of:

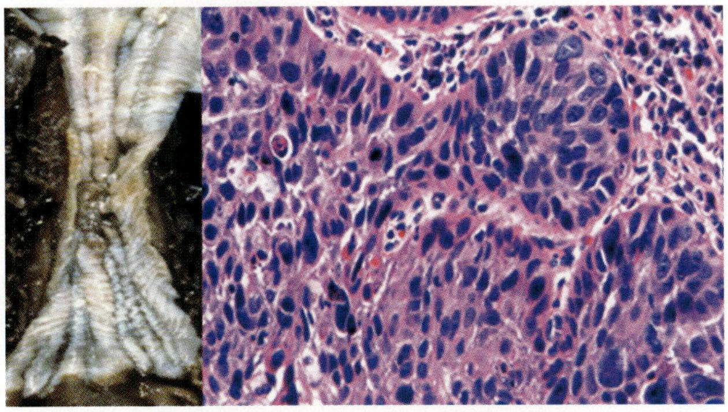

a) Squamous cell carcinoma of esophagus
b) Adenocarcinoma of esophagus
c) Metastasis
d) Gastroesophageal Reflux Disease

60. Gross and microscopic photographs confirm the diagnosis of:

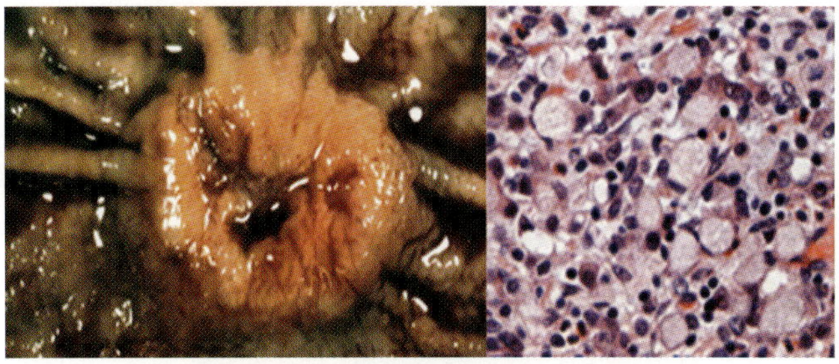

a) Adenocarcinoma
b) Squamous cell carcinoma
c) Non-Hodgkin disease
d) MALToma

61. Solitary, well-circumscribed, fleshy mass in stomach indicates:

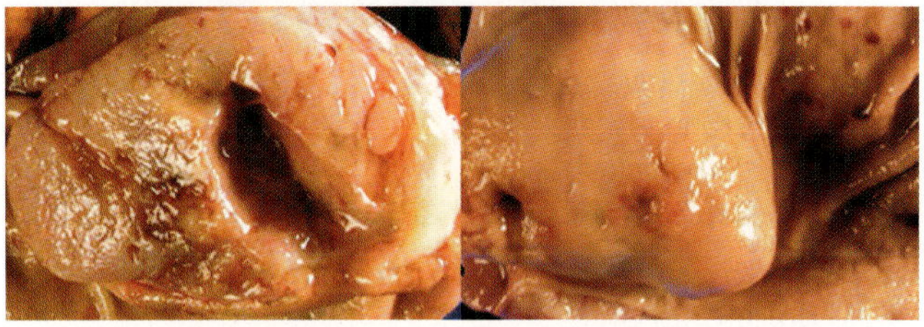

a) Gastrointestinal stromal tumor
b) Carcinoid tumor
c) Lymphoma
d) Necrotizing enterocolitis

62. Small intestinal segment shows the following pathology:

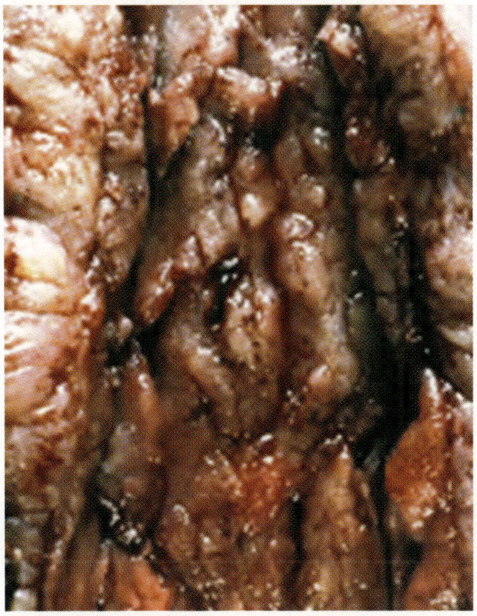

a) Crohn disease
b) Tuberculosis
c) Ulcerative colitis
d) Whipple disease

63. Pan-colectomy specimen shows the following pathology:

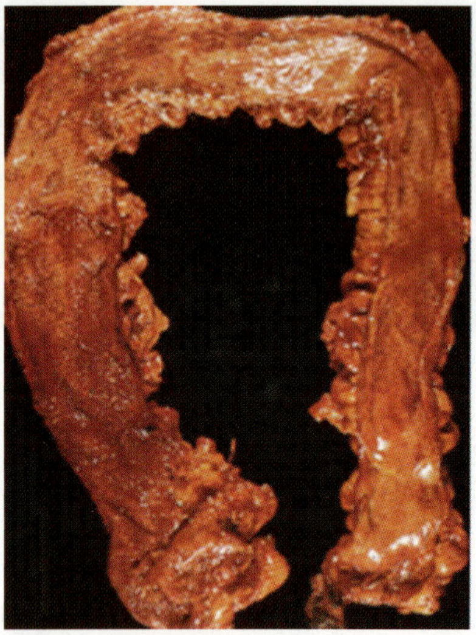

a) Ulcerative colitis
b) Crohn disease
c) Tuberculosis
d) Carcinoma colon

64. Following gross photograph indicates a diagnosis of:

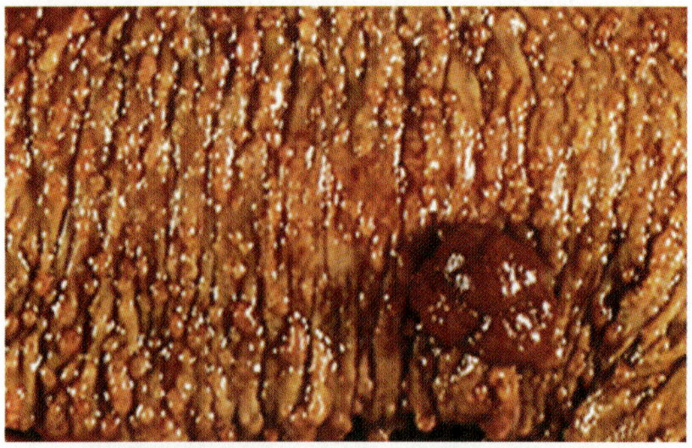

a) Familial adenomatosis polyposis
b) Adenocarcinoma
c) Crohn disease
d) Ulcerative colitis

CHAPTER 18

65. Cut section of the liver shows following pathology:

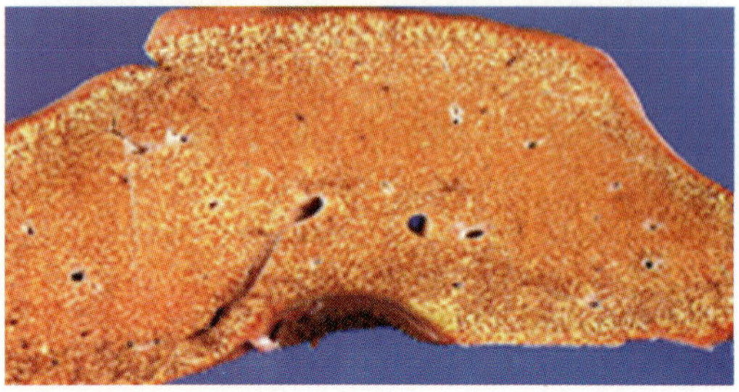

a) Hepatic necrosis b) Cirrhosis
c) Fatty liver d) Chronic venous congestion

66. Photograph shown below depicts the following pathology:

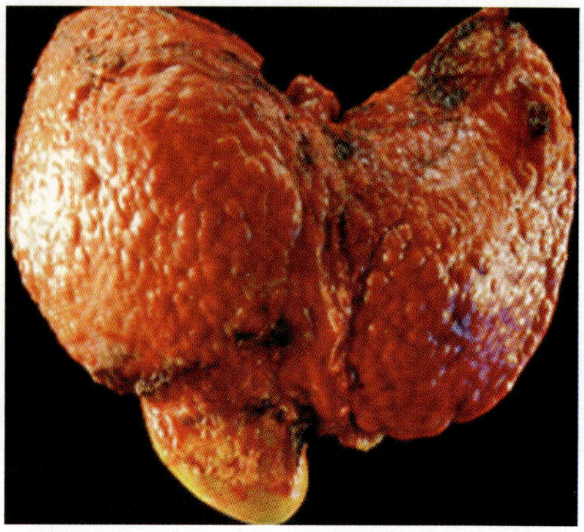

a) Cirrhosis b) Nutmeg liver
c) Fatty liver d) Hepatic nodules

67. Ground glass hepatocytes seen in the microphotograph shown below, indicates:

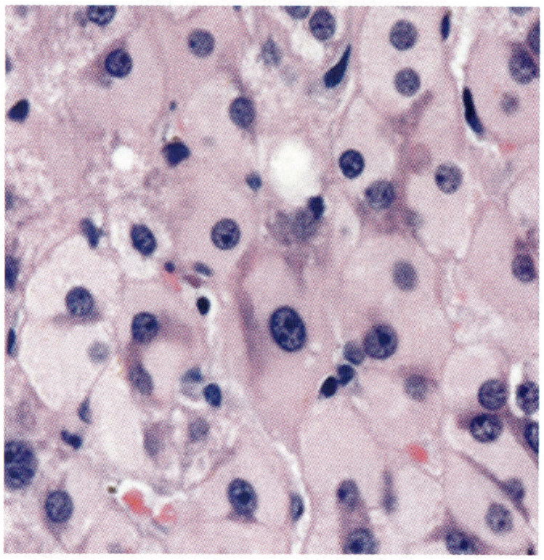

a) Hepatitis A b) Hepatitis B
c) Hepatitis C d) Hepatitis D

68. Figure point towards a diagnosis of:

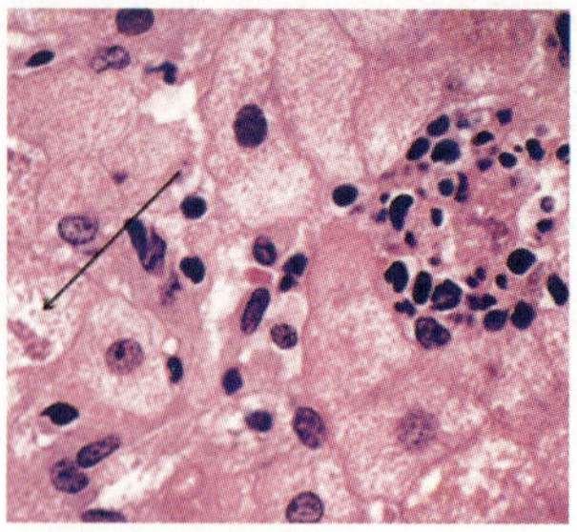

a) Alcoholic hepatitis
b) Hepatitis C

c) Non-alcoholic steatohepatitis
d) Alcoholic cirrhosis

CHAPTER 20

69. Microphotograph shown below, gives a clue towards following diagnosis?

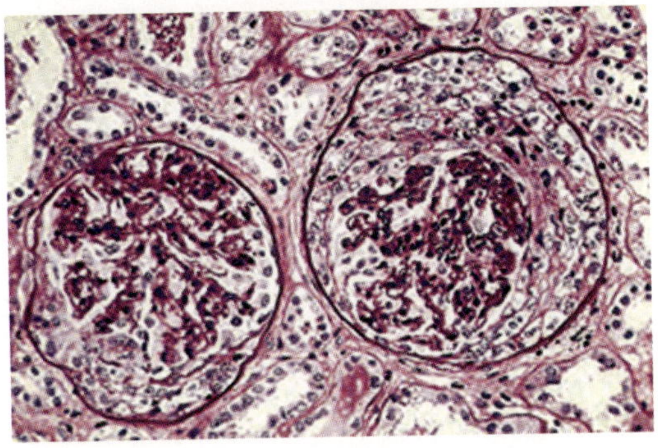

a) Crescentic Glomerulonephritis
b) Membranous nephropathy
c) Membranoproliferative Glomerulonephritis
d) Post-infectious glomerulonephritis

70. Photograph below depicts the following diagnosis:

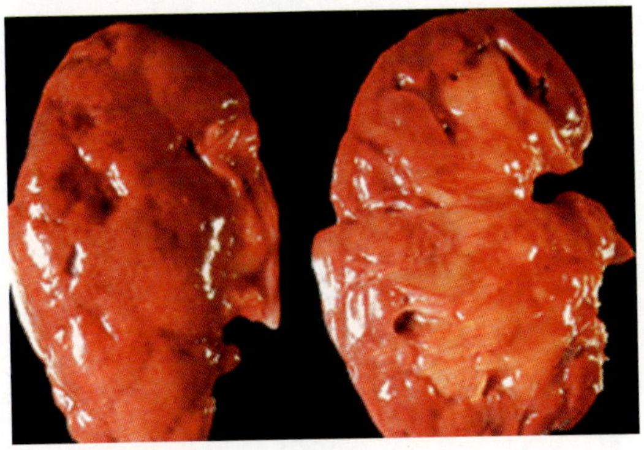

a) Chronic pyelonephritis
b) Acute pyelonephritis
c) Xanthogranulomatous pyelonephritis
d) Papillary necrosis

71. Kidney in the photograph below shows features of:

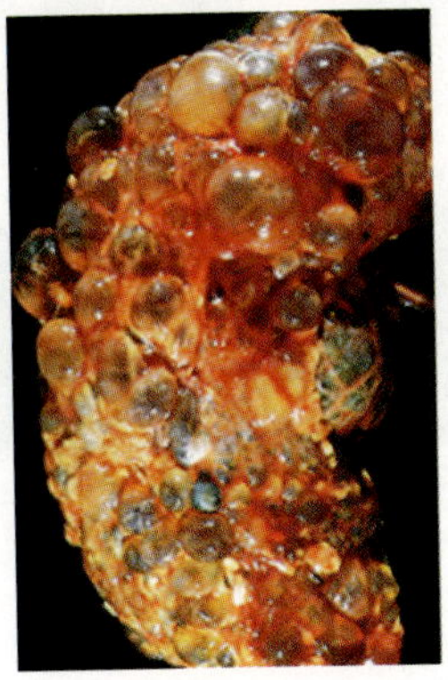

a) Polycystic kidney disease
b) Medullary sponge kidney
c) Medullary cystic disease
d) Multicystic renal dysplasia

72. Following gross photograph depicts:

a) Hydronephrosis
b) Pyelonephritis
c) Nephrolithiasis
d) Cystic kidney disease

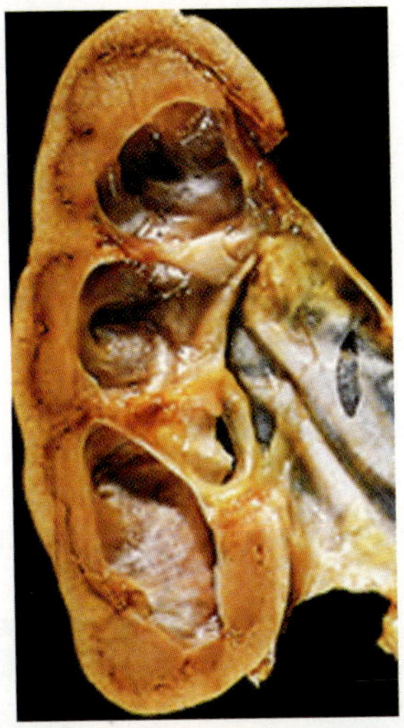

73. Photograph of the cut surface of the kidney shows:

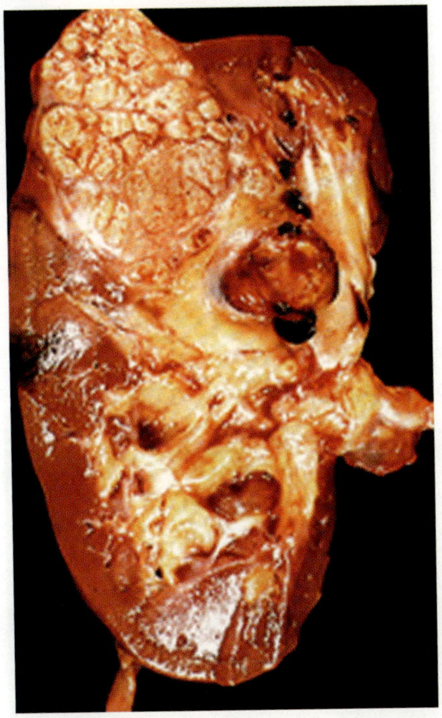

a) Renal cell carcinoma
b) Xanthogranulomatous pyelonephritis
c) Urothelial carcinoma of renal pelvis
d) Angiomyolipoma

CHAPTER 21

74. Microphotograph below depicts the following pathology:

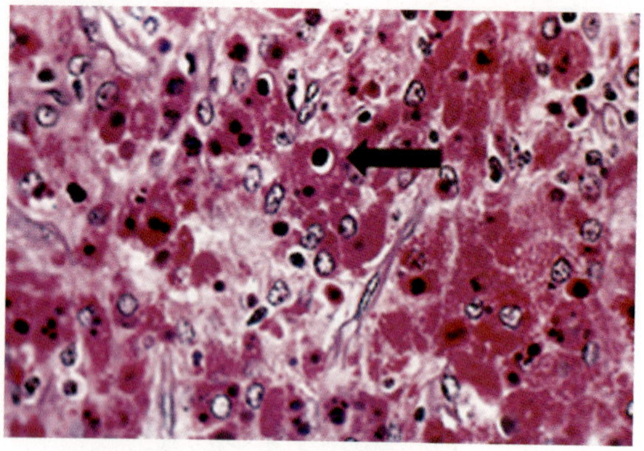

a) Malakoplakia
b) Cystitis cystica
c) Nephrogenic adenoma
d) Urothelial tumor

75. Gross photograph is of following testicular tumour:

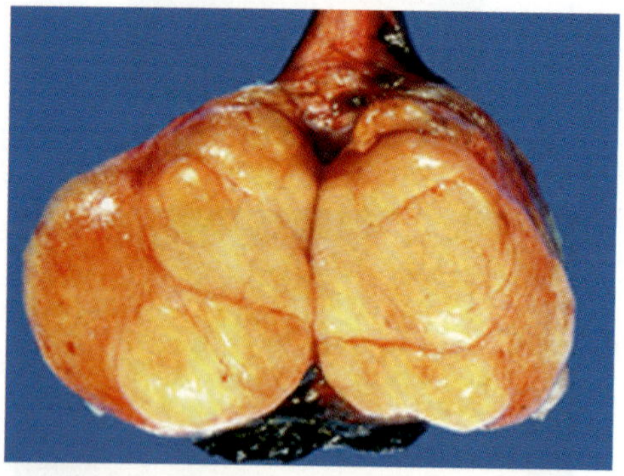

a) Seminoma of testes
b) Teratoma of testes
c) Choriocarcinoma
d) Embryonal carcinoma

76. Gross photograph depicts the following tumor:

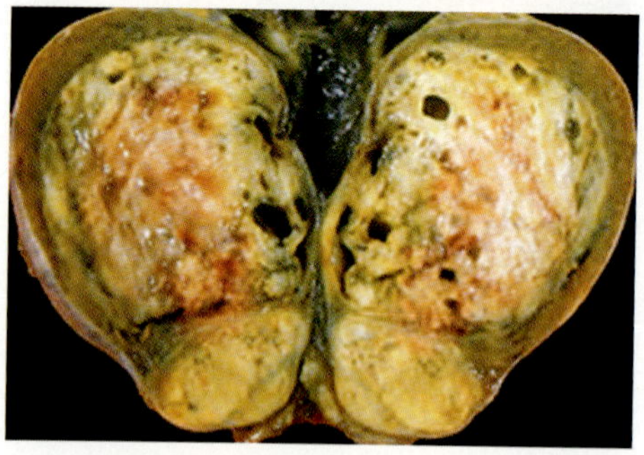

a) Teratoma of testes
b) Seminoma of testes
c) Choriocarcinoma
d) Embryonal carcinoma

CHAPTER 22

77. Intra-cytoplasmic viral inclusions suggests following infection:

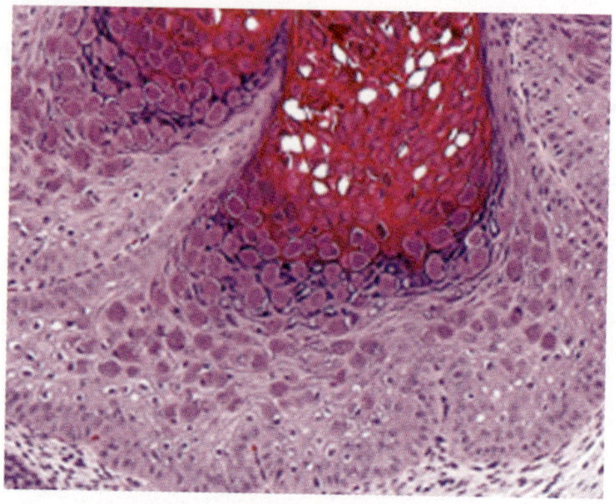

a) Molluscum contagiosum
b) Herpes simplex
c) Cytomegalovirus
d) Human papilloma virus

78. Following microphotograph depicts:

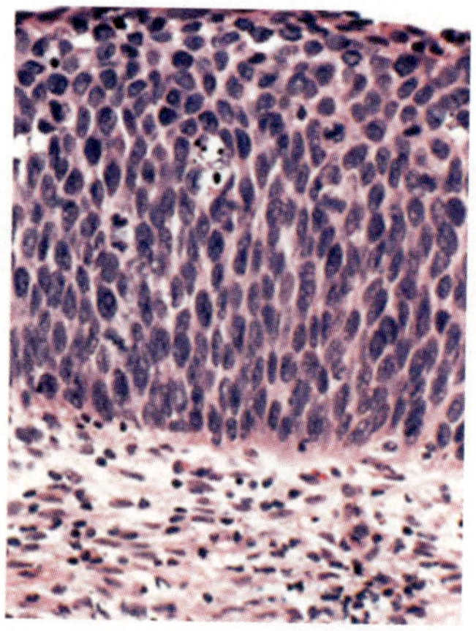

a) CIN I
b) CIN II
c) CIN III
d) Carcinoma in-situ

79. Photograph shows the following ovarian tumor:

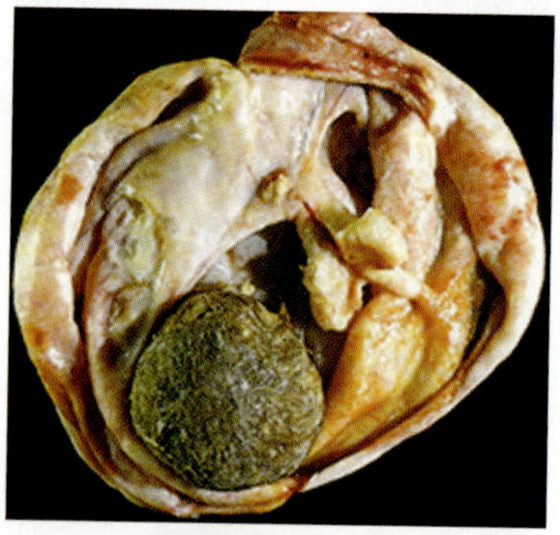

a) Ovarian teratoma
b) Serous cystadenoma
c) Mucinous cystadenoma
d) Brenner tumor

80. **Schiller-Duval Body as shown in microphotograph is seen in:**

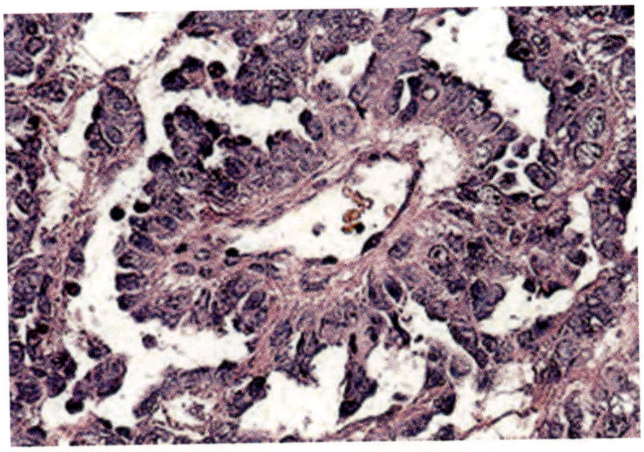

a) Yolk sac tumor
b) Teratoma
c) Brenner tumor
d) Serous cystadenoma

CHAPTER 24

81. **Giant cells in thyroid glands are seen in:**

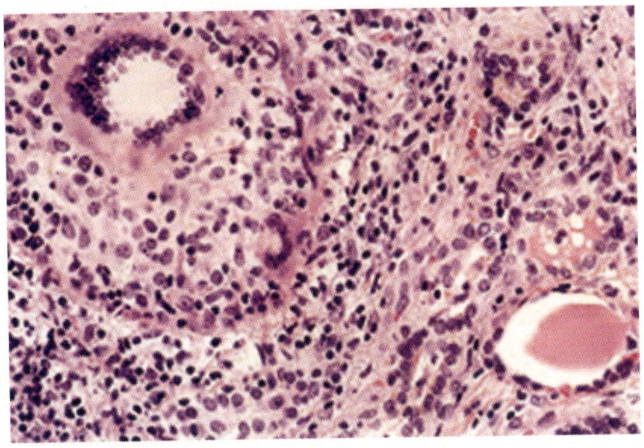

a) Tuberculosis
b) De Quervain thyroiditis
c) Graves disease
d) Hashimoto's thyroiditis

82. **Gross appearance of the cut surface of thyroid is seen in:**

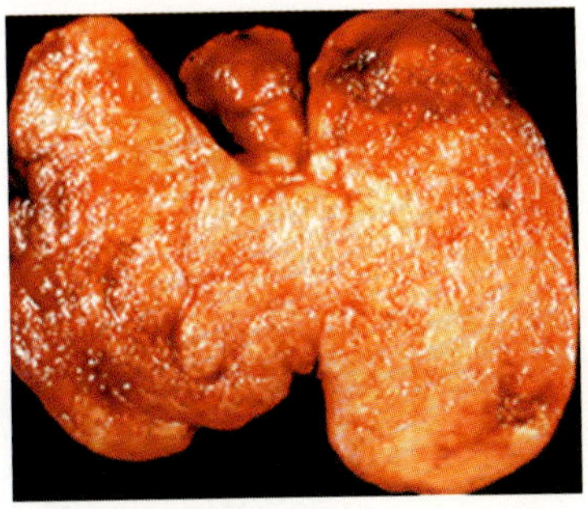

a) Graves disease
b) Multinodular goiter
c) Follicular adenoma
d) Hurthle cell neoplasm

83. **Following microphotograph of diabetic patient indicates:**

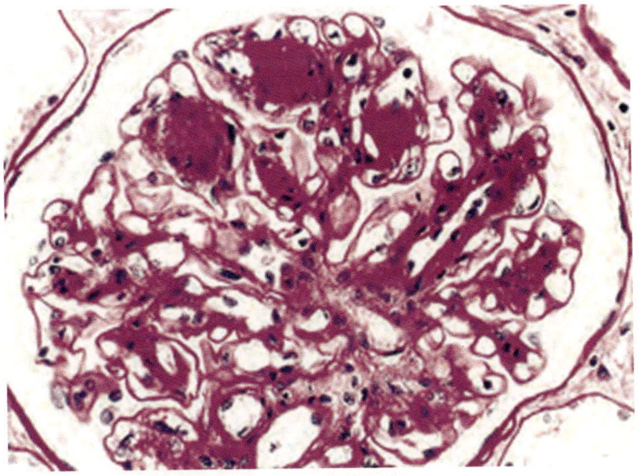

a) Nodular glomerulosclerosis
b) Membranous nephropathy
c) Mesangiocapillary glomerulonephritis
d) Nephrosclerosis

CHAPTER 25

84. **Following photograph depicts diagnosis as:**

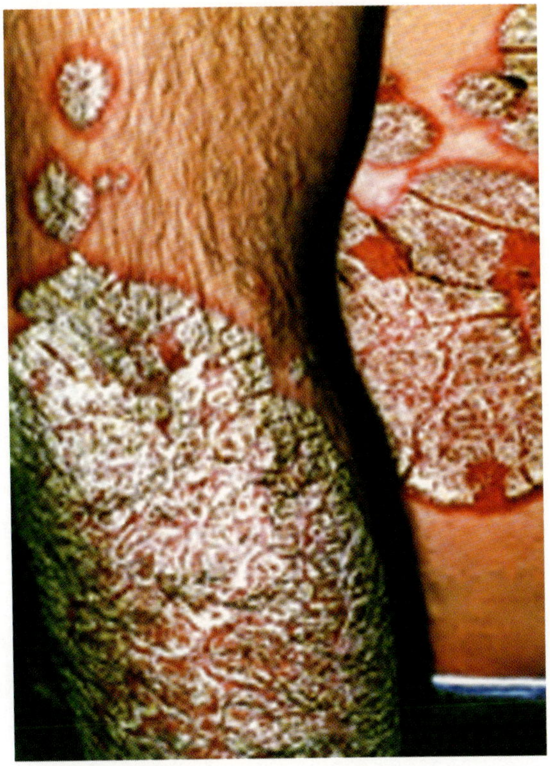

a) Psoriasis
b) Lichen planus
c) T-cell leukemia
d) Kaposi sarcoma

CHAPTER 28

85. Following microphotograph indicate towards the diagnosis of:

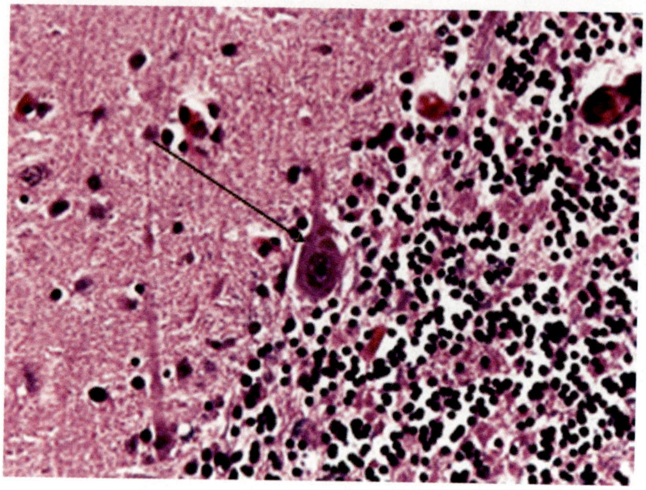

a) Rabies
b) HSV
c) CMV
d) HIV

86. Microphotograph shows a dural based tumor:

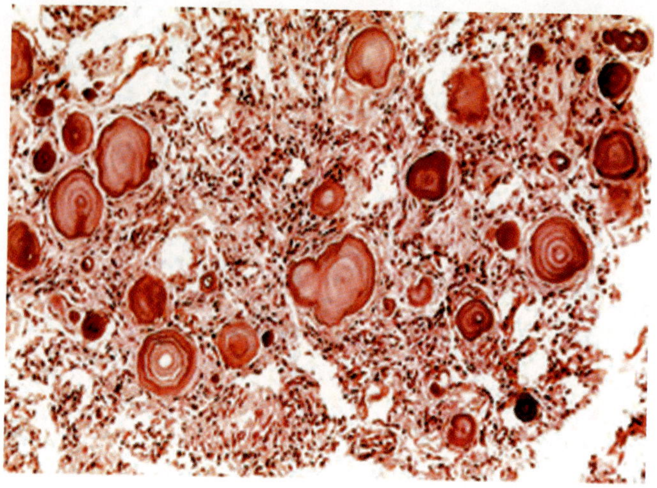

a) Meningioma
b) Metastasis
c) Glioblastoma
d) Ependymoma

ANSWERS

CHAPTER 2

Ans. 1) a. Metaplasia of columnar epithelium (left) to squamous epithelium (right) in a bronchus
Ans. 2) a. Coagulative necrosis
Ans. 3) a. Caseous necrosis
Ans. 4) a. The wall of the artery shows circumferential bright pink area of necrosis with inflammation
Ans. 5) a. Fat saponification
Ans. 6) a. Steatosis

CHAPTER 3

Ans. 7) a. Tuberculosis
- Tubercular granuloma showing an area of central necrosis surrounded by multiple Langhans-type giant cells, epitheloid cells and lymphocytes

CHAPTER 4

Ans. 8) d. Nutmeg liver
- Central areas are red and depressed compared with surrounding tan viable parenchyma, forming "nutmeg liver" pattern

Ans. 9) a. Mural thrombi
Ans. 10) b. White infarct

CHAPTER 5

Ans. 11) a. Gaucher's disease

CHAPTER 6

Ans. 12) b. Antibody to Sm antigen
- Figure shows **speckled pattern** of **ANA on Immunofluorescence,** which is representative of antibodies to **Sm antigen, Ribonucleoprotein** and **SS-A and SS-B reactive antigens**

Ans: 13) d. Class IV (Diffuse lupus nephritis) produces **wire loop structures** in the kidney on light microscopy
Ans: 14) b. Libman-Sack's endocarditis
Ans. 15) a. Congo-Red B

CHAPTER 7

Ans. 16) a. Carcinoma in-situ
- Epithelium is entirely replaced by atypical dysplastic cells. There is no orderly differentiation of squamous cells. The basement membrane is intact, and there is no tumor in the sub-epithelial stroma

Ans. 17) a. Metastasis

CHAPTER 9

Ans. 18) a. Measles
- **Warthin-Finkeldey cells** are multinucleate giant cells which have eosinophilic nuclear and cytoplasmic inclusion bodies

Ans. 19) a. CMV
- CMV infection shows prominent **intra-nuclear** and **cytoplasmic basophilic inclusions**

Ans. 20) a. EBV infection
- In, **Infectious mononucleosis**, peripheral smear shows atypical lymphocytes, with abundant cytoplasm, an oval, indented, or folded nucleus, and scattered cytoplasmic azurophilic granules

Ans. 21) a. Tuberculosis
- **Acid Fast stain**, in immunocompromised patient, shows sheets of foamy macrophages packed with mycobacteria

Ans. 22) a. Miliary tuberculosis
Ans. 23) a. Candidiasis
Ans. 24) a. Aspergillus
- Septate hyphae with acute-angle branching, as shown by Gomori methenamine-silver (GMS) stain here, suggests **Aspergillus species**

Ans. 25) a. Leishmania Donovani
- Macrophage showing Leishmania donovani parasites

Ans. 26) a. Trypanosoma

Ans. 27) a. Babesiosis

- How to differentiate between Babesia and Plasmodium Falciparum rings?
- Babesia organisms resembles *P. falciparum* ring stages, but lack hemozoin pigment
- Babesia forms characteristic **tetrads (Maltese cross),** which are **diagnostic**

Ans. 28) a. Plasmodium vivax

- Trophozoite stage of Plasmodium Vivax

CHAPTER 10

Ans. 29) a. Plasmodium falciparum

- Banana shaped gametocytes of P. falciparum

Ans. 30): a) Neuroblastoma

- **Gross:** Partially encapsulated tumor replacing whole kidney
- **Microscopy:** Tumor composed of small cells embedded in a finely fibrillar matrix.

Ans. 31) a. Wilm's tumor

- **Gross:** Wilm's tumor in the lower pole of the kidney with characteristic tan color and well-circumscribed margins

CHAPTER 11

Ans. 32) a. Hyaline arteriosclerosis

- Arteriolar wall is thickened and appears hyalinized, with the lumen being markedly narrowed

Ans. 33) a. Hyperplastic arteriosclerosis

- Onion skin appearance of arterioles with luminal narrowing

Ans. 34) a. Atherosclerotic plaque

Ans. 35) a. Leukocytoclastic vasculitis

- Microscopic polyangiitis with fragmentation of neutrophils in and around blood vessel walls

Ans. 36): a) Kaposi sarcoma

CHAPTER 12

Ans. 37) a. Calcified aortic stenosis

Ans. 38) a. Atrial myxoma

CHAPTER 13

Ans. 39) a. B-ALL

- Lymphoblasts with condensed nuclear chromatin, high N:C ratio and scant agranular cytoplasm

Ans. 40) a. Diffuse large B-cell lymphoma

Ans. 41) a. Burkitt lymphoma

Note: Macrophages with clear cytoplasm gives this tumor a characteristic starry-sky appearance

Ans. 42) a. Multiple myeloma

- In Multiple myeloma, normal marrow cells are replaced by plasma cells, which might show cells with multiple nuclei, prominent nucleoli and cytoplasmic droplets containing IgG

Ans. 43) a. Hairy cell leukemia

- Tumor cells with fine hairlike cytoplasmic projections, round nuclei and modest amounts of pale blue, agranular cytoplasm

Ans. 44) a. Hodgkin disease

- **Note:** Characteristic cell shown in the figure–Reed-Sternberg cell, which are seen in Hodgkin disease

Ans. 45): Acute myeloid leukemia (AML)-M3

- **Note: Acute promyelocytic leukemia** shows **t (15; 17) translocation** (FAB M3 subtype). One of the cells shows multiple **needle-like Auer Rods**

Ans. 46) Langerhans cell histiocytosis (LCH). Grooved nuclei with eosinophils and Bireback granules confirms diagnosis of LCH

Ans. 47) a. Spherocytes

- Diagnosis is Hereditary Spherocytosis. Howell-Jolly bodies are seen within few of the erythrocytes

Ans. 48) a. Sickle cells

Ans. 49) a. Thalassemia

- Crew-cut appearance of skull, seen in thalassemia

Ans. 50) a. Megaloblastic anemia.

- Hyper-segmented neutrophils with macrocytes in background suggests macrocytic anemia

CHAPTER 15

Ans. 51) a. Emphysema

Ans. 52) a. Bronchiectasis

- Cut surface of lung shows markedly distended peripheral bronchi filled with mucopurulent secretions

Ans. 53) a. Asbestosis

- **Asbestos bodies**–Golden brown, fusiform or beaded rods, consisting of asbestos fibers coated with an iron-containing proteinaceous material

Ans. 54) a. Asbestosis

- **Gross:** Large, discrete fibrocalcific plaques seen on the pleural surface of the diaphragm

Ans. 55) a. Lobar pneumonia

Ans. 56) a. Mesothelioma

- Thick, firm, white pleural tumor tissue that ensheathes the lung

CHAPTER 17

Ans. 57) a. Viral esophagitis

- **Gross:** Shows esophagus with herpetic ulcers
- **Microscopy:** Shows keratinized squamous cells with herpes viral nuclear inclusions

Ans. 58) a. Barrett esophagus

Ans. 59) a. Squamous cell carcinoma of esophagus

- **Note:** Esophageal squamous cell carcinoma usually involves **middle one-third** of esophagus and on microscopy–tumor is composed of **nests of malignant cells**

Ans. 60) a. Adenocarcinoma

- **Note:** Signet ring cell type of adenocarcinoma is seen in the microscopic figure

Ans. 61) a. Gastrointestinal stromal tumor

- Cut surface: Whorled texture is evident within white, fleshy tumor

Ans. 62) a. Crohn disease

- **Note:** Linear mucosal ulcers, which impart a cobblestone appearance to the mucosa

Ans. 63) a) Ulcerative colitis

- **Note:** Cecum (left) appears red and granular, whereas the rest of colonic mucosa appears atrophic and smooth

Ans. 64) a. Familial Adenomatosis Polyposis

- **Note:** Hundreds of small polyps are present throughout the colon with a single large polyp

CHAPTER 18

Ans. 65) a. Hepatic necrosis

Ans. 66) a. Cirrhosis

Ans. 67) a. Hepatitis B

- Ground-glass hepatocytes in chronic hepatitis B infection

Ans. 68) a. Alcoholic hepatitis

- **Note:** Mallory-Denk body (as shown by an arrow in the figure) hint towards Alcoholic hepatitis

CHAPTER 20

Ans. 69) a. Crescentic Glomerulonephritis

- **Note:** Collapsed glomerular tufts and crescent-shaped mass of proliferating parietal epithelial cells and leukocytes inside to the Bowman capsule

Ans. 70) a. Chronic Pyelonephritis

- Renal surface is scarred (left), whereas cut surface of the kidney (right) reveals blunting and loss of papillae

Ans. 71) a. Polycystic kidney disease

Ans. 72) a. Hydronephrosis

- There is marked dilation of the pelvis and calyces and thinning of the renal parenchyma

Ans. 73) a. Renal cell carcinoma

- **Note:** In the figure, cut surface of the kidney shows yellowish, spherical neoplasm in the upper pole of the kidney

CHAPTER 21

Ans. 74) a. Malakoplakia

- Photomicrograph show **macrophages** with round **Michaelis-Gutmann bodies**, surrounded by artifactual cleared holes (arrow)

Ans. 75) a. Seminoma of testes

- Well circumscribed, pale, fleshy, homogenous mass

Ans. 76) a. Teratoma of the testes

- Variegated cut surface with cysts

CHAPTER 22

Ans. 77) a. Molluscum Contagiosum

Ans. 78) c. CIN III

- High grade Squamous Intraepithelial Lesion (Cervical Intraepithelial Neoplasia III) shows diffuse atypia, loss of maturation, and immature basal cells are seen up to the epithelial surface

Ans. 79) a. Ovarian Teratoma

Ans. 80) a. Yolk sac tumor

- Schiller-Duval body is seen in yolk sac tumor

CHAPTER 24

Ans. 81) b. De Quervain thyroiditis

- Granulomatous thyroiditis: Thyroid parenchyma shows chronic inflammatory infiltrate with a multinucleate giant cell

Ans. 82) a. Graves' disease

- Cut-surface appears beefy red in Grave's disease

Ans. 83) a. Nodular glomerulosclerosis

- There occurs diffuse increase in mesangial matrix

CHAPTER 25

Ans. 84) a. Psoriasis

- Erythematous lesions which are covered by a characteristic silver-white scale

Ans. 85) a. Rabies

- **Note:** In Rabies, there is eosinophilic **Negri body**, which is seen in **Purkinje cell**

Ans. 86) a. Meningioma

- Microscopy shows a whorled pattern of cell growth and numerous psammoma bodies

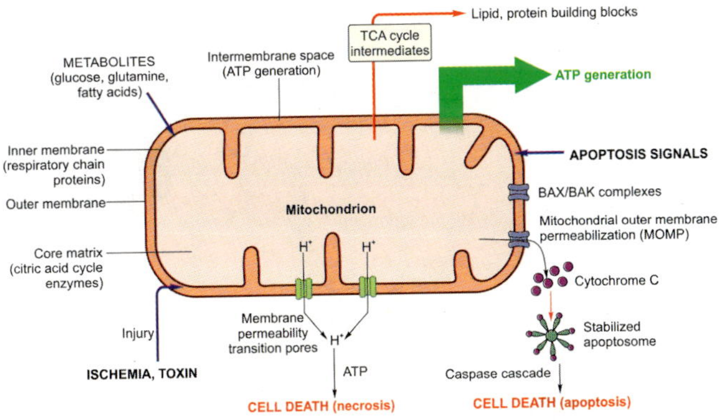

Q. 33, page 7

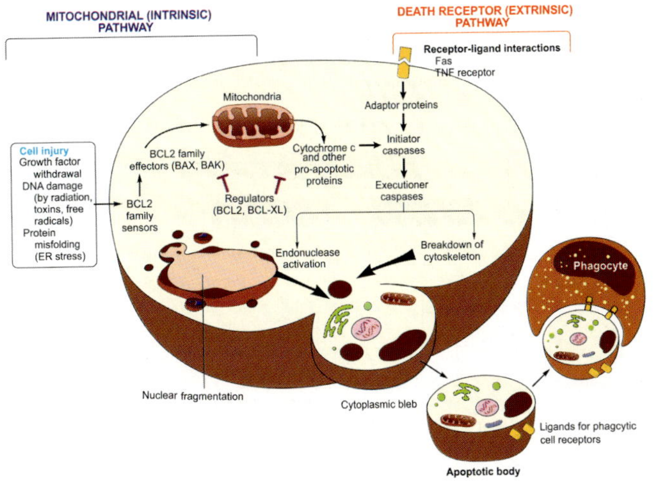

Q. 16, page 23

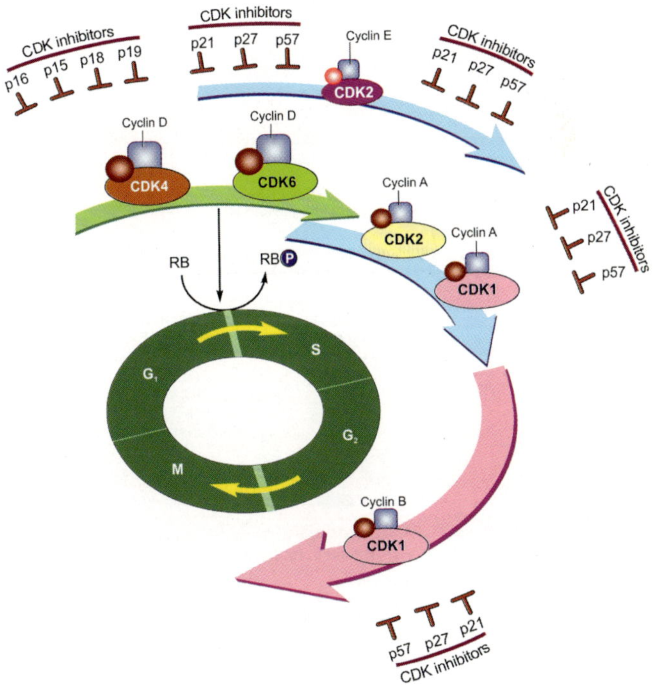

Q. 44, page 11

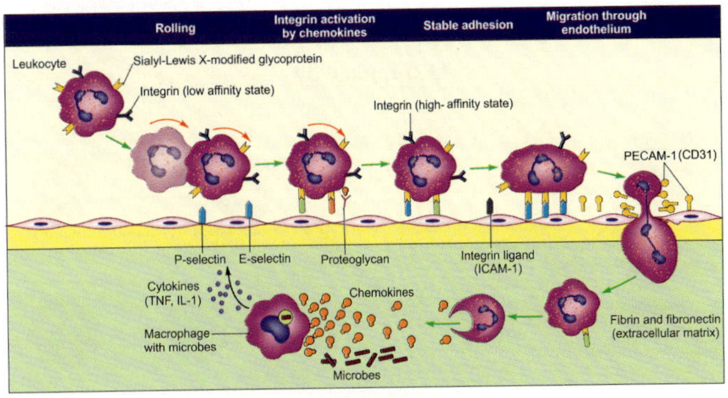

Q. 3, page 35

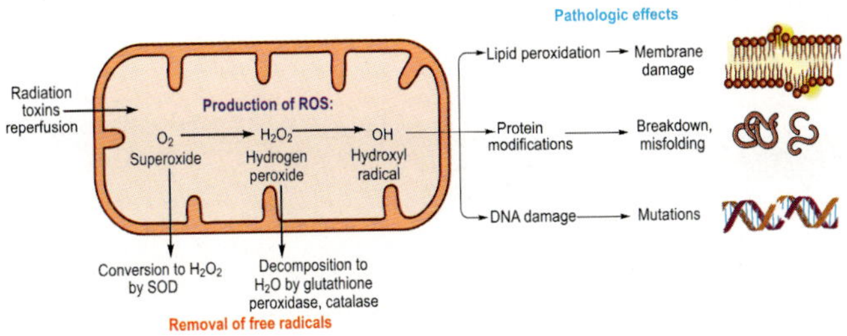

Q. 12, page 22

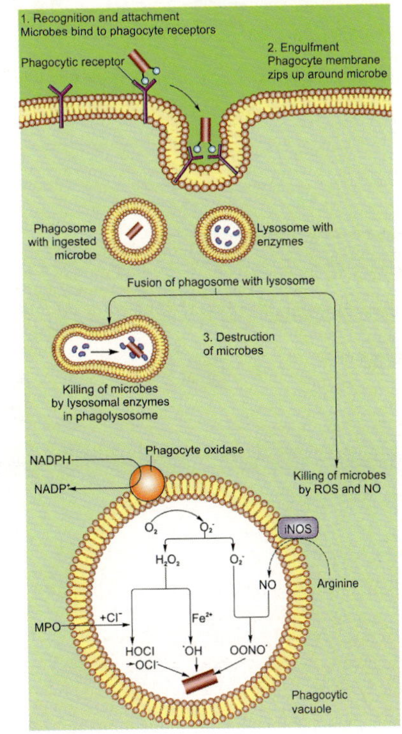

Q. 11, page 37

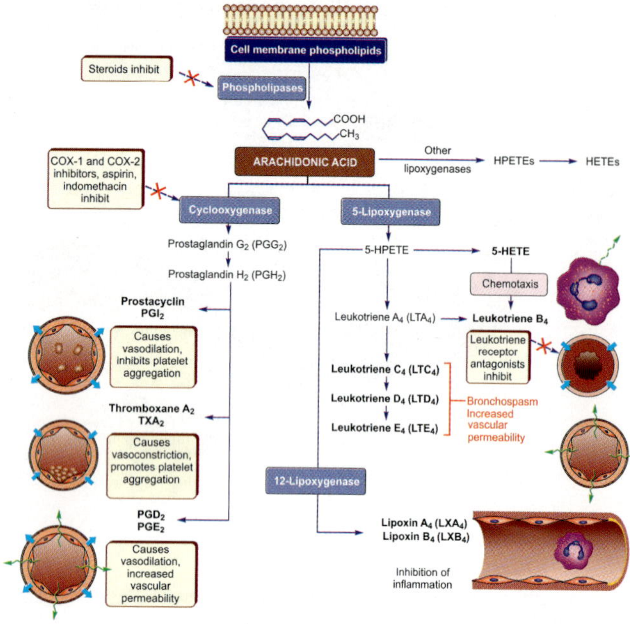

Q. 14, page 39

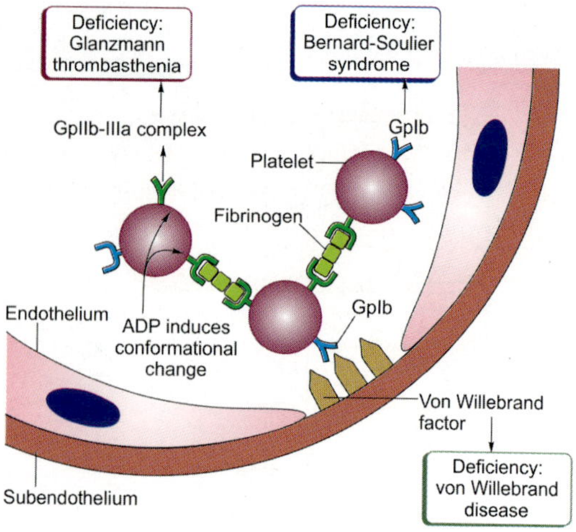

Q. 7, page 55

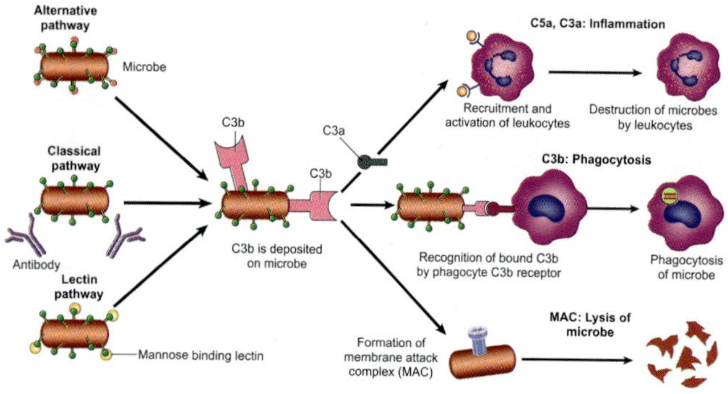

Q. 24, page 42

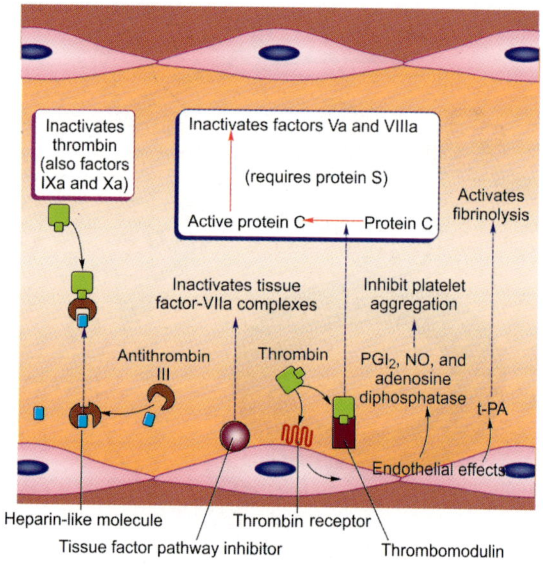

Q. 10, page 56

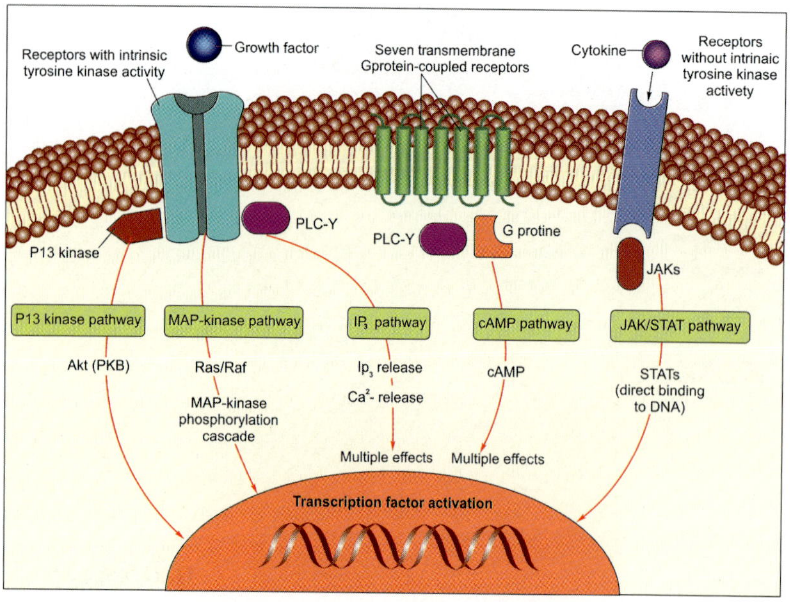

Q. 36, page 46

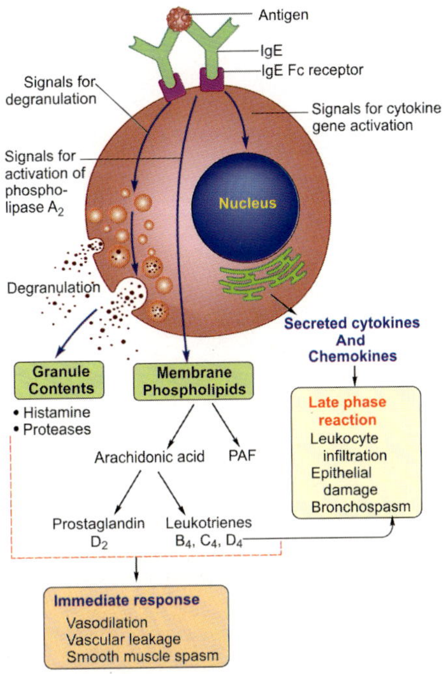

Q. 12, page 89

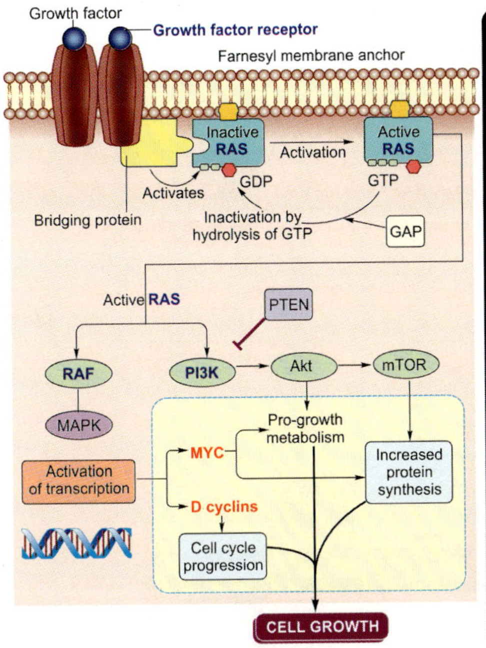

Q. 20, page 112

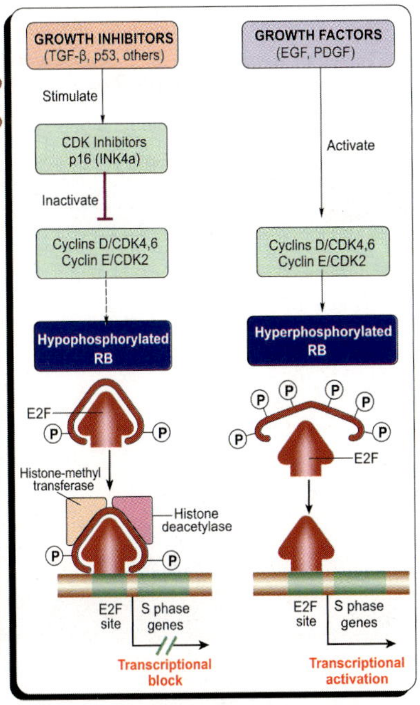

Q. 21, page 113

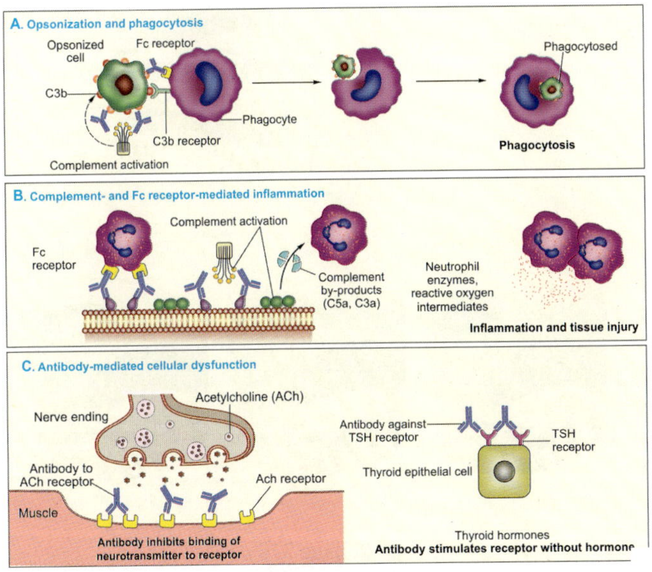

Q. 14, page 90

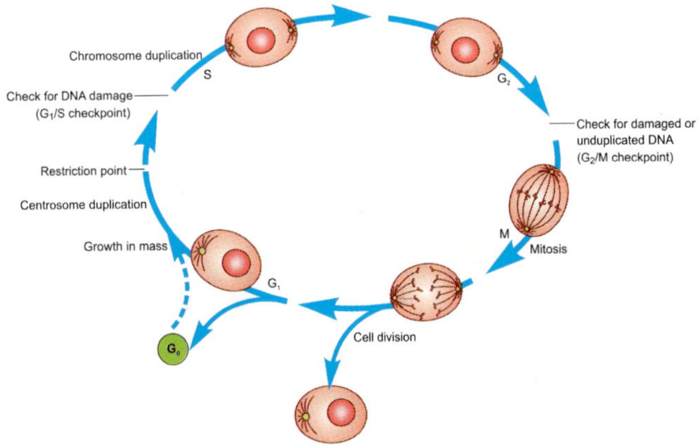

Q. 22, page 114

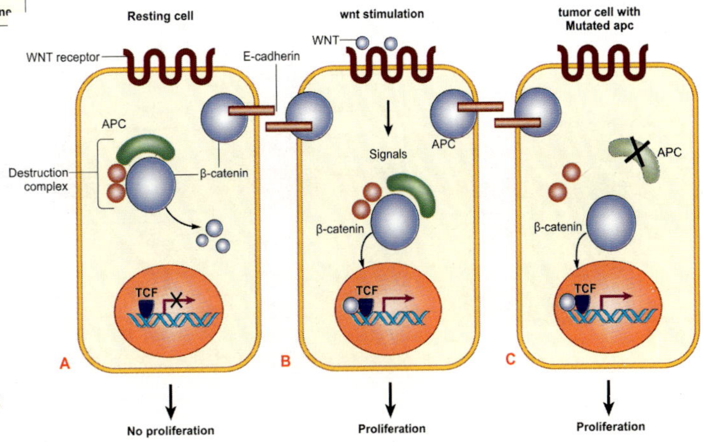

Q. 26, page 116

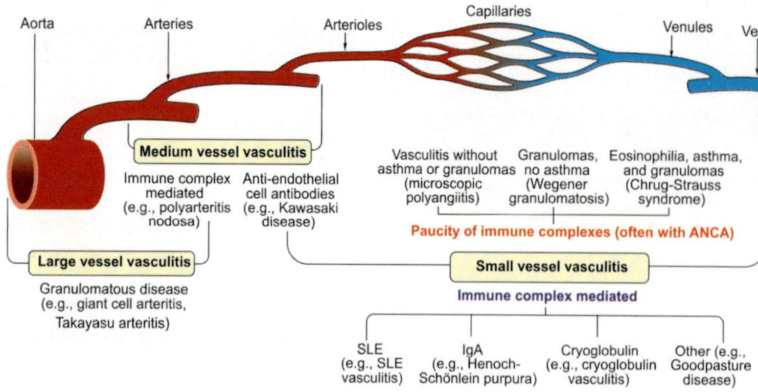

Q. 12, page 156

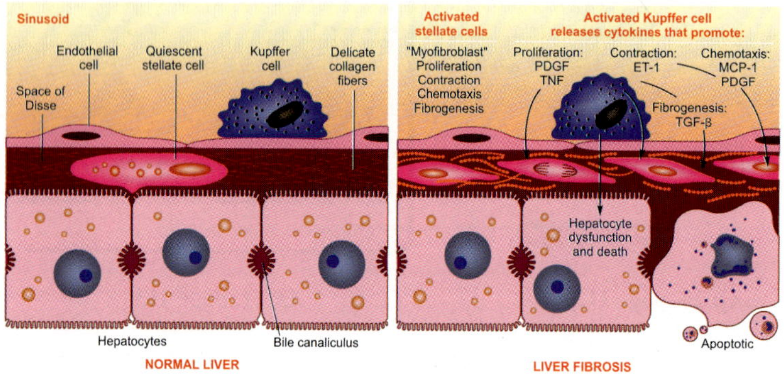

Q. 7, page 244

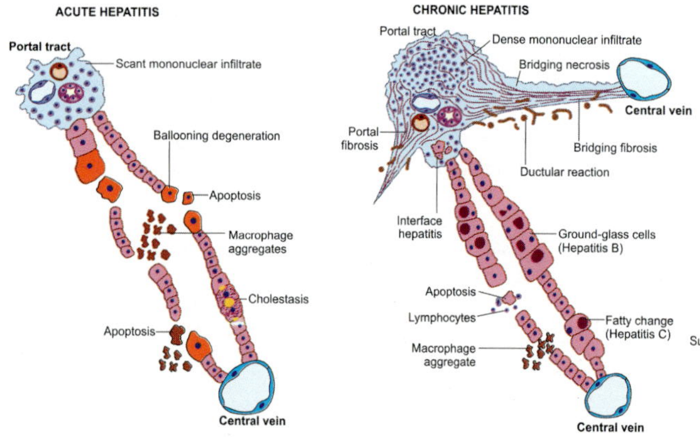

Q. 37, page 250

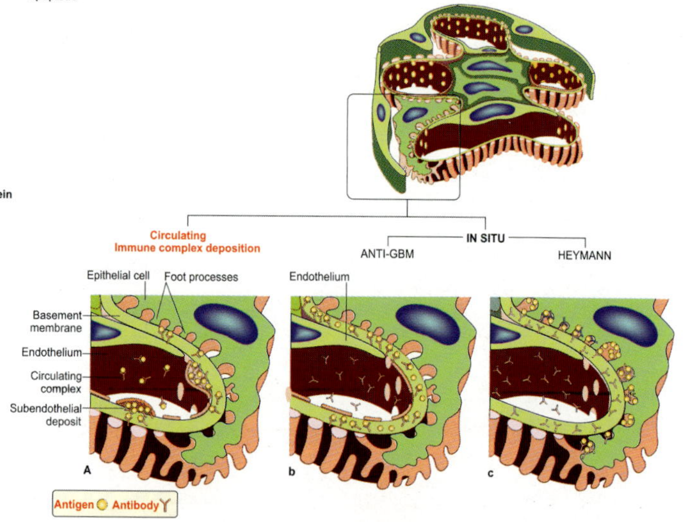

Q. 9, page 275

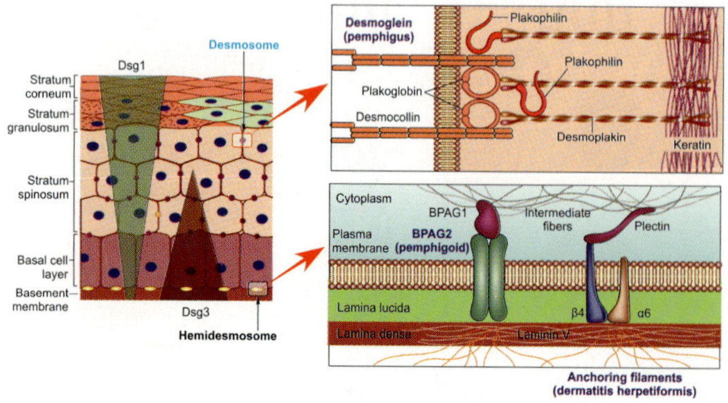

Q. 19, page 342

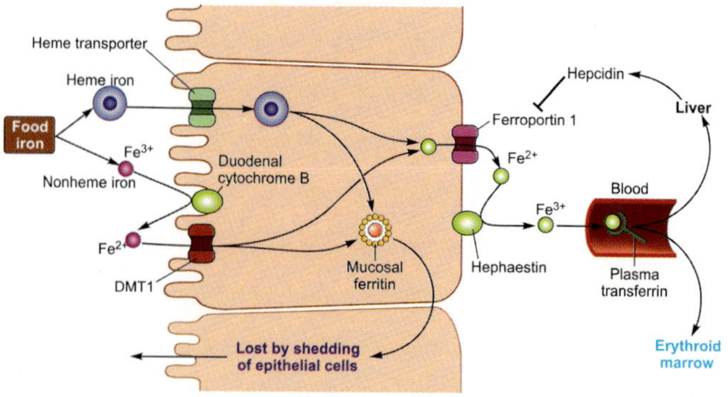

Q. 68, page 437

Contents

1 Cell as a Unit of Health and Disease

How to go about this chapter?

- **This chapter has been a new addition in 9 ed. Robbins and since than from last year, even single lines from this chapter has been picked up and asked as MCQs**
- **Be thorough with all the MCQs in this chapter, as each one of it is important, as being a topic of recent advance in pathology**
- **All topics covered are equally important and one should be thorough with all of them**

THE GENOME

1) **Human genome contains:**
   a) 3.2 billion DNA base pairs
   b) 2.3 billion DNA base pairs
   c) 3.2 million DNA base pairs
   d) 2.3 million DNA base pairs

2) **Protein-encoding genes comprises what percentage of genome?**
   a) 1.5% b) 5%
   c) 95% d) 98.5%

3) **Jumping genes take part in:**
   a) Gene regulation
   b) Chromosomal aberrations
   c) Gene movement in a species
   d) Amplification

4) **Most common form of DNA variation is:**
   a) Single nucleotide pleomorphism
   b) Copy number variations
   c) Transposons
   d) Mutations

5) **.....% of single nucleotide polymorphisms which occurs in coding region:**
   a) 1% b) 2%
   c) 3% d) 4%

6) **Linkage disequilibrium in relation to Single Nucleotide Pleomorphism (SNP) occurs when:**
   a) Disease causing genes are not co-inherited with SNP
   b) Inherited SNP but not with the disease causing genes
   c) Genetic mutations
   d) Co-inherited with the disease causing gene

7) **TRUE about human cell DNA:**
   a) Naked DNA is 1.8 m long
   b) DNA can be packed into nucleus of 7-8 micrometers
   c) Euchromatin is transcriptionally active chromatin
   d) All of the above

8) **Heritable genetic changes not caused by alterations in DNA sequence is:**
   a) Genetics b) Epigenetics
   c) Mutations d) Transposons

9) **Epigenetic factors refers to:**
   a) Histone methylation
   b) Histone phosphorylation
   c) DNA methylation
   d) All of the above

10) **Gene silencing RNA:**
    a) r-RNA b) t-RNA
    c) miRNA d) None of the above

11) **Function of miRNA:**
    a) Post-transcriptional silencing of gene expression
    b) Post-transcriptional modification of gene expression
    c) Translation of proteins
    d) All of the above

12) **miRNA has average of ..... nucleotides.**
    a) 11 b) 22
    c) 33 d) 44

13) **Human genome encodes ..... miRNA.**
    a) 10 b) 100
    c) 1000 d) 2000

14) **Function of peroxisomes is:**
    a) Protein synthesis
    b) Carbohydrate metabolism
    c) Generating H_2O_2
    d) DNA replication

15) All of the following can detect epigenetic modifications EXCEPT:
a) Chip-on-chip
b) Bi-sulphite method
c) HPLC
d) Methylation specific PCR

16) Coding DNA constitutes what proportion of total DNA?
a) 0.02
b) 0.1
c) 0.25
d) 0.4

17) GWAS stands for:
a) Genome wide association syndrome
b) Genome wide association studies
c) Genome wide array studies
d) Gene wide amplication studies

18) Genetic polymorphisms include all EXCEPT:
a) Single nucleotide polymorphisms
b) Microsatellites
c) Minisatellites
d) Mutation

19) Function of miRNA includes all EXCEPT:
a) Gene silencing
b) Transcription inhibition
c) Translation repression
d) Breaking of messenger RNA

20) Most abundant glycoprotein present in basement membrane is:
a) Laminin
b) Fibronectin
c) Collagen type IV
d) Heparin sulphate

21) Gene silencing RNA:
a) siRNA
b) mRNA
c) SnRNA
d) HnRNA

CELLULAR HOUSEKEEPING

22) Lifespan of mitochondria is:
a) 10 days
b) 20 days
c) 30 days
d) 40 days

23) Following are expressed on the outer surface of plasma membrane EXCEPT:
a) Phosphatidylcholine
b) Sphingomyelin
c) Glycolipids
d) Phosphatidylserine

24) Cytosolic enzymes function at pH of:
a) 7.4
b) 5
c) Less than 5
d) Any of the above

25) Movement of small and large molecules in a cell occurs by:
a) Endocytosis
b) Exocytosis
c) Transcytosis
d) Any of the above

26) Receptor mediated endocytosis is noted in transport of:
a) LDL
b) Transferrin
c) VLDL
d) Both a and b

27) Major class of cytoskeletal proteins include:
a) Actin
b) Intermediate filaments
c) Microtubules
d) All of the above

28) Which of the following statement is NOT TRUE?
a) Cytokeratin is the marker of muscle cells
b) Vimentin is used for fibroblasts
c) Neurofilaments are present in neurons
d) Desmin can be used as a marker for muscle cells

29) Transmembrane protein that mediate cell-cell interactions:
a) Occludin
b) Claudin
c) Zonulin
d) All of the above

30) Gap junctions comprise:
a) Catenins
b) Cadherins
c) Connexins
d) Claudin

31) Destruction of proteins is brought about by:
a) Ubiquitin
b) Chaperones
c) Ligases
d) Any of the above

MITOCHONDRIAL FUNCTION

32) Mitochondrial DNA is.......inherited.
a) Maternally
b) Paternally
c) Epigenetically
d) Any of the above

33) TRUE about mitochondria:
a) Inner membrane contains enzymes of respiratory chain
b) Inter-membrane space is the site for ATP synthesis
c) Outer membrane is studded with porin proteins
d) All of the above

CELL ACTIVATION

34) Secreted molecules helpful in cell signaling include(s):
a) Growth factors
b) Cytokines
c) Hormones
d) Any of the above

35) Signaling pathway by which the molecule secreted by one cell affects that same cell:
a) Paracrine
b) Autocrine
c) Synaptic
d) Endocrine

GROWTH FACTORS AND RECEPTORS

36) All of the following are functions of TGF-β EXCEPT:
a) Chemotactic for PMN's

b) Stimulates angiogenesis
c) Stimulates production of Matrix Metallo-proteinase (MMP's), fibronectin
d) Stimulates TIMP synthesis

37) All of the following are true about TGF-α EXCEPT:
a) Anti-inflammatory
b) Causes fibrosis
c) Tumor suppressor gene
d) Anti-angiogenic

INTERACTION WITH EXTRA-CELLULAR MATRIX

38) All are the components of basement membrane EXCEPT:
a) Laminin
b) Heparin sulphate
c) Rhodopsin
d) Proteoglycans

39) Most abundant collagen in body:
a) Type I b) Type II
c) Type III d) Type IV

40) FACIT collagen is:
a) Type I b) Type III
c) Type IX d) Type XI

41) Collagen present in cornea:
a) Type 1 b) Type 2
c) Type 4 d) Type 7

42) Tensile strength of fibrillar collagens is due to activity of:
a) Lysyl oxidase b) Hydroxylase
c) Protease d) Ligase

43) Most abundant glycoprotein in basement membrane:
a) Laminin b) Fibronectin
c) Integrin d) Type IV collagen

MAINTAINING CELL POPULATION

44) All are true about cyclin and its inhibitors EXCEPT:
a) Cyclin D/CDK4 acts in G1-S phase
b) Cyclin B/CDK1 acts on G2-M phase
c) p16 inhibits cyclin B/CDK1
d) p21 can inhibit all CDK's

45) Oval cells are seen in: (NEET 2013)
a) Skin b) Cornea
c) Liver d) Bone

46) Stem cells are taken from all EXCEPT:
a) Liver
b) Bone marrow
c) Blood
d) Adipose tissue

47) Embryonic stem cells can give rise to:
a) Neurons b) Cardiac muscle
c) Hepatocytes d) All of the above

48) Mesenchymal stem cells can give rise to:
a) Chondrocytes b) Osteocytes
c) Adipocytes d) All of the above

49) TRUE about stem cell niches:
a) Skin stem cells are located in bulge area of hair follicle
b) Small intestinal stem cells are located near base of crypt
c) Liver stem cells are located in canals of Herring
d) All of the above

50) Following cell(s) doesn't elicit any rejection reaction:
a) Mesenchymal stem cell
b) Embryonic stem cell
c) Induced pluripotent stem cell
d) Tissue stem cell

51) Following enzyme is used to alter/correct DNA sequences:
a) Cas 9 b) Caspase 9
c) Caspase 6 d) Any of the above

52) What generates intracellular signals when cells are subjected to shear stress? (NEET 2014)
a) Cadherin
b) Selectins
c) Integrins
d) Focal adhesion molecules

53) Collagen typical of basement membrane: (AIIMS May 2015)
a) Type I b) Type V
c) Type IV d) Type III

54) Mutation in COL4A5 leads to: (AIIMS Nov 2015)
a) Alport's syndrome
b) Good pasture's syndrome
c) Hereditary Non-polyposis colon cancer
d) Xeroderma pigmentosum

55) Real time polymerase chain reaction is done for: (AIIMS Nov 2013)
a) DNA detection only
b) RNA detection only
c) Both RNA and DNA detection
d) Monitoring amplification of target nucleic acid

56) In genomic imprinting, DNA is modified by: (AIIMS Nov 2015)
a) Acetylation
b) Methylation
c) Phosphorylation
d) Deamination

General Pathology – Answers

CHAPTER 1: CELL AS A UNIT OF HEALTH AND DISEASE

Ans. 1) A. 3.2 billion DNA base pairs (Ref: 9 ed. Robbins p 1)

- **Genome** refers to the **genetic material**[Q] of an organism
- **Human genome** contains roughly **3.2 billion DNA base pairs**[Q]

Ans. 2) A. 1.5% (Ref: 9 ed. Robbins p 1)

- In **human genome** there are about **20,000 protein-encoding genes**, which comprises around **1.5%**[Q] of the genome

Ans. 3) A. Gene regulation (Ref: 9 ed. Robbins p 2)

Jumping genes:

- Mobile genetic elements, called **transposons**[Q]
- Segments can move around the genome, exhibiting wide variation in number and positioning
- Implicated in **gene regulation** and **chromatin organization**[Q]

Ans. 4) A. Single nucleotide pleomorphism (Ref: 9 ed. Robbins p 3)

- **Two most common forms** of **DNA variation** in the **human genome** are **single nucleotide polymorphisms (SNPs)** and **copy number variations (CNVs)**[Q]

Single nucleotide polymorphisms[Q]**:**

- Variations at single nucleotide positions
- Always **bi-allelic**[Q]
- Can occur in **exons**, introns, intergenic regions, and coding regions
- Only **1% of SNPs**[Q] occur in **coding regions**

Ans. 5) A. 1% (Ref: 9 ed. Robbins p 3)

- About **1%** of **SNPs** occur in **coding regions**[Q]

Ans. 6) D. Co-inherited with the disease causing gene (Ref: 9 ed. Robbins p 3)

Linkage disequilibrium in relation to SNP:

- **Neutral SNP's:** When SNP's has no effect on gene function
- Neutral SNP's can act as useful marker, if **co-inherited** with the actual disease causing gene
- Hence, SNP and causative genetic factor occurs in **linkage disequilibrium**

Ans. 7) D. All of the above (Ref: 9 ed. Robbins p 3, f-1-1)

- **Naked DNA** of a human cell is about **1.8 meters long**[Q]
- DNA can be **packed** into a **nucleus** as **small as 7 to 8 micrometers**[Q] in diameter (width of lymphocyte)
- **Nuclear chromatin** exists in **two basic forms**:
  a) Cytochemically dense and transcriptionally **inactive heterochromatin**[Q]
  b) Cytochemically dispersed and transcriptionally **active euchromatin**[Q]

Ans. 8) B. Epigenetics (Ref: 9 ed. Robbins p 3-4)

- **Epigenetics**: Heritable changes in **gene expression**[Q] which are not caused by alterations in **DNA sequence**

Epigenetic factors[Q] include:

- Histone and histone modifying factors like **histone methylation, acetylation** and **phosphorylation**[Q]
- DNA methylation
- Chromatin organizing factors

Ans. 9) D. All of the above (Ref: 9 ed. Robbins p 3-4)

- **Refer to answer 6**

Ans. 10) C. miRNA (Ref: 9 ed. Robbins p 4-5, f-1-3)

Generation of microRNA (miRNA) and **their mode of action**[Q]:

- Transcription of **miRNA** → **Primary miRNA** →(in presence of enzyme **DICER**) primary miRNA is converted to **single stranded miRNAs + RNA induced silencing complex (RISC)** → induces **miRNA cleavage** or **repress its translation** → **Post transcriptional silencing**[Q] of target mRNA

Ans. 11) A. Post transcriptional silencing of gene expression (Ref: 9 ed. Robbins p 4-5, f-1-3)

Mechanism of **gene regulation** in all **eukaryotes**[Q]:

- **Post transcriptional silencing**[Q] of **gene expression** by **miRNA**

Ans. 12) B. 22 (Ref: 9 ed. Robbins p 5, f-1-3)

- **miRNA** are **short RNAs** with **22 nucleotides**[Q] on average

Ans. 13) C. 1000 (Ref: 9 ed. Robbins p 5)

- **Human genome**, contains **20,000 protein-encoding genes**[Q]
- **Human genome** encodes **1000 miRNA genes**[Q] **(20-fold less** than the **number of protein-coding genes)**

Ans. 14) C. Generating H_2O_2 (Ref: 9 ed. Robbins p 6-7)

Function of important cell organelles[Q]:

Lysosomes – digestion of **proteins, polysaccharides, lipids, nucleic acids**
Proteasomes – removal of denatured proteins
Peroxisomes[Q] – **breakdown of fatty acids**, thus producing **hydrogen peroxide**

Ans. 15) C. HPLC (Ref: 9 ed. Robbins p 3-4)

Methods used to detect epigenetic modifications[Q]:

- **Sequencing**
- **Microarray technology** (chip on chip)
- **Polymerase chain reaction (PCR)**
- **Bi-sulphite** method

Ans. 16) A. 0.02 (Ref: 9 ed. Robbins p 1)

- **Coding DNA** constitutes **0.02 or 1.5-2%** of **total DNA**[Q]

Ans. 17) B. Genome wide association studies (Ref: 9 ed. Robbins p 179)

- **GWAS** refers to **"Genome wide association studies"**[Q]
- In **GWAS**, genome of **large number of individuals**, with and without disease are examined for **common genetic variants or polymorphisms**[Q]

Ans. 18) D. Mutation (Ref: 9 ed. Robbins p 3)

- **Two types of genetic polymorphisms: Single nucleotide polymorphisms (SNP's)**[Q] and **repeat length polymorphisms**[Q]

Repeat length polymorphisms are of two types:

- **Mini-satellite (1-3 kb)**[Q] or **Micro-satellite repeats (<1 kb)**[Q]

Ans. 19) B. Transcription inhibition (Ref: 9 ed. Robbins p 4-5)

Functions of miRNA[Q] include:

- **Gene silencing**
- **Translation repression**
- **Breaking** of **messenger RNA**

Ans. 20) A. Laminin (Ref: 9 ed. Robbins p 24-25)

Major constituents of **Basement membrane include**[Q]:

- Amorphous **non-fibrillar type IV collagen**
- **Laminin (most abundant glycoprotein in basement membrane)**
- **Nidogen 1 and 2, entactin, proteoglycan** and **fibronectin**

Ans. 21) A. siRNA (Ref: 9 ed. Robbins p 4-5)

Small interfering RNAs (siRNAs)[Q]:

- Short **RNA sequences introduced experimentally**[Q] into the cells
- Their action is similar to **endogenous miRNAs**[Q]
- Synthetic **siRNAs** are **targeted against specific mRNA**
- **Useful laboratory tools** to **study gene function (knockdown technology)**[Q]
- Might act as therapeutic agents to **silence pathogenic genes**, such as **oncogenes**[Q]

Ans. 22) A. 10 days (Ref: 9 ed. Robbins p 6)

- **Macromolecules** and **organelles** have **finite lifespans**
- For example – **mitochondria**, life span is for only about **10 days**[Q]

Ans. 23) D. Phosphatidylserine (Ref: 9 ed. Robbins p 7-8, f-1-6)

Plasma membrane organization:

- **Phosphatidylcholine, Sphingomyelin** and **Glycolipids** are present on the **outer leafletQ** of the plasma membrane
- **Phoshatidylserine** and **phosphatidylethanolamine**[Q] are predominantly found on the **inner leaflet** of plasma membrane

Ans. 24) A. 7.4 (Ref: 9 ed. Robbins p 7-8, f-1-7)

- Most **cytosolic enzymes** works at **pH 7.4**[Q]
- **Lysosomal enzymes** function best at **pH 5 or less**[Q]

Ans. 25) D. Any of the above (Ref: 9 ed. Robbins p 9-10, f-1-7)

- **Endocytosis**[Q]: Uptake of fluids or macromolecules by the cell
- **Exocytosis**[Q]: Process by which large molecules are exported from cells
- **Transcytosis**[Q]: Movement of **endocytosed vesicles** between the apical and basolateral compartments of cells

Ans. 26) D. Both a and b (Ref: 9 ed. Robbins p 10, f-1-7)

- **Receptor-mediated endocytosis** is noted in transport of **transferrinQ** and **low-density lipoprotein (LDL)**[Q]

Ans. 27) D. All of the above (Ref: 9 ed. Robbins p 10-11, f-1-8)

Three major classes[Q] of **cytoskeletal proteins:**

a) Actin microfilaments:

- 5-9 nm diameter fibrils
- **G-actin**[Q] is the **most abundant** cytosolic proteins in the cell

b) Intermediate filaments: (refer answer 28)

- 10nm diameter fibrils

c) Microtubules[Q]**:**

- **25-nm-thick fibrils** composed of dimers of **α-** and **β-tubulin**

- Acts as **molecular motor proteins** that use **ATP** to move vesicles, organelles, or other molecules around cells along **microtubules**

Ans. 28) A. Cytokeratin is the marker of muscle cells (Ref: 9 ed. Robbins p 11)

Intermediate filaments[Q]	Tissue[Q]
Lamin A, B and C	Nuclear lamina of all cells
Vimentin	**Mesenchymal cells** (fibroblasts, endothelium)
Desmin	**Muscle cells**
Neurofilaments	Axons of neurons, imparting strength and rigidity
Glial fibrillary acidic protein	Glial cells around neurons
Cytokeratins	Acidic (type 1) and neutral/basic (type II). Used as **cell markers**

Ans. 29) D. All of the above (Ref: 9 ed. Robbins p 11, f-1-8)

- **Transmembrane proteins** that mediate **cell-cell interactions** includes **occludin, claudin, zonulin**, and **catenin**[Q]

Ans. 30) C. Connexins (Ref: 9 ed. Robbins p 12)

Communicating junctions (Gap junctions)[Q]**:**

- Mediate the passage of **chemical** or **electrical signals** from **one cell to another**[Q]
- **Gap junctions** comprises **1.5-2 nm pores** called **connexons**[Q]
- Pores are formed of transmembrane proteins called **connexins**[Q]

Ans. 31) A. Ubiquitin (Ref: 9 ed. Robbins p 14, f-1-9)

- **Proteasomes** play an important role in **degrading cytosolic proteins**[Q]
- **Proteins** destruction occurs by **protein** called **ubiquitin**[Q]

Ans. 32) A. Maternally (Ref: 9 ed. Robbins p 14)

- **Ovum** contributes the majority of **cytoplasmic organelles** to the **fertilized zygote**, hence **mitochondrial DNA**[Q] is entirely **maternally inherited**[Q]

Ans. 33) D. All of the above (Ref: 9 ed. Robbins p 14-15, f-1-10)

Mitochondrion has two **separate** and **specialized membranes:**

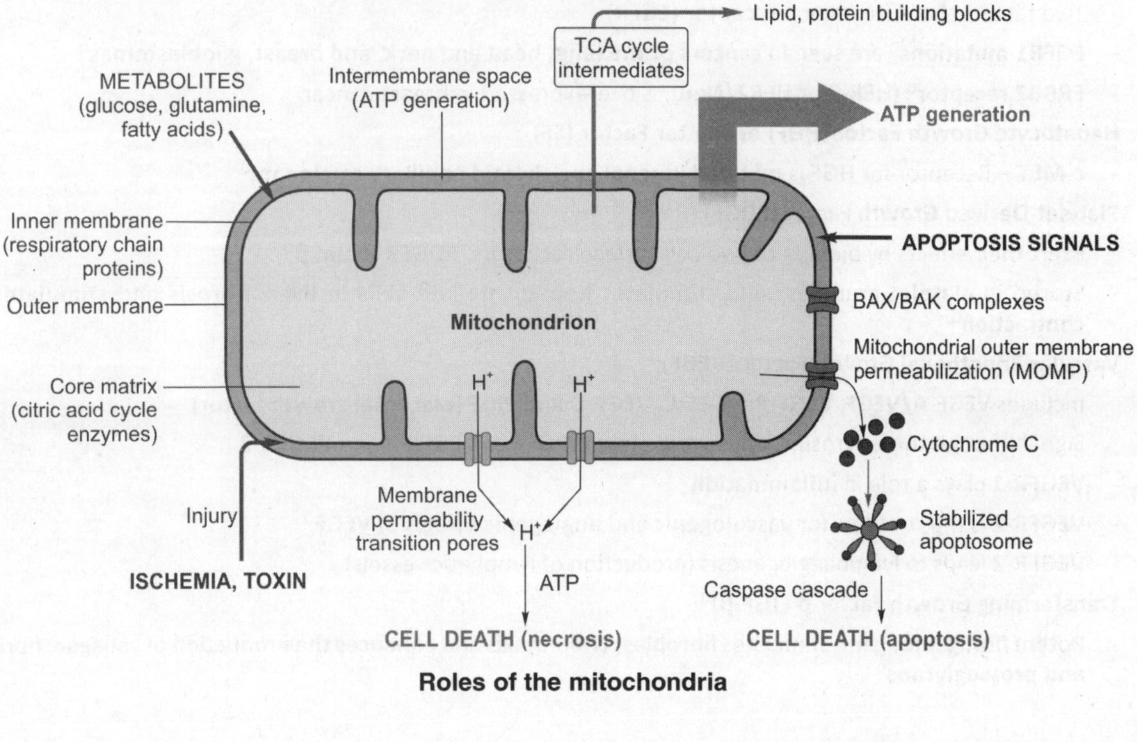

Roles of the mitochondria

Inner membrane[Q]

- Contains the **enzymes of respiratory chain** folded into **cristae**[Q]
- Has **core matrix space**, which contains the enzyme of **citric acid cycle**[Q]

Inter-membrane space

- Space outside the **inner membrane** and is the site of **ATP synthesis**[Q]

Outer membrane[Q]

- Contains **porin proteins**, that form **aqueous channels** permeable to small molecules

Ans. 34) D. Any of the above (Ref: 9 ed. Robbins p 16)

Secreted molecules[Q] which help in **cell signaling** include:

- **Growth factors**
- **Cytokines**
- **Hormones**

Ans. 35) B. Autocrine signaling (Ref: 9 ed. Robbins p 16)

Extracellular cell-cell signaling pathways[Q] are classified into:

Paracrine signaling[Q]:

- Cells in the immediate vicinity are affected

Autocrine signaling[Q]:

- Occurs when molecules secreted by a cell affect that same cell

Synaptic signaling[Q]:

- Activated neurons secrete **neurotransmitters** at specialized cell junctions **(synapses)** onto target cells

Endocrine signaling[Q]:

- A mediator is released into the **bloodstream** and **acts on target cells** at a **distance**

Ans. 36) C. Stimulates production of MMP's, fibronectin (Ref: 8 ed. Robbins p.87-92, 9 ed. p. 19-20, t-1-1)

Growth Factors:

Epidermal Growth Factor (EGF) and **Transforming Growth Factor α (TGF-α)**[Q]:

- Two factors share a common receptor **(EGFR)**
- **EGFR1 mutations**[Q] are seen in **cancers of the lung, head and neck, and breast, glioblastomas**[Q]
- **ERBB2 receptor**[Q] **(HER-2 or HER2/Neu)**, is overexpressed in **breast cancer**

Hepatocyte Growth Factor (HGF) or Scatter Factor (SF)

- **c-MET** – Receptor for **HGF** is mutated in **renal** and **thyroid papillary carcinoma**[Q]

Platelet-Derived Growth Factor (PDGF)[Q]

- Exert their effects by binding to two cell surface receptors, **PDGFR α and β**[Q]
- Stored in **platelet granules**[Q] and stimulates **hepatic stellate cells** in **liver, fibrosis** and **stimulate wound contraction**[Q]

Vascular Endothelial Growth Factor (VEGF)[Q]

- Includes **VEGF-A/VEGF**, **VEGF-B**, **VEGF-C**, **VEGF-D** and **PIGF (placental growth factor)**
- Signal through three tyrosine kinase receptors: **VEGFR-1**, **VEGFR-2** and **VEGFR-3**
- **VEGFR-1** plays a role in **inflammation**
- **VEGFR-2** is the receptor for **vasculogenic** and **angiogenic effects** of **VEGF**[Q]
- **VEGFR-3** leads to lymphangiogenesis (production of lymphatic vessels)

Transforming Growth Factor β (TGF-β)[Q]

- **Potent fibrogenic agent,** stimulates **fibroblast chemotaxis** and **enhances the production of collagen, fibronectin, and proteoglycans**[Q]

- Inhibits **collagen degradation** by **decreasing matrix proteases**[Q] and **increasing tissue inhibitors of proteinases (TIMPs)**[Q] , thus leading to development of **fibrosis**[Q]
- **High TGF-β expression** – seen in **hypertrophic scars, systemic sclerosis** and **Marfan syndrome**[Q]

Thus, **TGF-β** decreases the **level of MMP's** and doesn't increase them

Growth Factors Involved in Regeneration and Repair

Growth Factor	Functions
Epidermal growth factor (EGF)	1. Mitogenic for keratinocytes and fibroblasts 2. Stimulates keratinocyte migration 3. Stimulates formation of granulation tissue
Transforming growth factor-α (TGF-α)	1. Stimulates proliferation of hepatocytes and many other epithelial cells
Hepatocyte growth factor (HGF) (scatter factor)	1. Enhances proliferation of hepatocytes 2. Increases cell motility
Vascular endothelial growth factor (VEGF)	1. Stimulates proliferation of endothelial cells 2. Increases vascular permeability
Platelet-derived growth factor (PDGF)	1. Chemotactic for neutrophils, macrophages, fibroblasts and smooth muscle cells 2. Activates and stimulates proliferation of fibroblasts, endothelial and other cells 3. Stimulates ECM protein synthesis
Fibroblast growth factors (FGFs)	1. Chemotactic and mitogenic for fibroblasts 2. Stimulates angiogenesis and ECM protein synthesis
Transforming growth factor- β (TGF-β)	1. Chemotactic for leukocytes and fibroblasts 2. Stimulates ECM protein synthesis 3. Suppresses acute inflammation
Keratinocyte growth factor (KGF) (i.e., FGF-7)	1. Stimulates keratinocyte migration, proliferation and differentiation

Ans. 37) D. Anti-angiogenic (Ref: 9 ed. Robbins p 20)

Functions of TGF-α[Q]:

- **Anti-inflammatory**
- Stimulates the production of **collagen**
- Leads to scar formation and **fibrosis**
- **Tumor suppressor** and plays a role in **angiogenesis**

Ans. 38) C. Rhodopsin (Ref: 8 ed. Robbins p 94-98, 9 ed p 20-24, f-1-12-14)

Three groups of macromolecules include:

- **Fibrous structural proteins**[Q] (collagen and elastin)
- **Adhesive glycoproteins**[Q]
- **Proteoglycans and hyaluronan**[Q]

These **three macromolecules** assemble to form two basic forms of ECM: **interstitial matrix** and **basement membrane**[Q]

Interstitial matrix[Q]

- Found in spaces between epithelial, endothelial, smooth muscle cells and in connective tissue
- Consists of collagen, elastin, fibronectin, proteoglycans and hyaluronan

Basement membranes

- Consists of **non-fibrillar collagen (type IV)**[Q], **laminin, heparin sulfate**, and **proteoglycans**

Hence, **rhodopsin** doesn't form a component of **basement membrane** and thus the answer here

Ans. 39) A. Type I (Ref: 9 ed. Robbins p 20-23)

- **Collagen I** is the **most abundant collagen**[Q] in the body
- **Collagen I** is the **main component**[Q] of organic part of bone
- **Collagen II** is the **most abundant in cartilage**[Q]

Ans. 40) C. Type IX (Ref: 9 ed. Robbins p 20-23)

- **Type IX collagen**[Q] in cartilage help regulate **collagen fibril diameters** or **collagen-collagen interactions** via Fibril-Associated Collagen with Interrupted Triple helices **(FACIT's)**[Q]

Ans. 41) A. Type 1 (Ref: 9 ed. Robbins p 20-23)

Major types of collagen and **disorders** associated with them:

Type[Q]	Seen in[Q]	Disorders[Q]
I	Bone, **cornea**, cartilage, scar tissue, tendons, skin, artery walls, endomysium of myofibrils, fibrocartilage, teeth	Osteogenesis imperfecta, Ehlers-Danlos syndrome, Caffey's disease
II	Hyaline cartilage, vitreous humor of eye	Collagenopathy
III	Granulation tissue, reticular fiber, artery wall, skin, intestines and uterus	Ehlers-Danlos syndrome
IV	Basement membrane, eye lens, glomerular basement membrane	Alport syndrome **(COL4α5)** Good pasture's syndrome **(COL4α3)**

Ans. 42) A. Lysyl oxidase (Ref: 9 ed. Robbins p. 23, f-1-16)

- **Tensile strength** of the **fibrillar collagen** occurs due to **lateral cross-linking** of **triple helices**, facilitated by the activity of **lysyl oxidase**[Q]

Ans. 43) A. Laminin (Ref: 9 ed. Robbins p. 24, f- 1-16)

- **Laminin** is the **most abundant glycoprotein** in **basement membrane**[Q]

Ans. 44) C. p16 inhibits cyclin B/CDK1 (Ref: 8 ed. Robbins p 86, 284-86, 9 ed. p. 25-26, f-1-17,18)

- Cell cycle is regulated by **activators** and **inhibitors**[Q]
- **Cell cycle progression** is driven by proteins called **cyclins** and cyclin-associated enzymes called **cyclin dependent kinases (CDKs)**[Q]
- **Cyclins D, E, A and B** are important **cyclins**, which bind to **CDKs**[Q]
- **Cyclin dependent kinase inhibitors (CDKIs)**[Q] regulate the cell cycle check points
- **CDKIs** – includes one family of **p 16, p 15, p 18, p 19** and other of **p 21, p 27, and p 57**[Q]

Salient features of Cyclin, CDKs and CDKI's:

- **Cyclin D-CDK4**, **cyclin D-CDK6** and **cyclin E-CDK2** regulate the **G1-to-S transition**[Q]
- **Cyclin A-CDK2** and **cyclin A-CDK1** are active in the **S phase**[Q]
- **Cyclin B-CDK1** is essential for the **G2-to-M transition**[Q]

Cyclin dependent kinase inhibitors:

- **INK4 inhibitors**, composed of **p 16, p 15, p 18 and p 19**, act on **cyclin D-CDK4** and **cyclin D-CDK6**[Q]
- **p 21, p 27, and p 57**, can inhibit all **CDKs**[Q]

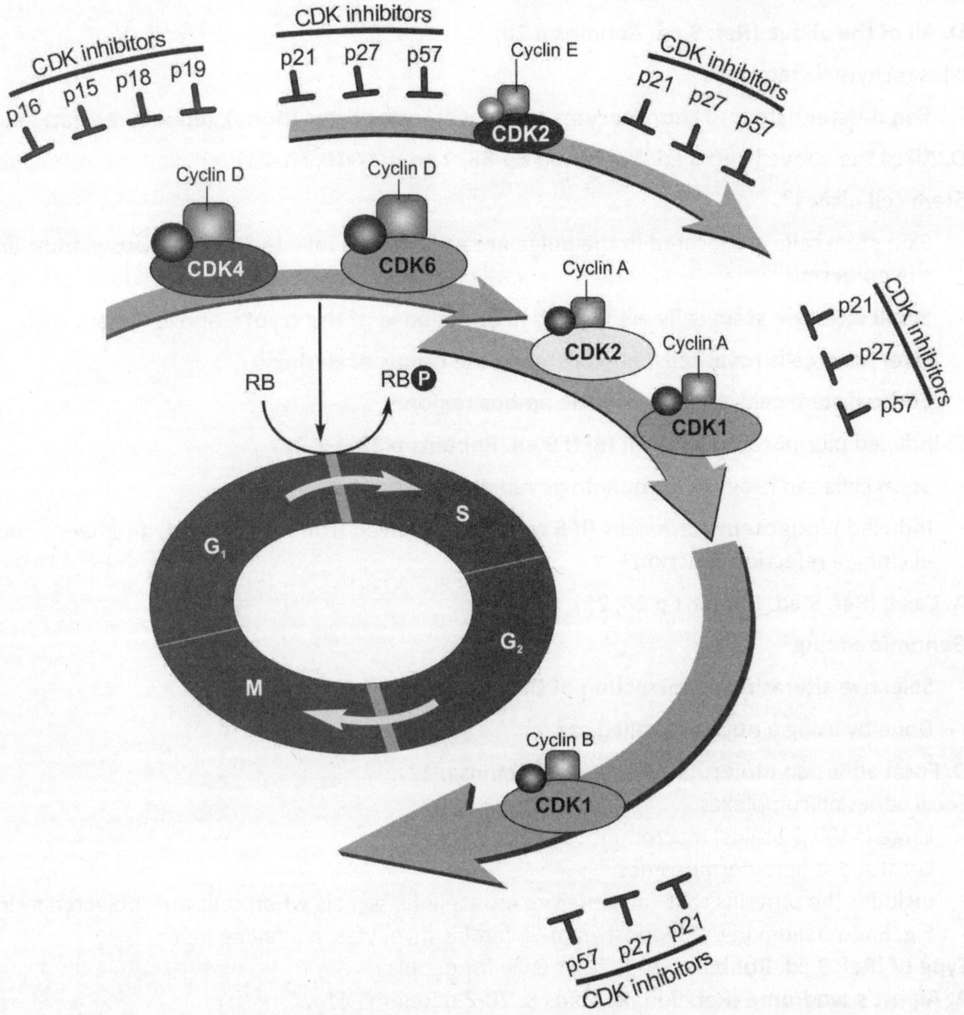

Cell cycle inhibitors

Ans. 45) C. Liver (Ref: 9 ed. Robbins p 27-28)

- **Liver stem cells (Oval cells)** are **found in canals of Hering**[Q]

Ans. 46) D. Adipose tissue (Ref: 9 ed. Robbins p 27-28)

Blood and **bone marrow** are **two important sources**[Q] of stem cells

Other sources of stem cells are:

Stem cell niches[Q]	Location[Q]
Skin stem cells	**Hair follicle bulge, sebaceous glands, interfollicular areas** of epidermis
Small intestine stem cells[Q]	Base of a crypt, above Paneth cells
Liver stem cells (Oval cells)[Q]	Canals of Hering[Q]
Corneal stem cells	Limbus region

Ans. 47) D. All of the above (Ref: 8 ed. Robbins p 83-84, 9 ed p. 27, f-1-20)

Embryonic stem cells (ES cells):

- Have **limitless cell renewal capacity** and can give rise to **every cell** in the body **(totipotent)**[Q]
- Can give rise to cells of all **three germ cell layers** including **neurons, cardiac muscle, liver cells** and **pancreatic islet cells**[Q]

Ans. 48) D. All of the above (Ref: 9 ed. Robbins p 28)

Mesenchymal stem cells[Q]:

- Can differentiate into **chondrocytes (cartilage), osteocytes (bone), adipocytes (fat),** and **myocytes (muscle)**[Q]

Ans. 49) D. All of the above (Ref: 8 ed. Robbins p 83-86, 9 ed p 27-28, f-1-21)

Stem cell niches[Q]:

- **Skin stem cells** are located in the **bulge area** of the **hair follicle**, in **sebaceous glands**, and in the lower layer of the **epidermis**[Q]
- **Small intestine stem cells** are located near the **base of the crypt**[Q], above Paneth cells
- **Liver stem cells (oval cells)** are located in the **canals of Hering**[Q]
- **Corneal stem cells** are found in the **limbus region**[Q]

Ans. 50) C. Induced pluripotent stem cell (Ref: 9 ed. Robbins p 28, f-1-22)

- **Stem cells** can provoke **immunologic reaction** in the host
- **Induced pluripotent stem cells (iPS cells)**[Q] are derived from the **patient**, and hence can be engrafted without eliciting a **rejection reaction**[Q]

Ans. 51) A. Cas 9 (Ref: 9 ed. Robbins p 28, 29)

Genomic editing[Q]

- Selective **alteration or correction** of **DNA sequences**[Q]
- Done by using a **nuclease** called **cas 9**[Q]

Ans. 52) D. Focal adhesion molecules (Ref: 9 ed. Robbins p 12)

Focal adhesion complexes:

- Large (>100 proteins) macromolecular complexes
- Localized at hemidesmosomes
- Includes the proteins that can generate intracellular signals when cells are subjected to increased shear stress
- E.g. Endothelium in the bloodstream or cardiac myocytes in a failing heart

Ans. 53) Type IV (Ref: 9 ed. Robbins p 4-5) Refer Q 20 for details

Ans. 54) A. Alport's syndrome (Ref: 9ed. Robbins p. 20-23) Refer Q 41

Ans. 55) A. Monitoring amplification of target nucleic acid (Ref: Harper 28 ed. p 395, Lippincott 3rd p 459)

Polymerase Chain Reaction:

a. A cell free, test tube method used for amplifying a target sequence of DNA

b. Much faster and more sensitive than cell based cloning

c. Used to amplify specific regions of DNA strand (target DNA)

d. It can amplify DNA fragments up to 10 kilobase pairs

e. Materials:

1. Two primers: Each of 20-35 bases along with sequence complimentary to sequence immediately adjacent to DNA segment of interest (flanking sequence)
2. DNA polymerase (Taq polymerase): Heat stable Taq polymerase obtained from thermas aquaticus, an organism found in hot springs
3. Free deoxynucleotides (dNTPs): Building blocks from which DNA polymerase synthesizes a new DNA strand
4. Target DNA fragment
5. Buffer solution: Provides a suitable chemical environment for optimum activity and stability of DNA polymerase
6. Divalent cations
7. Monovalent cations

f. Procedure:

1. Heat denaturation: DNA sample to be amplified is first heated to separate two steps
2. Annealing: Primers bind to the two separate strands of DNA flanking target sequence
3. Extension: Each strand is copied by DNA polymerase starting at primer site. Two new DNA strands serve as a template for synthesis of new DNA from two primers
4. Above three steps are repeated again and again leading to exponential increase in amount of target DNA, amplifying it by million fold to a billion fold

g. Advantages:

1. DNA sequence present only in trace amounts can be amplified to become predominant sequence
2. Speed
3. Less technically difficult

h. Disadvantages:

1. To synthesize primers flanking sequence of DNA segment of interest should be known
2. Applies only to short DNA fragments typically less than 10 kbs

Ans. 56) B. Methylation (Ref: 9 ed. Robbins p 3-4) Refer Q 8 for details

For genomic imprinting details refer Chapter 7

2 Cellular Responses to Stress and Toxic Insults: Adaptation, Injury and Death

How to go about this chapter?

- **One should have clear concepts about Necrosis, Apoptosis, free radical injury, which are asked repeatedly**
- **Chapter deals with important topics, asked in exams, so be thorough with each question and answer, so that the repeat MCQs can be dealt easily**
- **Recent advance topics–Pyroptosis and Necroptosis, will be a favorite topic of examiners in coming years**

ADAPTATIONS OF CELLULAR GROWTH AND DIFFERENTIATION

1) **All are true about Hypertrophy EXCEPT:**
   a) PI3K/AKT pathway and down streaming of G-PCR are involved
   b) Induction of embryonic/fetal genes is seen
   c) Cardiac hypertrophy is associated with re-induction of ANF gene expression
   d) Barbiturates leading to hypertrophy of smooth endoplasmic reticulum in hepatocytes leads to reduced amount of cytochrome P-450 levels

2) **Physiological hyperplasia and hypertrophy are seen simultaneously in:**
   a) Uterus in pregnancy
   b) Cardiac muscle in cardiomegaly
   c) Breast at puberty
   d) Skeletal muscle in athlete

3) **Compensatory hyperplasia is seen in:**
   a) Liver b) Breast
   c) Endometrium d) Prostate

4) **Brown atrophy is due to:**
   a) Melanin b) Lipofuscin
   c) Hemosiderin d) Any of above

5) **Most common epithelial metaplasia:**
   a) Columnar to squamous
   b) Squamous to columnar
   c) Cuboidal to squamous
   d) Squamous to cuboidal

6) **In Barrett esophagus following metaplasia is seen:**
   a) Columnar to squamous
   b) Squamous to columnar
   c) Cuboidal to squamous
   d) Squamous to cuboidal

MORPHOLOGIC ALTERATIONS IN CELL INJURY

7) **All of the following statements are true regarding reversible cell injury EXCEPT:**
   a) Formation of amorphous densities in mitochondrial matrix
   b) Diminished generation of adenosine triphosphate
   c) Formation of blebs in plasma membrane
   d) Detachment of ribosomes from the granular endoplasmic reticulum

8) **A 49 year-old male suffers an acute myocardial infarction because of sudden occlusion of left anterior descending artery. The areas within the ventricle of myocardial necrosis can be best described as:**
   a) Coagulative necrosis
   b) Liquefactive necrosis
   c) Fibrinoid necrosis
   d) Caseous necrosis

9) **Fibrinoid necrosis may be observed in all of the following EXCEPT:**
   a) Malignant hypertension
   b) Polyarteritis nodosa
   c) Diabetic glomerulosclerosis
   d) Acute rheumatic fever (Aschoff's nodule)

10) **A 41-year-old malnourished male, chronic alcoholic reported to the emergency with history of severe abdominal pain. Plain X-ray abdomen showed small fluffy white shadows. Serum**

amylase was elevated. These white shadow are due to:
a) Fat necrosis
b) Fat saponification
c) Metastatic calcification
d) Renal stones

11) **A 7 year-old boy developed jaundice and deep red colored urine after taking chloroquine tablets. He was diagnosed as homozygous G6PD deficiency and the red cell damage was attributed to free radical damage. The defect lies in:**
a) Excess production of ROS
b) Deficiency of antioxidant enzyme glutathione peroxidase
c) Deficiency of glutathione
d) All of the above

12) **Fenton reaction leads to free radical generation when:**
a) Radiant energy is absorbed by water
b) Hydrogen peroxide is formed by myeloperoxidase
c) Ferrous ions are converted to ferric ions
d) Nitric oxide is converted to peroxynitrite anion

CLINICOPATHOLOGIC CORRELATIONS: SELECTED EXAMPLES OF CELL INJURY AND NECROSIS

13) **About ischemia-reperfusion injury which is/are correct:**
a) After reperfusion, injury is paradoxically activated
b) Damage is mediated by ROS
c) Ischemic injury is associated with inflammation and complement system activation
d) All of the above

APOPTOSIS

14) **Ladder pattern of DNA electrophoresis in apoptosis is caused by the action of the following enzyme:**
a) Endonuclease
b) Transglutaminase
c) DNAse
d) Caspase

15) **Annexin V is a marker of:**
a) Apoptosis
b) Necrosis
c) Atherosclerosis
d) Inflammation

16) **All of the following are initiator caspases EXCEPT:**
a) Caspase 8 b) Caspase 9
c) Caspase 10 d) Caspase 3

17) **Intracellular accumulation of abnormally folded protein is a feature of:**
a) Alzheimer's disease
b) Huntington's disease
c) Parkinson's disease
d) All of the above

18) **TRUE about necroptosis:**
a) Also called as programmed necrosis
b) Does not result in caspase activation
c) Triggered by ligation of TNFR1
d) All of the above

19) **Which of the following plays a role in Pyroptosis?**
a) IL-1 b) Caspase-1
c) Caspase-11 d) All of the above

20) **Necroptosis is associated with cell death in:**
a) Steatohepatitis
b) Acute pancreatitis
c) Reperfusion injury
d) All of the above

AUTOPHAGY

21) **All of the following are true about autophagy EXCEPT:**
a) A process in which cell eats its own content
b) Autophagic vacuole fuses with lysosome to form autophagolysosome
c) Autophagy triggers cell death similar to apoptosis
d) Regulated by a set of autophagy genes

INTRACELLULAR ACCUMULATIONS

22) **All are used to identify fat histologically EXCEPT:**
a) Oil Red-O b) Sudan IV
c) PAS d) Frozen section

23) **Which of the following pigment is the tell-tale sign of free radical injury and lipid peroxidation?**
a) Lipofuscin b) Melanin
c) Bilirubin d) Hematin

PATHOLOGIC CALCIFICATION

24) **Which of the following is not a common site for metastatic calcification?**
a) Gastric mucosa b) Kidneys
c) Aorta d) Parathyroid

CELLULAR AGING

25) **Which of the following is associated with aging?**
a) Reduced cross linkages in collagen
b) Increased free radical injury
c) Decreased somatic mutations in DNA
d) Increased superoxide dismutase levels

26) **Fatty liver is due to accumulation of: (NEET 2014)**
a) Triglycerides b) LDL
c) Lipoprotein A d) VLDL

27) **Caspases are involved in: (NEET 2014, AIPGMEE 2010)**
a) Apoptosis b) Pinocytosis
c) Cell signaling d) Cell injury

28) **Execution caspases of apoptosis are: (NEET 2014)**
a) Caspase 1 and 3 b) Caspase 3 and 5
c) Caspase 1 and 5 d) Caspase 3 and 7

29) **Trauma to breast causes which type of necrosis? (NEET 2014)**
a) Coagulative necrosis
b) Liquefactive necrosis
c) Caseous necrosis
d) Fat necrosis

30) **Characteristic feature of apoptosis on light microscopy is: (NEET 2014)**
a) Cellular swelling
b) Nuclear compaction
c) Intact cell membrane
d) Cytoplasmic eosinophilia

31) **Lipid peroxidation of polyunsaturated lipids of subcellular membranes produces: (NEET 2014)**
a) Lipofuscin
b) Hemosiderin
c) Both of above
d) None of above

32) **Perforin: (NEET 2014)**
a) NK cell b) Cytotoxic T cell
c) Plasma cell d) Monocyte

33) **Enzyme that protects the brain from free radical injury is: (NEET 2014)**
a) Myeloperoxidase
b) MAO
c) Superoxide dismutase
d) Hydroxylase

34) **What happens in hypertrophy? (NEET 2014)**
a) Increase number of cells
b) Increase size of cells
c) Increase protein in cells
d) Decrease in cell number

35) **Metastatic calcification is characterized by: (NEET 2014)**
a) Hypercalcemia
b) Hypocalcemia
c) Eucalcemia
D) None of the above

36) **All of the following organs likely undergo coagulative necrosis EXCEPT: (NEET 2014)**
a) Spleen b) Heart
c) Kidney d) Brain

37) **Fenton reaction leads to free radical generation when: (NEET 2014)**
a) Radiant energy is absorbed by water
b) H_2O_2 is formed by myeloperoxidase
c) Ferrous ion converted to ferric ion
d) Nitric oxide is converted to peroxynitrite

38) **Cellular swelling with blebs and myelin figures are the changes seen in: (NEET 2014)**
a) Reversible cell injury
b) Irreversible cell injury
c) Metaplasia
d) Anaplasia

39) **Pro-inflammatory cytokines include all of the following EXCEPT: (NEET 2013)**
a) Interleukin 1
b) Interleukin-10
c) Interleukin 6
d) TNF- Alpha

40) **In apoptosis, cytochrome C acts through: (NEET 2013)**
a) Apaf 1 b) Bcl-2
c) FADD d) TNF

41) **True about Psammoma bodies are all EXCEPT: (NEET 2013)**
a) Seen in meningioma
b) Concentric whorled appearance
c) Contains calcium deposits
d) Seen in teratoma

42) **In cell death, myelin figures are derived from: (NEET 2013)**
a) Nucleus b) Cell membrane
c) Cytoplasm d) Mitochondria

43) **In myocardium, in reperfusion injury maximum effect is due to: (NEET 2013)**
a) Neutrophil b) Monocytes
c) Eosinophils d) Free radicals

44) **Irreversible cell injury: (NEET 2013)**
a) Mitochondrial densities
b) Cellular swelling
c) Blebs
d) None

45) **Actions of Bradykinin include all of the following, EXCEPT: (AIPGMEE 2010)**
a) Vasodilatation
b) Bronchodilatation
c) Increased vascular permeability
d) Pain

46) **What is the most important role of Bradykinin in acute inflammation? (AIPGMEE 2010)**
a) Increase in vascular permeability
b) Vasodilatation
c) Mediation of pain
d) Bronchoconstriction

47) All of the following are features of apoptosis, EXCEPT: (AIPGMEE 2010)
a) Cellular swelling
b) Nuclear compaction
c) Intact cell membrane
d) Cytoplasmic eosinophilia

48) Principle organelle involved in the execution of apoptosis is: (AIPGMEE 2011)
a) Nucleus
b) Lysosome
c) Mitochondria
d) Endoplasmic reticulum

49) All are involved in generating free oxygen radical for killing of bacteria EXCEPT: (AIPGMEE 2011)
a) Superoxide dismutase
b) Fenton's reaction
c) NADPH oxidase.
d) Glutathione peroxidase

50) Not a disorder of protein misfolding: (AIPGMEE 2012)
a) Alzheimer's disease
b) Tuberculosis
c) Cystic fibrosis
d) CJD

51) Which of the following suggests irreversible cell injury? (AIIMS May 2012)
a) Mitochondrial swelling
b) Amorphous density in mitochondria
c) Ribosomal detachment from ER
d) Formation of phagolysosome

52) Which of the following is not seen in apoptosis? (AIIMS May 2013)
a) Cell shrinkage
b) Nuclear condensation
c) Inflammation
d) All of the above

53) CD 95 is a marker of:
a) Intrinsic pathway of apoptosis
b) Extrinsic pathway of apoptosis
c) Monocyte
d) Leucocyte

54) Which of the following induces apoptosis in a cell? (AIIMS Nov 2013)
a) Oleic acid
b) Glucocorticoids
c) Isoprenoids
d) Myristic acid

CHAPTER 2: CELLULAR RESPONSES TO STRESS AND TOXIC INSULTS: ADAPTATION, INJURY AND DEATH

Ans. 1) **D. Barbiturates leading to hypertrophy of smooth endoplasmic reticulum in hepatocytes leads to reduced amount of cytochrome P-450 levels (Ref: 8 ed. Robbins p 7-8, 9 ed. p 34-35, f-2-3,4)**

Hypertrophy:

- **Barbiturates** leads to **hypertrophy** of the **smooth endoplasmic reticulum (ER)** in hepatocytes, leading to the increased amount of **cytochrome P-450**
- Cytochrome P-450 enzyme, **detoxify the drugs** and over time, patients respond less to this drug
- Two main biochemical pathways involved in muscle hypertrophy–**phosphoinositide 3-kinase/Akt**[Q] pathway and **G protein-coupled receptors**
- Associated with induction/expression of fetal genes, e.g. **atrial natriuretic factor (ANF)**[Q]
- Cardiac hypertrophy is associated with **re-induction of ANF**[Q] **gene expression**

Ans. 2) **A. Uterus in pregnancy (Ref: 8 ed. Robbins p. 6-9, 9 ed. p 34-35, f-2-3,4)**

- Both physiological **hypertrophy and hyperplasia**, are best seen in a **pregnant uterus**[Q]
- Hypertrophy and hyperplasia can be **physiological or pathological**
- **Most common** stimulus for **hypertrophy of muscle** is **increased workload**

Physiologic hyperplasia[Q] can be divided into:

- **Hormonal hyperplasia**, e.g. – Proliferation of the glandular epithelium of female breast at puberty and during pregnancy
- **Compensatory hyperplasia** – Increased tissue mass after damage or partial resection, e.g. – Liver, which has a capacity to regenerate

Pathological hyperplasia[Q]

- Seen in **endometrial hyperplasia** or in **benign prostatic hyperplasia**
- Leads to a fertile soil in which **cancer can** arise

Ans. 3) **A. Liver (Ref: 8 ed. Robbins p 6-9, 9 ed. p 36)**

- **Compensatory hyperplasia** is most commonly seen in **liver**[Q]

Ans. 4) **B. Lipofuscin (Ref: 8 ed. Robbins p 9-10, 9 ed. p 36-37)**

Atrophy:

- Results from **decreased protein synthesis** or **increased protein degradation** in cells
- Protein degradation occurs by **ubiquitin-proteasome pathway**

Autophagy ("self-eating")[Q] (can be **accompanied by atrophy**):

- Mechanism by which the starved **cell eats its own components** in an attempt to find the nutrients and survive
- **Autophagic vacuoles** are **membrane-bound vacuoles,** which contain fragments of cell components, some of which resist cell degradation and persist as residual bodies
- **Lipofuscin granules**[Q] – Example of **residual bodies**, which impart a brown discoloration to the tissue **(brown atrophy)**[Q]

Ans. 5) **A. Columnar to squamous (Ref: 8 ed. Robbins p. 10, 9 ed. p 37-38, f-2-6)**

- **Metaplasia**[Q] – **Reversible change** in which **one differentiated cell type** (epithelial or mesenchymal) is replaced by **another cell type**
- **Most common epithelial metaplasia** is **columnar** to **squamous**[Q]
- **Example** – In **cigarette smoker**, the normal **ciliated columnar epithelial cells** of the trachea and bronchi are replaced by **stratified squamous** epithelial cells[Q]

Ans. 6) **B. Squamous to columnar (Ref: 8 ed. Robbins p 10-11, 9 ed. p 38)**

- In **Barrett esophagus**[Q] – **Squamous epithelium is replaced by columnar type epithelium**[Q]

Ans. 7) **A. Formation of amorphous densities in mitochondrial matrix (Ref: 8 ed. Robbins p 12-14, 9 ed. p 38-41, t-2-2, f-2-8)**

- **Cellular swelling**[Q] is the first manifestation of cell injury

Ultra-structural changes of **reversible cell injury** include:

a. **Plasma membrane alterations - blebbing,** blunting, and loss of microvilli
b. **Mitochondrial changes**, include **swelling** and **appearance** of **small amorphous densities**
c. **Dilation of the Endoplasmic Reticulum** and intra-cytoplasmic **myelin figures**
d. **Nuclear alterations**, with disaggregation of **granular** and **fibrillar elements**
    - Morphologic changes are associated with **decreased generation of ATP**
    - **Large amorphous densities**[Q] are a feature of **irreversible cell injury**

Differences between Necrosis and Apoptosis

Feature	Necrosis	Apoptosis
Cell size	Enlarged (swelling)	Reduced (shrinkage)
Nucleus	Pyknosis → karyorrhexis → karyolysis	Fragmentation into nucleosome size fragments
Plasma membrane	Disrupted	Intact
Cellular contents	Can leak out of cell	Intact
Adjacent inflammation	Common	No
Physiologic or pathologic role	Pathologic (culmination of irreversible cell injury)	Physiologic – Eliminates unwanted cells; Pathologic – After cell injury

Ans. 8) **A. Coagulative necrosis (Ref: 8 ed. Robbins p 14-17, 9 ed. p 41-44, f-2-11-15)**

- In myocardial ischemia, cardiac muscle undergoes **coagulative necrosis**

Points to remember about necrosis:

a) Necrotic cell may have a more **glassy homogeneous appearance**

b) Dead cells may be replaced by **myelin figures**[Q] that are derived from damaged cell membranes

c) **Electron microscopy** – Marked dilation of mitochondria with the appearance of large **amorphous densities**, intra-cytoplasmic **myelin figures** and amorphous debris

d) **Nuclear changes**[Q]:

- **Karyolysis** – Basophilia of the nuclear chromatin may fade due to **enzymatic degradation** of DNA by **endonucleases**
- **Pyknosis** – Characterized by **nuclear shrinkage** and increased basophilia
- **Karyorrhexis** – Pyknotic nucleus undergoes fragmentation

Patterns of Tissue Necrosis:

a) Coagulative necrosis

- Ischemia caused by obstruction in a vessel, seen in **all organs except the brain**
- **Infarct** – Localized area of coagulative necrosis

b) Liquefactive necrosis

- Characterized by **digestion of dead cells**, resulting in transformation of the tissue into a **liquid viscous mass**
- **Examples** – Hypoxic death of cells within the **central nervous system** [Q]; **bacterial** or **fungal infections**, resulting in the formation of **pus**

c) **Gangrenous necrosis**

- Seen in lower limb, that has lost its blood supply and has undergone necrosis (typically **coagulative necrosis)**
- Superimposed **bacterial infection** leads to **liquefactive necrosis** (giving rise to so-called **wet gangrene)**[Q]

d) **Caseous necrosis**[Q]

- Most commonly seen in **tuberculous infection**
- Characteristic microscopic feature of "**caseous" (cheese like)** necrosis is **'granuloma'**

e) **Fat necrosis**

- Seen in **acute pancreatitis**
- **Fat saponification'**[Q]: Released fatty acids from the pancreas combine with calcium to produce chalky-white areas

f) **Fibrinoid necrosis**[Q]

- Special form of necrosis usually seen in **immune reactions**[Q] involving blood vessels

Ans. 9) C. Diabetic glomerulosclerosis (Ref: 8 ed. Robbins p 16-17, 514, 566, 9 ed. p 41-44, f-2-11-15)

Fibrinoid necrosis

- Occurs when complexes of antigens and antibodies are deposited in the walls of arteries
- These **"immune complexes",** together with fibrin; result in a bright pink and **amorphous appearance** in **H&E** stains, called **"fibrinoid" (fibrin-like)**[Q]

Examples:

A) Classic PAN

- Characterized by **transmural inflammation**[Q] of the arterial wall with a mixed infiltrate of neutrophils, eosinophils, and mononuclear cells
- Frequently accompanied by **fibrinoid necrosis**

B) Acute Rheumatic Fever

- **Aschoff bodies** [Q] – Consist of a foci of lymphocytes, occasional plasma cells and plump activated macrophages called **Anitschkow cells (pathognomonic for RF)**[Q]
- Inflammation of the endocardium and the left-sided valves results in **fibrinoid necrosis**

C) Malignant hypertension:

- Results in increased permeability of the small vessels, endothelial injury, focal death of cells of the vascular wall and platelet deposition
- Leads to the appearance of **fibrinoid necrosis** of **arterioles** and **small arteries**

D) Nodular/Diabetic Glomerulosclerosis or **Kimmelstiel-Wilson disease**[Q]

- Characterized by oval or spherical glomerular lesions, but are **not associated** with fibrinoid necrosis

Ans. 10) B. Fat saponification (Ref: 8 ed. Robbins p. 16, 9 ed. p.41-44, f-2-11-15)

- Diagnosis here is **acute pancreatitis**
- **Activated pancreatic lipases,** in acute Pancreatitis, are released into the substance of the pancreas, leading to fat destruction
- Fluffy white material in X-ray is due to **fat saponification** [Q] which occurs when fatty acids, combine with **calcium** to produce grossly visible chalky-white areas

Ans. 11) B. Deficiency of antioxidant enzyme glutathione peroxidase (**Ref: 8 ed. Robbins p 20-23, 644, 9 ed. p 47-49, t-2-3, f-2-20)**

Free radical injury in cellular pathology can be discussed in three phases:

1) **Generation of free radicals** (reactive oxygen species–**ROS)**
2) **Removal of free radicals and**

3) Pathological effects of free radical injury

1) Generation of free radicals can occur in the following ways:

- Reduction-oxidation reactions – leads to production of **superoxide anion (O_2^-), H_2O_2 and hydroxyl ions (OH^-)**[Q]
- Absorption of radiant energy (e.g., **ultraviolet light, X-rays)**
- Rapid bursts of ROS are produced in activated leukocytes during **inflammation**
- Enzymatic metabolism of exogenous chemicals or drugs **(e.g. CCl_4 can generate CCl_3)**
- Transition metals such as iron and copper as seen in **Fenton reaction**
- **Nitric oxide (NO)**, generated by endothelial cells, macrophages, neurons [Q] can be converted to **peroxynitrite anion ($ONOO^-$), NO_2** and **NO_3^-**

2) Removal of free radicals occur by:

- **Antioxidants** – Block the initiation of free radical formation or inactivate free radicals, examples–**Vitamin E and A, Ascorbic acid** and **Glutathione**[Q]
- **Iron and copper** can catalyze the formation of ROS
- Enzymes which act as **free radical–scavenging systems:**

a) **Catalase** (in **peroxisomes)**

b) **Superoxide dismutase (SOD)**[Q], includes **manganese–SOD**, which is localized in **mitochondria**, and **copper-zinc–SOD**, which is found in the **cytosol**

c) **Glutathione peroxidase**[Q] which catalyze **free radical breakdown** (H_2O_2 + 2GSH → GSSG [glutathione homodimer] + $2H_2O$, or 2OH + 2GSH → GSSG + $2H_2O$).

Note: Intracellular ratio of **oxidized glutathione (GSSG)** to **reduced glutathione (GSH)** is an important indicator of the cell's ability to detoxify ROS

3) Pathological effects of free radical injury[Q]:

- **Lipid peroxidation in membranes**, leading to extensive membrane damage
- **Oxidative modification of proteins**, disrupting the conformation of structural proteins
- **Lesions in DNA**

G6PD deficiency (X-linked recessive trait[Q]**):**

- Due to abnormalities in **HMP shunt** or **glutathione metabolism**, RBCs are prone to oxidative damage, which leads to **hemolysis**

Ans. 12) C. Ferrous ions are converted to ferric ions (Ref: 8 ed. Robbins p 21, 9 ed. p 47-48, f-2-20)

- **Fenton reaction**[Q] – **H_2O_2 + Fe^{2+} → Fe^{3+} + OH + OH^-**
- Intracellular free iron is in ferric (**Fe^{3+}**) form and must be reduced to ferrous (**Fe^{2+}**) form to participate in Fenton reaction
- This reduction reaction can be enhanced by **$O_2^{\bullet}$**

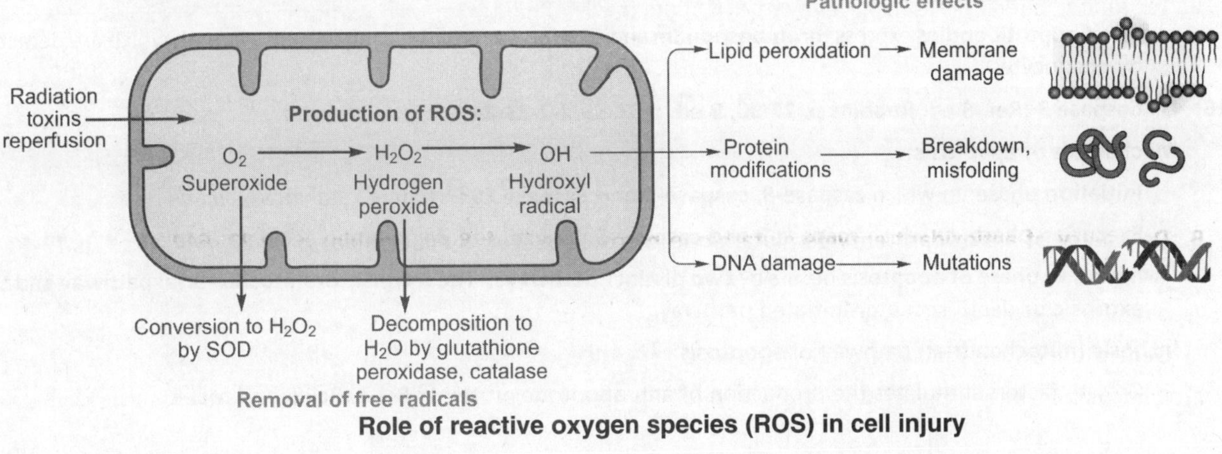

Role of reactive oxygen species (ROS) in cell injury

Ans. 13) **D. All of the above (Ref: 8 ed. Robbins p 24, 9 ed. p 51)**

Ischemia reperfusion injury:

- Restoration of blood flow to ischemic tissues can promote recovery of cells if they are **reversibly** injured
- In certain circumstances, when blood flow is restored to ischemic cells, injury is paradoxically exacerbated and occurs at a faster rate

Mechanisms proposed for **reperfusion injury** includes:

- Increased generation of **reactive oxygen** and **nitrogen species** Q
- **Inflammation** due to production of **cytokines** and increased expression of **adhesion molecules**, which recruit circulating neutrophils to re-perfused tissue
- Activation of the **complement system**

Ans. 14) **A. Endonuclease (Ref: 8 ed. Robbins p. 25-30, 9 ed. p 53-56)**

Apoptosis:

- Mechanism in which cells destined to die activate enzymes that degrade the cells own nuclear DNA
- Apoptotic cells break up into **apoptotic bodies**
- Plasma membrane of the apoptotic cell remains **intact**
- Contents of cell don't leak out, thus, it **does not elicit an inflammatory reaction**Q

Morphologic features of apoptosis:

- **Cell shrinkage**Q (in other forms of cell injury, an early feature is cell swelling)
- **Chromatin condensation**Q
- **Formation of cytoplasmic blebs and apoptotic bodies**Q
- **Phagocytosis of apoptotic cells or cell bodies**Q

Biochemical Features of Apoptosis:

- **Activation of Caspases**: Two groups—**Initiator** (include **caspase-8** and **caspase-9**) Q and **executioner (caspase-3** and **caspase-6**)Q
- **DNA and Protein Breakdown**: cleavage of DNA by **endonucleases**Q into fragments which may be visualized by electrophoresis as **DNA "ladders"** Q.
- In contrast, a **"smeared" pattern on electrophoresis** is indicative of **necrosis**

Thus, **endonucleases**, is responsible for **DNA "ladder" pattern** on electrophoresis

Ans. 15) **A. Apoptosis (Ref: 8 ed. Robbins p. 27, 30, 9 ed. p 53-58)**

- In apoptosis, the apoptotic cell is recognized by phagocytes for its removal
- Phagocytes recognize **phospholipids** (most commonly **phoshatidylserine**)Q on the surface of the apoptotic cell
- Phospholipids are recognized by a protein called **Annexin V**Q and thus **Annexin V staining** is commonly used to identify apoptotic cells
- Also **Apoptotic bodies** express **thrombospondin** and **C1q** (proteins of the complement system), which are detected by phagocytes

Ans. 16) **D. Caspase 3 (Ref: 8 ed. Robbins p. 27-30, 9 ed. p 53-55, f-2-23-24)**

Mechanism of apoptosis:

- **Initiation phase**: In which **caspase-8, caspase-9 and caspase 10**Q become catalytically active
- **Execution phase**: In which **caspase-3 and caspase-6** Q trigger the degradation cellular contents
- **Initiation phase of apoptosis** occurs by **two distinct pathways**: **The intrinsic or mitochondrial pathway** and the **extrinsic or death receptor-initiated pathway**

Intrinsic (mitochondrial) pathway of **apoptosis**:

- Growth factors stimulates the production of anti-apoptotic proteinsQ **Bcl-2, Bcl-x, and Mcl-1**

- When **cells are deprived of survival signals** or cell DNA is damaged, **"BH3-only proteins"** or **pro-apoptotic proteins** are activated, which include **Bim, Bid and Bad** [Q]
- **Induction of apoptosis** by **mitochondrial pathway** induces leakage of mitochondrial proteins especially **Cytochrome c**[Q]
- **Cytochrome c (in cytosol) binds to protein called Apaf-1**[Q] (apoptosis activating factor-1), which forms the **apoptosome**[Q]
- This complex is able to bind **caspase-9 (critical initiator caspase** of the **mitochondrial pathway)**

Extrinsic (Death Receptor–Initiated) pathway of **apoptosis**:

- Initiated by **death receptors** on cell surface
- **Best-known death receptors** are **Type 1 TNF receptor (TNFR1)**[Q] and a related protein called **Fas (CD95)**[Q]
- **Inactive form of caspase-8** and **caspase-10** are brought into **active form**
- Extrinsic pathway is **inhibited** by a protein called **FLIP**[Q]

Execution Phase of Apoptosis:

- **Mitochondrial pathway** leads to activation of the initiator **caspase-9**
- **Death receptor pathway** leads to activation of initiators **caspase-8 and -10**[Q]
- Both pathways leads to activation of the **executioner caspases** i.e. **caspase-3 and 6**[Q]
- Executioner caspases bring about cleavage of DNA into nucleosome-sized pieces

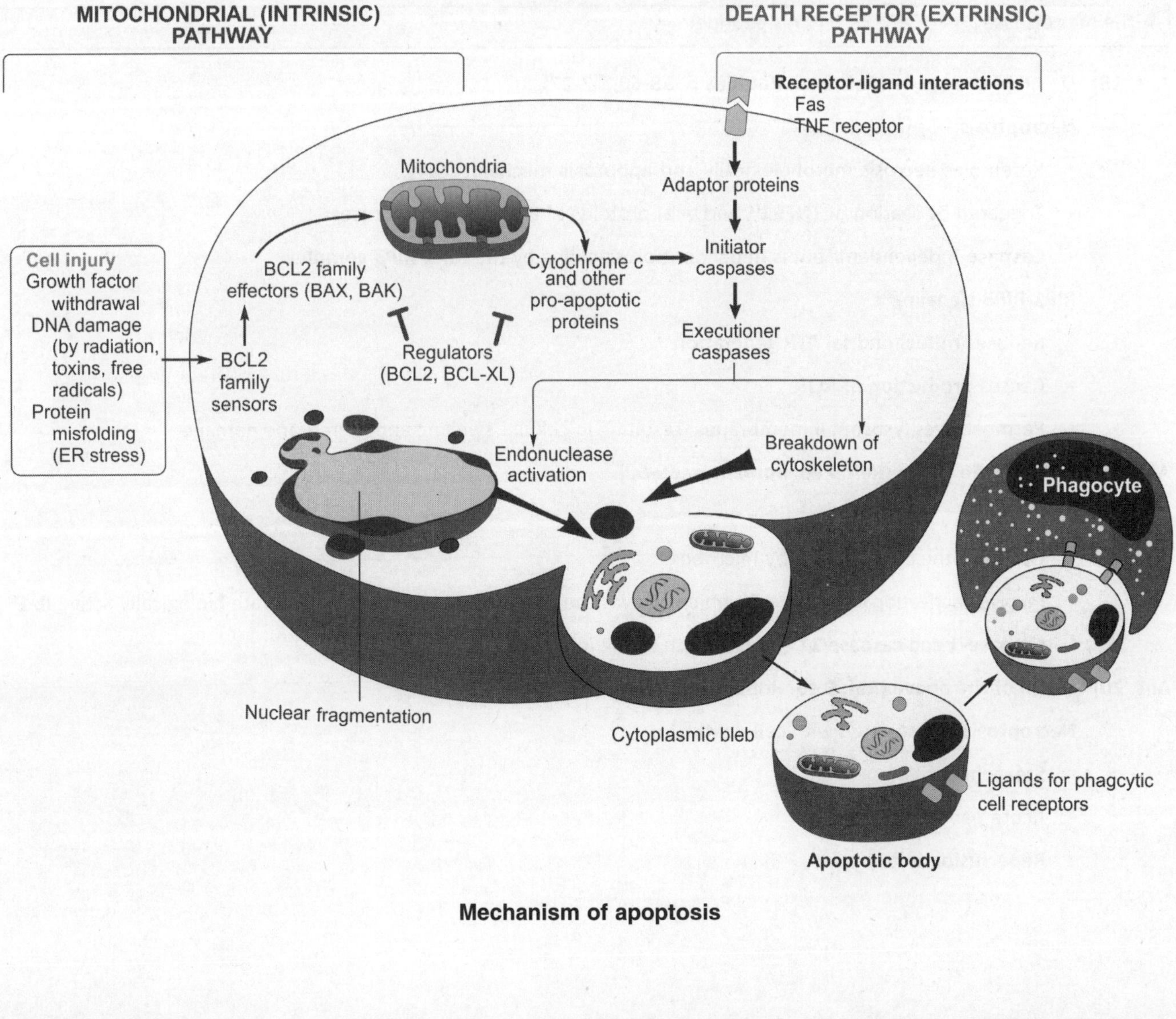

Mechanism of apoptosis

Ans. 17) D. All of the above (**Ref: 8 ed. Robbins p 30-31, 9 ed. p 57-58, f-2-26**)

Protein misfolding[Q]

- **Chaperones/heat shock proteins (HSP70)**[Q] in the endoplasmic reticulum (ER) results in proper folding of newly synthesized proteins
- **Unfolded protein response (UPR)**[Q]: Occurs when **unfolded or misfolded proteins** accumulate in the Endoplasmic Reticulum, because of **inherited mutations** or stress
- Unfolded protein response reduces the load of misfolded proteins in the cell
- **ER stress** – When UPR is unable to cope with the accumulation of misfolded proteins, the cell activates caspases and induces **apoptosis**
- **Intracellular accumulation of abnormally folded proteins**[Q]: Occurs in **neurodegenerative diseases e.g. Alzheimer**[Q], **Huntington**[Q] **and Parkinson disease**[Q] and possibly **Type II diabetes**[Q]

Examples of Diseases Caused by Misfolding of Proteins:

Disease	Affected protein
Cystic fibrosis	Cystic fibrosis trans-membrane conductance regulator (CFTR)
Familial hypercholesterolemia	LDL receptor
Tay-Sachs disease	Hexosaminidase β subunit
Alpha-1-antitrypsin deficiency	α1-antitrypsin
Creutzfeldt-Jacob disease	Prions
Alzheimer disease	Aβ peptide

Ans. 18) D. All of the above (Ref: 9 ed. Robbins p. 58-60, f-2-27)

Necroptosis:

- Resembles **necrosis** morphologically and **apoptosis** mechanistically
- Triggered by ligation of **TNFR1**[Q], and viral proteins of **RNA** and **DNA viruses**
- **Caspase-independent**[Q] but is dependent on signaling by the **RIP1-RIP3 complex**

RIP1-RIP3 signaling[Q]:

- Reduces **mitochondrial ATP generation**
- Causes **production of ROS**
- Permeabilizes **lysosomal membranes**, resulting in cellular swelling and membrane damage

Ans. 19) D. All of the above (Ref: 9 ed. Robbins p. 59-60)

Pyroptosis[Q]:

- Occurs in the cells infected by **microbes**[Q]
- Involves activation of **caspase-1**[Q] which cleaves the precursor form of **IL-1** to generate biologically active **IL-1**[Q]
- **Caspase-1** and **caspase-11**[Q] brings death of the infected cell

Ans. 20) D. All of the above (Ref: 9 ed. Robbins p 59)

Necroptosis is associated with **cell death**[Q] in:

- **Steatohepatitis**
- Acute pancreatitis
- **Reperfusion injury**

- Neurodegenerative diseases such as **Parkinson disease**
- In host defense against certain viruses (e.g. **cytomegalovirus**)

Ans. 21) C. Autophagy triggers cell death similar to apoptosis (Ref: 8 ed. Robbins p. 32, 9 ed. p 60-61, f-2-28)

Autophagy[Q]:

- Is a process in which a cell eats its own contents and it **triggers cell death**
- Occurs in **nutrient deprivation**, when the starved cell survives by cannibalizing itself
- Intracellular organelles are sequestered from the cytoplasm in an autophagic vacuole
- Autophagic vacuole fuses with lysosome to form an **autophagolysosome**
- Cellular components are digested by **lysosomal enzymes**[Q]
- Regulated by **"autophagy genes"**

Ans. 22) C. PAS (Ref: 8 ed. Robbins p 34)

For identification of fat:

- **Frozen tissue**[Q] sections should be made
- Sections are stained with **Sudan IV or Oil Red-O**[Q] (both of which impart an **orange-red color**[Q] to the lipid)

Note:

Periodic Acid-Schiff (PAS)[Q] or **Best Carmine**[Q] stain is used to identify **glycogen**[Q], which gives **rose to violet**[Q] color to glycogen vacuoles

Ans. 23) A. Lipofuscin (Ref: 8 ed. Robbins p 36, 9 ed. p 64, f-2-33)

Endogenous Pigments:

A) Lipofuscin (brown lipid)[Q]

- **Insoluble pigment**, also known as **lipochrome** or **wear-and-tear pigment**
- Is a **telltale sign of free radical injury**[Q]
- Prominent in the **liver and heart**[Q] of aging patients and in patients with severe malnutrition and cancer cachexia

B) Bilirubin

- Normal major pigment found in bile and is derived from **hemoglobin**

C) Hemosiderin

- Hemoglobin-derived, **golden yellow-to-brown**[Q], granular or crystalline pigment
- Serves as one of the major storage forms of iron
- **Hemosiderosis** is **systemic overload** of iron hemosiderin

Causes of Hemosiderosis:

- **Increased absorption of dietary iron**
- **Hemolytic anemia**[Q]
- **Repeated blood transfusions**[Q]

D) Melanin[Q]

- Endogenous **brown-black pigment**

Note:

Homogentisic acid:

- Black pigment that occurs in patients with **alkaptonuria**[Q]
- Pigment is **deposited in the skin, connective tissue and cartilage** and this **pigmentation is known as ochronosis**[Q]

Ans. 24) D. Parathyroid (Ref: 8 ed. Robbins p 38-39, 9 ed. p 65-66)

There are **two forms of pathologic calcification:**

Dystrophic Calcification[Q]:

- Deposition of calcium occurs locally in **dying tissues**
- **Serum levels** of calcium are **normal**
- Occurs in the absence of derangements in calcium metabolism
- Seen in **atheroma**[Q], **aging or damaged heart valves**[Q] and in **tuberculous lymph node**

Metastatic calcification[Q]:

- Deposition of calcium salts in normal tissues
- Seen in patients with **hypercalcemia**

Sites – Interstitial tissues of **gastric mucosa**[Q], **kidneys**[Q], **systemic arteries**[Q] **and pulmonary veins**[Q]

Causes

- **Increased secretion of PTH**
- Destruction of bone tissue due to **multiple myeloma**[Q] or **metastasis from breast cancer**[Q]
- Accelerated bone turnover in **Paget's disease**[Q] or **immobilization**
- **Vitamin D related disorders**[Q] including **vitamin D intoxication**
- **Sarcoidosis**
- **Renal failure**

Ans. 25) B. Increased free radical injury (Ref: 8 ed. Robbins p 39-41, 9 ed. p 66-68, f-2-35-36)

Cellular aging:

- Occurs due to progressive decline in cellular function due to genetic abnormalities
- Occurs due to accumulation of cellular and molecular damage
- **Werner syndrome** patients show premature aging, and the defective gene product is **DNA helicase**
- Most effective way of **prolonging life span** is **calorie restriction**[Q]
- **Effect of calorie restriction** is mediated by **sirtuins**[Q]
- **Increased levels of reactive oxygen species (ROS)** are associated with **aging**

Note:

- Red wine contains **resveratrol** [Q], which activates **Sir2 (sirtuins)** [Q] family of enzymes, and thus increasing the life-span

Ans. 26) A. Triglycerides (Ref. 9th ed. Robbins p 64)

- **Steatosis (fatty change)**: Abnormal accumulation of triglyceride within parenchymal cells

Ans. 27) A. Apoptosis (Ref: 9th ed. Robbin's p 53-55) Refer Q 16 for details

Ans. 28) D. Caspase 3 & 7 (Ref: 9th ed. Robbin's p 53-55) Refer Q 16 for details

Ans. 29) D. Fat necrosis (Ref: 9 ed. Robbins p 44-45)

Traumatic fat necrosis

- Occurs due to trauma
- Is seen in subcutaneous tissue of breast, thigh and abdomen

Ans. 30) C. Intact cell membrane (Ref: 9 ed. Robbins p 53-56) Refer Q 14 for details

Ans. 31) A. Lipofuscin (Ref: 9 ed. Robbins p 64) Refer Q 23 for details

Lipofuscin:

- Composed of polymers of lipids and phospholipids in complex with protein
- Derived from lipid peroxidation of polyunsaturated lipids of subcellular membranes

Ans. 32) B. Cytotoxic T cell (Ref: 9 ed. Robbins p 58)

- Cytotoxic T-cells secretes perforin, which promotes the entry of granzymes

Ans. 33) C. Super oxide dismutase (Ref: 9 ed. Robbins p 48)

Ans. 34) B. Increase in size of cells (Ref: 9 ed. Robbins p 34)

Ans. 35) A. Hypercalcemia (Ref: 9 ed. Robbins p 65-66) Refer Q 24 for details

Ans. 36) D. Brain (Ref: 9 ed. Robbins p 43) Refer Q 8 for details

Ans. 37) C. Ferrous ions converted to ferric ions (Ref: 9 ed. Robbins p 47-48) Refer Q 12 for details

Ans. 38) A. Reversible cell injury (Ref: 9 ed. Robbins p 38, 40-41) Refer Q 7 for details

Ans. 39) B. Interleukin-10

Anti-inflammatory cytokines – Interleukin-10, IL-5, IL-4

Ans. 40) A. Apaf 1(Ref: 9 ed. Robbins p 53-55) Refer Q 16 for details

Ans. 41) D. Seen in teratoma (Ref: 9 ed. Robbins p 602-03)

Psammoma Bodies

- Represent a process of dystrophic calcification

Are Seen in:

- Papillary carcinoma of thyroid
- Renal cell carcinoma
- Serous cyst adenoma of ovary
- Meningioma
- Malignant mesothelioma
- Somatostatinoma
- Prolactinoma
- Endometrial papillary serous cystadenocarcinomas

Ans. 42) B. Cell membrane (Ref: 9 ed. Robbins p 41-44) Refer Q 8 for details

Ans. 43) D. Free radicals (Ref: 9 ed. Robbins p 51) Refer Q13 for details

Ans. 44) A. Mitochondrial densities (Ref: 9 ed. Robbins p 38-41) Refer Q 7 for details

Ans. 45) B. Bronchodilation (Ref: 8 ed. Robbins p 64-66) Refer Q 26 for details

Ans. 46) A. Increase in vascular permeability (Ref: 8 ed. Robbins p 64-66) Refer Q 26 for details

Ans. 47) A. Cellular swelling (Ref: 9 ed. Robbins p 53-56) Refer Q 7 and 14 for details

Ans. 48) C. Mitochondria (Ref: 9 ed. Robbins p 53-55) Refer Q 16 for details

Ans. 49) D. Glutathione peroxidase (Ref: 8 ed. Robbins p 20-23, 644, 9 ed. p 47-49) Refer Q 11 for details

Ans. 50) B. Tuberculosis (Ref: 9 ed. Robbins p 57-58) Refer Q 17 for details

Ans. 51) B. Amorphous density in mitochondria Refer Q7 for details

Ans. 52) C. Inflammation (Ref: Robbins 9 ed. p 53-56) Note: Refer Q 14 for details

Ans. 53) B. Extrinsic pathway of apoptosis (Ref: 9 ed. Robbins p 53-55) Refer Q 16 for details

Ans. 54) B. Glucocorticoids (Ref: Underwood Pathology 5th ed. p 78)

1. **Inducers of apoptosis:**
   - Growth factor withdrawal
   - Detachment from matrix
   - Glucocorticoids
   - Cytotoxic drugs
   - Immune cytolysis
2. **Oleic acid induces autophagy**

3

Inflammation and Repair

How to go about this chapter?

- **Repeated MCQs are being asked from:**
  - **Mediators of inflammation**
  - **Integrins**
  - **Chemokines**
  - **Complement system**
  - **Coagulation pathways**
  - **Growth factors and receptors**
- **One should have thorough knowledge of all the figures of Robbins, mentioned in references**
- **Recent advances – Inflammasome and stem cell receptors are favorite MCQ topics**

OVERVIEW OF INFLAMMATION

1) **Four cardinal signs of inflammation were first described by:**
a) Virchow
b) Celsus
c) Elie Metchnikoff
d) John Hunter

ACUTE INFLAMMATION

2) **Endothelial contraction response in acute inflammation is:**
a) Early, reversible, short lived
b) Early, irreversible, long lived
c) Delayed, reversible, long lived
d) None of the above

3) **Transient adherence of leucocytes to the endothelium is called:**
a) Margination b) Rolling
c) Adhesion d) None of above

4) **ICAM-1 belongs to which category of adhesion proteins?**
a) Integrins b) Selectins
c) Immunoglobulin d) Glycoprotein

5) **Increased avidity of Integrins on leucocytes is mediated by:**
a) Histamine b) Thrombin
c) TNF d) Chemokines

6) **Transmigration is mediated by:**
a) E-selectin
b) PECAM-1(CD31)
c) Sialyl-Lewis X
d) None of the above

7) **Defect in Leucocyte adhesion Deficiency type-1 (LAD-1), lies in:**
a) Fucose metabolism
b) Sialyl-Lewis X
c) Beta-2 (CD11/CD18) Integrins
d) None of the above

8) **Absence of Sialyl Lewis X causes:**
a) LAD type 1
b) LAD type 2
c) Chronic granulomatous disease
d) Any of the above

9) **Most common type of leucocyte found at 2-4 days of pseudomonas infection is:**
a) Neutrophils b) Monocytes
c) Eosinophils d) Basophils

10) **Which of these is not an opsonin?**
a) IgG b) C3b
c) IgM d) Mannan binding lectin

11) **Most efficient bactericidal system in neutrophils is:**
a) H_2O_2 production b) HOCL production
c) OH^- ions d) O^-

12) **In Chediak- Higashi Syndrome there is a defect in:**
a) Leucocyte adhesion
b) Neutrophil specific protein deficiency
c) Defective fusion of phagosomes and lysosomes in phagocytes
d) Defective oxidative burst

13) **Which of the following is associated with chronic granulomatous disease?**
a) Leucocyte adhesion
b) Neutrophil specific protein deficiency
c) Defective fusion of phagosomes and lysosomes in phagocytes
d) Defective oxidative burst

14) **Arachidonic acid metabolism is caused by activation of:**
a) Phospholipase A_2
b) Phospholipase C
c) Phospholipase D
d) Lipoxygenase

15) **Serotonin is released by:**
a) Platelets b) Mast cells
c) Leucocytes d) Endothelium

16) **Vasodilation is mediated by all EXCEPT:**
a) Prostacyclin b) Thromboxane A_2
c) PGE_1 d) PGE_2

17) **Thromboxane A_2 formation is seen in:**
a) Lipoxygenase pathway
b) Cyclooxygenase pathway
c) Both
d) None

18) **Lipoxins belong to the following family of chemical mediators of inflammation:**
a) Kinin system
b) Cytokines
c) Chemokines
d) Arachidonic acid metabolites

19) **Which of the following is responsible for fever in acute inflammation?**
a) IL-6 b) TNF
c) IL-12 d) Chemokines

20) **All are true regarding inflammasome EXCEPT:**
a) Has an association with amyloidosis
b) Familial Mediterranean fever is related to inflammasome
c) Inflammation is partly mediated by IL-6
d) IL-1 antagonists are effective in treating this disorder

21) **54-year-old farmer has past history of allergy to dust. Also during harvesting season the farmer develops dyspnea and wheezing. Bronchial fluid cytology shows large number of eosinophils. Factor responsible for chemotactic motility of eosinophil is:**
a) α chemokine b) β chemokine
c) γ chemokine d) CX_3C chemokine

22) **RANTES and eotaxin belong to:**
a) α chemokine b) β chemokine
c) γ chemokine d) CX_3C chemokine

23) **Which of these nitric oxide synthase is not constitutively expressed?**
a) eNOS b) nNOS
c) iNOS d) None of the above

24) **Complement system proteins are found in highest concentration in:**
a) Neutrophils b) Mast cells
c) Plasma d) Extracellular matrix

25) **Which of these complements act as anaphylotoxins?**
a) C3b b) C5-9
c) C3a,C5a d) C4b

26) **Activated Hageman factor (Factor XIIa) can initiate the following system/s in acute inflammation:**
a) Kinin system b) Clotting system
c) Fibrinolytic system d) All of the above

CHRONIC INFLAMMATION

27) **Chronic inflammation is characterized by all EXCEPT:**
a) Infiltration with mononuclear cells
b) Vascular changes, edema, neutrophilic infiltration
c) Tissue destruction
d) Fibrosis

28) **Tissue macrophages seen in central nervous system are:**
a) Kupffer cells
b) Sinus histiocytes
c) Alveolar macrophages
d) Microglia

29) **Eosinophils are toxic to parasites because of:**
a) Eatoxin b) Major basic protein
c) Lysozyme d) Proteases

30) **All of the following shows granuloma formation EXCEPT:**
a) T.B.
b) Cat scratch disease
c) Ulcerative colitis
d) Crohn disease

SYSTEMIC EFFECTS OF INFLAMMATION

31) **All of the following are acute phase proteins EXCEPT:**
a) ESR
b) Fibrinogen
c) CRP
d) SAA (serum amyloid associated protein)

32) **Leucopenia is seen in all EXCEPT:**
a) Typhoid
b) Rickettsia

c) Protozoa
d) Infectious mononucleosis

TISSUE REPAIR

33) All of the following are labile cells EXCEPT:
a) Bone marrow
b) Intestinal mucosa
c) Epithelium of skin
d) Fibroblasts

34) Pluripotency of the stem cells depends on the following factors EXCEPT:
a) Oct 3/4 b) Sox-2
c) C-myc d) Nanog

35) Which of the following statements is not correct regarding stem cell?
a) Development elasticity
b) Trans-differentiation
c) Can be harvested from embryo
d) Somatic stem cells reside in special micro-environments called *niche*

36) All of the following acts by G-protein coupled receptors EXCEPT:
a) Parathyroid hormone
b) Calcitonin
c) Vitamin D
d) Corticotropin

37) All of the following acts by steroid hormone receptors EXCEPT:
a) Thyroid hormone
b) Parathyroid hormone
c) Retinoids
d) Steroids

38) All are true about liver regeneration EXCEPT:
a) Occurs by compensatory hyperplasia
b) Brought about by TGF-α, HGF, IL-6
c) Intrahepatic stem/progenitor cells play a role in compensatory growth
d) Inhibited/terminated by TGF-β

39) All are true about collagen and its disorders EXCEPT:
a) Type IV is the main component of basement membrane
b) Type II is associated Ehlers-Danlos Syndrome
c) Type VII is associated with dystrophic epidermolysis Bullosa
d) Vitamin C is required for the hydroxylation of procollagen

40) All are true about hyaluronic acid (HA) EXCEPT:
a) Found abundant in heart valves, skin, synovium, vitreous, umbilical cord
b) Produced at the plasma membrane by hyaluronan synthases
c) Concentration decreases in rheumatoid arthritis, osteoarthritis, psoriasis
d) LMW-HA attaches to CD44 receptor on leukocytes and promotes the recruitment of leukocytes to the sites of inflammation

41) Which of the following is the most important fibrogenic agent?
a) IL-1 b) FGF
c) TGF-β d) PDGF

42) Wound strength reaches a plateau of 70-80% of tensile strength of normal unwounded skin in:
a) 2 months b) 3 months
c) 4 months d) 5 months

43) Cell producing collagen in liver cirrhosis is:
a) Myofibroblasts b) Stellate cells
c) Kupffer cells d) Endothelial cells

44) Cytokine for activating macrophage and converting to epithelioid cell or giant cell: (NEET 2014)
a) IL2 b) IL 17
c) TNF alpha d) IFN gamma

45) Which acute phase reactant induces Rouleaux formation? (NEET 2014)
a) C-reactive protein b) Fibrinogen
c) Serum amyloid A d) IL 1

46) Which of the following is responsible for respiratory burst and production of superoxide ions: (NEET 2014)
a) Hydrolase b) Catalase
c) Peroxidase d) NADPH oxidase

47) Fibrosis is due to: (NEET 2014)
a) TGF beta b) TNF alpha
c) IL7 d) IL10

48) Increased vascular permeability in acute inflammation is due to: (NEET 2014)
a) Histamine b) IL 2
c) TGF beta d) FGF

49) Leukocyte adhesion to endothelium is mediated by all EXCEPT: (NEET 2014)
a) L selectin b) E selectin
c) VCAM-1 d) VCAM-4

50) Matrix metalloproteinases is: (NEET 2014)
a) Cathepsin
b) Zn metalloproteinase
c) Cu metalloproteinase
d) Cd metalloproteinase

51) True about wound healing with primary intention is: (NEET 2014)
a) By day 5 epidermis recovers its normal thickness
b) Intense inflammatory reaction
c) Wound contraction occurs
d) Abundant granulation tissue grows

52) Leukocyte migration to the site of injury occurs due to:
a) LTB4 b) C3b
c) IL 10 d) LTB

53) The definition of exudate is: (NEET 2014)
a) Extravascular fluid that has a high protein concentration and contains cellular debris
b) Extravascular fluid that has a low protein concentration
c) Extravascular fluid with high glucose concentration
d) Extravascular fluid with low glucose concentration

54) Endothelial molecule participating in rolling is: (NEET 2014)
a) CD 34 b) CD 65
c) CD 56 d) CD 100

55) In tuberculosis the cytokine causing fever is: (NEET 2014)
a) IL-1 b) IL-2
c) IL-3 d) IL-4

56) Which of the following is not a free radical scavenger? (NEET 2014)
a) Glutathione peroxidase
b) Superoxide dismutase
c) Catalase
d) Xanthine oxidase

57) All belong to family of selectins except: (NEET 2013)
a) P selectin b) L selectin
c) A selectin d) E selectin

58) Cell matrix adhesions are mediated by: (NEET 2013)
a) Cadherins b) Integrins
c) Selectins d) Calmodulin

59) Most important for diapedesis: (NEET 2013)
a) PECAM
b) Selectin
c) Integrin
d) Mucin like glycoprotein

60) Most important source of histamine: (NEET 2013)
a) Mast cells
b) Eosinophil
c) Neutrophil
d) Macrophages

61) Tensile strength of a wound after laparoscopic cholecystectomy in 30 years old woman depends upon: (AIIMS Nov 2013)
a) Replacement of type 3 collagen
b) Extensive cross linking of tropocollagen
c) Macrophage activity/invasion
d) Granulation tissue

62) When a cell transforms itself into different lineage the ability is known as: (NEET 2013)
a) De-differentiation
b) Re-differentiation
c) Trans-differentiation
d) Sub-differentiation

63) PAF causes all EXCEPT: (NEET 2013)
a) Bronchoconstriction
b) Vasodilation
c) Increased vascular permeability
d) Vasoconstriction

64) Maximum collagen in wound healing is seen at: (NEET 2013)
a) End of first week
b) End of second week
c) End of third week
d) End of 2 months

65) Which of the following helps in generating oxygen burst in the neutrophils? (AIPGMEE 2011)
a) Superoxide dismutase
b) NADPH oxidase
c) Peroxidase
d) Glutathione reductase

66) Which among the following is the hallmark of acute inflammation? (AIPGMEE 2011)
a) Vasoconstriction
b) Stasis
c) Vasodilation and increase in permeability
d) Leukocyte margination

67) Which complement component is first common point between involved classical and alternate pathway? (AIPGMEE 2011)
a) C1 b) C2
c) C3 d) C4

68) Bradykinin in acute inflammation causes (AIIMS May 2012)
a) Vasoconstriction
b) Pain at the sight of inflammation
c) Bronchodilatation
d) Decreased vascular permeability

69) In Lewis Triple Response, redness when skin is scratched with a pointed object is seen due to: (AIIMS May 2012)
a) Axon reflex causing vasoconstriction
b) Histamine release due to local injury to mast cells by pointing device
c) Free nerve endings
d) Endothelial damage leading to increase in permeability

70) Most important function of epithelioid cells in tuberculosis is: (AIIMS May 2014)
a) Phagocytosis b) Secretory
c) Antigenic d) Healing

71) In cellular event of acute inflammation all are seen EXCEPT: (AIIMS May 2014)

a) Complement involved in chemotaxis
b) ICAM – Adhesion of leukocytes
c) PECAM – Activation of leukocytes
d) Selectins – Margination

72) Incisional wound contains new collagen fibril network and epithelial layer. Age of wound: (AIIMS May 2015)

a) 12 to 24 hours
b) 24 to 72 hours
c) 4 to 5 days
d) 1 week

73) In acute inflammation, endothelial cells retraction due to cytoskeleton re-organization causes: (AIIMS Nov 2011)

a) Immediate transient increase in permeability
b) Delayed prolonged increase in permeability
c) Early permanent increase in permeability
d) Late permanent increase in permeability

CHAPTER 3: INFLAMMATION AND REPAIR

Ans. 1) **B. Celsus (Ref: 8 ed. Robbins p. 44, 9 ed. p. 71)**

Celsus listed the **four cardinal signs** [Q] of inflammation:

- **Rubor (redness)**
- **Tumor (swelling)**
- **Calor (heat)**
- **Dolor (pain)**
- **Loss of function (functio laesa)** [Q]: **Fifth clinical sign**, was added by **Rudolf Virchow** [Q]

Note:

John Hunter noted that **inflammation is not a disease** but a nonspecific response

Elie Metchnikoff [Q] discovered the process of **phagocytosis**

Ans. 2) **A. Early, reversible, short lived (Ref: 8 ed. Robbins p. 47, 9 ed. 74-75, f. 3-3)**

Vascular leakage:

- Hallmark of **acute inflammation** and leads to escape of a **protein-rich exudate** into the extravascular tissue, causing **edema**
- **Contraction of endothelial cells – most common** mechanism of vascular leakage
- Endothelial cell contraction is **mediated by histamine** [Q], **bradykinin** [Q], leukotriene, neuropeptide substance P
- Occurs as **immediate transient response** [Q]
- Occurs rapidly after exposure to the mediator and is usually **short-lived (15–30 minutes)** [Q]

Delayed prolonged leakage [Q]:

- Seen after **burns**, **irradiation** or **ultraviolet radiation**, and exposure to certain bacterial toxins
- Vascular leakage occurs after a **delay of 2 to 12 hours**, and lasts for several hours or even days
- Caused by **contraction of endothelial cells or mild endothelial damage** [Q]

Ans. 3) **B. Rolling (Ref: 8 ed. Robbins p. 48-51, 9 ed. 75-78, f. 3-4, t-3-3)**

Role of Neutrophils in Acute Inflammation:

Recruitment of Leukocytes occurs in following steps:

1. **In the lumen of vessel**:
   - **Margination, rolling and adhesion** to endothelium
   - In **inflammation,** endothelial **activation** and binding to **leukocytes**
2. **Migration** across the **endothelium and vessel wall**
3. **Migration** in the **tissues** toward a **chemotactic stimulus**

Leukocyte Adhesion to Endothelium:

A) Margination:

- In normal flowing blood in venules, **red cells** are confined to the center column, and **leukocytes** toward the **vessel wall**
- As inflammation leads to **stasis**, more white cells assume a peripheral position along the endothelial surface
- The process of **leukocyte redistribution** is called **Margination**

B) Rolling:

- Leukocytes adhere transiently to the endothelium, detach and bind again
- Initial **rolling interactions** are mediated by **selectins**

- **Types of selectins: L-selectin** – expressed on **leukocytes** [Q], **E-selectin** [Q] – on **endothelium** and **P-selectin – on platelets and endothelium**

Role of Selectins:

- Expression of selectins and their ligands is regulated by **cytokines (TNF and IL-1)** [Q]
- Redistribution of **P-selectin** from endothelial cell granules (**Weibel-Palade bodies**) to cell surface is brought about by **histamine, thrombin and platelet-activating factor (PAF)**
- Leukocytes express **L-selectin** [Q] at the tips of their microvilli and also express ligands for E- and P-selectins

Role of Integrins [Q]**:**

- Help in binding leukocytes firmly to the **endothelium**
- **TNF** and **IL-1** induce endothelial expression of ligands for **integrins**

Examples:

- Vascular cell adhesion molecule 1 (**VCAM-1) – ligand for the VLA-4 integrin** [Q]
- Intercellular adhesion molecule 1 (**ICAM-1) – ligand for the LFA-1 and Mac-1 integrins**[Q]

Note:

- Leukocytes normally express **integrins** in a **low-affinity state**
- **Chemokines** helps **integrins** in order to attain a high affinity state

Chemokines:

- Leads to conversion of **VLA-4 and LFA-1 integrins** on the leukocytes to a **high-affinity state**
- High affinity state results in firm **integrin-mediated binding** of the leukocytes to the endothelium at the site of inflammation

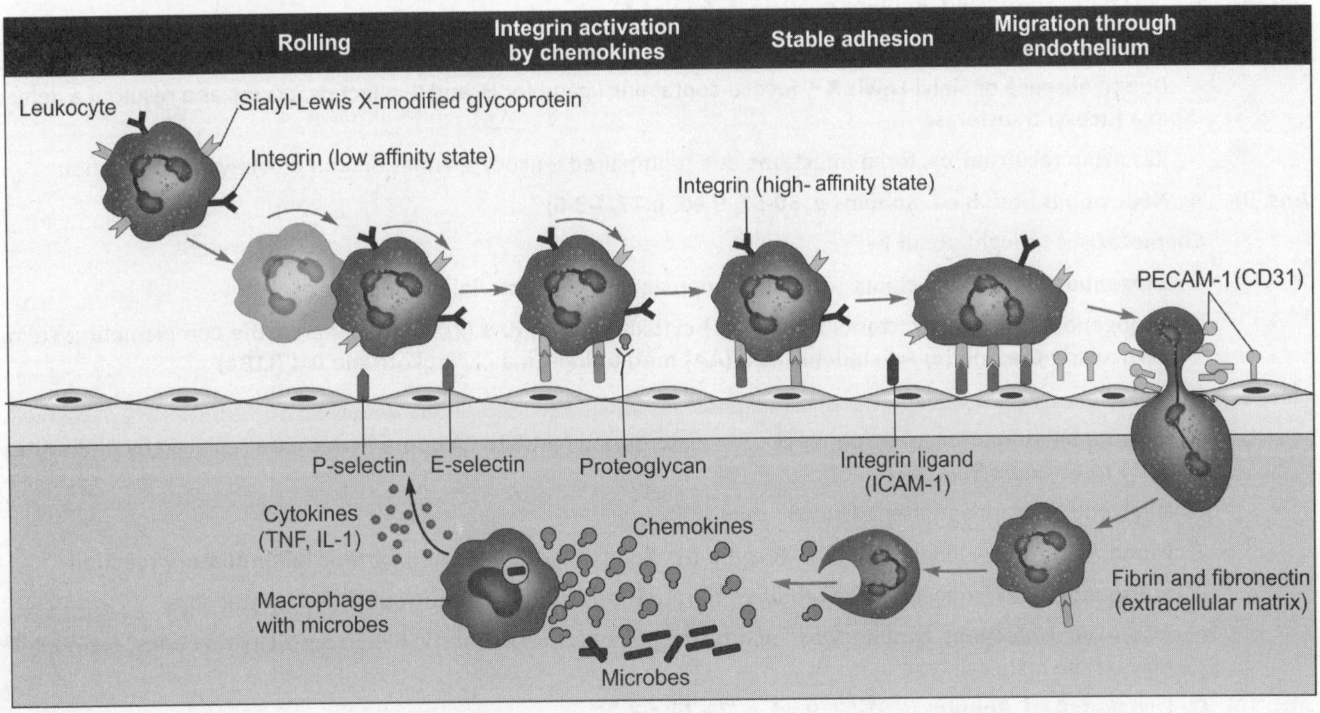

Complex process of leukocyte migration through blood vessels

Ans. 4) C. Immunoglobulin (**Ref: 8 ed. Robbins p. 49, 9 ed. p. 76-77, t/3-3**)

Role of Endothelial-Leukocyte Adhesion Molecules in inflammation:

- **ICAM-1** and **VCAM-1** belong to **immunoglobulin** Q families which are **endothelial molecules**
- **ICAM-1** binds to **CD11/CD18 (β2) integrins / (LFA-1, Mac-1)** Q and brings adhesion, arrest, transmigration of neutrophils, monocytes, lymphocytes
- **VCAM-1** binds to **VLA-4 (β1) integrin** Q and brings **adhesion** of eosinophils, monocytes, lymphocytes.

Ans. 5) **D. Chemokines (Ref: 8 ed. Robbins p. 49-50, 9 ed. p. 75-78, f-3-4, t-3-3)**

- Conversion of **VLA-4 and LFA-1 integrins** on the leukocytes **to a high-affinity state** is brought by **activation by chemokines**

Ans. 6) **B. PECAM-1 (CD31) (Ref: 8 ed. Robbins p. 48-50, 9 ed. 76-77, f-3-4)**

Transmigration or Diapedesis:

- Process of migration of leukocytes through the **endothelium**
- **Occurs mainly in post-capillary venules** Q
- **Migration of leukocytes** is brought about by **adhesion molecules** present in the **intercellular junctions** between endothelial cells
- Adhesion molecules include a member of the immunoglobulin superfamily called **PECAM-1 (platelet endothelial cell adhesion molecule) or CD31** Q

Ans. 7) **C. Beta-2 (CD11/CD18) Integrins (Ref: 8 ed. Robbins p. 50,56, t-3-3)**

Leukocyte adhesion deficiency type 1 (LAD 1):

- Defect in the biosynthesis of the **β2 chain** which is shared by the **LFA-1** and **Mac-1 integrins** Q
- Patient presents as **recurrent bacterial infections** Q as a consequence of **impaired leukocyte adhesion** and defective inflammation

Ans. 8) **B. LAD type 2 (Ref: 8 ed. Robbins p. 50,56. f-2-4, t-3-3)**

Leukocyte adhesion deficiency type 2 (LAD 2):

- Due to **absence of Sialyl-Lewis X** Q, fucose-containing ligand for **E- and P-selectins**, occurs as a result of a defect in a **fucosyl transferase**
- Results in **recurrent bacterial infections** due to impaired leukocyte adhesion and defective inflammation

Ans. 9) **A. Neutrophils (Ref: 8 ed. Robbins p. 50-51, 9 ed. p.77, f-3-6)**

Chemotaxis is brought about by:

- **Exogenous chemo attractants** – most common agents are **bacterial products** or
- **Endogenous chemo attractants** include: (1) **cytokines**, e.g., **IL-8** (2) components of the complement system, particularly **C5a** and (3) **Arachidonic acid (AA) metabolites**, mainly **leukotriene B 4 (LTB4)**

Note:

- In **acute inflammation**, **neutrophils** predominate during first **6 to 24 hours** Q which are replaced by **monocytes** in **24 to 48 hours** Q
- Neutrophils disappear after 24 to 48 hours
- **Monocytes** survive longer and thus become the dominant population in **chronic inflammatory reactions** Q
- In **Pseudomonas** Q infection, the cellular infiltrate is dominated by **neutrophils** for several days
- Also, **in viral infections, lymphocytes** Q may be the first cells to arrive and in **hypersensitivity reactions, eosinophil**Q may be the main cell type

Ans. 10) **C. IgM (Ref: 8 ed. Robbins p. 51-52, 9 ed. p. 78-79, f-3-7)**

Opsonization:

- Process of coating a particle to target it for ingestion (phagocytosis)
- Substances responsible for this are called **opsonins** and includes **antibodies, complement proteins and lectins**
- Coating the particles with **IgG antibodies** Q leads to increased phagocytosis of the particles

- **Components of the complement system**, especially **C3** Q are **potent opsonins**
- **Plasma lectins: Mannan-binding lectin** Q bind to the bacteria and deliver them to leukocytes

Ans. 11) A. H_2O_2 production (Ref: 8 ed. Robbins p. 53-54, 9 ed. p. 79-80, f-3-8)

Phagocytosis involves **three sequential steps:**

- **Recognition and attachment** of the particle to be ingested by the leukocyte;
- **Engulfment**, with subsequent formation of a **phagocytic vacuole**; and
- **Killing or degradation** of the ingested material
- Efficiency of phagocytosis is enhanced when the microbes are opsonized by specific proteins **(opsonins)**
- **Microbial killing** occurs due to **reactive oxygen species** (ROS) and **reactive nitrogen species**, mainly derived from **NO**

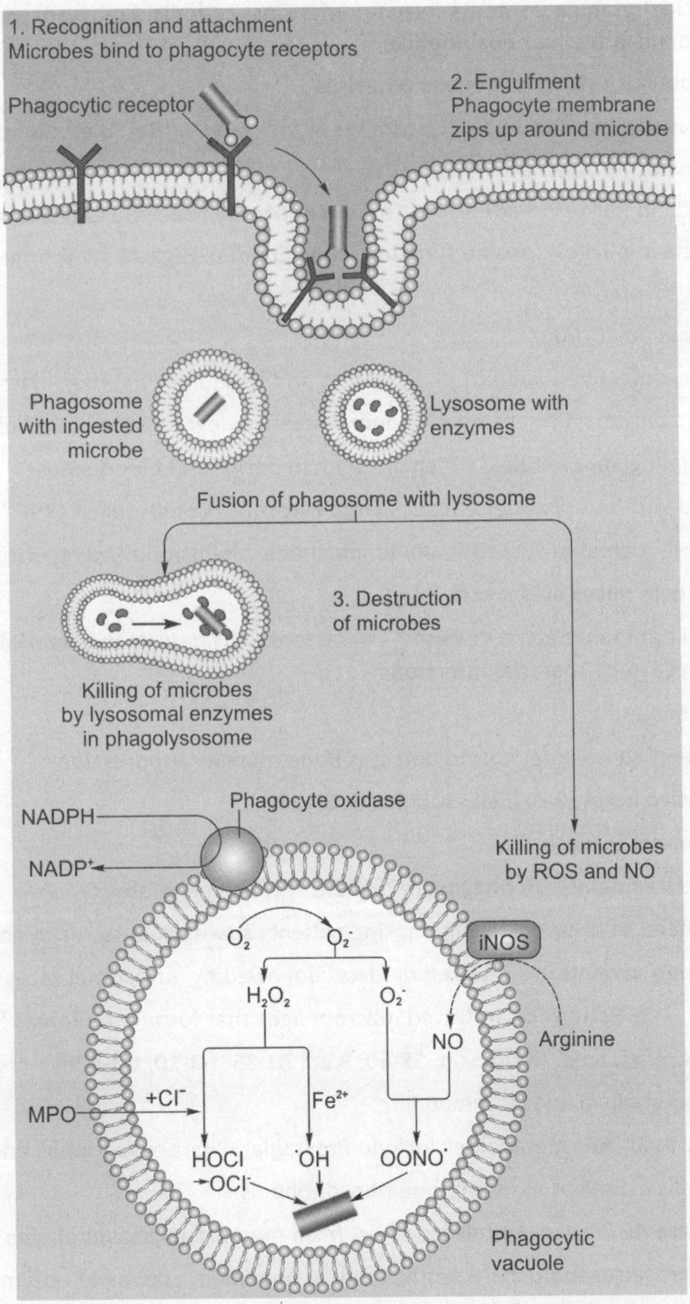

Phagocytosis and intracellular destruction of microbes

- Generation of ROS occurs due to **NADPH oxidase** ^q^, also called **phagocyte oxidase** ^q^, which oxidizes **NADPH** and, in the process, reduces **oxygen to superoxide anion (O^{2-})**
- In neutrophils, this rapid oxidative reaction is called as **respiratory burst** ^q^
- **ROS** are produced within the lysosome where O^{2-} is converted into **hydrogen peroxide (H_2O_2)**, which is not able to efficiently kill microbes by itself
- However, the **azurophilic granules** of **neutrophils** contain the enzyme **myeloperoxidase (MPO)** ^q^ which, in the presence of **halide** such as Cl^-, converts H_2O_2 to **hypochlorite ($OCl^{\bullet}$)**
- **HOCl** is a potent antimicrobial agent that destroys microbes
- **H_2O_2-MPO-halide system** ^q^ is the **most efficient bactericidal system** of neutrophils
- **Leukocyte granules** contain various enzymes, e.g. elastase, which induces microbial killing.
- Other **microbicidal granule contents** include **defensins, cathelicidins, lysozyme, lactoferrin** and **major basic protein** ^q^ (a cationic protein of **eosinophils**) ^q^
- Major basic protein is cytotoxic to many **parasites**

Ans. 12) C. Defective fusion of phagosomes and lysosomes in phagocytes (Ref: 8 ed. Robbins p. 55, t-2-3)

Impairments in Leukocyte function includes:

a) Inherited defects in leukocyte adhesion – examples of which include **LAD-1 and LAD-2**

b) Inherited defects in phagolysosome function – e.g. **Chédiak-Higashi syndrome** ^q^

Chédiak-Higashi Syndrome ^q^**:**

- **Autosomal recessive** disorder
- Characterized by **defective fusion of phagosomes and lysosomes** in phagocytes
- Main leukocyte abnormalities are **neutropenia**, defective degranulation and delayed microbial killing
- Leukocytes contain **giant granules**, which are seen in **peripheral blood smears**
- Gene associated with this disorder encodes **large cytosolic protein** called **LYST** ^q^
- **Clinical features** – Increased susceptibility to infections, **albinism**, bleeding disorders

c) Inherited defects in microbicidal activity:

Example: Chronic granulomatous disease ^q^, characterized by **defects in bacterial killing,** thus patients are more susceptible to **recurrent bacterial infections**

d) Acquired deficiencies:

- **Most frequent** cause of leukocyte defect is **bone marrow suppression**

Ans. 13) D. Defective oxidative burst (Ref: 8 ed. Robbins p. 55-56)

Chronic Granulomatous Disease:

- Due to **inherited defects** in **phagocyte oxidase** ^q^, which generates O_2^-
- Leads to defects in bacterial killing, making patients **susceptible to recurrent bacterial infection**
- **Most common variants** are **X-linked defects** ^q^ followed by **autosomal recessive defects**
- Microscopy – **Collections of activated macrophages** that form **granulomas** ^q^

Ans. 14) A. Phospholipase A_2 (Ref: 8 ed. Robbins p. 58-60, 9 ed. 83-85, f-3-10, t-3-4,5)

Arachidonic acid metabolism and its metabolites:

- **Arachidonic Acid (AA)** metabolites include **Prostaglandins, Leukotrienes and Lipoxins**
- **AA** is normally esterified in **membrane phospholipids**
- **Phospholipase A2** ^q^: Leads to release of **AA from membrane phospholipids**

AA derived mediators (eicosanoids) are synthesized by **two major classes** of enzymes:

- **Cyclooxygenases** ^q^ (which generate **prostaglandins and TxA_2**) and **lipoxygenases** ^q^ (which produce **Leukotrienes and lipoxins**)

a) **Prostaglandins (PGs):**

- Produced by **mast cells, macrophages, endothelial cells**
- Produced by actions of two **cyclooxygenases, COX-1** and the **COX-2**
- E.g.: **PGE_2, PGD_2, $PGF_{2\alpha}$, PGI_2 (prostacyclin), and TxA_2 (thromboxane)**
- **TxA_2 – Major product** derived from enzyme **thromboxane synthetase** in the platelets and is a potent **platelet-aggregating agent** [Q] and **vasoconstrictor** [Q]
- **Prostacyclin** is a **vasodilator**, a **potent inhibitor** of **platelet aggregation**
- **PGD_2 and PGE_2** are secreted by **mast cells** and causes **vasodilation**
- **PGF2α** [Q] stimulates the contraction of uterine and bronchial smooth muscle and small arterioles
- **PGD_2** is **chemo attractant for neutrophils** [Q]
- **PGE_2** is **hyperalgesic** [Q] and makes the skin hypersensitive to painful stimuli

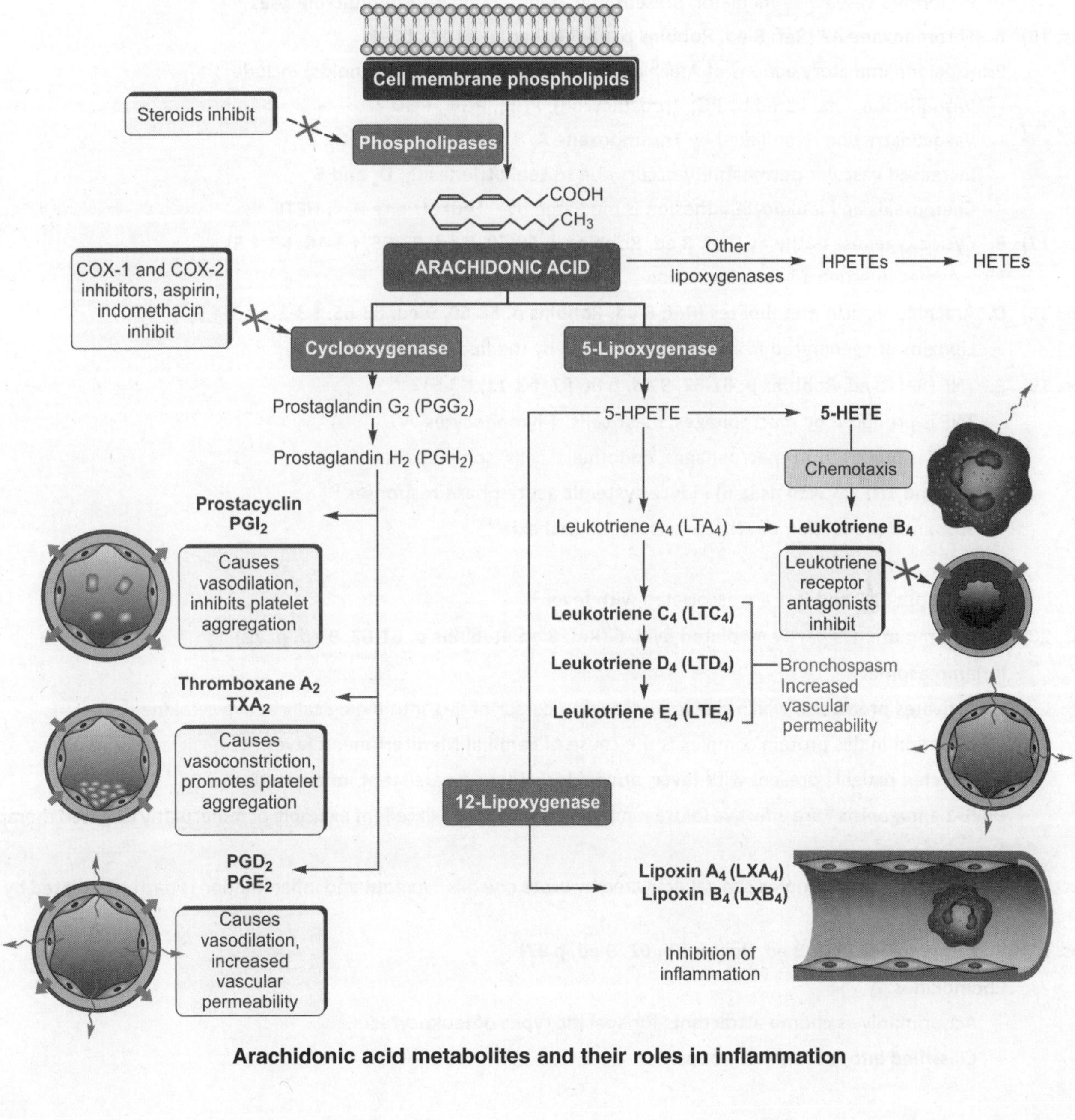

Arachidonic acid metabolites and their roles in inflammation

b) Leukotrienes (LTs):

- **Lipoxygenase enzymes** are responsible for the production of **leukotrienes**
- **LTB_4** Q is a **potent chemotactic agent** Q and **activator of neutrophils**
- **LTC_4, LTD_4, LTE_4** cause **intense vasoconstriction, bronchospasm and increased vascular permeability**

c) Lipoxins:

- Are also generated from AA by **lipoxygenase pathway**
- Are inhibitors of inflammation Q
- **Inhibits leukocyte recruitment** Q and cellular components of inflammation Q
- Play a role in resolution of inflammation

Ans. 15) A. Platelets (Ref: 8 ed. Robbins p. 57-58, 9 ed. p. 84)

Serotonin (5-hydroxytryptamine):

- Preformed vasoactive mediator, present in **platelets** Q and **neuroendocrine cells** Q

Ans. 16) B. Thromboxane A2 (Ref: 8 ed. Robbins p. 58-59, 9 ed. p 84-85, t-3-5)

Principal inflammatory actions of Arachidonic Acid Metabolites **(Eicosanoids)** include:

- **Vasodilation** – mediated by **PGI_2 (prostacyclin), PGE_1, PGE_2, PGD_2**
- **Vasoconstriction** – mediated by **Thromboxane A_2** Q, Leukotrienes C_4, D_4, E_4
- **Increased vascular permeability** occurs due to **Leukotrienes C_4, D_4 and E_4**
- **Chemotaxis** and **leukocyte adhesion** is mediated by – **Leukotriene B_4** Q, **HETE**

Ans. 17) B. Cyclooxygenase pathway (Ref: 8 ed. Robbins p. 58-60, 9 ed. 83-85, f-3-10, t-3-4,5)

Please refer question 14 for explanation

Ans. 18) D. Arachidonic acid metabolites (Ref: 8 ed. Robbins p. 58-60, 9 ed. 83-85, f-3-10, t-3-4,5)

- **Lipoxins** are generated from **Arachidonic Acid** by the **lipoxygenase pathway** Q

Ans. 19) B. TNF (Ref: 8 ed. Robbins p. 61-62, 9 ed. p 86-87, f-3-11, t-3-6)

- **TNF** is produced by **macrophages, mast cells, T-lymphocytes**
- **IL-1** Q is produced by macrophages, endothelial cells, some epithelial cells
- **IL-1 and TNF (as well as IL-6)** induce **systemic acute-phase responses** Q
- Sustained production of TNF contributes to **cachexia** Q

Note:

Hence, both **TNF and IL-1** are associated with **fever** Q

Ans. 20) C. Inflammation is partly mediated by IL-6 (Ref: 8 ed. Robbins p. 61-62, 9 ed. p. 72)

Inflammasome:

- Activates **proteases**, which cleaves inactive precursor of **IL-1** into biologically active cytokine
- Mutation in this protein complex is the cause of **Familial Mediterranean fever**
- Affected patients present with **fever, amyloidosis** (due to **persistent inflammation**)
- **IL-1 antagonists** Q are effective for treating these disorders, an **excellent example** of **molecularly targeted therapy** Q

Note:

- **Inflammasome complex** can get activated by **urate crystals** Q in **gout** and inflammation is partly **mediated by IL-1** Q

Ans. 21) B. β chemokine (Ref: 8 ed. Robbins p. 62, 9 ed. p 87)

Chemokines:

- Act primarily as **chemo attractants** for **specific types of leukocytes**
- **Classified into four major groups**:

A) **C-X-C chemokines (α chemokines)**

- Acts primarily on **neutrophils** [Q]
- **E.g.: IL-8** [Q]
- Causes **activation** and **chemotaxis of neutrophils** [Q]
- **Most important** inducers – **microbial products, IL-1**[Q] **and TNF** [Q]

B) **C-C chemokines (β chemokines)**

- Includes **monocyte chemo attractant protein (MCP-1)** [Q], **eotaxin** [Q], **macrophage inflammatory protein-1α (MIP-1α)** [Q] **and RANTES** [Q]
- **Attract monocytes, eosinophils, basophils and lymphocytes** but not neutrophils
- **Eotaxin** [Q] selectively recruits **eosinophils** [Q]

C) **C chemokines (γ chemokines)**

- Includes **lymphotactin** [Q] which is relatively specific for **lymphocytes** [Q]

D) **CX3C chemokines**

- E.g. **Fractalkine** [Q]
- Promotes strong **adhesion of monocytes** [Q] **and T cells**

Note:

Chemokine receptors – CXCR-4 [Q], **CCR-5** [Q] act as **co-receptors** for viral envelope glycoprotein of **HIV-1** [Q]

- As in the question, **bronchial fluid** shows **eosinophils**, which is mainly mediated by the action of **β chemokines** mainly **eotaxin**

Ans. 22) B. β chemokine (Ref: 8 ed. Robbins p. 62, 9 ed. p 87)

- **RANTES** (regulated and normal T-cell expressed and secreted) and **eotaxin** belong to **β chemokine** group of chemokine [Q]

Ans. 23) C. iNOS (Ref: 8 ed. Robbins p. 60-61, f-2-12)

Nitric Oxide (NO):

- Produced by **endothelial cells, macrophages** and **neurons** [Q]
- **Three different types** of NOS: endothelial **(eNOS)**, neuronal **(nNOS)** and inducible **(iNOS)**
- **eNOS and nNOS** are rapidly activated by an increase in **cytoplasmic Ca^{2+}**
- **iNOS**, is **induced** when **macrophages** are **activated by cytokines (e.g., TNF, IFN-γ)** or by **microbial products**

NO have **dual actions** in inflammation:

- **Relaxes vascular smooth muscle** [Q]
- Promotes **vasodilation** and is an **inhibitor** of inflammatory responses [Q]

Ans. 24) C. Plasma (Ref: 8 ed. Robbins p. 63-64, 9 ed. p. 88-89, f-3-12)

Complement System:

- **Critical step in complement activation** is **cleavage** of **C3** (most abundant component)

Cleavage of C3 can occur by **one of the three pathways**:

- **Classical pathway** is triggered by **fixation of C1** to **antibody (IgM or IgG)** that has combined with antigen
- **Alternative pathway**: Triggered by **microbial surface molecules** (e.g., endotoxin or LPS), **complex polysaccharides**, cobra venom
- **Lectin pathway**: Plasma **mannose-binding lectin** binds to carbohydrates on microbes and directly activates C1
- All three pathways, leads to formation of an **active enzyme called C3 convertase**, which **splits C3 into C3a and C3b**

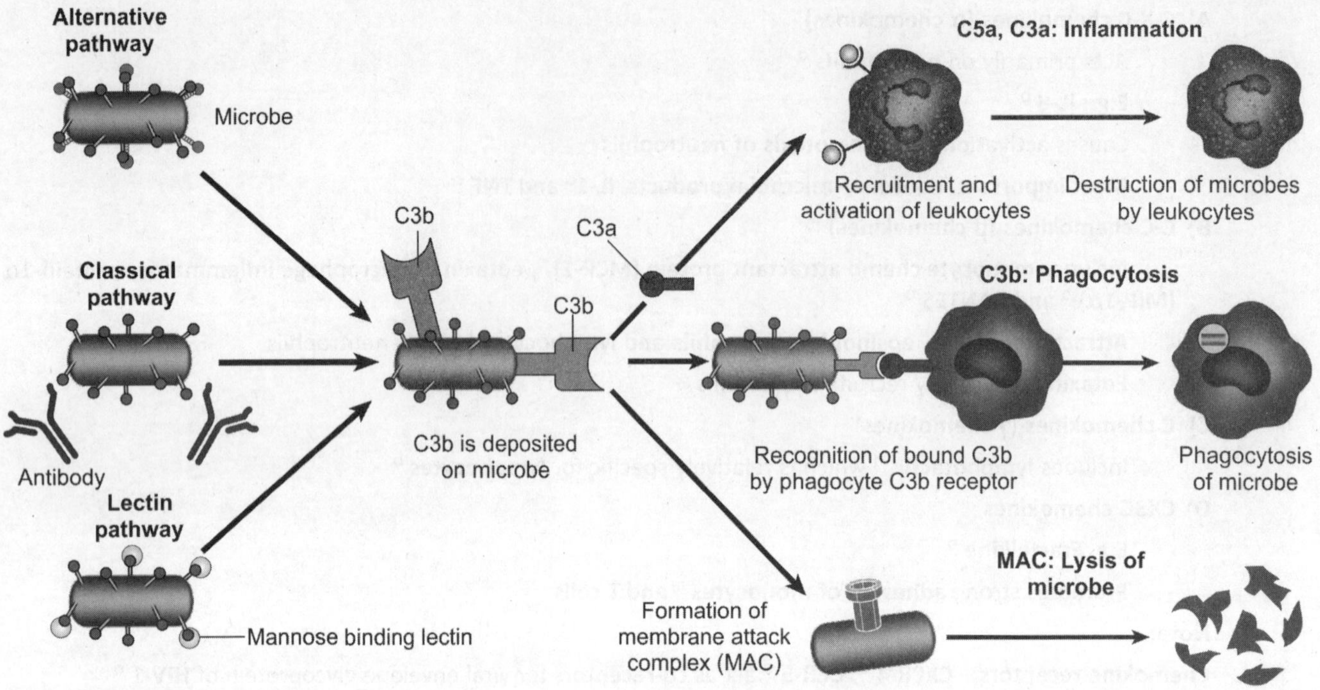

Functions of complement system

Ans. 25) C. C3a,C5a (Ref: 8 ed. Robbins p. 63-64, 9 ed. p. 88-89, f-3-12)

Functions of Complement System:

a) Inflammation –

- **C3a, C5a** and **C4a** stimulate **histamine release** from **mast cells** [Q], which leads to **increased vascular permeability** and cause **vasodilation**
- **C3a, C5a** and **C4a** are called as **anaphylotoxins** [Q] as they produce similar effects of **mast cell mediators** that are involved in **anaphylaxis**
- **C5a** – Powerful **chemotactic agent** [Q] for neutrophils, monocytes, eosinophils and basophils

b) Phagocytosis – C3b, act as **opsonins** [Q] and **promote phagocytosis** [Q] by **neutrophils and macrophages**

c) Cell lysis – Deposition of **Membrane Attack Complex (MAC)** on the cells makes them permeable to water and ions and results in death of the cells

Ans. 26) D. All of the above (Ref: 8 ed. Robbins p. 64-66, f-2-15)

Activated Hageman Factor (factor XIIa) initiates the **four systems** involved in the inflammatory response:

- **Kinin system**, which produces vasoactive kinins
- **Clotting system**, which induces formation of thrombin, fibrinopeptides and factor X
- **Fibrinolytic system**, which produces plasmin and degrades fibrin
- **Complement system**, which produces **anaphylotoxins**

Important Points to Remember:

Kinin system:

- **Factor XIIa**, converts plasma **prekallikrein** to **kallikrein**, which cleaves, **high molecular weight kininogen**, to produce **bradykinin** [Q]

Bradykinin:

- Increases **vascular permeability** [Q]
- Causes contraction of smooth muscle, dilation of blood vessels and **pain**

- **Action of bradykinin** is **short-lived**, as it is quickly **inactivated** by **kininase** [Q] or **lung** by **angiotensin converting enzyme in lung**[Q]

Clotting system:

- Divided into **two pathways**, resulting in **activation of thrombin** and **formation of fibrin** [Q]

Fibrinolytic system [Q]

- **Factor XIIa** activates fibrinolytic system by cleaving fibrin and solubilizing the clot
- **Kallikrein**, as well as **plasminogen activator** cleaves **plasminogen** to generate **plasmin**
- Plasmin **lyses fibrin** to form **fibrin split products** [Q]
- **During inflammation**, plasmin also cleaves the **complement protein C3** to produce **C3 fragments** [Q]

Ans. 27) B. Vascular changes, edema, neutrophilic infiltration (Ref: 8 ed. Robbins p. 70, 9 ed. 93-94)

Vascular changes, edema, and predominantly neutrophilic infiltration [Q] are manifestations of **acute inflammation** [Q]

Chronic inflammation is **characterized by**:

- Infiltration with **mononuclear cells**, i.e. **macrophages, lymphocytes** and **plasma cells**
- **Tissue destruction** and **healing of damaged tissue** by proliferation of **small blood vessels (angiogenesis)** and **fibrosis**

Ans. 28) D. Microglia (Ref: 8 ed. Robbins p. 71-72, 9 ed. p. 88-89, f-3-19-21)

Role of Macrophages in Chronic Inflammation:

- **Mononuclear phagocyte system** includes **blood monocytes** and **tissue macrophages**
- Tissue macrophages in different organs are named by different names:
  - In **Liver – Kupffer cells** [Q]
  - In **spleen and lymph nodes – sinus histiocytes**
  - In **lungs – alveolar macrophages**
  - In **central nervous system – microglia** [Q]

Note:

- **Half-life** of blood **monocytes** is about **1 day**, whereas **life span of tissue macrophages** is several **months or years**

Ans. 29) B. Major basic protein (Ref: 8 ed. Robbins p. 72, 9 ed. p. 96-97, f-3-22)

- Eosinophils are **abundant** in immune reactions mediated by **IgE** and in **parasitic infections**
- **Eotaxin** is the **most important chemokine** responsible for **eosinophil recruitment** [Q]
- Eosinophil granules contain **major basic protein** [Q], that is **toxic to parasites**

Ans. 30) C. Ulcerative colitis (Ref: 8 ed. Robbins p. 73-74, 9 ed. p. 97-98, f-3-23, t-3-8)

Granuloma:

- **Cellular attempt** to contain the offending agent in which there is activation of **T-lymphocytes** leading to **macrophage activation**

Examples:

- **Tuberculosis** [Q] (is the prototype of the **granulomatous diseases**)
- **Sarcoidosis** [Q]
- **Cat-scratch disease** [Q]
- **Lymphogranuloma inguinale**
- **Leprosy** [Q]
- **Brucellosis**
- **Syphilis**
- **Mycotic infections, Berylliosis, reactions of irritant lipids**

Note:

- In **Crohn disease** [Q], we see **microgranulomas** [Q]
- **Ulcerative colitis** is **not** associated with **granuloma formation**

Ans. 31) A. ESR (Ref: 8 ed. Robbins p. 75, 9 ed. p. 99-100)

Acute-phase proteins are **plasma proteins**, synthesized in **liver** [Q] and include:

- **C-reactive protein (CRP)**
- **Fibrinogen**
- **Serum amyloid A (SAA) protein**

Important Points to Remember:

- **CRP** and **SAA** bind to **microbial cell walls** and act as **opsonins**
- **Fibrinogen binds** to **red cells** and causes them to form **stacks (rouleaux)**, that forms the basis for measuring **erythrocyte sedimentation rate**
- **ESR** itself is **not an acute phase protein** [Q], as it is dependent on **fibrinogen**
- Prolonged production of these proteins (especially **SAA**) in states of **chronic inflammation** causes **secondary amyloidosis** [Q]
- **Elevated CRP** levels leads to **increased risk of myocardial infarction** [Q] in patients with **coronary artery disease**
- **Hepcidin** [Q] – **Acute phase reactant** whose elevated plasma concentration is responsible for **anemia associated with chronic inflammation** [Q]

Ans. 32) D. Infectious mononucleosis (Ref: 9 ed. Robbins p.99)

Causes of:

Neutrophilia (increased neutrophil count) [Q] – Bacterial infections

Lymphocytosis [Q] – Viral infections, such as infectious mononucleosis, mumps, German measles

Eosinophilia – Allergies and parasitic infestations

Leukopenia (decreased number of circulating white cells) [Q] – Typhoid fever, viral, rickettsial, and certain protozoal infections

Ans. 33) D. Fibroblasts (Ref: 8 ed. Robbins p. 81-82, 9 ed. p. 101)

Tissues on the basis of their **proliferative activity** are divided into **three groups:**

A) Continuously dividing (labile tissues):

Cells which proliferate throughout life and include **surface epithelia e.g.**

- **Stratified squamous epithelia** of skin, oral cavity, vagina and cervix
- Lining mucosa of all the excretory ducts of the glands
- **Columnar epithelium** of the GI tract and uterus
- **Transitional epithelium** of the urinary tract
- **Cells of the bone marrow and hematopoietic tissues**

B) Quiescent (stable tissues):

Have low level of **replication** but can replicate in response to stimuli or injury

Examples include:

- Parenchymal cells of liver, kidneys and pancreas
- Mesenchymal cells such as **fibroblasts** and **smooth muscle**
- **Vascular endothelial cells, lymphocytes** and other **leukocytes**

C) Non-dividing (permanent tissues):

Cells that **cannot undergo mitotic division** in postnatal life

Examples include:

- **Neurons** [Q]**, skeletal and cardiac muscle cells**

Ans. 34) D. Nanog (Ref: 8 ed. Robbins p. 84, f-3-6)

Pluripotency:

- Cells which are taken from one cell, can be transformed/ induced into certain other cell population in human body i.e. **Induced Pluripotent cells**

Transcription factors responsible for **induced pluripotent cells (iPS)**:

- **Oct3/4**
- **Sox2**
- **C-myc**
- **Klf4**

However, **homeobox protein Nanog**[Q] acts to **prevent differentiation**

Ans. 35) A. Development elasticity (Ref: 8 ed. Robbins p.82-85, f-3-4, 5)

Trans-differentiation [Q]:

- A change in the differentiation of a cell from one type to another

Developmental plasticity [Q]:

- The capacity of a cell to trans-differentiate into diverse lineages

Note:

- Stem cell doesn't show development elasticity

Ans. 36) C. Vitamin D (Ref: 8 ed. Robbins p. 90-92, 9 ed. p. 16-18, f-1-11)

Common receptors involved in signal transduction pathway:

A) Receptors with intrinsic tyrosine kinase activity:

- Growth factors such as EGF, TGF-α, HGF, PDGF, VEGF, FGF, c-KIT ligand and insulin

B) Receptors lacking intrinsic tyrosine kinase activity:

- **IL-2, IL-3, interferon α, β and γ, erythropoietin, granulocyte colony-stimulating factor**, growth hormone and prolactin

C) G protein–coupled receptors [Q]:

- E.g.: Chemokines, vasopressin, serotonin, histamine, epinephrine and norepinephrine, **calcitonin**, glucagon, **parathyroid hormone**, **corticotropin** and rhodopsin

D) Steroid hormone receptors [Q]:

- Located in the **nucleus** [Q]

Examples:

- **Steroid hormones, thyroid hormone, vitamin D** and **retinoids**
- **Peroxisome proliferator-activated receptors:** Involved in **adipogenesis, inflammation and atherosclerosis**

Hence, Vitamin D belongs to **steroid family of receptors** and not G-PCR's

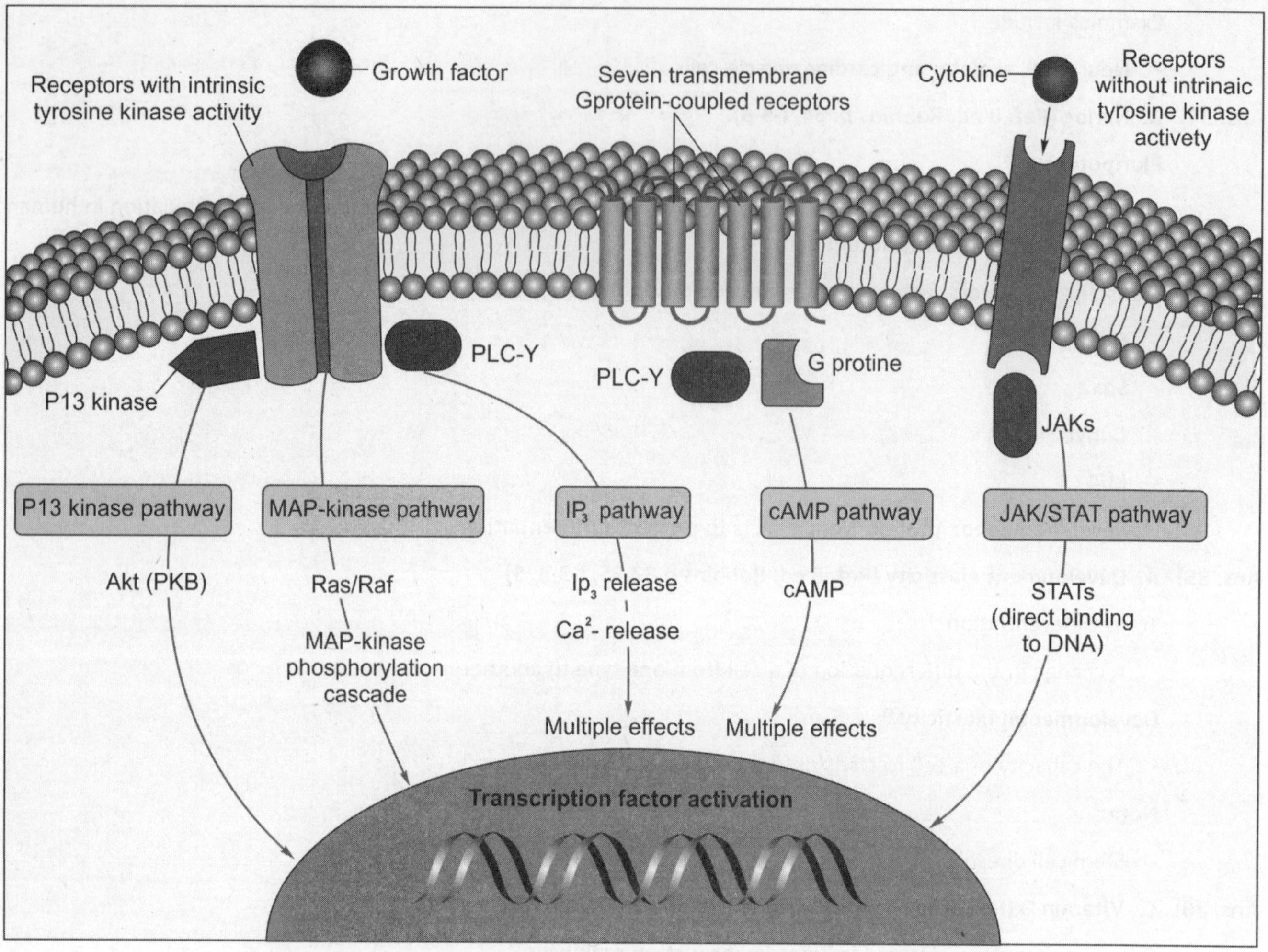

Cell surface receptors and their principal signal transduction pathways

Ans. 37) B. Parathyroid hormone (Ref: 8 ed. Robbins p.90-92, 9 ed. p. 16-18, f - 1-11)

- Refer to the above question for details

Ans. 38) C. Intrahepatic stem/progenitor cells play a role in compensatory growth (Ref: 8 ed. Robbins p. 93-94, 9 ed. p 102-03, f-3-25)

Compensatory growth or **Compensatory Hyperplasia**:

- Human liver has a remarkable capacity to regenerate after **partial hepatectomy**
- Occurs due to **enlargement of the remaining lobes** after hepatectomy
- Cells responsible for this regrowth include **Kupffer cells** [Q], **endothelial cells** and **stellate cells** [Q]
- **Hepatocyte proliferation** is triggered by **TGF-α**, **HGF** and **IL-6** [Q]
- **TGF-β** [Q] **(Growth inhibitor)** inhibits the **hepatocyte replication**
- **Intrahepatic stem** or **progenitor cells** do not play a role in **compensatory growth** [Q]

Ans. 39) B. Type II is associated Ehlers - Danlos Syndrome (Ref: 8 ed. Robbins p. 95-96, 9 ed. p 20-24, f – 12-15)

Collagen and Its Disorders:

- Collagen is composed of **three chains** in the shape of a **triple helix**
- **Types I, II, III and V, and XI** are the **fibrillar collagens**
- **Type IV collagen** is major components of **basement membrane** [Q], together with **laminin**

- **Type VII** collagen forms the **anchoring fibrils** between **epidermis** and **dermis**
- Genetic deficiency of **Type I collagen** results in **Osteogenesis imperfecta; Ehlers - Danlos syndrome—type I** Q
- **Type IV collagen deficiency** results in **Alport syndrome** Q
- **Type VII collagen** deficiency (dermal epidermal junction) results in **Dystrophic epidermolysis bullosa** Q
- **Vitamin C** Q is required for **hydroxylation** of **pro-collagen**, which explains inadequate wound healing in **scurvy**

Ans. 40) C. Concentration decreases in rheumatoid arthritis, osteoarthritis, psoriasis (Ref: 8 ed. Robbins p. 97-98, 9 ed. p. 23-24)

Four structurally distinct families of **Glycosaminoglycan's (GAGs):**

- **Heparan sulfate**
- **Chondroitin/dermatan sulfate**
- **Keratan sulfate**
- **Hyaluronan (HA)**

Hyaluronan:

- Produced at the **plasma membrane** by enzyme **hyaluronan synthases** Q
- Is abundant in **heart valves, skin and skeletal tissues, synovial fluid, the vitreous of the eye** and **umbilical cord**Q
- Concentration **increases** Q in **inflammatory diseases** such as **rheumatoid arthritis, scleroderma, psoriasis, and osteoarthritis** Q
- **Hyaluronidases** fragment HA into lower molecular weight molecules (LMW HA)
- **LMW HA** binds to **CD44 receptor** Q on leukocytes and promotes the recruitment of leukocytes to the sites of inflammation

Ans. 41) C. TGF-β (Ref: 8 ed. Robbins p. 102-106, 9 ed. p. 106-08, f-3-29-30)

Three phases of cutaneous wound healing include: **inflammation**, **proliferation** and **maturation**

Healing by **primary union** Q or by **first intention**:

- Healing of clean, **uninfected** surgical incision approximated by **surgical sutures**

Healing by **secondary union** Q or by **second intention**:

- Is seen in **excisional wounds** that create **large defects** on the skin surface and results in **scar** Q formation

Sequence of events in wound healing:

a) Formation of Blood Clot
  - Within 24 hours, **neutrophils** Q appear at the margins of the incision

b) Formation of Granulation Tissue
  - **Fibroblasts** Q and **vascular endothelial cells** proliferate in **24 to 72 hours** Q and forms **granulation tissue** (which is a **hallmark** of tissue repair)

c) Cell Proliferation and Collagen Deposition
  - Neutrophils are largely replaced by **macrophages** Q in **48 to 96 hours**
  - **TGF-β** is the most important **fibrogenic agent** Q

d) Scar Formation – occurs by the end of the **first month** Q

e) Wound Contraction
  - Occurs in large surface wounds
  - Seen in wounds which heal by **secondary union** Q
  - Brought about by **myofibroblasts** Q

f) Connective Tissue Remodeling

g) Recovery of Tensile Strength

Ans. 42) B. 3 months (Ref: 8 ed. Robbins p. 102-106, 9 ed. p. 108-09)

- **Type I collagen** [Q] is essential for the development of strength in healing wounds
- At the end of the **first week**, wound strength is **10%** that of unwounded skin
- Wound strength **increases rapidly** over the next **4 weeks**
- At the end of **third month**, it reaches a plateau at about **70% to 80%** of the tensile strength of unwounded skin

Ans. 43) B. Stellate cells (Ref: 8 ed. Robbins p. 108, 9 ed. p. 109, f-3-31)

- In **lung and kidney** fibrosis, **myofibroblasts** [Q] are the main source of collagen
- **Stellate cells** [Q] are the **major collagen producers** in **liver cirrhosis**
- **Osteopontin (OPN)** [Q] is strongly expressed in fibrosis of the heart, lung, liver, kidney

Ans. 44) D. IFN gamma (Ref: 9 ed. Robbins p. 97)

- Helper T-cells are activated by IL-2 and produce IFN-γ (interferon gamma)

Interferon gamma

- Major cytokine of granulomatous inflammation
- Induces formation of granuloma by conversion of activated macrophages into epithelioid cells and formation of giant cells by fusion of epithelial cells

Ans. 45) B. Fibrinogen (Ref: 9 ed. Robbins p. 98-99) Refer Q 31 for details

Ans. 46) D. NADPH oxidase (9 ed. p. 79-80) Refer Q 11 for details

Ans. 47) A. TGF-beta (Ref: 9 ed. Robbins p. 94-95)

- Growth factors and TGF- beta from activated macrophages brings about tissue repair and fibrosis

Ans. 48) A. Histamine (Ref: 9 ed. Robbins p. 83)

- Histamine causes dilation of arterioles and increases the permeability of venules

Ans. 49) D. VCAM 4 (Ref: 9 ed. Robbins p. 75) Refer Q 2 and 3 for details

Ans. 50) C. Zn metalloproteinase (Ref: 9 ed. Robbins p. 105)

- Degradation of collagens is brought by a family of matrix metalloproteinase (MMPs)
- Metals ions (e.g., zinc) are required for their activity

Ans. 51) A. By day 5 epidermis recovers its normal thickness (Ref: 9 ed. Robbins p. 106-07)

Healing by primary intention (By day 5)

- Incisional space is filled with granulation tissue
- Neovascularization is maximum
- Collagen fibrils become more abundant and begin to bridge the incision
- Epidermis recovers its normal thickness

Ans. 52) A. LTB4 (Ref: 9 ed. Robbins p. 77) Refer Q 9 for details

Ans. 53) A. Extravascular fluid that has a high protein concentration and contains cellular debris (Ref: 9 ed. Robbins p. 73)

- Exudate – Is an extravascular fluid that has a high protein concentration and contains cellular debris

Ans. 54) A. CD 34 (9 ed. Robbins p. 75-78)

Ans. 55) A. IL-1 (Ref: 9 ed. Robbins p. 86-87) Refer Q19 for details

Ans. 56) D. Xanthine oxidase (Ref: 9 ed. Robbins p. 80) Refer Q 11 for details

Ans. 57) C. A selectin (Ref: 9 ed. Robbins p. 76) Refer Q 3 for details

Ans. 58) B. Integrins (Ref: 9 ed. Robbins p. 75-78)

- Cell-matrix adhesions are mediated by integrins
- Cell-cell adhesions in anchoring junctions are mediated by cadherins

Ans. 59) **A. PECAM (Ref: 9 ed. Robbins p. 76-77)** Refer Q 6 for details

Ans. 60) **A. Mast cells (Ref: 9 ed. Robbins p. 88-89)** Refer Q 25 for details

Ans. 61) **A. Extensive cross linking of tropocollagen (Ref: Robbins 8 ed p. 105-106)**

Wound Strength:

1. At the end of 1st week, wound strength is approximately 10% of that of unwounded skin
2. Wound strength increases rapidly over the next 4 weeks
3. At 3rd month, it reaches a plateau of 70-80% of the tensile strength of unwounded skin
4. Recovery of tensile strength results from the excess of collagen synthesis over collagen degradation, during the first two months of healing and later from structural modification of collagen fibers

Ans. 62) **C. Trans-differentiation (Ref: 8 ed. Robbins p. 82-85)** Refer Q 35 for details

Ans. 63) **B. Vasodilation (Ref: 9 ed. Robbins p. 89)**

Platelet-Activating Factor (PAF):

- Elaborated by platelets, basophils, mast cells, neutrophils, macrophages and endothelial cells
- Leads to platelet aggregation, vasoconstriction and bronchoconstriction, increased venular permeability

Ans. 64) **C. End of third week (Ref: 9 ed. Robbins p. 108-09)** Refer Q 41, 42 for details

Ans. 65) **B. NADPH oxidase (Ref: 9 ed. Robbins p. 79-80)** Refer Q 11 for details

Ans. 66) **C. Vasodilation and increase in permeability (Ref: 9 ed. Robbins p. 74-75)** Refer Q 2 and 27 for details

Ans. 67) **C. C3 (Ref: 9 ed. Robbins p. 88-89)** Refer Q 24, 25 for details

Ans. 68) **B. Pain at the sight of inflammation (Ref: 8 ed. Robbins p. 64-66, f-2-15)** Refer Q 26 for details

Ans. 69) **B. Histamine release due to local injury to mast cells by pointing device (Ref: 9 ed. Robbins p. 83)**

Histamine:

- Is stored and released from mast cells in response to a stimulus
- Causes dilation of arterioles and increases the permeability of venules

Ans. 70) **B. Secretory (Ref: 9 ed. Robbins p. 56)**

- Epithelioid cells are activated macrophages
- Most important role of epithelioid histiocytes is not phagocytosis
- Epithelioid cells secrete lysozyme and a variety of enzymes

Granulomatous Inflammation

- In H&E preparations, epithelioid cells in granulomas have pink, granular cytoplasm with indistinct cell boundaries
- Aggregates of epithelioid macrophages are surrounded by a collar of lymphocytes
- Multinucleate giant cells, 40 to 50 micrometers in diameter are found in granulomas
- Such cells consists a large mass of cytoplasm and many nuclei, due to the fusion of multiple activated macrophages

Ans. 71) **C. PECAM-activation of leukocytes (Ref: 9 ed. Robbins p. 35, 36)** Refer Q 4 and 6 for details

Cellular Events – PECAM, has no role in leucocyte activation and it is involved in transmigration

Ans. 72) **B. 24 to 72 hours (Ref: 9 ed. Robbins p. 106-08)** Refer Q 41 for details

Ans. 73) **A. Immediate transient increase in permeability (Ref: 9 ed. Robbins p. 74-75)** Refer Q 2 for details

4 Hemodynamic Disorders

How to go about this chapter?

- **Be thorough with following topics:**
  - **Endothelial function**
  - **Hemostasis**
  - **Thrombosis**
  - **Coagulation cascade**
  - **Embolism**
  - **Shock**
  - **Disseminated intravascularcCoagulation**

EDEMA AND EFFUSIONS

1) **Edema results from:**
   a) Increased capillary hydrostatic pressure and diminished plasma oncotic pressure
   b) Increased capillary hydrostatic pressure and increased plasma oncotic pressure
   c) Decreased capillary hydrostatic pressure and increased plasma oncotic pressure
   d) Decreased capillary hydrostatic pressure and decreased plasma oncotic pressure

2) **Increased blood volume in a tissue is known as:**
   a) Hyperemia
   b) Congestion
   c) Both of the above
   d) Purpura

HEMOSTASIS AND HEMORRHAGIC DISORDERS

3) **Minute 1- to 2-mm hemorrhages into skin, mucous membranes, or serosal surfaces are:**
   a) Petechiae b) Hematoma
   c) Purpura d) Ecchymosis

4) **All are TRUE about normal hemostatic mechanism EXCEPT:**
   a) Endothelin brings about vasodilation
   b) Platelets are responsible for primary hemostasis
   c) Tissue factor plays a role in secondary hemostasis
   d) t-PA limits the formation of hemostatic plug

5) **Endothelium after injury to endothelial cells exhibit the following properties:**
   a) Fibrinolytic
   b) Anticoagulant
   c) Procoagulant
   d) Antiplatelet

6) **α-Granules of platelets contain all EXCEPT:**
   a) Fibrinogen
   b) Fibronectin
   c) Calcium
   d) Factors V and VIII

7) **Genetic deficiency of von Willebrand factor results in:**
   a) Bernard-Soulier syndrome
   b) Von Willebrand disease
   c) Glanzmann thrombasthenia
   d) Platelet aggregation defect

8) **Glanzmann thrombasthenia occurs due to deficiency of:**
   a) vWF b) GpIb
   c) GpIIb-IIIa d) GpIXb

9) **Extrinsic pathway is mediated by:**
   a) Factor XII b) Factor III
   c) Thrombin d) Factor X

10) **Endogenous anticoagulants include all EXCEPT:**
   a) Anti-thrombin
   b) Protein C and S
   c) Factor V
   d) Tissue factor pathway inhibitor

THROMBOSIS

11) **Virchow's triad include all EXCEPT:**
a) Endothelial injury
b) Laminar blood flow
c) Stasis
d) Hypercoagulability

12) **All are TRUE about Heparin induced thrombocytopenia syndrome EXCEPT:**
a) Occurs due to administration of unfractionated heparin
b) Increases risk of bleeding
c) Newer low-molecular weight heparin preparations are at lower risk
d) None of the above

13) **All are TRUE about Antiphospholipid antibody syndrome (APAS) EXCEPT:**
a) Repeated miscarriages, thrombosis, cardiac valve vegetation, thrombocytopenia
b) Antibodies give frequently a false positive serological test for syphilis
c) Individuals with autoimmune diseases are designated as primary APAS
d) Anti-phospholipid antibodies can be seen in apparently normal individuals

14) **Characteristic feature of antemortem clot is:**
a) Lines of Zahn
b) Gelatinous appearance
c) Yellow chicken fat appearance
d) Not attached to the underlying wall

EMBOLISM

15) **All of the following are TRUE about fat embolism EXCEPT:**
a) Rarely symptomatic
b) Characterized by pulmonary insufficiency, anemia, thrombocytopenia
c) Petechial rash is a useful diagnostic feature
d) Fat micro globules are easily demonstrated on paraffin embedding sections

16) **All are TRUE about air embolism EXCEPT:**
a) >100 cc of air is required to have a clinical effect
b) Decompression sickness occurs when individuals experience sudden decreases in atmospheric pressure
c) Caisson disease is an acute form of decompression sickness
d) Acute decompression sickness is treated by placing the individual in a high pressure chamber

INFARCTION

17) **White infarcts are seen in all EXCEPT:**
a) Heart b) Spleen
c) Kidney d) Lung

18) **All are the features of infarct EXCEPT:**
a) Are wedge-shaped
b) Liquefactive necrosis is the dominant histologic feature
c) In lung, hemorrhagic infarcts are seen
d) Are replaced by scars

SHOCK

19) **All are the features of septic shock EXCEPT:**
a) Peripheral vasodilation and pooling of blood
b) Disseminated intravascular coagulation
c) Failure of myocardial pump resulting from intrinsic myocardial damage
d) Activation of cytokine cascades

20) **Laboratory findings in fat embolism consist of the following EXCEPT: (NEET 2014)**
a) Thrombocytopenia
b) Fat globules in urine
c) Hypercalcemia
d) Anemia

21) **White infarct is seen in: (NEET 2014)**
a) Lung
b) Intestine
c) Liver
d) Ovary

22) **Increased accumulation of fluid in the interstitial space is described as: (NEET 2014)**
a) Edema
b) Effusion
c) Transudate
d) Exudate

23) **Most important growth factors in angiogenesis: (NEET 2014)**
a) PDGF b) TGF alpha
c) TGF beta d) Ang 1

24) **Necrosis with cell bodies retained as ghost cells is: (NEET 2014)**
a) Coagulative necrosis
b) Liquefactive necrosis
c) Caseous necrosis
d) Gangrenous

25) **Following injury to a blood vessel, immediate haemostasis is achieved by: (NEET 2013)**
a) Fibrin deposition
b) Vasoconstriction
c) Platelet adhesion
d) Thrombosis

26) **Nutmeg liver is seen in: (NEET 2013)**
a) Right sided heart failure
b) Left sided heart failure
c) Increased pulmonary pressure
d) Decreased pulmonary pressure

27) Cells most sensitive to hypoxia are: (NEET 2013)
- a) Myocardial cells
- b) Neurons
- c) Hepatocytes
- d) Renal tubular epithelial cells

28) Lines of Zahn occur in: (NEET 2013)
- a) Postmortem clot
- b) Infarct
- c) Embolus
- d) Antemortem thrombus

29) All are TRUE about blood coagulation EXCEPT: (AIPGMEE 2011)
- a) Factor X is a part of both intrinsic and extrinsic pathway
- b) Extrinsic pathway is activated by contact with plasma and negatively charged proteins
- c) Calcium is very important for coagulation
- d) Intrinsic pathway can be activated in vitro

CHAPTER 4: HEMODYNAMIC DISORDERS

Ans. 1) **A. Increased capillary hydrostatic pressure and diminished plasma oncotic pressure (Ref: 8 ed. Robbins p. 111-113, 9 ed. 113-15, f-4-1-2, t-4-1)**

- Outflow of fluid from the **arteriolar end** into the interstitium is in equal proportion to the **inflow at the venular end**
- **Increased capillary pressure** Q or **diminished colloid osmotic pressure** Q result **in increased interstitial fluid**
- **Edema** – Abnormal increase in interstitial fluid within tissues
- **Transudate** Q – Protein-poor fluid due to **increased hydrostatic pressure or reduced plasma protein. E.g. – heart failure, renal failure, hepatic failure, malnutrition**
- **Exudate** Q **– Inflammatory edema** (protein-rich fluid due to **increased vascular permeability**)

Ans. 2) **C. Both of the above (Ref: 8 ed. Robbins p.113-114, 9 ed. 115-16, f-4-3)**

- **Hyperemia and congestion** are terms used for **increased blood volume**
- **Hyperemia** – Active process in which **arteriolar dilatation** leads to **increased blood flow**
- **Congestion – Passive process**, resulting from reduced outflow of blood from a tissue

Examples:

- In lung, **hemosiderin laden macrophages** Q or **heart failure cells** Q are seen **in chronic pulmonary congestion** Q
- **Nutmeg liver** Q **– Chronic passive congestion** Q **of liver**

Ans. 3) **A. Petechiae (Ref: 8 ed. Robbins p.114, f-4-4)**

Definitions to remember:

- **Hematoma** – Accumulation of blood at any site
- **Petechiae – 1- to 2-mm** hemorrhages into skin, mucous membranes, or serosal surfaces. E.g. thrombocytopenia
- **Purpura** – Slightly larger **(>3 mm)** hemorrhages, secondary to **trauma, vasculitis, or increased vascular fragility (e.g. in amyloidosis)**
- **Ecchymosis** – Larger **(1 to 2 cm)** subcutaneous hematomas **(i.e. bruises)**

Ans. 4) **A. Endothelin brings about vasodilation (Ref: 8 ed. Robbins p.114, 9 ed. 116-17, f-4-4)**

Normal hemostasis:

- **Endothelin** Q (a potent **endothelium-derived vasoconstrictor**): Brings arteriolar vasoconstriction

Primary hemostasis:

- **Endothelial injury exposes** highly thrombogenic **sub-endothelial** extracellular matrix (ECM) which leads to **platelet adherence and activation**
- Within minutes the secreted products recruit additional platelets **(aggregation)** to form a **hemostatic plug**

Secondary hemostasis:

- **Tissue factor** Q or **factor III / thromboplastin** Q is exposed at the site of injury, which is synthesized by **endothelial cells** Q
- **Tissue factor** along with **factor VII** acts as initiator of **coagulation cascade,** leading to the **thrombin** generation
- **Thrombin** cleaves **fibrinogen** into **insoluble fibrin**, creating a **fibrin meshwork**
- Consolidates the initial platelet plug

Note: Tissue plasminogen activator (t-PA): limit the hemostatic plug formation at the site of injury

Ans. 5) **C. Pro-coagulant (Ref: 8 ed. Robbins p.115-17, 9 ed. p. 121, f-4-10)**

Endothelial cells:

- Exhibit **antiplatelet, anticoagulant** and **fibrinolytic properties** Q

- However, after injury or activation, acquire **pro-coagulant** [Q] properties
- Endothelium can be activated by trauma, infectious agents, hemodynamic forces, plasma mediators and cytokines

Important Properties of Endothelium

a) Antithrombotic Properties [Q]**:**

Antiplatelet effects:

- **Non-activated platelets** do not adhere to endothelial cells
- **Prostacyclin (PGI2)** [Q] **and nitric oxide (NO)** [Q] produced by the endothelial cells **inhibit** [Q] platelet adhesion and platelet aggregation and are **potent vasodilators** [Q]
- Endothelial cells also elaborate **adenosine diphosphatase,** which degrades **adenosine diphosphate (ADP)** and further **inhibits platelet aggregation**

Anticoagulant effects [Q] **:**

- Mediated by endothelial membrane associated **heparin-like molecules, thrombomodulin** and **tissue factor pathway inhibitor**

Fibrinolytic effects [Q]**:**

- Endothelial cells synthesize **tissue-type plasminogen activator (t-PA)** [Q], which cleaves **plasminogen** to **plasmin;** which in turn, cleaves fibrin to degrade thrombi

b) Prothrombotic Properties [Q]**:**

Platelet effects:

- After **endothelial injury,** platelets come into contact with the underlying extracellular matrix
- **von Willebrand factor (vWF)** [Q] – Produced by normal endothelial cells leads to subsequent adhesion

Pro-coagulant effects [Q]**:**

- In response to **cytokines** or **bacterial endotoxin,** endothelial cells synthesize **tissue factor** which activates **extrinsic clotting cascade**

Anti-fibrinolytic effects [Q] **:**

- Endothelial cells secrete **inhibitors of plasminogen activator,** which limit fibrinolysis and favors thrombosis

Ans. 6) **C. Calcium (Ref: 8 ed. Robbins p. 117, 9 ed. p. 117)**

- Platelets contains two types of granules – α- **Granules** and **Dense (or δ) granules**

α- Granules:

- Have adhesion molecule **P-selectin** on their membranes
- Contain **fibrinogen, fibronectin, factors V and VIII, platelet factor 4,** platelet-derived growth factor (PDGF) and transforming growth factor-β (TGF-β)

Dense (or δ) Granules:

- Contain **ADP** [Q] **and ATP** [Q], **ionized calcium** [Q], histamine, serotonin and epinephrine

Ans. 7) **B. von Willebrand disease (Ref: 8 ed. Robbins p. 117-18, 9 ed. p. 117-18, f -4-5)**

von Willebrand Factor:

- Mediates platelet adhesion to Extra Cellular Matrix (ECM)
- Acts as a bridge between platelet surface receptors **(i.e. glycoprotein Ib [GpIb])** and exposed collagen
- **Genetic deficiency of vWF** results in **von Willebrand disease** [Q] and its receptor (i.e. GpIb) deficiency results in **Bernard-Soulier syndrome** [Q]

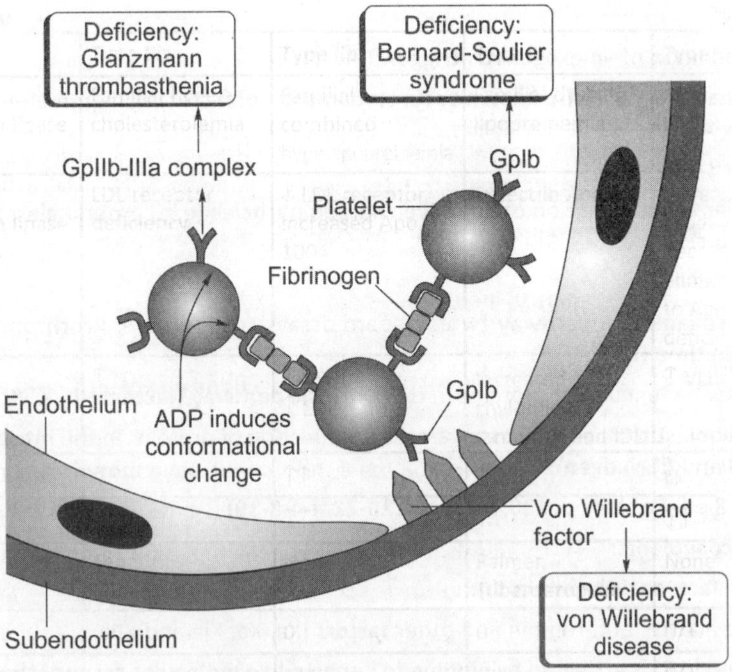

Platelet adhesion and aggregation

Ans. 8) **C. GpIIb-IIIa (Ref: 8 ed. Robbins p. 118, 9 ed. p. 117-18, f-4-5)**

- **Glanzmann thrombasthenia** Q– due to inherited deficiency of **GpIIb-IIIa**
- **Platelet adhesion** to the **endothelial surface** is brought about by **vWF-GpIb interactions** Q
- **Platelet aggregation** Q is brought by fibrinogen bridging **GpIIb-IIIa receptors** Q on different platelets

Ans. 9) **B. Factor III (Ref: 8 ed. Robbins p. 118-20, 9 ed. 118-20, f-4-6-8)**

- Blood coagulation is classified into **extrinsic and intrinsic pathways** that converge on the activation of **factor X** Q

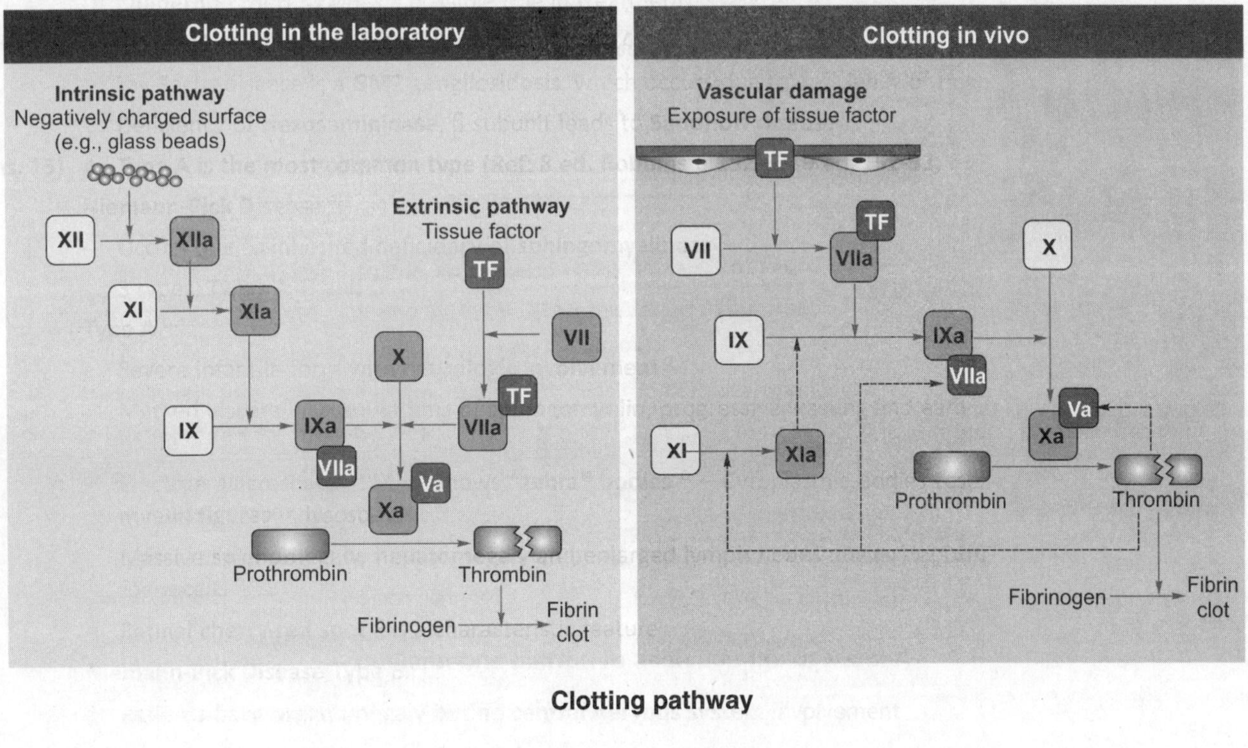

Clotting pathway

Extrinsic pathway [Q]

- Requires the addition of an **exogenous trigger** [Q]
- **Activated** by **tissue factor** [Q] **(also known as thromboplastin or factor III),** membrane-bound lipoprotein expressed at sites of injury

Intrinsic pathway [Q]

- Clotting is initiated with addition of **negative charged particles (e.g., ground glass)** [Q] which activates **factor XII (Hageman factor)** [Q]

Also Remember:

- To assess the **coagulation pathway** two standard assays required are: **Prothrombin time (PT)** [Q] and **partial thromboplastin time (PTT)** [Q]
- **PT assay** assess the function of proteins in the **extrinsic pathway (factors VII, X, II, V and fibrinogen)** [Q]
- **Partial thromboplastin time (PTT) assay** assess the function of proteins in the **intrinsic pathway (factors XII, XI, IX, VIII, X, V, II and fibrinogen)**

Ans. 10) C. Factor V (Ref: 8 ed. Robbins p. 120, 9 ed. p. 120-21, f-4-8-10)

Endogenous anticoagulants:

A) Anti-thrombin (e.g. anti-thrombin III):

- Inhibit the activity of thrombin and other factors IXa, Xa, XIa and XIIa
- **Anti-thrombin III is activated** by binding to **heparin-like molecules on endothelial cells,** which signifies the administration of heparin to **minimize thrombosis**

B) Proteins C and S:

- **Vitamin K–dependent** [Q] proteins that **inactivates factors Va and VIIIa**

C) Tissue factor pathway inhibitor (TFPI):

- Protein produced by the **endothelium** that inactivates **tissue factor–factor VIIa complexes** [Q]

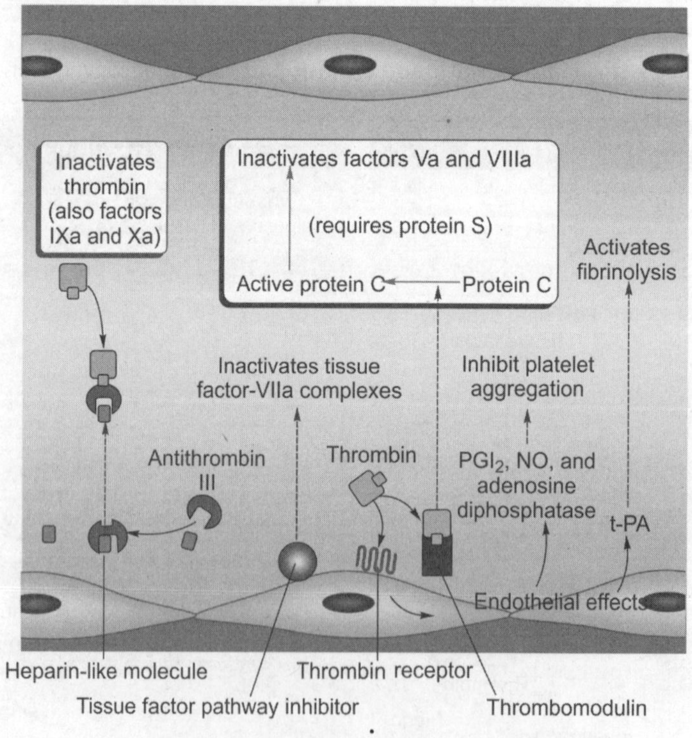

Anticoagulant activities of normal endothelium

Ans. 11) B. Laminar blood flow (Ref: 8 ed. Robbins p.121-25, 9 ed. p.122-23, f-4-12, t-4-2)

Virchow's triad [Q]**:**

Three primary abnormalities that lead to **thrombus formation:**

- Endothelial injury
- Stasis or turbulent blood flow
- Hypercoagulability of the blood

A) Endothelial dysfunction:

Causes – Hypertension, turbulent blood flow, bacterial endotoxins, radiation injury, homocystinemia or hypercholesterolemia, cigarette smoke

B) Alteration in Normal Blood Flow:

- Normal blood flow is **laminar** [Q]
- **Turbulent blood flow** leads to arterial and cardiac thrombosis by causing endothelial injury or dysfunction
- **Stasis** is a major contributor in the development of venous thrombi

C) Hypercoagulability:

Inherited (genetic) causes:

- **Factor V gene** mutation (called as ***Leiden*** **mutation)** [Q]
- **Prothrombin gene** mutation
- **Elevated levels** of **homocysteine** [Q] contribute to arterial and venous thrombosis
- **Anti-thrombin III, Protein C or Proteins S** [Q] **deficiency**

Acquired causes:

- Prolonged bed rest or immobilization, Myocardial infarction, Atrial fibrillation
- Tissue injury (surgery, fracture and burn), Cancer, Prosthetic cardiac valves
- Disseminated intravascular coagulation, Heparin-induced thrombocytopenia
- Anti-phospholipid antibody syndrome

Ans. 12) B. Increases risk of bleeding (Ref: 8 ed. Robbins p. 123, 9 ed. p. 124)

Heparin-induced thrombocytopenia (HIT) syndrome:

- Occurs following the administration of **unfractionated heparin** [Q]
- **Unfractionated heparin** induces the formation of antibodies against complexes of **heparin and platelet factor 4** [Q]
- Binding of antibodies to platelets results in **thrombocytopenia**
- This leads to **prothrombotic state,** even in face of heparin administration low platelet counts
- **Low-molecular weight heparin** [Q] preparations are at **lower risk** to induce antibody formation
- Other anticoagulants such as **fondaparinux** [Q] **(inhibitor of factor X** [Q]**)** rarely cause HIT-like syndrome

Ans. 13) C. Individuals with autoimmune diseases are designated as primary APAS (Ref: 8 ed. Robbins p. 123-24, 9 ed. p. 124-25)

Antiphospholipid antibody syndrome (lupus anticoagulant syndrome):

- Present with **recurrent thrombosis, repeated miscarriages, cardiac valve vegetations** and **thrombocytopenia**
- **Fetal loss** occurs due to antibody-mediated inhibition of **tissue Plasminogen activator (t-PA)** [Q], that helps in **trophoblastic invasion** of the uterus
- **Antibodies** frequently give a **false-positive serologic test for syphilis** [Q] as the antigen in the standard assay is embedded in **cardiolipin**
- **Two types:**

A) Primary antiphospholipid syndrome – Presence of a hypercoagulable state without any evidence of other autoimmune disorders

B) **Secondary Antiphospholipid syndrome (lupus anticoagulant syndrome)** [Q] – Individuals have a well-defined autoimmune disease, such as **SLE**

Ans. 14) **A. Lines of Zahn (Ref: 8 ed. Robbins p. 123-24, 9 ed. p. 125, f-4-13)**

Ante mortem thrombi [Q]**:**

- Shows **Lines of Zahn**[Q], which represent pale platelet and fibrin deposits alternating with darker **red cell–rich layers**
- Lines of Zahn signify that the thrombus has formed in the **flowing blood**
- Are **firm** and **focally attached** [Q]

Postmortem clots [Q]**:**

- Are **gelatinous** [Q] with **dark red portion** where red cells have settled by gravity and a **yellow "chicken fat" upper portion** [Q]
- Are **not attached** to the underlying wall

Ans. 15) **D. Fat micro globules are easily demonstrated on paraffin embedding sections (Ref: 8 ed. Robbins p. 126-27, 9 ed. p. 128, f-4-16)**

Fat embolism:

- Occurs in 90% of individuals with **severe skeletal injuries**

Fat embolism syndrome:

- Symptomatic patients of fat embolism
- Characterized by **pulmonary insufficiency, neurologic symptoms, anemia and thrombocytopenia**
- Fatal in about 5% to 15% of cases

Clinical features:

- Sudden onset of **tachypnea, dyspnea** and **tachycardia;** irritability and restlessness, 1 to 3 days after injury
- **Diffuse petechial rash** [Q] due to rapid onset of thrombocytopenia is a diagnostic clue

Lab findings:

- **Thrombocytopenia** – due to the platelet adhesion to fat globules
- Anemia can result from **red cell aggregation and/or hemolysis**
- **Frozen sections** and **stains for fat** are **special techniques** to diagnose as **lipids**
- **Paraffin embedding** cannot diagnose **fat** as they are **dissolved out** of the tissue preparations by the **solvents**

Ans. 16) **C. Caisson disease is an acute form of decompression sickness (Ref: 8 ed. Robbins p. 127, 9 ed. 128-29)**

Air embolism [Q]**:**

- **>100 cc** [Q] of air is required to have a clinical effect in the pulmonary circulation

Causes:

- During bypass surgery
- Introduced into the **cerebral circulation** by neurosurgery in the "sitting position"
- During obstetric or laparoscopic procedures
- As a consequence of chest wall injury

Decompression sickness [Q]**:**

- When individuals experience sudden decreases in atmospheric pressure
- Seen in **scuba** and **deep sea divers,** underwater construction workers and individuals in unpressurized aircraft in rapid ascent
- During deep sea dive, when air is breathed at high pressure, increased amounts of gas **(nitrogen)** are dissolved in the blood and tissues
- When the driver ascends **(depressurizes) too rapidly,** nitrogen comes out of solution in the tissues and the blood

Caisson disease [Q]:

- **Chronic form** [Q] of **decompression sickness**
- **Ischemic necrosis** – Seen in **femoral heads, tibia and humeri** due to persistence of gas emboli in the skeletal system

Ans. 17) **D. Lung (Ref: 8 ed. Robbins p. 127-28, 9 ed. p. 129-30, f-4-18)**

White (anemic) infarcts:

- Occurs due to **arterial occlusions** [Q] in **solid organs** with **end arterial circulation** [Q] (e.g., **heart, spleen and kidney)** [Q]

Red (hemorrhagic) infarcts:

- Occurs with venous occlusions (e.g. **ovary)**[Q], in loose tissues (e.g., **lung**)[Q], in tissues with **dual circulations** [Q] (e.g. **lung and small intestine)**
- When the flow is re-established to a site of **previous arterial occlusion** and **necrosis** (e.g., following **angioplasty** of an **arterial obstruction**)

Ans. 18) **B. Liquefactive necrosis is the dominant histologic feature (Ref: 8 ed. Robbins p. 128-9, 9 ed. p. 129-131)**

Infarcts:

- Are **wedge-shaped**
- Results from **arterial occlusions in organs** without a dual blood supply
- In the lung, **hemorrhagic infarcts** are the **rule**
- Dominant histology of infarction is **ischemic coagulative necrosis** [Q] except in **central nervous system infarction, which results in liquefactive necrosis** [Q]
- Most of the infarcts are ultimately replaced by **scar**

Note:

- **Neurons** [Q] **and myocardial cells** [Q] undergo **irreversible damage** when their blood supply is deprived of for **3 to 4 minutes** [Q] and **20 to 30 minutes** [Q], respectively

Hence the answer here is **'B'** as ischemic **coagulative necrosis** is seen in most of infarcts

Ans. 19) **C. Failure of myocardial pump resulting from intrinsic myocardial damage (Ref: 8 ed. Robbins p. 129-33, 9 ed. p. 131-34, f- 4-20, t-4-3)**

Classification of Shock:

Cardiogenic shock [Q]

- Results from **low cardiac output** due to **myocardial pump failure**
- Occurs due to **infarction, ventricular arrhythmias, cardiac tamponade** and pulmonary embolism

Hypovolemic shock [Q]

- Results from **low cardiac output,** due to loss of blood or plasma volume
- Due to **massive hemorrhage or fluid loss** from **severe burns**

Septic shock [Q]

- **Results from vasodilation and peripheral pooling of blood**
- **Causes** – Systemic response to bacterial or fungal infections, **endothelial activation/injury, disseminated intravascular coagulation** [Q]

Neurogenic shock [Q]

- Can occur during anesthetic accident or a spinal cord injury

Anaphylactic shock [Q]

- Due to **systemic vasodilation and increased vascular permeability**
- **IgE–mediated hypersensitivity reaction**

Important Points to Remember About Shock:

- Shock affects predominantly **brain, heart, lungs, kidneys, adrenals and gastrointestinal tract**

- **Adrenal changes** [Q] in shock: **Cortical cell lipid depletion** [Q]
- **Kidneys** exhibit **acute tubular necrosis** [Q]
- **Diffuse alveolar damage/ shock lung** may develop, when shock is caused by **bacterial sepsis** or **trauma**

DIC In Septic Shock:

- Develops due to widespread deposition of **fibrin-rich micro thrombi** [Q]
- Can affect brain, heart, lungs, kidney, adrenal glands and gastrointestinal tract
- Consumption of platelets and coagulation factors leads to the appearance of **petechial hemorrhages** [Q]

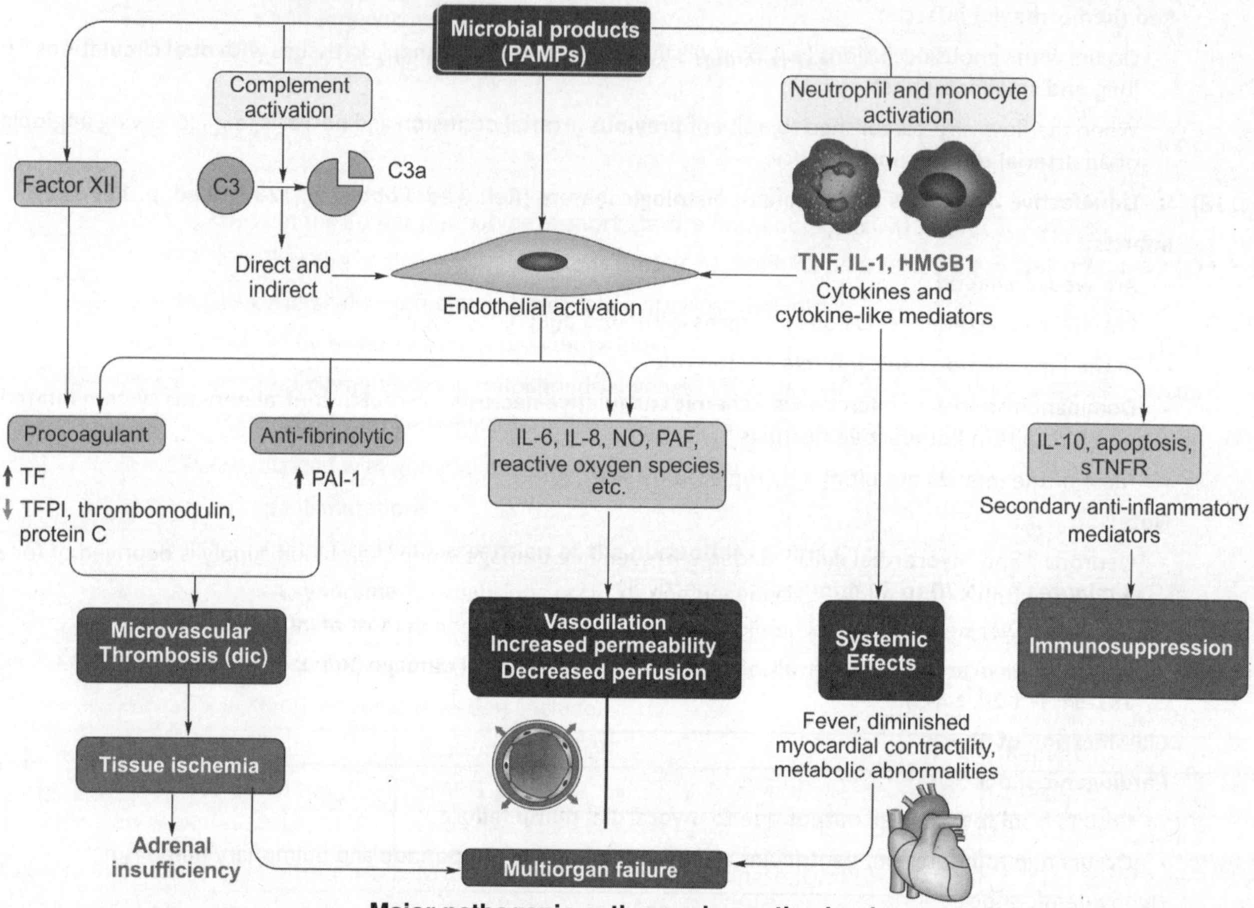

Major pathogenic pathways in septic shock

Ans. 20) **C. Hypercalcemia (Ref: 9th ed. Robbins p. 128) Refer Q 15 for details**

Ans. 21) **C. Liver (Ref: 9 ed. Robbins p. 129-30) Refer Q 17 for details**

Ans. 22) **A. Edema (Ref: 9 ed. Robbins p. 113)**

Edema: Accumulation of fluid in the interstitial space

Ans. 23) **D. Ang I (Ref: 9 ed. Robbins p. 104)**

Angiopoietins 1 and 2 (Ang 1 and Ang 2) are growth factors that play a role in angiogenesis and the structural maturation of new vessels

Ans. 24) **A Coagulative necrosis (Ref: 9 ed Robbins p. 130)**

Ans. 25) **B. Vasoconstriction (Ref: 9 ed. Robbins p. 116-17) Refer Q 4 for details**

Ans. 26) **A. Right sided heart failure (Ref: 9 ed. Robbins p. 115-16) Refer Q 2 for details**

Ans. 27) **B. Neurons (Ref: 9 ed. Robbins p. 129-131) Refer Q 18 for details**

Ans. 28) **D. Antemortem thrombus (Ref: 9ed. Robbins p. 125) Refer Q 14 for details**

Ans. 29) **B. Extrinsic pathway is activated by contact with plasma and negatively charged proteins (Ref: 9 ed. Robbins p. 118-20) Refer Q 9 for details**

5 Genetics

How to go about this chapter?

- **One should be thorough with the following topics:**
  - **Mutations and diseases associated with them**
  - **Mendelian disorders**
  - **Autosomal dominant and recessive disorders**
  - **X-linked disorders**
  - **Lysosomal storage disorders**
  - **Hyperlipidemias**
  - **Chromosomal disorders**
  - **Single gene disorders with non-classical disorders**
  - **Recent advances in molecular genetic diagnosis**

GENES AND HUMAN DISEASES

1) Proteomics is:
a) Study of all DNA sequences
b) Measurement of all proteins in a cell or tissue
c) Computer based techniques that can manage vast collections of data
d) None of the above

MENDELIAN DISORDERS

2) Sickle cell anemia occurs due to the following mutation:
a) Glutamic acid to valine
b) Valine to glutamic acid
c) Any of the above
d) None of the above

3) Co-dominance is seen in:
a) Histocompatibility
b) Pleotropism
c) Genetic hetrogenity
d) Sickle cell anemia

4) All are TRUE about Autosomal Dominant disorders EXCEPT:
a) Manifested in a heterozygous state
b) Both males and females are affected
c) Few proportion of patients do not have affected parents
d) Gain of function mutations affecting regulatory proteins is more common

5) All are autosomal dominant disorders EXCEPT:
a) Marfan syndrome
b) Hereditary spherocytosis
c) Acute intermittent porphyria
d) Cystic fibrosis

6) All are TRUE about autosomal recessive disorders EXCEPT:
a) Occurs only when both alleles at a given gene locus are mutated
b) Trait does not usually affect the parents of the affected individual
c) Incomplete penetrance is common
d) Onset is frequently early in life

7) All are TRUE about X-linked disorders EXCEPT:
a) All sex linked disorders are X-linked, and almost all recessive
b) An affected male can transmit the disease to his son
c) Heterozygous female usually does not express the full phenotypic change
d) An illustrative example is G-6PD deficiency

8) Tay-Sachs disease occurs due to following enzyme deficiency:
a) Hexosaminidase
b) Adenosine deaminase
c) Phenylalanine hydroxylase
d) α1-Antitrypsin

9) All are TRUE about Marfan Syndrome EXCEPT:
a) Autosomal dominant disorder, 70-85% cases are familial

b) Myofibrils are abundant in aorta, ligaments and ciliary zonules
c) FBN-2 mutations are most common
d) Loss of microfibrils leads to activation of TGF-β

10) Most frequent cause of death in Marfan syndrome is:
a) Mitral valve prolapse
b) Aortic dissection
c) Mitral regurgitation
d) Cardiac failure

11) Disorder(s) resulting from mutation affecting collagen synthesis include:
a) Ehler-Danlos syndrome
b) Osteogenesis imperfecta
c) Alport syndrome
d) All of the above

12) Class II LDL receptor mutation results in failure of the following:
a) Synthesis of LDL receptor
b) Transport of LDL receptor
c) Binding of the LDL receptor
d) Clustering of LDL receptor

13) Molecular chaperon therapy can be helpful for which Lysosomal storage disorder:
a) Tay-Sachs disease
b) Metachromatic leucodystrophy
c) Krabbe disease
d) Fabry disease

14) All are TRUE about Tay-Sachs disease EXCEPT:
a) Is a G_{M1} gangliosidosis
b) Is due to Hexosaminidase A deficiency
c) Affects neurons and retina
d) On EM, there is a whorled configuration within the lysosomes

15) All are TRUE about Niemann-Pick disease EXCEPT:
a) Type A is the most common type
b) Occurs due to deficiency of sphingomyelinase
c) Type A involves the neurons and has worse prognosis
d) Type B have organomegaly but no CNS involvement

16) All are TRUE for Niemann-Pick disease EXCEPT:
a) An example of epigenetic silencing (paternal gene is silenced)
b) EM shows concentric lamellated myelin figures/ zebra bodies
c) EM shows onion skin layers of membranes
d) Massive enlargement of spleen is seen

17) All are TRUE about Gaucher disease EXCEPT:
a) Most common form of Lysosomal storage disorder
b) Occurs due to glucocerebrosidase deficiency
c) Type I–non-neuronopathic disease
d) Macrophages and cytokines don't play a role in pathogenesis

18) TRUE about Gaucher disease is/are:
a) Type II has a good prognosis
b) Gaucher cells have a vacuolated cytoplasm
c) Gaucher cells have a fibrillary cytoplasm which on EM shows stacks of bilayers due to stored lipids
d) Gaucher cells are seen in Robin-Virchow spaces in cerebrum
e) Both C and D

19) Replacement therapy with recombinant enzymes is a mainstay of therapy in:
a) Niemann-Pick disease
b) Gaucher disease
c) Tay-Sach's disease
d) Sandhoff disease

20) Glycosaminoglycan that accumulate in Mucopolysaccharidoses (MPS's):
a) Dermatan sulfate
b) Heparin sulfate
c) Chondroitin sulfate
d) All of the above

21) All are TRUE about Mucopolysaccharidoses EXCEPT:
a) Hurler's syndrome is due to deficiency of α–L-iduronidase
b) Coarse facial features, clouding of cornea, joint stiffness, mental retardation are seen
c) Cardiac complications are the most common cause of death in Hurler's syndrome
d) All MPS's are autosomal recessive disorders except Hurler's syndrome

22) All are TRUE about Von-Gierke's disease EXCEPT:
a) Due to deficiency of glucose 6-phosphatase
b) Also called as Type I glycogenosis
c) Hepatomegaly and renomegaly are commonly seen
d) Hyperglycemia is a common association

23) Mc-Ardle syndrome is due to deficiency of:
a) Glucose 6-phosphatase
b) Muscle phosphorylase
c) Branching enzyme
d) De-branching enzyme

24) All are TRUE about Pompe's disease EXCEPT:
a) Glycogen storage disorder
b) Acid maltase is the deficient enzyme
c) Also called as Type I glycogenosis
d) Cardiac complications leads to early death

25) All are TRUE about Alkaptonuria EXCEPT:
a) Due to deficiency of homogentisic acid oxidase
b) Methylacetoacetic acid deposits in the tissues
c) Ochronosis is most serious complication
d) Intervertebral disc is the most common site affected in vertebral column
e) Small joints of hand and feet are spared

26) **A couple with a family history of beta thalassemia major in a distant relative has come for counseling. The husband has HbA_2 of 4.5% and the wife has HbA_2 of 2.1%. The risk of having a child with beta thalassemia major is:**
a) 50% b) 25%
c) 5% d) 0%

27) **TRUE statement about inheritance of X-linked recessive trait is:**
a) 50% of boys of carrier mother are affected
b) 50% of girls of diseased father are carrier
c) Father transmits the disease to son
d) Mother transmits the disease to daughter

CHROMOSOMAL DISORDERS

28) **All are TRUE about Karyotyping EXCEPT:**
a) Dividing cells are arrested in metaphase
b) G-banding is most common staining method
c) After staining chromosomes are analyzed under a microscope and photographed
d) Chromosomes are arranged in pairs and in increasing order of length

29) **Down syndrome is caused by:**
a) Maternal non-disjunction
b) Paternal non-disjunction
c) Translocation
d) Mosaicism

30) **Down syndrome is associated with:**
a) Congenital heart disease
b) Acute leukemia
c) Early onset Alzheimer's disease
d) All of the above

31) **Velocardiofacial abnormality is characterized by all of the following EXCEPT:**
a) Also known as DiGeorge syndrome/22q11.2 deletion syndrome
b) Associated with resultant T-cell immunodeficiency
c) Associated with parathyroid hyperplasia
d) Can be diagnosed by FISH

32) **Chromosomal analysis reveals 47, XYY karyotype. Which of the following description best fits this abnormality?**
a) Autosomal trisomy
b) Sex chromosomal aneuploidy
c) A female with Turner's syndrome
d) Sex chromosomal triploidy

33) **All are TRUE about Turner syndrome EXCEPT:**
a) 45 X karyotype
b) Phonotypical females are affected
c) Mental retardation is commonly seen
d) SHOX gene abnormality is noted

SINGLE-GENE DISORDERS WITH NON-CLASSIC INHERITANCE

34) **All are TRUE about Fragile X syndrome EXCEPT:**
a) Due to triple nucleotide repeat mutation at Xq27.3
b) CGG repeats located FMR 1 gene
c) CGG expansions occur during oogenesis
d) Expansions affect the coding region i.e. exons

35) **Two siblings with Osteogenesis imperfecta, but their parents are normal, mechanism of inheritance is explained by:**
a) Anticipation
b) Genoming imprinting
c) Germ line mosaicism
d) New mutation

MOLECULAR GENETICS IN DIAGNOSTIC PATHOLOGY

36) **All are TRUE about Array CGH EXCEPT:**
a) Used for known genetic loci
b) Both duplication and deletion can be studied
c) Can detect multiple abnormalities at the same time
d) Uses array hybridization technology

37) **Known gene loci is diagnosed by:**
a) FISH
b) Comparative gene hybridization
c) PCR
d) Chromosomal painting

38) **Resolution of light microscope for viewing chromosome:**
a) 5 kb b) 500 kb
c) 5 mb d) 50 mb

39) **Real time polymerase chain reaction is done for:**
a) DNA detection only
b) RNA detection only
c) Both RNA and DNA detection
d) Monitoring amplification of target nucleic acid

40) **Karyotyping is done in which phase of cell cycle?**
a) Anaphase b) Metaphase
c) Telophase d) S phase

41) **Microarray is:**
a) Study of multiple genes
b) Study of diseases
c) Study of organisms
d) Study of blood group

42) **Which of the following procedures is routine technique for karyotyping using light microscopy?**
a) C-banding b) G-banding
c) Q-banding d) Brd V-staining

43) Karyotyping is useful in diagnosis of:
a) Autosomal recessive disorders
b) X-linked recessive disorders
c) Chromosomal abnormalities
d) Biochemical abnormalities

44) In-situ DNA nick end labeling can quantitate:
a) Fraction of cells in apoptotic pathways
b) Fraction of cells in S-phase
c) p53 gene produce
d) bcr/abl gene

45) Gene or protein deficient in Marfan syndrome: (NEET 2014)
a) Fibrillin I b) Fibrillin II
c) Collagen d) Elastin

46) Neurofibromatosis shows which of the following mode of inheritance? (NEET 2014)
a) AD
b) AR
c) X-linked dominant
d) X-linked recessive

47) Following statement is true for hemophilia patients: (NEET 2014)
a) All females are carriers and all males are affected
b) All males are carriers and all females are affected
c) Females are mostly carriers and all males are affected
d) Males are mostly carriers and all females are affected

48) Barr body is absent in: (NEET 2014)
a) Klinefelter
b) Turner
c) Super female
d) None of the above

49) Ring chromosome is a result of: (NEET 2014)
a) Deletion b) Inversion
c) Duplication d) Translocation

50) SRY gene is located on: (NEET 2014)
a) Short arm of X chromosome
b) Long arm of X chromosome
c) Short arm of Y chromosome
d) Long arm of Y chromosome

51) Boys are more likely to be affected by which? (NEET 2014)
a) AD
b) AR
c) X-linked dominant
d) X-linked recessive

52) Phenylketonuria is: (NEET 2014)
a) AD
b) AR
c) X-linked dominant
d) X-linked recessive

53) Decreased T cell immunity is a feature of: (NEET 2014)
a) Di George syndrome
b) Hyper IgM syndrome
c) Severe congenital neutropenia
d) Chronic granulomatous disease

54) Which of the following is not a feature of Down's syndrome? (NEET 2014)
a) Clinodactyly
b) Pigmented birth marks
c) Hypotonia
d) Respiratory tract infections

55) Following are TRUE about Turners syndrome EXCEPT: (NEET 2014)
a) External genitilia are normal
b) Biscuspid aortic valve
c) Swelling of nape of neck
d) Short stature

56) Decreased T cell immunity is a feature of: (NEET 2014)
a) Di George syndrome
b) Hyper IgM syndrome
c) Severe congenital neutropenia
d) Chronic granulomatous disease

57) Which of the following is not a feature of Down's syndrome? (NEET 2014)
a) Clinodactyly
b) Pigmented birth marks
c) Hypotonia
d) Respiratory tract infections

58) One of the following disorders is due to maternal disomy:
a) Prader-Willi syndrome
b) Angelman syndrome
c) Hydatidiform mole
d) Klinefelter syndrome

59) Mitochondrial chromosomal abnormality leads to: (NEET 2013)
a) Lebers hereditary optic neuropathy
b) Angelman syndrome
c) Prader-Willi syndrome
d) Myotonic dystrophy

60) Duchenne muscular dystrophy is inherited as: (NEET 2013)
a) X-linked
b) Autosomal dominant
c) Autosomal recessive
d) Co-dominant

61) True statement about inheritance of an X-linked recessive trait is: (NEET 2013)
a) 50% of boys of carrier mother are affected
b) 50% of girls of diseased father are carrier
c) Father transmits disease to the son
d) Mother transmits the disease to the daughter

62) Genomic imprinting is seen in: (NEET 2013)
a) Klinefelter syndrome
b) Down's syndrome
c) Angelman syndrome
d) Hydatidiform mole

63) Cystic medical necrosis is seen in: (NEET 2013)
a) Marfan
b) Friedreich ataxia
c) Downs
d) Kawasaki

64) Pataus syndrome due to: (NEET 2013)
a) Trisomy 21 b) Trisomy 18
c) 18p deletion d) Trisomy 13

65) Klinefelter no of chromosomes: (NEET 2013)
a) 47 b) 46
c) 45 d) 44

66) Microarray is: (NEET 2013)
a) Study of multiple genes
b) Study of disease
c) Study of organisms
d) Study of blood group

67) Thymic hypoplasia is seen in: (NEET 2013)
a) Wiskott-Aldrich syndrome
b) DiGeorge syndrome
c) IgA deficiency
d) Agammaglobulinemia

68) Inheritance of Huntington's chorea: (NEET 2013)
a) AD b) AR
c) XR d) XD

69) Karyotyping is done in which phase of cell cycle? (NEET 2013)
a) Anaphase b) Metaphase
c) Telophase d) S phase

70) Centrosome duplication takes place in: (NEET 2013)
a) M phase b) GO phase
c) S phase d) G2 phase

71) Male to male transmission is seen in: (NEET 2013)
a) Autosomal dominant diseases
b) Autosomal recessive
c) X-linked dominant
d) Mitochondrial disease

72) Female is affected, male is not. Disease is autosomal dominant, what is the chance in children? (NEET 2013)
a) 50% affected b) 25% affected
c) 75% affected d) All affected

73) Number of chromosomes in Turner syndrome: (NEET 2013)
a) 45 b) 46
c) 45 d) 42

74) Number of chromosomes in Klinefelter syndrome: (NEET 2013)
a) 47 b) 46
c) 45 d) 44

75) Down's syndrome is most commonly caused by: (AIPGMEE 2010)
a) Maternal non-disjunction
b) Paternal non-disjunction
c) Translocation
d) Mosaicism

76) Cystic fibrosis is inherited as an autosomal recessive condition. A normal couple has one daughter affected with the disease. They are now planning to have another child. What is the chance of her sibling being affected by the disease? (AIPGMEE 2010)
a) 0 b) ½
c) ¼ d) ¾

77) Males are more commonly affected than females in: (AIPGMEE 2010)
a) Autosomal dominant
b) Autosomal recessive
c) X-linked dominant
d) X-linked recessive

78) If a chromosome divides in an axis perpendicular to usual axis of division it is going to form: (AIIMS May 2013)
a) Ring chromosome
b) Isochromosome
c) Acrocentric
d) Sub-telocentric

79) What is used for diagnosis of fragment of chromosomes? (AIIMS May 2013)
a) FISH b) CGH
c) PCR d) RFLP

80) A man has hepatosplenomegaly with pancytopenia. On biopsy of liver large cells are seen with a crumpled tissue paper appearance of nuclei. Which of the following may be deficient in this patient? (AIIMS May 2013)
a) Glucocerebrosidase
b) Sphingomyelinase
c) L-Iduronase
d) Hexosaminidase

81) Inheritance of blood groups AB: (AIIMS May 2015)
a) Co-dominance b) Dominant
c) Recessive d) None

82) The phenomenon where subsequent generations are at risk of earlier and more severe disease is known as: (AIIMS May 2015)
a) Genetic anticipation
b) Dominance
c) Pleiotropy
d) Dominance

83) Resolution of chromosomes in karyotyping is: (AIIMS Nov 2013)

a) 5 Kb
b) 500 Kb
c) 5 mb
d) 50 mb

84) Cancers are usually associated with: (AIIMS Nov 2014)

a) Loss of heterozygosity
b) Hypo-methylation of oncogenes
c) Hyper-methylation of tumor suppression genes
d) Mutation in introns

85) An Afro-American boy of 6 years of age presented with abdominal pain, chronic hemolysis and abnormal RBC shape on peripheral smear. Most likely disorder responsible for this condition: (AIIMS Nov 2014)

a) Tri-nucleotide repeats
b) Point mutation
c) Antibodies against RBC membrane
d) Genetic imprinting

86) Identify the disease shown in the karyotype: (AIIMS Nov 2014)

a) Bloom syndrome
b) Cri-du-chat syndrome
c) Prader-Willi syndrome
d) Down's syndrome

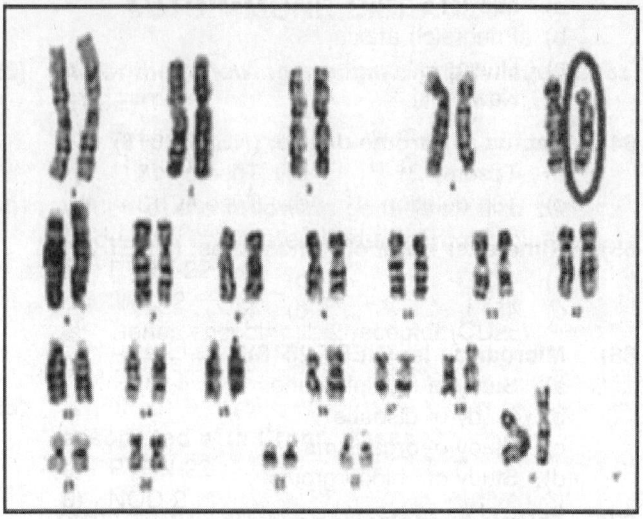

CHAPTER 5: GENETICS

Ans. 1) **B. Measurement of all proteins in a cell or tissue (Ref: 8 ed. Robbins p.136-37)**

- **Genetics** ^{Q} – Study of single or few genes and their phenotypic effects
- **Genomics** ^{Q} **– Study of all the genes** in the genome and their interactions
- **Proteomics** ^{Q} **– Measurement of all proteins** expressed in a cell or tissue
- **Bioinformatics** ^{Q} – Can manage **vast collections** of data, including expression of involving **thousand of genes** and **proteins**

Ans. 2) **A. Glutamic acid to valine (Ref: 8 ed. Robbins p.138-39, 9 ed. p. 140)**

Point mutation – Alter the **code** in a **triplet of bases** and lead to the replacement of one amino acid by another

A) Missense mutations ^{Q}:

- Alter the meaning of the sequence of the **encoded protein**
- **Example – Sickle cell mutation** affecting **β-globin chain** of hemoglobin
- **In sickle cell anemia,** nucleotide triplet **CTC (or GAG in mRNA)**, which encodes **glutamic acid** ^{Q}, is changed to **CAC (or GUG in mRNA)**, which encodes **valine** ^{Q}

B) Nonsense mutation:

- **Point mutation** may change an **amino acid codon** to a **stop codon e.g. UAG**
- **E.g.** β^{0} **– thalassemia** ^{Q} – There is **premature termination** of **β-globin gene translation**

Ans. 3) **A. Histocompatibility (Ref: 8 ed. Robbins p.140, 9 ed. p. 140)**

Co-dominance ^{Q}:

- When both alleles of a gene pair contribute to the phenotype
- Examples – **Histocompatibility** ^{Q} **and blood group antigens** ^{Q}

Pleiotropism ^{Q}:

- If a single **mutant gene** may lead to many end effects
- **Example – Sickle cell anemia** ^{Q} **– Point mutation** in the gene can give rise to **HbS**, which predisposes **red cells to hemolysis** ^{Q}
- In **sickle cell anemia,** abnormal red cells occlude lumen of small vessels, leading to splenic fibrosis, **organ infarcts** and bone changes

Genetic Heterogeneity ^{Q}:

- Mutations at several genetic loci may produce the same trait
- Examples – **Diabetes mellitus** and **profound childhood deafness**

Ans. 4) **D. Gain of function mutations affecting regulatory proteins is more common (Ref: 8 ed. Robbins p.140-41, 9 ed. p. 140-41, t-5-1)**

Autosomal Dominant (AD) Disorders:

- Manifested in a **heterozygous state** ^{Q}, so at least one parent is affected
- Both **males and females are affected** ^{Q} and both can transmit the condition
- When an affected person marries an unaffected one, every child has **one chance in two** ^{Q} of having the disease
- ***Incomplete penetrance*** ^{Q} – In which few individuals inherit the mutant gene but are phenotypically normal
- **Mutation,** when leads to reduced production of a gene product is called as **loss-of-function mutations** ^{Q}
- Less commonly, **gain-of-function mutations** ^{Q} can be seen, e.g. in **Huntington disease** ^{Q}

Ans. 5) **D. Cystic fibrosis (Ref: 8 ed. Robbins p.141-42, t-5-1, 9 ed. p. 140-41, t-5-1)**

Autosomal dominant disorders include:

System	Disorder
Nervous system	Huntington disease, Neurofibromatosis, Myotonic dystrophy, Tuberous sclerosis
Urinary system	Polycystic kidney disease
Gastrointestinal system	Familial polyposis coli
Hematopoietic system	Hereditary spherocytosis, von Willebrand disease
Skeletal system	Marfan syndrome, Ehlers-Danlos syndrome, Osteogenesis imperfecta, Achondroplasia
Metabolic causes	Familial hypercholesterolemia, acute intermittent porphyria

Note:

- **Cystic fibrosis** is an **autosomal recessive** Q **(AR) disorder**

Make a pneumonic, which you can reproduce at time of exams!!

Ans. 6) **C. Incomplete penetrance is common (Ref: 8 ed. Robbins p.141-42, 9 ed. p. 141, t-5-2)**

Autosomal Recessive (AR) Disorders:

- Results when both alleles at a **given gene locus** are **mutated**
- The parents **may not be affected**, but **siblings** can show the disease
- Risk of sibling being affected is **one chance in four** Q (the recurrence risk is **25%** for each birth)
- **Consanguineous marriage** increases the risk

Following features distinguish **AR** disorders from **AD** diseases:

- Uniform expression of the defect in **AR disorders**
- **Complete penetrance** Q is common
- Onset is frequently early in life
- **AR disorders** includes **inborn errors of metabolism**

Examples of **AR disorders** include:

System	Disorder
Metabolic causes	Cystic fibrosis, Phenylketonuria, Galactosemia, Homocystinuria, Lysosomal storage diseases, α1-Antitrypsin deficiency, Wilson disease, Hemochromatosis, Glycogen storage diseases
Hematopoietic causes	Sickle cell anemia, Thalassemia
Endocrine causes	Congenital adrenal hyperplasia
Skeletal causes	Ehlers-Danlos syndrome, Alkaptonuria
Nervous system	Neurogenic muscular atrophies, Friedreich ataxia, Spinal muscular atrophy

Make a pneumonic, which you can reproduce at time of exams!!

Ans. 7) **B. An affected male can transmit the disease to his son (Ref: 8 ed. Robbins p.142, 9 ed. p. 142, t-5-3)**

X-linked disorders: (mostly recessive)

- **Affected male does not** transmit the disorder to his **sons** Q
- All **daughters** are **carriers** Q
- Because of a "**paired normal allele**" heterozygous female **does not** express the full phenotypic change

Examples of **X-linked recessive** disorders include:

System	Disease
Musculoskeletal	Duchenne muscular dystrophy
Hematological	Hemophilia A and B, Chronic granulomatous disease, Glucose-6-phosphate dehydrogenase deficiency

Immunological	Agammaglobulinemia, Wiskott-Aldrich syndrome
Metabolic	Diabetes insipidus, Lesch-Nyhan syndrome
CNS	Fragile-X syndrome

Note:

Vitamin D - resistant rickets is an example of **X-linked dominant disorder** Q

Ans. 8) A. **Hexosaminidase (Ref: 8 ed. Robbins p.142, 9 ed. p. 151-52, f-5-11, t-5-6)**

- **Phenylalanine hydroxylase deficiency** leads to **Phenylketonuria** Q
- **Hexosaminidase deficiency** leads to **Tay-Sachs disease** Q
- **Adenosine deaminase** deficiency leads to **Severe combined immunodeficiency** Q
- **α1-Antitrypsin deficiency** leads to **Emphysema** Q and liver disease

Lysosomal Storage Diseases

Disease	**Enzyme Deficiency**	**Major Accumulating Metabolites**
Glycogenosis	Type 2—Pompe disease α-1,4-Glucosidase (lysosomal glucosidase)	Glycogen
Sphingolipidoses		
GM1 gangliosidosis Type 1—infantile, generalized Type 2—juvenile	β-galactosidase	GM1 ganglioside, galactose-containing oligosaccharides
GM2 gangliosidosis Tay-Sachs disease Sandhoff disease	 Hexosaminidase, α subunit Hexosaminidase, β subunit	 GM2 ganglioside GM2 ganglioside
Sulfatidoses		
Metachromatic leukodystrophy	Arylsulfatase A	Sulfatide
Krabbe disease	Galactosylceramidase	Galactocerebroside
Fabry disease	α-Galactosidase A	Ceramide trihexoside
Gaucher disease	Glucocerebrosidase	Glucocerebroside
Niemann-Pick disease: types A and B	Sphingomyelinase	Sphingomyelin
Mucopolysaccharidoses (MPSs)		
MPS I H (Hurler)	α-L-Iduronidase	Dermatan sulfate, heparan sulfate
MPS II (Hunter)	L-Iduronosulfate sulfatase	Dermatan sulfate, heparan sulfate
Wolman disease	**Acid lipase**	Cholesterol esters, triglycerides

Ans. 9) C. **FBN-2 mutations are most common (Ref: 8 ed. Robbins p. 144-45, 9 ed. p. 144-45)**

Marfan syndrome:

- **Autosomal Dominant** Q inheritance
- **Skeleton, eyes and cardiovascular system** are most commonly affected
- Due to **fibrillin-1** mutation, encoded by **FBN1 gene** mapped on chromosome 15q
- **FBN2 gene** Q **mutations** can give rise to **congenital contractual arachnodactyly**

- **Fibrillin** – Major component of **microfibrils**, which is abundant in **aorta, ligaments and ciliary zonules** that support the lens

Points to remember:

- **Ocular changes** [Q] – **Most characteristic** is **bilateral subluxation** [Q] or **dislocation** (usually **outward and upward**)[Q] of the lens, referred to as **ectopia lentis**
- **Cardiovascular lesions** [Q] – **Mitral valve prolapse** [Q], **aortic incompetence** (**cystic medionecrosis** [Q] leading to dilation of **ascending aorta**)

Ans. 10) **B. Aortic dissection (Ref: 8 ed. Robbins p. 145, 9 ed. p. 145)**

- **Most common cause of death** in Marfan – **rupture of aortic dissections** [Q], followed by **cardiac failure**
- **Floppy valve** [Q] – Due to loss of connective tissue support in the mitral valve leaflets
- **Valvular lesions** can lead to **mitral regurgitation**

Ans. 11) **D. All of the above (Ref: 8 ed. Robbins p. 145-147, 9 e. p. 145-46, t-5-5)**

Disorders resulting from mutations affecting collagen synthesis:

- **Ehlers-Danlos Syndromes (EDS)** [Q]
- **Osteogenesis imperfecta** [Q]
- **Alport syndrome** [Q]
- **Epidermolysis bullosa** [Q]

Ehlers-Danlos Syndromes (EDS) [Q]

- Abnormal collagen fibers lack adequate tensile strength, due to which, skin is **hyper extensible** and the joints are **hypermobile**

Most Common Types:

- **Classical (I/II)** [Q] type – **AD**, due to mutation in ***COL5A1, COL5A2*** [Q]
- **Vascular (IV)** type – **Arterial or uterine rupture** are seen commonly, **AD** form occurs due to mutation in ***COL3A1***
- **Kyphoscoliosis (VI)** type – Most common **AR** form, due to **mutation** in **Lysyl hydroxylase**

Ans. 12) **B. Transport of LDL receptor (Ref: 8 & 9 ed. Robbins p.147-49, f-5-6-8)**

Molecular genetics of **familial hypercholesterolemia** can be classified into **five groups**:

- **Class I mutations** (uncommon), lead to complete **failure of synthesis** of the receptor protein **(null allele)**
- **Class II mutations** are **common** and occur due to folding defects in **LDL receptor**, which affects **transportation** of **LDL receptor** to the **Golgi complex**
- **Class III mutations** affect **LDL binding domain** of the receptor
- **Class IV mutations** results in **defective internalization** of **bound LDL**
- **Class V mutation** leads to failure of the **dissociation of the receptor** and **bound LDL**

Hence, **in Type II mutation,** there is defect in **transport of LDL receptor**

Hyperlipidemias: (See Table)

Ans. 13) **A. Tay-Sachs Disease (Ref: 8 ed. Robbins p.149-52, , 9 ed. 151-52, f-5-11, t-5-6)**

Tay-Sachs Disease:

- Most common form of **G_{M2} gangliosidosis** [Q]
- Results from severe deficiency of **hexosaminidase A**
- G_{M2} ganglioside accumulates in many tissues (e.g., **heart, liver, spleen**)
- Involvement of **neurons** [Q] and **retina** [Q] dominates the clinical picture

Table Ans. 12 Hyperlipidemias:

	Type I	Type IIa	Type IIb	Type III	Type IV	Type V
Nomenclature	Familial lipoprotein lipase deficiency	Familial hyper-cholesterolemia	Familial combined hyperlipopreinemia	Familial dysbeta lipopreinemia	Familial hyper-triglyceridemia	Endogenous hyper-triglyceridemia
Problem	Decreased lipoprotein lipase or Apo C-II	LDL receptor deficiency	↓ LDL receptor, increased Apo B-100	Defect in Apo-E	Increased VLDL production and decreased elimination (Due to Apo V deficiency)	Same as in type IV, but more severe
Lipoprotein	Elevated chylomicrons (also VLDL)	↑ LDL	↑ VLDL ↑ LDL	Increased chylomicron remnants and IDL	↑ VLDL	↑ VLDL and chylomicron
Cholesterol	↑↑	↑↑↑	↑↑	↑↑	N	↑↑↑
Triglyceride	↑↑↑↑	N	↑↑	↑↑	↑↑	↑↑↑
Xanthomas	Eruptive	Tendon, Tuberous	None	Palmer, Tuberoeruptive	None	Eruptive
Pancreatitis	+++	0	0	0	0/+	+++
Coronary atherosclerosis	0	+++	+++	+++	0/+	0/+
Peripheral atherosclerosis	0	+	+	++	0/+	0/+

- **Electron microscopy** Q – shows **whorled configurations** Q within lysosomes composed of **onion-skin layers** Q of membranes
- **Cherry-red spot** Q in the **macula** is a **characteristic finding**
- Due to the deficiency of **hexosaminidase α gene**, protein folding is affected and **misfolded proteins** trigger **'unfolded protein' response (UPR)** Q leading to **apoptosis**
- **Chaperone therapy** Q has a possible role in treatment

Ans. 14) A. Is a GM1 gangliosidosis (Ref: 8 ed. Robbins p.149-52, 9 ed. 151-52)

- Tay-Sachs disease is a **GM2 gangliosidosis**, which occurs due to deficiency of **Hexosaminidase**, α subunit Q
- Deficiency of **Hexosaminidase**, β subunit leads to **Sandhoff disease** Q

Ans. 15) A. Type A is the most common type (Ref: 8 ed. Robbins p.152-53, 9 ed. 152-53, f-5-12)

Niemann-Pick Disease Q:

- Occurs due to inherited deficiency of **sphingomyelinase** Q
- 3 types: Types A, B and C

Type A Q:

- Severe infantile form with **neurologic involvement** Q
- Marked **visceral accumulations** of **sphingomyelin**, progressive wasting and early death within the **first 3 years** of life
- **Electron Microscopy (EM)** – Shows **"zebra" bodies** Q – Cytoplasmic bodies resembling concentric lamellated **myelin figures** in lysosomes
- Massive **splenomegaly, hepatomegaly** and enlarged lymph nodes due to deposition of **lipid-laden phagocytic foam cells** Q
- Retinal **cherry-red spot** Q is a characteristic feature

Niemann-Pick Disease Type B

- **Patients** have **organomegaly** but **no central nervous system** involvement

Niemann-Pick Disease Type C Q

- More common than type A and B
- Associated with **NPC1 and NPC2** mutations, with **NPC1** Q being responsible for 95% of cases

Ans. 16) C. EM shows onion skin layers of membranes (Ref: 8 ed. Robbins p.152-53, 9 ed. 152-53, f-5-12)

Electron microscopy findings in Niemann-Pick disease:

- **Zebra bodies** Q – Lysosomes containing membranous cytoplasmic bodies resembling concentric **lamellated myelin figures**

Electron microscopy findings in Tay-Sach's disease Q

- **Whorled configurations** Q within lysosomes, composed of **onion-skin layers of membranes** Q

Ans. 17) D. Macrophages and cytokines does not play a role in pathogenesis (Ref: 8 & 9 ed. Robbins p.153-54, f-5-13)

Gaucher Disease:

- **Most common form of lysosomal storage disorder**
- **AR** Q **disorder**, occurs due to mutation in the gene encoding **glucocerebrosidase** Q
- Glucocerebroside accumulates in the phagocytes and **central nervous system** Q
- **Activation of macrophages** and secretion of cytokines such as **IL-1, IL-6** and **TNF** Q are important for pathogenesis

Three Clinical Subtypes:

A) Type 1 or **chronic non-neuronopathic form** Q:

- Most common form
- **Glucocerebrosides** accumulate in the **mononuclear phagocytes** throughout the body
- **Central Nervous System is spared** Q

B) Type 2 or **acute neuronopathic** Q:

- No detectable glucocerebrosidase activity in the tissues
- **Hepatosplenomegaly** is seen
- **Central nervous system** Q involvement leads to death at an early age

C) Type 3 is intermediate between Type 1 and 2

Ans. 18) E. Both C and D (Ref: 8 & 9 ed. Robbins p.153-54, f-5-13)

Gaucher Cells:

- Distended phagocytic cells, found in spleen, liver, bone marrow, lymph nodes, tonsils, thymus and Peyer's patches
- Have **fibrillary cytoplasm** Q similar to **crumpled tissue paper** Q and dark, eccentrically placed nuclei
- **Periodic acid–Schiff (PAS) stain** is **positive**
- **Electron microscopy** Q – Fibrillary cytoplasm can be seen as elongated, distended lysosomes, containing the **stored lipid in stacks of bilayers**
- Gaucher cells are seen in the **Virchow-Robin spaces**, in patients with cerebral involvement

Ans. 19) B. Gaucher's disease (Ref: 8 & 9 ed. Robbins p.153-54)

Diagnosis of Gaucher Disease:

- By measuring the **glucocerebrosidase activity** in peripheral blood **leukocytes** or in cultured skin **fibroblasts**
- **Mutations** in **glucocerebroside gene** – detection of **heterozygotes**

Treatment of Gaucher disease:

- **Replacement therapy** with **recombinant enzymes** (treatment of choice)
- **Bone marrow transplantation**

Ans. 20) D. All of the above (Ref: 8 & 9 ed. Robbins p.154-55)

Mucopolysaccharidoses:

- Results from the **genetic deficiencies** of **lysosomal enzymes** involved in the degradation of mucopolysaccharides (**MPS or glycosaminoglycans**)
- Glycosaminoglycans that accumulate include **dermatan sulfate, heparan sulfate, keratan sulfate and chondroitin sulfate**

Ans. 21) D. All MPS's are autosomal recessive disorders except Hurler's syndrome (Ref: 8 & 9 ed. Robbins p.154-55)

Mucopolysaccharidoses (MPS):

- **7 types – MPS I to MPS VII**, results from the deficiency of one specific enzyme
- Inherited as **Autosomal Recessive** [Q] trait
- **Hunter syndrome** [Q] is inherited as **X-linked recessive trait** [Q]
- Characterized by **coarse facial features, clouding of the cornea, joint stiffness and mental retardation.**

Hurler Syndrome (MPS I):

- **Most severe form** of **MPS** and **most commonly** seen in children
- Children are normal at birth and develop **hepatosplenomegaly** by age **6 to 24 months**
- **Cardiovascular complications** [Q] leads to death by the age of 6 to 10 years

Ans. 22) D. Hyperglycemia is a common association (Ref: 8 & 9 ed. Robbins p.155-57, f-5-14,15, t-5-7)

Glycogenoses is divided into three major subgroups:

- Hepatic
- Myopathic
- Miscellaneous forms

Hepatic form [Q]:

- Liver plays an important role in **glycogen metabolism** and contains the enzymes for synthesis and degradation of **glycogen** into free glucose
- **Inherited deficiency** of hepatic enzymes, leads to storage of glycogen in the liver and **thus, hypoglycemia**

Example:

- **Von Gierke disease, or type I glycogenoses** occurs due to the deficiency of the enzyme **glucose-6-phosphatase** [Q]

Ans. 23) B. Muscle phosphorylase (Ref: 8 & 9 ed. Robbins p.157, t-5-7)

Myopathic form of glycogenosis:

- **Example: Type V glycogenosis** or **McArdle disease** [Q] occurs due to deficiency of **muscle phosphorylase** [Q]

Ans. 24) C. Also called as Type I glycogenosis (Ref: 8 ed. Robbins p.157, f-5-16, t-5-7)

Type II glycogenosis [Q] or **Pompe disease** [Q]:

- **Occurs** due to the deficiency of lysosomal enzyme **acid maltase** [Q]
- **Cardiomegaly** [Q] is the **most prominent** feature
- Leads to **cardiorespiratory failure** within **2 years** followed by death early in life

Ans. 25) B. Methylacetoacetic acid deposits in the tissues due to enzyme deficiency (Ref: 8 ed. Robbins p.155-56)

Alkaptonuria (Ochronosis):

- First human inborn error of metabolism
- **Autosomal Recessive disorder** [Q]
- Occurs due to lack of **homogentisic oxidase** [Q] which converts **homogentisic acid** to **methylacetoacetic acid** leading to accumulation of homogentisic acid
- **Excretion of homogentisic acid** imparts **black color** to the **urine** if allowed to stand, due to oxidation
- **Ochronosis**: **Blue-black pigmentation** of the tissues, as homogentisic acid binds to the collagen in connective tissues, tendons and cartilage

- **Vertebral column**, particularly **intervertebral disc** Q, is the **most common site**
- **Small joints** of the **hands and feet** Q are usually spared

Ans. 26) D. 0% (Ref: 8 ed. Robbins p.142, 9 ed. p. 141)

- Normal % of **HbA_2 is 1.5-3.5%** Q
- In the question, husband HBA_2 is elevated, consistent with the **Thalassemia minor** ($\beta\beta^+$) picture
- Thalassemia, being an **Autosomal Recessive disorder**, does not affect any of the off springs
- Hence, the risk of having a child with thalassemia major is **0%**

Ans. 27) A. 50% of boys of carrier mother are affected (Ref: 8 ed. Robbins p.141-142, 9 ed. p. 142)

X-linked disorders Q:

- As **male** has only one **X-chromosome**, he will always manifest the disease
- As female has **XX-chromosome**, heterozygous female will be a carrier
- 50% boys of **carrier mothers** are affected Q
- **Father will transmit** the **defective X-chromosome** to all **daughters** and hence all daughters of affected father will be carrier
- Father does not transmit the disease to the son as boys don't inherit **X-chromosome from father** Q

Ans. 28) D. Chromosomes are arranged in pairs and in increasing order of length (Ref: 8 & 9 ed. Robbins p.158-59, f-5-17)

Karyotyping Q:

- **Study of chromosomes**
- Somatic cells of human contain **46 chromosomes**, which comprise **22 pairs** of **autosomes** and **two sex chromosomes, XX** in the female and **XY** in the male

Procedure:

- **Dividing cells** are arrested in metaphase with **mitotic spindle inhibitors** (e.g. **colchicine**) followed by **staining of the chromosomes**
- Most common stain used is **Giemsa stain** Q and is hence called **G banding** Q
- **Chromosomes** are **arranged in pairs** and **in decreasing order of length**
- **Short arm** of chromosome is designated **p (for petit)** and the **long arm** is referred to as **q** (the next letter of the alphabet)

Ans. 29) A. Maternal nondisjunction (Ref: 8 & 9 ed. Robbins p.161-63, f-5-19, 20)

Be thorough with the **following basic terms**:

- **Euploid** Q: Humans have **23 pairs** of **chromosome** and any exact multiple of the haploid number i.e. 23X2 etc. is called euploid
- **Aneuploidy** Q: When a cell acquires **chromosome complement** that is not an exact multiple of 23 and which occurs due to error in meiosis or mitosis
- Causes for **aneuploidy: Nondisjunction** Q and **anaphase lag** Q

Nondisjunction Q:

- Occurs during **gametogenesis** and the gametes formed have either an **extra chromosome (n + 1)** or one less chromosome **(n −1)**
- **Fertilization** of such **gametes** by **normal gametes** results in two types of zygotes—**trisomic (2n + 1)** or **monosomic (2n − 1)**

Down syndrome:

- Major cause of **mental retardation**
- **95%** of affected individuals have **trisomy 21** Q, with chromosome count being **47**
- **Most common cause** of **trisomy** is **meiotic nondisjunction** Q
- **Maternal age** Q has a strong influence with Down syndrome

- In most cases, **meiotic nondisjunction** of **chromosome 21** occurs in the **ovum**
- In 95% of the cases with **trisomy 21** the **extra chromosome** is of **maternal origin** Q

Clinical Features:

- Flat facial profile, oblique palpebral fissures, epicanthic folds
- Congenital heart disease, most commonly **endocardial cushion** Q **defects**
- **Increased risk** of developing **acute lymphoblastic leukemia** and **acute myeloid leukemia** (most commonly **acute megakaryoblastic leukemia**) Q
- **Alzheimer disease** Q in all patients with trisomy 21 **older than 40 years**
- Predisposition to **serious infections** Q

Ans. 30) D. All of the above (Ref: 8 & 9 ed. Robbins p.161-63, f-5-19, 20)

Details of Downs syndrome are discussed in Q 29

Ans. 31) C. Associated with parathyroid hyperplasia (Ref: 8 ed. Robbins p.162-64, 9 ed. p. 163-64, f-5-21)

Chromosome 22q11.2 deletion syndrome

- Includes — **DiGeorge syndrome** and **velocardiofacial syndrome**

DiGeorge syndrome:

- **Thymic hypoplasia** with resultant T-cell immunodeficiency
- **Parathyroid hypoplasia** Q giving rise to hypocalcaemia
- Variety of **cardiac malformations** and **mild facial anomalies**

Velocardiofacial syndrome:

- Includes **facial dysmorphism**, **cleft palate**, **cardiovascular anomalies** and **learning disabilities**
- Increased risk for **psychotic illnesses**, such as **schizophrenia**, **bipolar disorders** and **attention deficit hyperactivity disorder**

Diagnosis by detection of the deletion by **FISH (Fluorescence in situ hybridization)** Q

Ans. 32) B. Sex chromosomal aneuploidy (Ref: 8 ed. Robbins p.165, 9 ed. p. 164-66)

Klinefelter syndrome:

- One of the most common causes of **hypogonadism** Q in male
- **47, XXY** is classical **karyotype** Q which results from **nondisjunction** Q during meiotic division

Clinical Features:

- Eunuchoid body habitus with abnormally long legs
- Small atrophic testes, lack of secondary male characteristics as deep voice, beard and male distribution of pubic hair, gynecomastia
- Mean IQ is lower than normal, but **mental retardation** is **not seen**
- Increased incidence of **type 2 diabetes** Q and **metabolic syndrome**
- **Mitral valve prolapse** Q is commonly seen in adults
- **FSH levels** are consistently **elevated** Q, with reduced **testosterone** levels Q
- Increased risk for **breast cancer** Q, **extra gonadal germ cell tumors** Q and autoimmune diseases like **SLE**

Note:

Higher number of **X chromosome** leads to greater likelihood of mental retardation

Ans. 33) C. Mental retardation is commonly seen (Ref: 8 ed. Robbins p.165-67, 9 ed. p. 166-67, f-5-22)

Turner syndrome:

- Results from **complete or partial monosomy** of the **X chromosome**
- Characterized by **hypogonadism** in phenotypic females
- Most common structural abnormality of **X chromosome** include **45, X**

Clinical Features:

In Infants:

- Presents with **edema** of the dorsum of the hand and foot due to lymph stasis
- Swelling of the nape of the neck **(cystic hygroma)** [Q]
- **Congenital heart disease – preductal coarctation of the aorta** [Q] and **bicuspid aortic valve** [Q]

Puberty:

- Failure to develop normal secondary sex characteristics
- **Short stature** and **amenorrhea** [Q]
- **Turner syndrome** is the **single most cause** of **primary amenorrhea**
- **Streak ovaries** [Q]
- **Hypothyroidism** [Q]

Note:

- Gene involved in the Turner phenotype is **short stature homeobox (SHOX)** [Q] gene at **Xp22.33**

Ans. 34) **D. Expansions affect the coding region i.e. exons (Ref: 8 ed. Robbins p.167-70, 9 ed. p. 168-171, f-5-23-28, t-5-8)**

Single-Gene Disorders with Non-classic Inheritance are classified into:

- Diseases caused by tri-nucleotide repeat mutations
- Disorders caused by mutations in mitochondrial genes
- Disorders associated with genomic imprinting
- Disorders associated with gonadal mosaicism

Tri-nucleotide-repeat mutations:

- Mutations are associated with **expansion of the nucleotides G and C**
- E.g. In **Fragile-X syndrome** [Q], expansions occur during **oogenesis** [Q], whereas in **Huntington disease** [Q] it occurs during **spermatogenesis** [Q]
- Affects the **Non coding regions**

Important Trinucleotide repeat disorders include:

Disease	Gene	Protein	Repeat
Fragile X syndrome	FMR-1	FMR-1 protein	CGG
Friedreich ataxia	FXN	Frataxin	GAA
Myotonic dystrophy	DMPK	Myotonic dystrophy protein kinase (DMPK)	CTG

Fragile-X syndrome [Q]

- **X-linked disorder** [Q]
- Gene mutated is **familial mental retardation-1 (FMR1)** [Q] **which is** located on **Xq27.3**
- **Mutation** leads to long repeating sequence of **three nucleotides (CGG)** [Q]
- **Second most common** genetic cause of **mental retardation**, after Down syndrome
- **FMR1 gene** [Q] mutation is diagnosed by **PCR** and **Southern blot analysis**

Also know about

Anticipation [Q]:

- Clinical features of fragile-X syndrome **worsen with each successive generation**

Ans. 35) **C. Germ line mosaicism (Ref: 8 ed. Robbins p.175, 9 ed. p. 174)**

Gonadal or germ line mosaicism [Q]:

- In **Autosomal Dominant** disorders e.g. **osteogenesis imperfecta** [Q], few patients have normal/unaffected parents
- Occurs when **gametes carry mutation** and somatic cells of the individual are completely **normal**

- Normal parent with **germ line mosaicism** can transmit the disease-causing mutation to the offspring through the mutant gamete

Also Know:

Genomic Imprinting Q:

- Each individual inherit **two copies** of **each autosomal gene**, from maternal and paternal chromosome
- Imprinting selectively inactivates either the **maternal** or **paternal** allele
- **Maternal imprinting** implies that **maternal allele** is **inactivated**
- **Paternal imprinting** implies that the **paternal allele** is **inactivated**
- **Imprinting** occurs in the ovum or the sperm, before fertilization and is transmitted to all somatic cells through mitosis

Examples:

a) Prader-Willi syndrome Q:

- Occurs due to **deletion** of **paternally derived chromosome 15** Q
- Characterized by mental retardation, short stature, hypotonia, profound hyperphagia, obesity, small hands and feet and hypogonadism

b) Angelman syndrome Q:

- Occurs due to **deletion** of **maternally derived chromosome 15** Q
- Characterized by mental retardation, ataxic gait, seizures and inappropriate laughter
- Because of their laughter and ataxia they have been referred to as **"happy puppets"** Q

Point to Remember:

- **Genomic imprinting** Q: Molecular basis of these two syndromes
- However both of these disorders can also result from **uniparental disomy** Q
- **Uniparental disomy** – Inheritance of both chromosomes of a pair from one parent

Ans. 36) A. Used for known Genetic loci (Ref: 8 ed. Robbins p.179-80, 9 ed. p. 177-78)

Array based Comparative genomic hybridization Q:

- Used for **unknown genetic loci** Q
- **Test DNA** and **reference DNA** are labeled with two **different fluorescent dyes**
- Can **detect multiple abnormalities at the same time**, by detecting difference in signal with duplication, deletion and normal genes

Ans. 37) A. FISH (Ref: 8 ed. Robbins p.179, 9 ed. p. 177)

Diagnostic tests with their **characteristic features:**

Fluorescent In-situ Hybridization (FISH) Q – For diagnosis of **known genetic loci**

Comparative genomic hybridization – Used for **unknown genetic loci**

PCR – Used for amplification and sequencing of DNA segments

Chromosomal painting Q:

- **Fluorescent labeled DNA probes** span entire chromosome
- To diagnose **chromosomal aberrations**
- **Spectral karyotyping** – Different mixtures of **five fluorochromes** in probes

Ans. 38) C. 5 mb (Ref: 8 ed. Robbins p.159, 9 ed. p. 158)

- Resolution of **light microscope** of viewing chromosome (**Karyotype**): **5 mb** Q
- Resolution of **FISH: 22 Kilobases (more sensitive than karyotype)** Q

Ans. 39) D. Monitoring amplification of target nucleic acid (Ref: 8 ed. Robbins p.174, 9 ed. p. 175-76)

Real Time PCR:

- To **monitor the frequency of cancer cells** [Q] with characteristic **genetic lesions** in blood or tissues
- Quantify the presence of particular **nucleic acid sequences** in **"real time"** [Q]

Ans. 40) B. Metaphase (Ref: 8 ed. Robbins p.159, 9 ed. p. 158)

Karyotype:

- Arranging each pair of **autosomes** according to the length, followed by **sex chromosomes** [Q]
- **Normal karyotype: 46XX (females) & 46XY (males)**

Method:

- Chromosomes are examined after arresting dividing cells in **metaphase** [Q] with mitotic spindle inhibitors (e.g. colchicine) and are stained
- Resolution of Karyotyping: **2 to 5 million base pairs** [Q]

Ans. 41) A. Study of multiple genes (Ref: 8 ed. Robbins p.179-180, 9 ed. p. 177-78)

Microarray:

- Study of **multiple genes**
- Detects **genomic abnormalities without prior knowledge** [Q] of the **genes involved**

Ans. 42) B. G-banding (Ref: 8 ed. Robbins p.159, 9 ed. p. 158)

- Routine technique for **karyotyping** using light microscopy – **G-banding** [Q]
- In **Q-banding, fluorescent** microscopy is used [Q]

(Note: **G – Geimsa stain, Q – Quinacrine** mustard stain)

Ans. 43) C. Chromosomal abnormalities (Ref: 8 ed. Robbins p.159, 9 ed. p. 158)

- **Karyotyping** is **useful** in **diagnosis** of **chromosomal abnormalities** [Q]

Ans. 44) A. Fraction of cells in apoptotic pathways

- **In-situ DNA nick end labeling** is used for detecting areas of DNA, that are nicked during **apoptosis** [Q]

Ans. 45) A. Fibrillin (Ref: 9th ed. Robbins p. 144-145) Refer Q 9 for details

Ans. 46) A. AD (ReF: 9 ed. Robbins p. 140-41) Refer Q 5 for details

Ans. 47) C. Females are mostly carriers and all males are affected (Ref: 9 ed. Robbins p.142) Refer Q 27 for details

Ans. 48) B. Turner (Ref: 9ed. Robbins p. 166-167)

- Barr body (sex chromatin) is derived from one of the two X-chromosomes which becomes inactivated
- Number of Barr bodies is thus one less than the number of X-chromosomes

Examples:

In Kleinefelter's syndrome (XXY), with two 'X' chromosomes, only 1 Barr body will be there

However, in Turner syndrome (XO), with only one 'X' chromosome, no Barr body will be seen

Ans. 49) A. Deletion (Ref: 9 ed. RoBbins p. 160)

Ring Chromosome:

Special form of deletion

- Produced when a break occurs at both ends of a chromosome with fusion of the damaged ends

Ans. 50) C. Short arm of Y chromosome (Ref: 9ed. Robbins p. 165)

SRY: Sex determining region Y gene:

- Gene that dictates testicular development
- Located on its distal short arm

Ans. 51) D. X-linked recessive (Ref: 9 ed. Robbins p. 142) Refer Q 27 for details

Ans. 52) B. AR (Ref: 9 ed. Robbins p. 141) Refer Q 6 for details

Ans. 53) **A. Di George syndrome (Ref: 9 ed. Robbins p. 163)** Refer Q 31 for details

Ans. 54) **B. Pigmented birth marks (Ref: 9 ed. Robbins p. 161-63)** Refer Q 29 for details

Ans. 55) **A. External genitalia are normal (Ref: 9 ed. Robbins p. 166)** Refer Q 33 for details

Ans. 56) **A. Di George syndrome (Ref: 9 ed. Robbins p. 163)** Refer Q 31 for details

Ans. 57) **B. Pigmented birth marks (Ref: 9 ed. Robbins p. 161-63)** Refer Q 29 for details

Ans. 58) **B. Angleman syndrome (Ref: 9 ed. Robbins p. 174)** Refer Q 35 for details

Ans. 59) **A. Lebers hereditary optic neuropathy (Ref: 9 ed. Robbins p. 171)**

- **Mitochondrial DNA is located outside of the nucleus and is always maternally inherited**
- **Leber hereditary optic neuropathy is a prototype of mitochondrial inheritance disorder**

Ans. 60) **A. X-linked (Ref: 9 ed. Robbins p. 142, 1242-43)**

Ans. 61) **A. 50% of boys of carrier mother are affected (Ref: 9 ed. Robbins p. 142)** Refer Q 59 for details

Ans. 62) **C. Angelman syndrome (Ref: 9 ed. Robbins p. 174)** Refer Q 35 for details

Ans. 63) **A. Marfan syndrome (Ref: 9 ed. Robbins p. 144-45)** Refer Q 9 for details

Ans. 64) **D. Trisomy 13 (Ref: 9 ed. Robbins p. 163)**

Ans. 65) **A. 47 (Ref: 9 ed. Robbins p. 164-66)** Refer Q 32 for details

Ans. 66) **A. Study of multiple genes (Ref: 9 ed. Robbins p. 177-78)** Refer Q 41 for details

Ans. 67) **B. DiGeorge syndrome (Ref: 9 ed. Robbins p. 163-64)** Refer Q 31 for details

Ans. 68) **A. AD (Refer: 9 ed. Robbins p. 140-41)** Refer Q 5 for details

Ans. 69) **B. Metaphase (Ref: 9 ed. Robbins p. 158-59)** Refer Q 28 for details

Ans. 70) **C. S phase (Ref: Internet)**

Centrosome duplication occurs during the G1 phase and S phase

Ans. 71) **A. Autosomal dominant disease**

Ans. 72) **A. 50% affected (Ref: 9 ed. Robbins p. 140-41)**

- **If any one affected parent marries normal parent, there is 50% chance of the child having the disease**
- **If both the parents are affected, the chance of having unaffected baby is 25%**

Ans. 73) **A. 45 (Ref: 9 ed. Robbins p. 166-67)** Refer Q 33 for details

Ans. 74) **A. 47 (Ref: 9 ed. Robbins p. 164-66)** Refer Q 32 for details

Ans. 75) **A. Maternal nondisjunction (Ref: 9 ed. Robbins p.161-63)** Refer Q 29 for details

Ans. 76) **C. ¼ (Ref: 9 ed. Robbins p. 141)** Refer Q 6 for details

Ans. 77) **D. X-linked recessive (Ref: 9ed. Robbins p. 142)** Refer Q 7 for details

Ans. 78) **B. Isochromosome (Ref: 9 ed. Robbins p. 160-61)**

Isochromosome

- **Is formed when the centromere divides transversely rather than longitudinally**
- **Shows loss of one arm with duplication of the other**
- **Most commonly, it consists of 2 long arms of X chromosome**
- **Accounts for 15% of all cases of Turner Syndrome**

Ans. 79) **A. FISH (Ref: 9th ed. Robbins p. 177) Note:** Refer Q 37 for details

Ans. 80) **A. Glucocerebrosidase (Ref: 9 ed. Robbins p.153-54)** Refer to Q 17 & 18 for details

Ans. 81) **A. Co-dominance (Ref: 9 ed. Robbins p. 140)** Refer Q 3 for details

Ans. 82) **A. Genetic Anticipation (Ref: 9 ed. Robbins p. 168-171)** Refer Q 34 for details

Ans. 83) **C. 5 mb (Ref: Internet)** Refer Q 38 for details

In Karyotyping, overall resolution is 5 mega bases (mb), breakpoint resolution is 5 to 15 mb

Different banding techniques:

- **G-banding**
- **Q-banding: Involves the use of fluorescent dye quinacrine**
- **C-banding**
- **R-banding or reverse banding**

Ans. 84) **C. Hyper-methylation of tumor suppression genes**

- **Hyper-methylation of tumor-suppressor genes is a common hallmark of all human cancers**

Ans. 85) **B. Point mutation (Ref: 9 ed. Robbins p.140)** Refer Q 2 & 3 for details

Ans. 86) **B. Cri-du-chat syndrome (Ref: Internet)**

- **Caused by a partial deletion of chromosome 5p**
- **Characterized by a distinctive, high-pitched, catlike cry in infancy with growth failure, microcephaly, facial abnormalities and mental retardation throughout life**

6 Immunity

How to go about this chapter?

- **Be thorough with the following topics:**
  - **Innate and adaptive immunity – T cells, B cells and NK cells**
  - **Major Histocompatibility Complex (MHC) molecules**
  - **Hypersensitivity reactions**
  - **Autoimmune diseases – SLE and antibodies associated with them**
  - **Rejection of Tissue Transplants**
  - **Immunodeficiency syndromes – SLE, leucocyte adhesion defects, Severe Combined Immunodeficiency**
  - **HIV infection**
  - **Amyloidosis**

INTRODUCTION

1) **Features of innate immunity are all EXCEPT:**
a) Recognizes foreign antigen in blood
b) Initial defense system against infections
c) Complement system is a part of innate immune system
d) Includes phagocytes and natural killer cells

2) **Toll like receptors are located on:**
a) Cell surface
b) Endosome
c) Both of the above
d) None of the above

3) **In innate immunity complement system is activated by:**
a) Classical pathway
b) Alternate pathway
c) Lectin pathway
d) Both b and c

4) **In adaptive immunity complement system is activated by:**
a) Classical pathway
b) Alternate pathway
c) Lectin pathway
d) Any of the above

5) **Toll like receptors, recognize bacterial products and stimulates immune response by:**
a) Perforin and granzyme mediated apoptosis
b) FADD ligand apoptosis
c) Transcription of nuclear factor mediated by NF-Kβ which recruits cytokines
d) Cyclin

6) **B-cell infectivity occurs due to:**
a) Type 2 complement receptor (CR2/CD21)
b) Fc receptor
c) CD40
d) None of the above

7) **All of the following statements about Natural Killer (NK) cells are true EXCEPT:**
a) They are derived from large granular cells
b) They comprise about 10-15% of human peripheral lymphoid cells
c) They are MHC restricted cytotoxic cells
d) CD 16 is used to identify NK cells

8) **MHC class III encodes:**
a) Complement component C1
b) TNF
c) IL-2
d) Beta-2 microglobulin

9) **T_H1 cells produce the following interleukins:**
a) IL-2
b) IFN-γ
c) Both a and b
d) IL-5

10) **TRUE about T_H2 cells:**
a) Produces IL-4, IL-5, IL-13
b) IL-4 stimulates B-cells to differentiate into IgE secreting plasma cells

c) IL-5 activates eosinophils, eliminates helminths
d) All of the above

11) T_H17 are powerful recruiters of:
a) Eosinophils
b) Neutrophils and monocytes
c) Lymphocytes
d) Plasma cells

HYPERSENSITIVITY REACTIONS

12) **Most important Ig mediating Type I Hypersensitivity reaction is:**
a) IgG b) IgA
c) IgE d) IgM

13) **Most potent eosinophil activating cytokine:**
a) IL-1 b) IL-4
c) IL-5 d) IL-13

14) **Type II hypersensitivity is mediated by:**
a) IgG b) IgM
c) Complement d) All of the above

15) **Type II hypersensitivity is seen in:**
a) Myasthenia gravis
b) Grave's disease
c) Autoimmune hemolytic anemia
d) All of the above

16) **Morphological feature of fibrinoid necrosis:**
a) Type I HS b) Type II HS
c) Type III HS d) Type IV HS

17) **All of the following are examples of Type III HS reactions EXCEPT:**
a) SLE
b) Post streptococcal glomerulonephritis
c) Mismatched blood transfusion
d) Polyarteritis nodosa

18) **Arthus reaction is the following HS reaction:**
a) Localized immune complex
b) Ag-Ab reaction
c) Complement mediated
d) Antibody mediated

19) **Delayed type HS reactions are seen in all EXCEPT:**
a) Contact dermatitis
b) Tuberculin test
c) Rheumatoid arthritis
d) Arthus reaction

20) **CD4 naive T cells differentiate into T_H1 subset in response to following cytokine:**
a) IL-1 b) IL-6
c) IL-12 d) IL-23

21) **Epithelial granuloma is caused by:**
a) Neutrophil
b) Cytotoxic (CD-8) T-cells
c) Helper (CD-4) T-cells
d) NK cells

22) **T-cell mediated killing of target involve(s) the following mediator(s):**
a) Perforins
b) Granzymes
c) Serglycin
d) All of the above

AUTOIMMUNE DISEASES

23) **All of the following are immune privileged sites EXCEPT:**
a) Eyes b) Testis
c) Thyroid d) Brain

24) **Which of the following gene is said to be most frequently implicated in autoimmune diseases?**
a) PTPN-22
b) NOD-2
c) Genes encoding IL-2 receptor (CD25)
d) Genes encoding IL-7 receptor α chain

25) **Which of the following gene polymorphism is associated with Crohn disease?**
a) PTPN-22
b) NOD-2
c) Genes encoding IL-2 receptor (CD25)
d) Genes encoding IL-7 receptor α chain

26) **Speckled pattern on fluorescence in SLE represents which antibody:**
a) Anti- Sm antibody
b) Anti-ds DNA antibody
c) Anti-histone antibody
d) Anti-chromatin antibody

27) **Following can be an LE cell:**
a) Neutrophil b) Macrophage
c) Both of the above d) Lymphocyte

28) **Hematoxylin bodies are seen in:**
a) SLE
b) RA
c) PAN
d) Wegener's granulomatosis

29) **Sub-endothelial deposits 'wire loop lesions' in SLE are seen most commonly in:**
a) Class I lupus b) Class III lupus
c) Class IV lupus d) Both b and c

30) **In kidney 'wire loop lesions' in SLE occurs due to …….. Ig and complement deposits.**
a) Sub epithelial
b) Sub endothelial
c) Any of the above
d) None of the above

31) **Antibodies most commonly seen in drug induced lupus:**
a) Anti-Rho b) Anti-histone antibody
c) Anti-Sm d) Anti-ds DNA

32) **Which of the following plasma protein antibody is responsible for false positive syphilis test in SLE patients?**
a) Prothrombin
b) Annexin V
c) β 2-glycoprotein
d) Protein C

33) **All are TRUE regarding Libman-Sacks endocarditis EXCEPT:**
a) Vegetation on one surface of valve leaflets
b) Warty deposits of 1-3 mm on either surface of leaflets
c) Characteristic feature of SLE
d) Was more common prior to the use of steroids

34) **All are TRUE about SLE EXCEPT:**
a) In skin, IF shows deposition of Ig and complement along the dermoepidermal junction
b) Erosive arthritis
c) Pleuritis and pleural effusions are most common pulmonary manifestation
d) LE or hematoxylin bodies are strongly indicative of SLE

35) **Most common disorder associated with secondary Sjogren's syndrome is:**
a) RA
b) SLE
c) Scleroderma
d) Polymyositis

36) **In Sjogren's which biopsy site is essential to make a diagnosis?**
a) Lip
b) Lacrimal gland
c) Submandibular gland
d) Any of the above

37) **Anti-centromere antibodies are seen most commonly in:**
a) Diffuse systemic sclerosis
b) Limited scleroderma–CREST syndrome
c) Mixed connective tissue disorder
d) Polymyositis

38) **Which of the following biopsies is most characteristic of scleroderma?**
a) A conjunctival biopsy that reveals noncaseating granulomas
b) A peripheral nerve biopsy that reveals rare acid-fast bacteria
c) A skin biopsy that reveals dermal fibrosis with an absence of adnexal structures
d) A subcutaneous fat biopsy that reveals an infiltrate of plasma cells and eosinophils

39) **Major cause of death in systemic sclerosis is:**
a) Pulmonary disease
b) Renal failure
c) Malignant hypertension
d) Cardiac dysfunction

REJECTION AND GRAFT VERSUS HOST DISEASE (GVHD)

40) **All are seen in histology of acute humoral rejection of renal transplant EXCEPT:**
a) Neutrophilic infiltration
b) Necrotizing vasculitis
c) Glomerular vasodilation
d) Proliferating smooth muscle cells in intima

41) **All are TRUE about GVHD EXCEPT:**
a) Occurs when host is immunocompromised
b) Occurs when donor cells are immune compromised
c) HLA typing/DNA sequencing methods reduces its incidence
d) A common cause is stem cell transplantation

42) **All are affected in Acute Graft-Versus host reaction (GVH) EXCEPT:**
a) Skin b) GIT
c) Liver d) Lung

43) **Most common organism causing pneumonitis due to BMT related immunodeficiency:**
a) Streptococcus b) Haemophilus
c) CMV d) Neisseria

44) **Mainstay of immunosuppression in increasing graft survival is:**
a) Cyclosporine b) Steroids
c) Rapamycin d) Azathioprine

IMMUNODEFICIENCY

45) **All are TRUE about Bruton's agammaglobulinemia EXCEPT:**
a) Loss of germinal centre in lymph nodes
b) Most commonly affects females
c) Presents with recurrent sinonasal and respiratory infections
d) T cell reactions are normal

46) **All are TRUE about Di-George syndrome EXCEPT:**
a) Absence of T-cells
b) Absence of B-cells
c) Deletion of gene located on chromosome 22q11
d) Presents with tetany

47) **Adenosine deaminase (ADA) deficiency is seen in the following:**
a) Combine variable immunodeficiency
b) Severe combined immunodeficiency
c) Chronic granulomatous disease
d) Nezelof syndrome

48) **All are TRUE about Wiskott-Aldrich Syndrome EXCEPT:**
a) Due to mutation affecting chromosomal region Xp11.23 (WAS protein)
b) IgG levels are normal

c) IgM are elevated
d) IgA and IgE levels are elevated

HIV

49) Which HIV subtype is seen most commonly in India?
a) HIV-1
b) HIV-2
c) Any of the above
d) None of the above

50) Risk of transmission of HIV infection following needle stick accidents is:
a) 0.3% b) 1%
c) 3% d) 30%

51) Which antigen is most readily detected antigen and target for antibodies in diagnosing HIV?
a) p 24 b) p 17
c) gp 120 d) gp 41

52) CD4 receptors are required for entry of HIV in all cells EXCEPT:
a) Macrophages b) Dendritic cells
c) Astrocytes d) Monocytes

53) Least common mode of transmission of HIV:
a) Homosexual contact
b) Heterosexual contact
c) I.V. drug abuse
d) Transfusion of blood products

54) Most common fungal opportunistic infection in AIDS:
a) Candidiasis
b) Cryptococcus
c) Coccidiomycosis
d) Histoplasma capsulatum

55) Kaposi sarcoma in HIV patients is caused by:
a) CMV b) EBV
c) HHV-8 d) HPV

56) Chorio-retinitis in AIDS occurs when CD4+ cell count:
a) <200/ml b) <100/ml
c) <50/ml d) None of the above

57) All of the following malignancies are seen in AIDS EXCEPT:
a) Carcinoma cervix
b) Kaposi sarcoma
c) Lung carcinoma
d) Lymphomas

AMYLOIDOSIS

58) AA protein is associated with:
a) Rheumatoid arthritis
b) Hodgkin lymphoma
c) Renal cell carcinoma
d) All of the above

59) All are TRUE about Familial Mediterranean Fever EXCEPT:
a) Associated with increased levels of IL-1
b) Characterized by fever and inflammation of serosal surfaces
c) Due to deposition of mutant ATTR fibrils
d) FMF genes encodes a protein named "Pyrin"

60) Transthyretin protein deposition is associated with all EXCEPT:
a) Familial amyloidotic neuropathies
b) Familial Mediterranean fever
c) Systemic Senile Amyloidosis
d) Senile cardiac amyloidosis

61) Lardaceous spleen is due to deposition of amyloid in:
a) Sinusoids of red pulp
b) White pulp
c) Pencilary artery
d) Splenic trabeculae

62) Activation of Naive B lymphocytes by protein antigens is: (NEET 2014)
a) T cell independent
b) NK cell dependent
c) NK cell independent
d) T cell dependent

63) Mantoux test/ Tuberculin reaction is based on which hypersensitivity? (NEET 2014)
a) Type 1 b) Type 2
c) Type 3 d) Type 4

64) HLA associated with rheumatoid arthritis is: (NEET 2014)
a) HLAB-27
b) HLADR-4
c) HLAB-19
d) HLADR-2

65) Which of the following interleukin is secreted by T helper 2 cells? (NEET 2014)
a) IL 11 b) IL 7
c) IL 1 d) IL 13

66) Atopy in hypersensitivity is: (NEET 2014)
a) Systemic type I hypersensitivity
b) Local type I hypersensitivity
c) Systemic type II hypersensitivity
d) Local type II hypersensitivity

67) NK cell shows presence of: (NEET 2014)
a) CD 44 b) CD 16
c) CD 54 d) CD 32

68) Which is the best marker of SLE? (NEET 2014)
a) Anti Sm antibodies
b) Anti ds DNA antibodies
c) Anti histone antibodies
d) Anti Ro Antibodies

69) Most common cause of death in amyloidosis is: (NEET 2014)
a) Heart failure
b) Renal failure
c) Sepsis
d) None

70) LE cell is seen in: (NEET 2014)
a) Lupus erythematosus
b) Lupus vulgaris
c) HNPCC
d) Medullary carcinoma of thyroid

71) Interleukin-2 is produced by: (NEET 2014)
a) T helper cells 1
b) T helper cells 2
c) Natural killer cells
d) Basophils

72) Plasma cells are derived from: (NEET 2014)
a) B lymphocytes
b) T lymphocytes
c) NK cells
d) Monocytes

73) Autoimmunity is caused by: (NEET 2014)
a) Pressure of forbidden clones
b) Expression of cryptic antigens
c) Negative selection of T-cells in thymus
d) Inappropriate expression of MHC proteins

74) Grafting done between genetically different individuals of same species is: (NEET 2014)
a) Autograft b) Allograft
c) Isograft d) Xenograft

75) Cells responsible for GVHD is: (NEET 2014)
a) Immunocompetent T cell donor
b) Immunocompetent T cell recipient
c) Immunocompetent B cell donor
d) Immunocompetent B cell recipient

76) Blood transfusion is which type of hypersensitivity reaction? (NEET 2014)
a) I b) II
c) III d) IV

77) In which of the following arthritis erosions are not seen? (NEET 2014)
a) RA b) SLE
c) Psoriasis d) Gout

78) Large granular lymphocytes are:
a) B cells b) NK cells
c) T cell d) Plasma cells

79) Activation of Naive B lymphocytes by protein antigens is: (NEET 2014)
a) T cell independent
b) NK cell dependent
c) NK cell independent
d) T cell dependent

80) TRUE about MHC is: (AIIMS May 2013)
a) Antigen presenting
b) Regulation of T-cell mediated immune response
c) Class II gene presents on T cells
d) Class I gene present on B cells

81) A female patient was on hemodialysis developed carpel tunnel. It was found to be due to amyloidosis. What is the type of amyloid form synovial fluid? (Nov 2011)
a) AA
b) AL
c) Beta 2 microglobulin
d) AL and AA

82) Immunity against cancer cells: (NEET 2013)
a) Basophils
b) Eosinophils
c) NK cells
d) Neutrophils

83) Most potent stimulator of Naive T-cells: (NEET 2013)
a) Mature dendritic cells
b) Follicular dendritic cells
c) Macrophages
d) B-cell

84) NK cells express: (NEET 2013)
a) CD 15, CD 55
b) CD 16, CD 56
c) CD 16, CD 57
d) CD 21, CD 66

85) Common variable hypogammaglobulinemia shows: (NEET 2013)
a) Decreased B cell count
b) Increased B cell count
c) Normal B cell count
d) Absent B cells

86) Cell mediated immunity is: (NEET 2013)
a) Type I b) Type II
c) Type III d) Type IV

87) Autoantibody specific for SLE: (NEET 2013)
a) ds DNA
b) Anti RO
c) Anti-centromere
d) Anti-topoisomerase

88) Least likely associated with SLE: (NEET 2013)
a) Anti ds DNA
b) Anti Sm
c) Anti topoisomerase
d) Anti histone

89) Which of the following is not seen in liver transplant rejection? (NEET 2013)
a) Inflammatory cells in portal tract
b) Endothelitis
c) Periportal fibrosis
d) Non-suppurative cholangitis

90) Preformed antibodies cause: (NEET 2013)
a) Hyper acute rejection
b) Acute rejection
c) Chronic rejection
d) Acute humoral rejection

91) Amyloidosis is most commonly seen in: (NEET 2013)
a) Maturity onset DM
b) Type I DM
c) Type II DM
d) HTN

92) Eosinophils are activated by: (NEET 2013)
a) IL-1 b) IL-5
c) IL-4 d) IL-6

93) MHC class I represented on: (NEET 2013)
a) All cells b) All nucleated cells
c) RBCs d) None

94) Hemodialysis associated with amyloid pattern: (NEET 2013)
a) AA
b) AL
c) Beta-2-microglobulin
d) ATTR

95) Which type of amyloidosis is caused by mutation of the transthyretin protein? (NEET 2013)
a) Familial Mediterranean fever
b) Familial amyloidotic polyneuropathy
c) Dialysis associated amyloidosis
d) Prion protein associated amyloidosis

96) SCID which is TRUE: (NEET 2013)
a) Adenosine deaminase deficiency
b) Decreased circulating lymphocytes
c) NADPH oxidase deficiency
d) C-1 esterase deficiency

97) A diabetic patient is undergoing dialysis. Aspiration done around knee joint would show: (NEET 2013)
a) A-Beta2 microglobulin
b) AA
c) AL
d) Lactoferrin

98) CD 8 cell: (NEET 2013)
a) T-cells b) B-cells
c) Null cells d) Macrophages

99) An 8-year-old boy completed 8 out of 10-day course of cefaclor. Now he developed a generalized erythematic rash which is mildly pruritic and lymphadenopathy. Diagnosis is: (AIPGMEE 2011)
a) Kawasaki disease
b) Type 3 hypersensitivity
c) Anaphylaxis
d) Infectious mononucleosis

100) Some antigen was injected into a rabbit. What antibody will it produce initially? (AIPGMEE 2011)
a) IgG b) IgM
c) IgA d) IgD

101) Most potent activator of T cells: (AIPGMEE 2011)
a) B cells
b) Follicular dendritic cells
c) Mature dendritic cells
d) Macrophages

102) Which of the following is not an autoimmune disorder? (AIIMS May 2015)
a) Ulcerative colitis
b) Grave's disease
c) Rheumatoid arthritis
d) SLE

CHAPTER 6: IMMUNITY

Ans. 1) **A. Recognizes foreign antigen in blood (Ref: 8 ed. Robbins p.184-85, 9 ed. p. 186-87, f-6-1)**

Major components of innate immunity Q:

- **Epithelial barriers** – Block the entry of microbes by **anti-microbial** molecules (e.g. **defensins)** Q
- **Phagocytic cells** (mainly neutrophils and macrophages)
- **Dendritic cells**
- Natural killer **(NK) cells**
- Several **plasma proteins**, including the proteins of the complement system

Note:

- In **innate immunity**, complement system is activated by microbes using **alternative** and **lectin pathways** Q
- In **adaptive immunity**, complement system is activated by **antibodies** using the **classical pathway** Q

Ans. 2) **C. Both of the above (Ref: 8 ed. Robbins p.184-85, 9 ed. p. 186-87, f-6-2)**

Toll-like Receptors (TLRs) Q:

- **Cellular receptors** through which leukocytes recognize molecules released by injured and necrotic cells
- Located on the **cell surface** and in **endosomes** Q
- Have ability to recognize and initiate cellular responses to extracellular and ingested microbes
- **TLRs signal** leads to the activation of **transcription factor NF-κB (nuclear factor κB)** Q

Ans. 3) **D. Both b and c (Ref: 8 ed. Robbins p.184, 9 ed. p. 186-88)**

- In **innate immunity**, the **complement system** is activated by the microbes using the **alternative** and **lectin pathways**

Ans. 4) **A. Classical pathway (Ref: 8 ed. Robbins p.184)**

- In **adaptive immunity**, complement system is activated by antibodies using the **classical pathway**

Ans. 5) **C. Transcriptions of nuclear factor mediated by NF-Kβ which recruits cytokines (Ref: 8 ed. Robbins p.184, 9 ed. p. 186-87)**

- Refer answer 2 for details

Ans. 6) **A. Type 2 complement receptor (CR2/CD21) (Ref: 8 ed. Robbins p.186-87, 9 ed. p. 191)**

B cell receptors:

- **Complement receptors**
- **Fc receptors**
- **CD40**
- **Type 2 complement receptor (CR2, or CD21)** Q

CR2/CD21 receptor is specific for **Epstein-Barr Virus (EBV)** Q and hence **EBV** readily infects **B cells**

Ans. 7) **C. They are MHC restricted cytotoxic cells (Ref: 8 ed. Robbins p.188, 9 ed. p. 192, f-6-7)**

Natural Killer (NK) Cells:

- Comprises **10% to 15%** of **peripheral blood lymphocytes**
- Also called as **large granular lymphocytes** Q
- Have the ability to kill **infected** and **tumor cells**, without prior exposure to or activation by these microbes or tumors
- Act as an **early line of defense** Q against **viral infections** and some tumors
- **CD16** Q and **CD56** Q, are commonly used to identify **NK cells**
- **NK cells** secrete **interferon-γ (IFN-γ)** Q, which activates the macrophages to destroy ingested microbes
- Activity of **NK cells** is regulated by **cytokines** – **Interleukins IL-2, IL-15 and IL-12** Q

Ans. 8) **B. TNF (Ref: 8 ed. Robbins p.191-92, 9 ed. 194-96, f-6-9)**

Major Histocompatibility Complex (MHC):

- Genes encoding **MHC molecules** are located on **chromosome 6** [Q] (**major histocompatibility complex**, or the **human leukocyte antigen (HLA) complex)**
- **MHC gene** products are **classified** into **three groups** –

A) Class I MHC molecules [Q]

- Expressed on all **nucleated cells** [Q] and **platelets** [Q]
- Encoded by three closely linked loci, designated **HLA-A, HLA-B and HLA-C**
- **CD8+ T cells** are called **class I MHC–restricted** [Q] because they recognize the **peptides** presented by **class I MHC molecules**

B) Class II MHC molecules [Q]

- Encoded in a region called **HLA-D** [Q], which has three sub-regions: **HLA-DP, HLA-DQ and HLA-DR**
- **CD4+ T cells** are called **class II MHC–restricted** [Q] because they recognize the **peptides** presented by **class II MHC molecules**

C) Class III MHC molecules [Q]

- Contains gene that encode **complement components (C2, C3)** [Q], **cytokines** – tumor necrosis factor **(TNF)** [Q], **lymphotoxin** [Q]

Ans. 9) **B. IFN-γ (Ref: 8 ed. Robbins p.195-96, 9 ed. p. 197-98, f-6-10, 11)**

- **CD4+ helper T cells** secrete cytokine **IL-2** [Q]
- Subset of differentiated **CD4+ helper cells** are the **T_H1 and T_H2 cells**

a) T_H1 cells secrete cytokine **IFN-γ** [Q], which is a potent **macrophage activator**

b) T_H2 cells produce:

- **IL-4** [Q] – which stimulates **B cells** to differentiate into **IgE-secreting plasma cells** [Q]
- **IL-5** – which activates **eosinophils** [Q]

c) T_H17 cells – secrete **IL-17** and are powerful **recruiters** of **neutrophils and monocytes**

Ans. 10) **D. All of the above (Ref: 8 ed. Robbins p.195-96, 9 ed. p. 198, f-6-11)**

Refer to answer 9

- Also know – **eosinophils** and **mast cells** bind to **IgE-coated microbes** such as helminthic parasites and function to eliminate helminths

Ans. 11) **B. Neutrophils and monocytes (Ref: 8 ed. Robbins p.195-96, 9 ed. p. 198, f-6-11)**

T_H17 cells:

- Powerful recruiters of **neutrophils and monocytes** [Q]
- Play a major role in several inflammatory diseases
- Important for defense against **bacterial** and **fungal infections**

Ans. 12) **C. IgE (Ref: 8 ed. Robbins p.197-201, 9 ed. p. 200-05, f-6-13-15, t-6-1,2)**

Immediate or Type I Hypersensitivity [Q]:

- **Immunologic reaction** occurring within **minutes**
- Occurs when **antigen** combines with the antibody bound to the **mast cells** in individuals previously sensitized to the antigen
- Mediated by **IgE antibody–dependent activation of mast cells** [Q]
- **Mast cells** can also be triggered by complement components **C5a** and **C3a** (called **anaphylatoxins)** [Q]

Two well-defined phases:

a) Immediate/initial reaction [Q]:

- Characterized by **vasodilation, vascular leakage, smooth muscle spasm**
- Occurs within **5 to 30 minutes** [Q] after exposure to an allergen and subside in **60 minutes** [Q]

b) Late-phase reaction Q:

- Occurs within **2 to 24 hours** Q and **last for several days**
- Characterized by **infiltration of tissues** with **eosinophils, neutrophils, basophils, monocytes** and **CD4+ T cells**

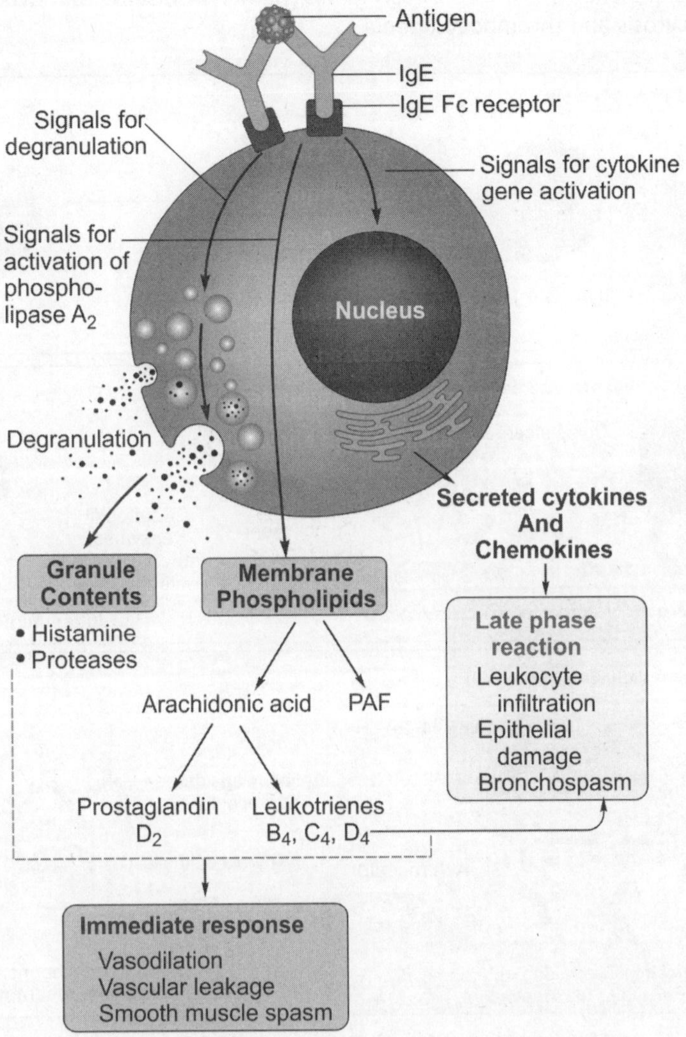

Mast cell mediators in Type I Hypersensitivity

Ans. 13) C. IL-5 (Ref: 8 ed. Robbins p.199, 9 ed. p. 202)

T_H**2 cells** Q:

- Play a role in **immediate hypersensitivity** reactions by stimulating **IgE production** and promoting **inflammation**
- **Produces IL-4, IL-5 and IL-13**
- **IL-4** Q acts on **B cells** to stimulate **IgE** Q production
- **IL-5** Q leads to activation of **eosinophils** Q
- **IL-13** enhances **IgE production** Q and acts on **epithelial cells** Q to stimulate mucus secretion

Points to Remember:

- **IL-5** is the most potent **eosinophil activating cytokine** Q
- Eosinophils liberate **major basic protein** Q and **eosinophil cationic protein** Q which are toxic to **epithelial cells** Q

Ans. 14) D. All of the above (Ref: 8 ed. Robbins p.201-204, 9 ed. p. 205-07, f-6-16, t-6-3)

(Type II) Antibody-Mediated Hypersensitivity Q:

- **Caused by antibodies** that react with **antigens** present on **cell surfaces** or in the **extracellular matrix**
- Antibodies include **IgM** [Q] and **IgG** [Q], which also activate **complement system** [Q] by the **classical pathway**
- **Phagocytosis** is responsible for **depletion of cells** coated with **antibodies**
- **Seen in:** Transfusion reactions, Erythroblastosis fetalis (Hemolytic disease of newborn), autoimmune hemolytic anemia, agranulocytosis and thrombocytopenia

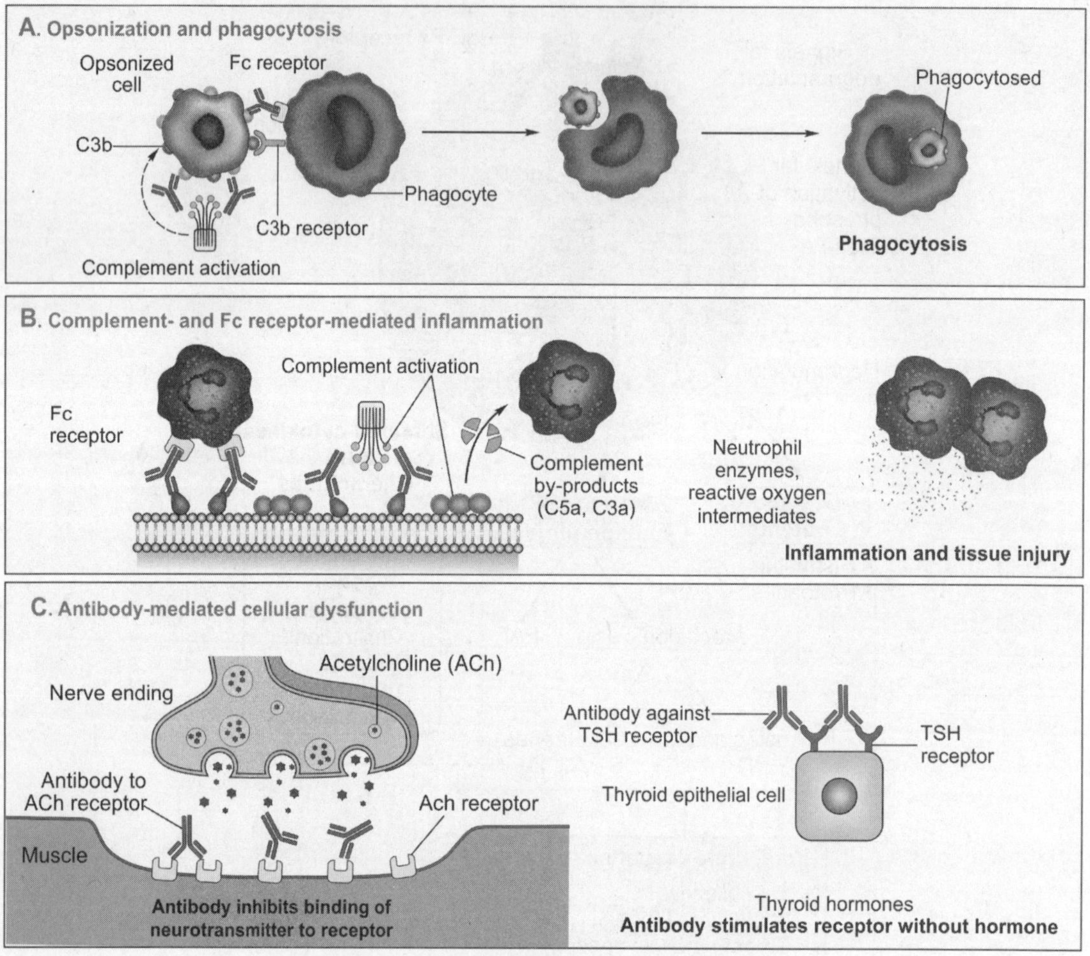

Mechanisms of antibody-mediated injury

Ans. 15) D. All of the above (Ref: 8 ed. Robbins p.201-204, 9 ed. p. 205-07, f-6-16, t-6-3)

Examples of **Type II hypersensitivity reaction** include:

- Pemphigus vulgaris [Q]
- Vasculitis caused by ANCA [Q]
- Goodpasture syndrome [Q]
- Acute rheumatic fever [Q]
- Myasthenia gravis [Q]
- Grave's disease [Q]
- Insulin resistant diabetes
- Pernicious anemia

Ans. 16) C. Type III HS (Ref: 8 ed. Robbins p.204-05, 9 ed. p. 207-08, f-6-17,18, t-6-4)

Type III/Immune Complex [Q] **mediated hypersensitivity:**

- Can be **systemic or localized** in which antigen-antibody complexes produce tissue damage
- Occurs when the antigen combines with antibody within the circulation **(circulating immune complexes)** and which are deposited in the vessel walls

a) Systemic Immune Complex Disease:

Pathogenesis can be divided into **three phases:**

- Formation of antigen-antibody complexes in the circulation
- Deposition of the immune complexes in various tissues
- Inflammatory reaction at the sites of **immune complex deposition**

Morphology:

- **Acute necrotizing vasculitis** Q **(fibrinoid necrosis)** – Necrosis of the **vessel wall** and **intense neutrophilic infiltration** Q

Example: Acute serum sickness Q is the **prototype**

b) Local Immune Complex Disease (Arthus Reaction) Q**:**

- **Localized area** Q of **tissue necrosis** resulting from **acute immune complex vasculitis**, seen in skin

Ans. 17) C. Mismatched blood transfusion (Ref: 8 ed. Robbins p. 204-05, 9 ed. p. 207-08, f-6-17,18, t-6-4)

Examples of Immune Complex-Mediated Diseases:

- SLE Q, Post Streptococcal glomerulonephritis Q, Polyarteritis nodosa Q, Reactive arthritis Q, Serum sickness Q and Arthus reaction Q

Ans. 18) A. Localized immune complex (Ref: 8 ed. Robbins p.204-05, 9 ed. p. 207-08, f-6-17, t-6-4)

- **Refer to answer 16 for details**

Ans. 19) D. Arthus reaction (Ref: 8 ed. Robbins p.205-08, 9 ed. p. 208-11, f-6-18-20, t-6-5)

T Cell–Mediated (Type IV) Hypersensitivity Q**:**

- Initiated by **antigen-activated CD4+ and CD8+ T-lymphocytes** Q

Examples of **Type IV HS reactions** Q are:

- Type 1 DM Q
- Multiple Sclerosis Q
- Rheumatoid Arthritis Q
- Crohn disease Q
- Peripheral neuropathy Q
- Contact dermatitis Q, hypersensitivity pneumonitis Q

Tuberculin Reaction Q:

- Example of **DTH (delayed type hypersensitivity)**
- Produced by **intra-cutaneous injection** of **purified protein derivative** Q **(PPD** or **tuberculin)**
- **Reddening and induration** at the site appears in **8 to 12 hours**, reach a peak in **24 to 72 hours** and thereafter slowly subside

Ans. 20) C. IL-12 (Ref: 8 ed. Robbins p.205-07, 9 ed. p. 209, f-6-20)

- **Antigen Presenting Cells (dendritic cells** and **macrophages)** produce **IL-12** Q which induces differentiation of **CD4+ T cells** to the **T_H1 subset** Q
- **Cytokines** such as **IL-1, IL-6** and **IL-23** from APCs will stimulate the differentiation of T cells to the **T_H17** subset

Ans. 21) C. Helper (CD4) T-cells (Ref: 8 ed. Robbins p.205-08, 9 ed. p. 210-11, f-6-19-20)

- **In tuberculosis, macrophages** tries to combat **tubercle bacilli** in lungs and other tissues
- These activated macrophages undergo **morphologic transformation into epithelium-like cells** also referred as **epithelioid cells** Q
- **Granuloma** Q – **Microscopic aggregation** of **epithelioid cells**, surrounded by a collar of lymphocytes

- This pattern of inflammation is called **granulomatous inflammation** Q
- **CD4+ T cells** Q activate **TNF** and **IFN-γ** which results in **epithelioid cell transformation**

Ans. 22) D. All of the above (Ref: 8 ed. Robbins p.207-08, 9 ed. p. 211)

CD8+ cytotoxic T lymphocytes (CTLs)

- Mediates tissue destruction in **type 1 diabetes**
- Play an important role in **graft rejection**
- Recognition and killing of **virus-infected cells**

Note:

- **T cell–mediated killing of target** occurs with the help of **perforins** Q, **granzymes** Q and a protein called **serglycin** Q

Ans. 23) A. C. Thyroid (Ref: 8 ed. Robbins p.211, 9 ed. p. 214)

- Few **antigens** are **hidden (sequestered)** Q from the **immune system**
- **Immune-privileged sites** Q: Tissues in which these hidden antigens are located and do not communicate with blood and lymph
- **Self-antigens** Q fail to elicit immune response in **testis** Q, **eye** Q **and brain** Q
- Following **trauma** or **infection**, these sites show prolonged **tissue inflammation** and **injury**
- Thus forms the mechanism for **post-traumatic orchitis** and **uveitis** Q

Ans. 24) A. PTPN-22 (Ref: 8 ed. Robbins p.212, 9 ed. p. 215-16, t-6-8)

- Most autoimmune diseases are **complex multi-genic disorders**. Recently described genetic associations:

a) PTPN-22 Q **polymorphisms:**

  - **PTPN-22** Q gene is most frequently implicated in autoimmunity
  - Associated with **rheumatoid arthritis** Q, **type 1 diabetes** Q

b) Polymorphisms in the gene for **NOD-2** Q is associated with **Crohn disease** Q

c) Genes encoding IL-2 receptor (CD25) and **IL-7 receptor α chains** are associated with **multiple sclerosis** and other autoimmune diseases

Ans. 25) B. NOD-2 (Ref: 8 ed. Robbins p. 212, 9 ed. p. 215-16, t-6-8)

- **NOD-2 polymorphisms** Q are associated with **Crohn disease** Q

Ans. 26) A. Anti- Sm antibody (Ref: 8 ed. Robbins p.214, 9 ed. 219-220, f- 6-24, t-6-10)

- **Indirect immunofluorescence (IIF)** – **Most widely** used method for detecting **ANAs** Q

Antinuclear Antibodies (ANAs) are divided into:

- Antibodies to DNA
- Antibodies to histones
- Antibodies to non-histone proteins bound to RNA
- Antibodies to nucleolar antigens

Four basic patterns recognized on **IIF**:

- **Homogeneous or diffuse nuclear staining** Q pattern, occurs due to the presence of **antibodies** to chromatin, histones and, double-stranded DNA
- **Rim or peripheral staining** Q pattern is indicative of antibodies to **double stranded DNA** Q
- **Speckled pattern** Q is seen due to the **presence of antibodies** to **Sm antigen** Q, ribonucleoprotein, SS-A and SS-B reactive antigens
- **Nucleolar pattern** Q refers to the presence of **few discrete spots** of fluorescence within the **nucleus** and is seen in patients with **systemic sclerosis** Q

Antibodies in Systemic Autoimmune Diseases:

Disease	Specificity for antibody	Association with
Systemic lupus erythematosus	Double-stranded DNA U1-RNP Smith (Sm) antigen (core protein of small RNP particles) Ro (SS-A)/La (SS-B) nucleoproteins Phospholipid-protein complexes (anti-PL)	Nephritis; specific for SLE Specific for SLE Congenital heart block; neonatal lupus Antiphospholipid syndrome
Systemic sclerosis	DNA topoisomerase 1 Centromeric proteins (CENPs) A, B, C RNA polymerase III	Systemic sclerosis Limited skin disease, ischemic digital loss Acute onset, scleroderma renal crisis, cancer
Sjögren syndrome	Ro/SS-A, La/SS-B	
Rheumatoid arthritis	CCP (cyclic citrullinated peptides)	Specific for rheumatoid arthritis

Ans. 27) C. Both of the above (Ref: 8 ed. Robbins p.217, 9 ed. p. 222)

LE bodies:

- In **SLE**, **ANAs** are involved in **immune complex formation**
- **ANAs** cannot **penetrate intact cells**
- But if the cell nuclei are exposed (due to cell damage), **ANAs** can bind to them
- Nuclei of **damaged cells** react with **ANAs** and appear **homogeneous**, to produce **LE bodies** [Q] or **hematoxylin bodies** [Q]

LE cell:

- Is seen when blood is **agitated in vitro**
- Is any **phagocytic leukocyte** i.e. blood **neutrophil** [Q] or **macrophage** [Q] which has engulfed denatured nucleus of an injured cell
- Test is now only for historical interest

Ans. 28) A. SLE (Ref: 8 ed. Robbins p.217, 9 ed. p. 222)

- Refer to answer 27 for details

Ans. 29) D. Both b and c (Ref: 8 ed. Robbins p. 217-219, 9 ed. p. 222-24, f-6-26-27)

Morphology of Kidney in Lupus Nephritis:

Five patterns are **recognized:**

- Minimal mesangial (class I)
- Mesangial proliferative (class II)
- Focal proliferative (class III)
- Diffuse proliferative (class IV)
- Membranous (class V)

Sub-endothelial [Q] deposits (between the endothelium and basement membrane):

- Seen in **proliferative types** [Q] **(classes III and IV)**
- These deposits create a **homogeneous thickening** of the **capillary wall**, which are seen by **light microscopy** as a **"wire-loop" lesion** [Q]
- **Wire loop lesions** are seen in **focal and diffuse proliferative (class III or IV)** [Q] lupus nephritis

Sub-epithelial [Q] **deposits** (between the basement membrane and visceral epithelial cells) are seen in **membranous lupus nephritis (class V)** [Q]

Ans. 30) B. Sub endothelial (Ref: 8 ed. Robbins p.217-219, 9 ed. p. 222-24, f-6-26-27)

- Refer to answer 29 for details.

Ans. 31) B. Anti-histone antibody (Ref: 8 ed. Robbins p.214-216, 221, t-6-9, 9 ed. p.226)

- Drugs inducing **lupus erythematosus–like** syndrome – **hydralazine, procainamide, isoniazid and D-penicillamine** Q
- In **drug induced lupus**, there is a **high frequency** of **antibodies specific for histone** Q
- Persons with **HLA-DR4** Q **allele** are at a greater risk of developing lupus erythematosus after administration of hydralazine

Ans. 32) C. β2-glycoprotein (Ref: 8 ed. Robbins p.215, 9 ed. p. 219)

Anti-Phospholipid Antibodies:

- Directed against **plasma proteins-phospholipid complex**
- E.g. **prothrombin, annexin V, β2-glycoprotein, protein S and protein C**

In SLE:

- Antibodies against **phospholipid – β2-glycoprotein complex** Q also bind to cardiolipin antigen, used in **syphilis serology**
- Hence, **lupus** patients may have **false-positive** Q **test** result for **syphilis**
- These **antibodies** interfere with in vitro clotting tests, such as **partial thromboplastin time** and are referred to as **lupus anticoagulant** Q

Ans. 33) A. Vegetation on one surface of valve leaflets (Ref: 8 ed. Robbins p.220, 9 ed. p. 224-25, f-6-28)

Libman-Sacks Endocarditis Q:

- Valvular abnormality in SLE
- Primarily affects **mitral** Q and **aortic valves** Q, with **diffuse leaflet thickening**
- Presents as a single or multiple **1- to 3-mm warty deposits** Q on **either surface of the leaflets**
- Common prior to the use of **steroids** Q
- Vegetations in **infective endocarditis** Q are **larger** Q
- Vegetations in **rheumatic heart disease** Q are **smaller** Q and seen on **lines of closure** of valve leaflets

Ans. 34) B. Erosive arthritis (Ref: 8 ed. Robbins p.218-220, 9 ed. p. 222-225, f-6-27)

Features of SLE:

- **Non-erosive synovitis**
- **Immunofluorescence (IF) microscopy** shows deposition of **immunoglobulin and complement** along the **dermo-epidermal junction** Q
- **Pulmonary manifestations** – Pleuritis and pleural effusions
- **LE** or **hematoxylin bodies** Q in the bone marrow or other organs are strongly indicative of SLE

Ans. 35) A. RA (Ref: 8 ed. Robbins p.221-223, 9 ed. p. 226-28, f- 6-29)

Sjögren Syndrome:

- Characterized by **dry eyes** (keratoconjunctivitis sicca), **dry mouth** (xerostomia)
- Occurs as a **primary form** (isolated disorder), also known as the **sicca syndrome** or as **secondary form** in association with other **autoimmune diseases**
- **Autoimmune diseases associated** includes **Rheumatoid arthritis (most common)**Q, SLE, polymyositis, scleroderma, vasculitis, mixed connective tissue disease, thyroiditis

Ans. 36) A. Lip (Ref: 8 ed. Robbins p.221-223, 9 ed. p. 226-28, f-6-29)

- **Biopsy of the lip** Q (to examine minor salivary glands) is **essential** for diagnosis of **Sjögren syndrome**
- **Mikulicz syndrome** Q: Inflammatory involvement of **lacrimal** and **salivary gland**
- **Mikulicz syndrome** association can occur in **Sjögren syndrome**, **sarcoidosis**, **leukemia**, **lymphoma** and other tumors

Ans. 37) B. Limited scleroderma - CREST syndrome (Ref: 8 ed. Robbins p.223-225, 9 ed. 228-31, f-6-30-31)

Systemic sclerosis is of two types:

A) Diffuse scleroderma:

- Characterized by widespread skin involvement and early visceral involvement
- Antibodies against **DNA topoisomerase I (anti-Scl 70)** [Q] is highly specific

B) Limited scleroderma:

- Skin involvement is often confined to fingers, forearms and face
- **CREST syndrome** [Q] i.e. calcinosis, Raynaud's phenomenon, esophageal dysmotility, sclerodactyly and telangiectasia is a common association
- **Anticentromere antibody** [Q] is found in 20% to 30% of patients

Ans. 38) C. A skin biopsy that reveals dermal fibrosis with an absence of adnexal structures (Ref: 8 ed. Robbins p.223-225, 9 ed. 228-31, f-6-30-31)

Morphology of Scleroderma:

- **Thinning of epidermis,** loss of **rete ridges,** marked **increase of collagen** in the dermis, **atrophy of the dermal appendages (adnexal structures)**
- **Hyaline thickening** of the walls of **dermal arterioles and capillaries**
- **Focal** and **diffuse subcutaneous calcifications**

Ans. 39) A. Pulmonary disease (Ref: 8 ed. Robbins p. 223-225, 9 ed. 228-31)

Systemic Sclerosis:

- **Pulmonary disease** [Q] is now the **major cause** of death
- **Malignant hypertension** [Q] is most dangerous manifestation which leads to **renal failure**

Ans. 40) C. Glomerular vasodilation (Ref: 8 ed. Robbins p.228-30, 9 ed. p. 233-34, f-6-34)

Acute humoral rejection (rejection vasculitis) [Q]:

- Mediated by **anti-donor antibodies**
- Manifested by **necrotizing vasculitis, neutrophilic infiltration**, deposition of **immunoglobulin**, complement and fibrin

Note:

- In vasculitis there is marked thickening of the intima with **proliferating fibroblasts** [Q], **myocytes** and **foamy macrophages** resulting in **infarction** or **renal cortical atrophy**

Ans. 41) B. Occurs when donor cells are immune compromised (Ref: 8 ed. Robbins p. 230, 9 ed. p. 236-37)

Graft Versus Host Disease:

- Occurs when **immunologically competent cells** [Q] are transplanted into **immunologically crippled recipients**
- Most commonly seen in setting of **bone marrow transplantation**
- To minimize GVH disease, transplants are done between **donor** and **recipient** that are **HLA-matched** using sensitive **DNA sequencing** [Q] methods

Ans. 42) D. Lung (Ref: 8 ed. Robbins p.230, 9 ed. p. 236)

Salient Features of Acute GVH Disease:

- Occurs within days to weeks after **allogeneic bone marrow transplantation**
- Major organs involved – **epithelia of the skin** [Q], **liver** [Q], **intestines** [Q] and immune system
- **Skin involvement** leads to **generalized rash** [Q] which may lead to desquamation
- **Jaundice** occurs due to destruction of small bile ducts
- Bloody diarrhea due to mucosal ulceration of the gut

Ans. 43) C. CMV (Ref: 8 ed. Robbins p.230, 9 ed. p. 236)

- **Immunodeficiency** is a frequent complication of **bone marrow transplantation**
- **Cytomegalovirus-induced pneumonitis** [Q] can be a **fatal complication** due to immunodeficiency

Ans. 44) A. Cyclosporine (Ref: 8 ed. Robbins p.230, 9 ed. p. 236)

- Except in the case of **identical twins, immunosuppressive therapy** is a necessity in **transplant recipients**
- Mainstay of immunosuppression is **cyclosporine** [Q]
- **Cyclosporine** works by blocking activation of a **transcription factor** called **nuclear factor of activated T cells (NFAT)** [Q]

Other drugs Used to Treat Rejection:

- **Azathioprine** (inhibits leukocyte development from bone marrow precursors)
- **Steroids** (which block inflammation)
- **Rapamycin** and **mycophenolate mofetil** (both of which inhibit lymphocyte proliferation)
- **Monoclonal anti–T-cell antibodies** (e.g. monoclonal anti-CD3)

Ans. 45) B. Most commonly affects females (Ref: 8 ed. Robbins p.231-233, 9 ed. p. 240-41, f-6-37)

X-Linked Agammaglobulinemia (Bruton's Agammaglobulinemia)[Q]:

- Characterized by the **failure of B-cell precursors** to develop into **mature B cells**
- Caused by mutations in **Bruton tyrosine kinase (Btk)** [Q]; located on the long arm of the X chromosome at **Xq21.22** [Q]
- Seen exclusively in **males** [Q] and becomes apparent after **6 months** of age

Clinical Features:

- **Recurrent bacterial infections** [Q] of **respiratory tract** – Acute and chronic pharyngitis, sinusitis, otitis media, bronchitis, pneumonia
- **Causative organisms – Haemophilus influenzae, Streptococcus pneumoniae, or Staphylococcus aureus**
- Increased susceptibility to **viral infections**, especially **enteroviruses** [Q] such as echovirus, poliovirus and coxsackievirus
- Protozoal infection with **Giardia lamblia** [Q] is also common

Salient Features:

- **B cells are absent or markedly reduced** [Q] with normal T cell–mediated reactions
- Underdeveloped germinal centers of lymph nodes, Peyer's patches, appendix and tonsils
- Absent plasma cells

Ans. 46) B. Absence of B-cells (Ref: 8 ed. Robbins p.234, 9 ed. p. 241, f-6-37)

DiGeorge syndrome:

- Results from failure of development of **third and fourth pharyngeal pouches** [Q]
- **3rd** and **4th** pharyngeal pouches give rise to the **thymus, parathyroid**, clear cells of the **thyroid** and ultimobranchial body
- **Absence of cell-mediated immunity** due to reduced **T-lymphocytes** in the blood
- **T-cell zones** of **lymphoid organs**—i.e. **Para cortical area** of **lymph nodes** and **periarteriolar sheaths of the spleen**—are depleted
- Results from the deletion of a gene on **chromosome 22q11** [Q]
- Is a component of ***22q11 deletion syndrome*** [Q]

Clinical Features:

- **Loss of T cell–mediated immunity** [Q] (due to hypoplasia or lack of thymus)
- **Tetany** (resulting from lack of the **parathyroid**)
- **Congenital defects** of heart and great vessels

Ans. 47) B. Severe combined immunodeficiency (Ref: 8 ed. Robbins p.234-35, 9 ed. p. 239-40, f-6-37)

Severe combined immunodeficiency (SCID):

Syndrome with defects in both **humoral** and **cell-mediated immune responses**

Two forms:

A) X-linked [Q]**:**

- Most common form
- More common in boys than in girls
- Occurs due to mutation in **cytokine receptors** [Q]

B) Autosomal recessive:

- Due to deficiency of the enzyme **adenosine deaminase (ADA)** [Q]

Clinical Features:

- Infants present with oral candidiasis, extensive diaper rash, failure to thrive
- Susceptibility to recurrent, severe infections including Candida albicans, P. jiroveci, Pseudomonas, cytomegalovirus, varicella

Treatment:

- **Bone marrow transplantation** [Q] is the **mainstay** of treatment
- **X-linked SCID** [Q] is the first human disease in which **gene therapy** [Q] has been successful

Ans. 48) C. IgM are elevated (Ref: 8 ed. Robbins p.235, 9 ed. p. 242)

Wiskott-Aldrich Syndrome:

- **X-linked recessive** [Q] **disease** characterized by **thrombocytopenia, eczema** and increased susceptibility to recurrent infections
- Occurs due to the mutation in the gene encoding **Wiskott-Aldrich syndrome protein (WASP)** [Q], located at **Xp11.23** [Q]
- **Low** [Q] serum **IgM levels**
- **Normal** [Q] **IgG** levels
- **Elevated** [Q] **IgA** and **IgE** levels
- Increased risk of developing **Non-Hodgkin B-cell lymphomas** [Q]

Ans. 49) B. HIV-2 (Ref: 8 ed. Robbins p. 237, 9 ed. p. 245)

AIDS:

- **Caused by HIV, human retrovirus** belonging to **lentivirus family**
- HIV has two genetically distinct forms called **HIV-1** and **HIV-2**
- **HIV-1** [Q] is the **most common** type associated with **AIDS** in the United States, Europe and Central Africa
- **HIV-2** [Q] is prevalent in **West Africa** and **India** [Q]

HIV-1 can be divided into three subgroups:

- **M (major), O (outlier)** and **N (neither M nor O)**
- **Group M viruses** [Q] is further divided into several subtypes, designated A through K and **subtype C** [Q] is the **fastest-spreading worldwide**, being present in **India**

Ans. 50) A. 0.3% (Ref: 8 ed. Robbins p. 237, 9 ed. p. 245)

- **Routes of transmission** of **HIV**: sexual contact (homosexuals), parenteral inoculation and from infected mothers to their newborns
- After accidental **needle-stick injury**, risk of transmission of HIV is about **0.3%** [Q]
- **Anti-retroviral therapy** given within **24 to 48 hours** of a needle stick can reduce the risk of infection eightfold

Point to remember:

- **Risk of transmission** for **Hepatitis B** after being accidentally exposed to **infected blood** is **30%** [Q]

Ans. 51) A. p24 (Ref: 8 ed. Robbins p.237, 9 ed. p. 245, f-6-38, 39)

Structure of HIV:

- **HIV-1 virion** is **spherical** and contains a **cone shaped core** surrounded by a **lipid envelope**
- **Virus core** contains:
  a) Major capsid protein **p24**
  b) Nucleocapsid protein **p7/p9**
  c) Two copies of **genomic RNA**
  d) **Three viral enzymes** (protease, reverse transcriptase and integrase)
- **p24** [Q]**:** Most commonly detected viral antigen and is the **target for antibodies** [Q] that are used for the **diagnosis of HIV infection**
- Viral core is surrounded by a **matrix protein** called **p17**
- Studding the **viral envelope** are **two viral glycoproteins, gp 120** and **gp 41**, which are critical for **HIV infection** of cells

Ans. 52) C. Astrocytes (Ref: 8 ed. Robbins p.238-39, 9 ed. p. 246-47, f-6-40)

- **HIV infects** the cell by using **CD4 molecule** [Q] as a **receptor** and **chemokine receptors** as **co-receptors**
- **Selective tropism** [Q]: Virus shows **tropism for CD4 + T-cells, monocytes/macrophages** and **dendritic cells**
- In addition to binding to **CD4 cells, HIV gp120** [Q] also bind to **chemokine co-receptors – CCR5** [Q] **and CXCR4** [Q] for entry into the cell

Ans. 53) D. Transfusion of blood products (Ref: 8 ed. Robbins p.236, 9 ed. p. 244)

Following are the **risk factors** for developing AIDS:

- **Homosexual or bisexual men** constitute the largest group (> **50%** [Q])
- **Intravenous drug abusers** constitute about **20%** [Q] of the affected individuals
- **Heterosexual contacts** constitute about **10%** of affected individuals
- Patients who have received **HIV-infected blood** or its products account for **1%** of **affected population**
- **Hemophiliacs**, with **transfusion of factor VIII** or **factor IX concentrate** make up **0.5%** [Q] of all cases

Ans. 54) A. Candidiasis (Ref: 8 ed. Robbins p.246, 9 ed. p. 252-53, t-6-16)

Candidiasis:

- **Most common fungal infection** in patients with **AIDS**
- Affects oral cavity, vagina and esophagus
- Other **opportunistic infections** include – fungus **Pneumocystis jiroveci** [Q], atypical mycobacteria / **M. avium-intracellulare** [Q]

Ans. 55) C. HHV-8 (Ref: 8 ed. Robbins p.246-48, 9 ed. p. 253-55, f-6-43)

Oncogenic DNA viruses are responsible for following tumors in AIDS patients [Q]:

- **Kaposi sarcoma – Most common, caused by Kaposi sarcoma Herpes virus** [Q]
- **Non-Hodgkin B-cell lymphoma** caused by **EBV** [Q]
- **Cervical cancer in women and anal cancer in men** caused by **HPV** [Q]

Points to Remember:

- **Kaposi sarcoma (most common neoplasm)** is caused by the **KS herpes virus (KSHV)**, also called **human herpes virus 8 (HHV8)** [Q]
- **KSHV infection** also leads to **body cavity-based primary effusion lymphoma** (rare **B-cell lymphoma)**

Ans. 56) C. <50/ml (Ref: 8 ed. Robbins p.246, 9 ed. 253, t-6-16)

- **Cytomegalovirus retinitis** [Q] occurs in patients with **CD4+ T cell** counts below **50 per microliter** [Q]

Ans. 57) C. Lung carcinoma (Ref: 8 ed. Robbins p.246-48, 9 ed. p. 253-55)

Malignancies in patients with AIDS:

- **AIDS-related lymphomas** [Q] are **aggressive B-cell tumors** [Q]

- **Primary central nervous system lymphoma** [Q] is **more common** in patients with AIDS
- Increased risk of **carcinoma cervix** and **anal cancer**, due to reactivation of latent **human papillomavirus (HPV)** [Q] infection

Ans. 58) D. All of the above (Ref: 8 ed. Robbins p.249-52, 9 ed. p. 256-59, f-6-44-45, t-6-17)

Physical Nature of Amyloid:

X-ray crystallography

- Shows a characteristic **cross-β-pleated sheet** [Q] conformation

Electron microscopy [Q]**:**

- Shows amyloid as continuous, nonbranching fibrils with diameter of **7.5 to 10 nm** [Q]
- This structure is responsible for **Congo red staining** and **birefringence of amyloid**

Chemical Nature of Amyloid:

Most common forms include:

A) **AL (amyloid light chain)** [Q] is produced from free Ig light chains secreted by a monoclonal population of **plasma cells**

B) **AA (amyloid-associated)** [Q]**:**
- Derived from precursor **SAA (serum amyloid–associated)** protein that is synthesized in the **liver**
- Increased in inflammatory states as part of **"acute phase response"**
- Associated with **chronic inflammation**
- Often called **secondary amyloidosis** [Q]

C) **Aβ amyloid** [Q] – Derived from amyloid precursor protein and is found in the **cerebral lesions** of **Alzheimer disease** [Q]

Note:

- **'AA protein'** is seen in **following conditions – Rheumatoid arthritis** [Q] (most common cause), **renal cell carcinoma**[Q], **Hodgkin lymphoma** [Q], tuberculosis, bronchiectasis, chronic osteomyelitis

Classification of Amyloidosis:

Clinicopathologic Category	Major Fibril Protein	Related Precursor Protein
Systemic (Generalized) Amyloidosis		
Immunocyte dyscrasias with amyloidosis (primary amyloidosis)	AL	Immunoglobulin light chains, chiefly λ type
Reactive systemic amyloidosis (secondary amyloidosis)	AA	SAA
Hemodialysis-associated amyloidosis	Aβ2m	β2-microglobulin
Hereditary Amyloidosis		
Familial Mediterranean fever	AA	SAA
Familial amyloidotic neuropathies (several types)	ATTR	Transthyretin
Systemic senile amyloidosis	ATTR	Transthyretin
Localized Amyloidosis		
Senile cerebral	Aβ	APP
Endocrine		
Medullary carcinoma of thyroid	A Cal	Calcitonin
Islets of Langerhans	AIAPP	Islet amyloid peptide
Isolated atrial amyloidosis	AANF	Atrial natriuretic factor

Ans. 59) C. Due to deposition of mutant ATTR fibrils (Ref: 8 ed. Robbins p.252-53, 9 ed. p. 259-60, t-6-17)

Other than **AL, AA and Aβ amyloid**, the most common forms of amyloid deposited are:

- **Transthyretin (TTR)** – **mutant form** of **TTR** is **deposited** in **familial amyloid polyneuropathies** [Q] and in the **heart of aged individuals** (**senile systemic amyloidosis**) [Q]
- **β2 - microglobulin** [Q] – **amyloid fibril subunit (Aβ2m)** is seen in patients on long-term **hemodialysis** [Q]

Familial Mediterranean Fever (FMF):

- **AR**, most common form of **Heredofamilial Amyloidosis**
- Due to increased production of cytokine **IL-1** [Q]
- Gene for FMF encodes a protein called **'Pyrin'** [Q]
- Amyloid deposited is composed of **AA proteins** [Q]

Ans. 60) B. Familial Mediterranean fever (Ref: 8 ed. Robbins p.252-53, 9 ed. 259-60, t-6-17)

- Normal **TTR molecules** [Q] **are** deposited in **senile systemic amyloidosis** [Q]/ **senile cardiac amyloidosis** [Q] and Familial amyloidotic neuropathies
- In **Familial Mediterranean fever**, the amyloid deposited is **AA protein** [Q]

Ans. 61) A. Sinusoids of red pulp (Ref: 8 ed. Robbins p.252-53, 9 ed. p. 261)

Amyloidosis of the spleen shows two patterns:

- Amyloid deposits in **splenic follicles** [Q] produces **tapioca-like granules** [Q] and is called as **sago spleen** [Q]
- Amyloid deposits in the walls of the **splenic sinuses** [Q] and in **red pulp** [Q], producing **large; map like areas** and is called as **lardaceous spleen** [Q]

Points to Remember About Amyloidosis:

- **Most common organs** involved: kidneys, liver, spleen, lymph nodes, adrenals and thyroid
- **Macroscopically**, affected organs are often enlarged and firm and have a **waxy appearance** [Q]
- **Congo red stain**, under **ordinary light** imparts a **pink** or **red color** to amyloid deposits, however under **polarized light** [Q], it shows a **green birefringence** [Q]

Ans. 62) D. T cell dependent (Ref: 9th ed. Robbins p. 198) Refer to Q 9 for details

Ans. 63) D. Type 4 (Ref: Robbins 9 ed. p. 208-11) Refer Q 19 for details

Ans. 64) B. HLA DR4 (Ref: 9th ed. Robbins p. 215)

HLA associated with the development of Rheumatoid arthritis:

- HLA-DR4, HLA-DR1, HLA-DR9

Ans. 65) D. IL 13 (Ref: 7th ed. Robbins. p. 198) Refer to Q 9 for details

Ans. 66) B. Local type I hypersensitivity (Ref. 9th ed. Robbins p. 201-204)

Type I Hypersensitivity is of following types:-

Anaphylaxis: Acute, potentially fatal and systemic

Atopy: Chronic, Nonfatal and localized

Ans. 67) B. CD 16 (Ref: Robbins 9th ed. p. 192) Refer Q 7 for details

Ans. 68) B. Anti ds-DNA antibodies (Ref: 9th ed. Robbins p. 219) Refer Q 26 for details

Ans. 69) B. Renal Failure (Ref: 9th ed. Robbin's p. 262)

- Renal failure is most common cause of death
- Cardiac conduction disturbances and arrhythmias, may prove fatal

Hence, it is clear from the above mentioned facts (as Robbins mention), that renal failure is the most common cause of death in patients with amyloidosis

Ans. 70) A. Lupus erythematousus (Ref: 9 ed. Robbins p. 222) Refer Q 29 for details

Ans. 71) A. T helper cells 1 (Ref: 9 ed. Robbins p. 9 ed. p. 197-98) Refer Q 9 for details

Ans. 72) **A. B lymphocytes (Ref: 9 ed. Robbins p. 191)**

After, stimulation by antigen, B cells develop into plasma cells

Ans. 73) **C. Negative selection of T cells in thymus (Ref: 9ed. Robbins p. 212-214)**

- Central deletion or Negative selection: Process which does not allow self-reactive cells to grow

Ans. 74) **B. Allograft (Ref: 9ed. Robbin's p. 231-233)**

Allografts: Grafts exchanged between individuals of the same species

Xenografts: Grafts from one species to another

Autograft (autogenic graft): Graft from self

Isograft (syngraft): Graft from genetically identical person, e.g. identical twin

Ans. 75) **A. Immunocompetent T-cell donor (Ref: 9 ed. Robbins p. 236)** Refer Q 41 and 42 for details

Ans. 76) **B. II. (Ref: 9 ed. Robbins p.205-207)** Refer Q 14 for details

Ans. 77) **B. SLE (Ref: 9 ed. Robbins p. 224)** Refer Q 35 for details

Ans. 78) **B. NK cells (Ref: 9 ed. Robbins p. 192)**

- NK cells are called as large granular lymphocytes (LGL), because they contain large azurophilic cytoplasmic granules

Ans. 79) **D. T cell dependent (Ref: 9th ed. Robbins p. 198)** Refer to Q 9 for details

Ans. 80) **A. Antigen presenting (Ref: Robbins 9 ed. 194-96) Note:** Refer Q 8 for details

Ans. 81) **A. Beta 2 microglobulin (Ref: 9ed. Robbins p. 256-59)** Refer Q 58 & 59 for details

Ans. 82) **C. NK cells (Ref: 9 ed. Robbins p. 192)** Refer Q 7 for details

Ans. 83) **A. Mature dendritic cells (Ref: 9ed. Robbins p. 191-92)**

- Dendritic cells are recruited to the T-cell zones of lymphoid organs, where they present antigens to T cells

Ans. 84) **B. CD16, CD56 (Ref: 9 ed. Robbins p. 192)** Refer Q 7 for details

Ans. 85) **C. Normal B cells count (Ref: 9 ed. Robbins p. 241-42)**

Common Variable Immunodeficiency:

- Patients have normal or near-normal numbers of B cells in the blood and lymphoid tissues
- B cells are not able to differentiate into plasma cells (which secrete antibodies)
- Clinical manifestations are caused by antibody deficiency

Ans. 86) **D. Type IV (Ref: 9 ed. Robbins p. 208-11)** Refer Q 19 for details

Ans. 87) **A. ds DNA (Ref: 9 ed. Robbins p. 219-220)** Refer Q 26 for details

Ans. 88) **C. Anti topoisomerase (Ref: 9 ed. Robbins p. 219-220)** Refer Q 26 for details

Ans. 89) **None (Ref: 9 ed. Robbins p. 865)**

Acute rejection in transplanted liver:

- Infiltration by mixed portal inflammatory infiltrate associated with bile duct injury and endothelitis

Chronic Rejection:

- Obliterative arteriopathy of small and large arteries
- Vanishing bile duct – Destruction of bile ducts due to immunologic attack and interruption of blood flow

Ans. 90) **A. Hyperacute rejection (Ref: 9 ed. Robbins p. 233)**

Hyperacute Rejection:

- Occurs when the preformed antidonor antibodies are present in the circulation of the recipient

Ans. 91) **C. Type II DM (Ref: 9 ed. p. 260)**

Endocrine Amyloidosis is associated with:

- Medullary carcinoma of the thyroid gland
- Islet tumors of pancreas

- Pheochromocytomas, undifferentiated carcinomas of the stomach and in the islets of Langerhans in individuals with type 2 diabetes mellitus (derived from islet amyloid polypeptide)

Ans. 92) B. IL5 (Ref: 9ed. Robbins p. 197-98) Refer Q 9 for details

Ans. 93) B. All nucleated cells (Ref: 9 ed. Robbins p. 194-96) Refer Q 8 for details

Ans. 94) C. Beta-2-microglobulin (Ref: 9 ed. Robbins p. 256-59) Refer Q 58

Ans. 95) B. Familial Amyloidotic Polyneuropathy (Ref: 9 ed. Robbins p. 259-60) Refer Q 59 for details

Ans. 96) A. Adenosine deaminase deficiency (Ref: 9 ed. Robbins p. 239-40) Refer Q 47 for details

Ans. 97) A. A-Beta 2 microglobulin (Ref: 9 ed. Robbins p. 259-60) Refer Q 58 & 59 for details

Ans. 98) A. T-cells (Ref: 9 ed. Robbins p. 211) Refer Q 22 for details

Ans. 99) B. Type 3 hypersensitivity (Ref: 9ed. Robbins p. 207-08) Refer Q 16 for details

Ans. 100) B. IgM

Ans. 101) C. Mature dendritic cells (Ref: 9 ed. Robbins p. 209) Refer Q 20 for details

Ans. 102) None of the above

Quote from Robbins:

Ulcerative colitis is associated with:

- Perinuclear anti-neutrophil cytoplasmic antibodies in 75% of individuals
- Polymorphisms in ECM1 (extracellular matrix protein 1), which inhibits matrix metalloproteinase 9

Grave's disease:

- Polymorphisms in the genes like CTLA4, PTPN22 and HLA-DR3 allele are seen

Rheumatoid arthritis:

- **Associated with Anti-CCP antibodies**

SLE:

- Anti-Double-stranded DNA antibodies are most specific for SLE

7 Neoplasia

How to go about this chapter?

- **Be thorough with the following topics:**
  - **Cell cycle and its regulators**
  - **Inherited cancer syndromes**
  - **Cancers associated with infectious agents and microbial agents**
  - **Proto-oncogenes and tumor suppressor genes**
  - **Chemical carcinogens**
  - **Clinical aspects of neoplasia**
  - **Paraneoplastic syndromes**
  - **Tumor markers**
  - **Recent advance topics – miRNA's, Uses of immunohistochemistry, DNA microarrays, Autophagy**

NOMENCLATURE

1) **Hamartoma is:**
   a) Benign appearing mass composed of cells indigenous to the particular site
   b) Heterotopic rest of cells
   c) Is similar to choristoma
   d) None of the above

2) **All are TRUE about dysplasia EXCEPT:**
   a) Characterized by loss of uniformity of cells
   b) Can progress to CIS and carcinoma
   c) Does not necessarily progress to cancer
   d) Completely reversible process

3) **All are the morphological features of malignancy EXCEPT:**
   a) Pleomorphism
   b) Mitosis
   c) Low N:C ratio
   d) Loss of polarity

RATES OF GROWTH

4) **Rate of growth of tumor is determined by all EXCEPT:**
   a) Doubling time of tumor cells
   b) Fraction of tumor cells that are in replicative pool
   c) Rate at which the cells shed or die
   d) Shortening of the cell cycle

5) **Implications for doing de-bulking surgery (or radiation) for any tumor before chemotherapy:**
   a) For tumors with high growth fraction
   b) For tumors containing large pools of dividing cells
   c) Tumor cells enter the cell cycle and become susceptible to drug therapy
   d) For improving the prognosis

6) **Factor responsible for high intrinsic resistance to conventional therapies in cancer stem cells is:**
   a) MDR 1 (Multiple drug resistance-1)
   b) T- ICs (Tumor initiator cells)
   c) BMI 1 (B-lymphoma Mo-MLV insertion region 1 homologue)
   d) WNT pathway

7) **All are TRUE about trans-differentiation EXCEPT:**
   a) When non-stem cells transform into a different cell type
   b) When stem cell transforms into a different cell type
   c) Type of metaplasia
   d) All trans-differentiation processes are metaplasia but not all metaplasia are trans-differentiation

LOCAL INVASION AND METASTASIS

8) **Most reliable feature that differentiates malignant from benign tumor is:**
   a) Invasion b) Metastasis
   c) Size d) None of the above

9) All of the tumors metastasize EXCEPT:
a) Renal cell carcinoma
b) Basal cell carcinoma
c) Urothelial carcinoma
d) Bronchogenic carcinoma

10) All are TRUE about the pathways of spread of tumor EXCEPT:
a) Lymphatic spread is the most common pathway for initial dissemination of carcinomas
b) Hematogenous spread is typical of carcinomas
c) Biopsy of sentinel nodes is often used to assess the presence of metastasis in lymph nodes
d) Liver and lungs are most frequently involved in hematogenous dissemination

11) All of the following tumors metastasize through peri-neural route EXCEPT:
a) Adenoid cystic carcinoma
b) Rhabdomyosarcoma
c) Prostatic carcinoma
d) Pancreatic carcinoma

GENETIC PREDISPOSITION TO CANCER

12) Following genes are associated with their respective inherited cancer syndromes EXCEPT:
a) PTCH – Nevoid basal cell carcinoma Syndrome
b) PTEN – Cowden syndrome
c) LKB-1 – Peutz Jeghers syndrome
d) p 16/ INK4a – Renal cell carcinoma

13) Mutations of BRCA-1 and BRCA-2 are seen in .... % of breast cancers.
a) 3% b) 5%
c) 8% d) 15%

14) Vinyl chloride is responsible for the following occupational cancer:
a) Lung cancer b) Mesothelioma
c) Leukemia d) Angiosarcoma

15) Cancers associated with infectious agents include all EXCEPT:
a) Cholangiocarcinoma
b) Gastric adenocarcinoma
c) Non Hodgkin lymphoma
d) Lung carcinoma

MOLECULAR BASIS OF CANCER

16) All are TRUE for molecular basis of cancer EXCEPT:
a) Non- lethal genetic damage lies at the heart of carcinogenesis
b) mi – RNA's a new class of regulatory molecules acts as either oncogenes/tumor suppressor genes
c) Tumors are polyclonal
d) Four classes of normal regulatory genes exist

17) All are TRUE for growth factor receptors EXCEPT:
a) RET – proto-oncogene is normally expressed in neuroendocrine cells
b) MEN 2A is associated with point mutation in extracellular domain
c) MEN 2B is associated with point mutation with intracellular domain
d) ERBB-1 is associated breast cancer

18) All proto-oncogenes belong to growth factor receptors family EXCEPT:
a) FLT3 b) SIS
c) RET d) KIT

19) H-RAS mutations are most commonly seen in:
a) Pancreatic adenocarcinomas
b) Cholangiocarcinoma
c) Bladder tumors
d) Leukemias

20) Which of the following prevents the uncontrolled RAS activity?
a) GAP's b) GTP
c) GDP d) Any of the above

21) All of the following are cell cycle regulators EXCEPT:
a) Cyclin D b) Cyclin E
c) C-MYC d) CDK4

22) All are TRUE about cell cycle check points EXCEPT:
a) G_1/S checkpoint checks for DNA damage
b) G_2/M checks whether the cell can safely initiate mitosis
c) Cells damaged by ionizing radiation activate G_1/S checkpoint
d) p53 is required for both the checkpoints

23) All are TRUE for "RB" EXCEPT:
a) Is first and the prototypic tumor suppressor gene
b) Loss of heterozygosity for RB gene is responsible for the development of cancer
c) RB exists in active hyper phosphorylated form in quiescent cells
d) Mutation of RB gene predisposes to osteosarcoma

24) All are TRUE about p53 EXCEPT:
a) Brings arrest of cell cycle (by inducing the transcription of p21)
b) Helps in DNA repair (by inducing transcription of GADD45)
c) Activity in the cell decreases following UV radiation and stimulated the cell cycle
d) Induces apoptosis by the activation of the BAX (apoptosis inducing gene)

25) p53 mutation makes tumor:
a) Resistant to chemotherapy
b) Responsive to chemotherapy

c) Any of the above
d) None of the above

26) All are TRUE about APC/β-Catenin Pathway EXCEPT:
a) APC is mapped at 5q21
b) APC down regulates β-Catenin
c) Mutation leads to hepatoblastoma and hepatocellular carcinoma
d) Pathway is located in nucleus of cell

27) All are TRUE about NF-1 gene EXCEPT:
a) Is a tumor suppressor gene
b) Encodes for a protein neurofibromin which is a GAP
c) Located on chromosome 17q11
d) Neurofibromin facilitates the conversion of RAS from an inactive to active stage

28) TRUE about NF2 gene is/are:
a) Located on chromosome 22q12
b) Is a cytoskeletal protein
c) Encodes a protein Neurofibromin 2 or merlin
d) All of above

29) Cancer cells rely on their nutrition on:
a) Aerobic glycolysis
b) Anaerobic glycolysis
c) Oxidative phosphorylation
d) Any of the above

30) All are TRUE regarding telomeres and telomerase EXCEPT:
a) Telomeres are short repeating sequences of DNA present at linear end of chromosomes
b) Telomeres shortening signals cell cycle arrest
c) Telomerase is a reverse transcriptase which is responsible for maintaining the length of telomers
d) In cancer cells telomerase activity is lost

31) All are TRUE about follicular lymphoma EXCEPT:
a) t(14;18) translocation
b) Juxtaposition of IgH causes overexpression of BCL2 on chromosome 18
c) Increase in BCL2/BCL-XL buffer protecting lymphocytes from apoptosis leading to accumulation of B-lymphocytes
d) BCL2 overexpressing lymphocytes arise due to explosive cell proliferation

32) All of the below are potent angiogenesis inhibitor EXCEPT:
a) Angiostatin b) Endostatin
c) Vasculostain d) b-FGF

33) Following chemokine receptors play an important role in metastasis of breast cancer:
a) CXCR4 b) CX3C
c) C-C d) C-X-C

34) Micrometastases is described in:
a) Melanomas
b) Breast cancer
c) Prostate cancer
d) Any of the above

35) Osteoclasts are activated by following:
a) PTHRP b) RANKL
c) IGF d) TGF

36) TRUE about metastasis includes all EXCEPT:
a) Prostatic carcinoma preferentially spreads to the bone
b) Bronchogenic carcinomas tend to involve the adrenals and the brain
c) Neuroblastomas spread to the liver and bones
d) Lung is the most common site of metastasis

37) All are true regarding breast cancer metastasis:
a) Epithelial-mesenchymal transcription (EMT) is the key feature in breast cancer
b) EMT is promoted by loss of E-cadherin
c) SNAIL and TWIST are transcriptional repressors that down-regulate E-cadherin
d) MiR 10b inhibits metastasis

38) TRUE about autophagy in relation to tumor cells:
a) Cells cannibalize their own organelles
b) Tumor suppressor genes promote autophagy
c) Tumor cells may go into a dormant state
d) All of the above

39) All are TRUE about chromosomal translocations EXCEPT:
a) t(9;22) – CML
b) t(9;22) – ALL
c) t(11;14) – Mantle cell lymphoma
d) t(14;18) – Burkitt lymphoma

40) Chromothrypsis is observed in:
a) Osteomas
b) Osteosarcomas
c) Chondroma
d) Any of the above

41) OncomiRs include(s):
a) miR-200
b) miR-15
c) miR-16
d) All of the above

CARCINOGENIC AGENTS AND THEIR CELLULAR INTERACTIONS

42) Following is considered to induce cutaneous cancers:
a) UV-A
b) UV-B
c) UV-C
d) None of the above

43) All of the following are TRUE about HTLV-1 EXCEPT:
a) Route of transmission is same as of HIV
b) Implicated in development of cancer in humans
c) HTLV-1 has tropism for CD4+ T cells
d) Gag, pol, env plays a role in cancer development

44) Following are TRUE about HPV infection EXCEPT:
a) Oncogenic RNA virus
b) Role in development of benign squamous papillomas/warts
c) HPV -16 and 18 associated with squamous cell carcinoma of cervix
d) Oncogenic potential due to HPV E6 and E7

45) Oncogene responsible for EBV induced B-cell Lymphoma is:
a) LMP-1
b) EBNA-2
c) Cyclin–D
d) None of the above

46) True about *H. Pylori*:
a) Responsible for chronic gastritis and gastric adenocarcinomas
b) Cag A gene is associated with gastric adenocarcinomas
c) Associated with increased risk of gastric lymphoma
d) All of the above

CLINICAL ASPECTS OF NEOPLASIA

47) Hypercalcemia is associated with all of the following EXCEPT:
a) Squamous cell carcinoma
b) Breast carcinoma
c) Renal carcinoma
d) Small-cell carcinoma of lung

48) Immunohistochemistry is useful in:
a) Categorization of undifferentiated malignant tumors
b) Determination of site of origin of metastatic tumors
c) Detection of molecules that have prognostic or therapeutic significance
d) All of the above

49) NextGen sequencing involves:
a) DNA sequencing
b) RNA sequencing
c) mRNA sequencing
d) Any of the above

50) All of the following are TRUE regarding tumor markers EXCEPT:
a) Calcitonin – Medullary carcinoma of thyroid
b) HCG – Seminoma
c) α-Fetoprotein – Liver cancer
d) CA -125 – Ovarian cancer

51) Normal upper limit of CA-125: (NEET 2014)
a) 25 U/ ml b) 45 U/ ml
c) 65 U/ ml d) 85 U/ ml

52) Replacement of columnar epithelium in respiratory tract to squamous epithelium is: (NEET 2014)
a) Hyperplasia
b) Hypoplasia
c) Metaplasia
d) None of the above

53) Which of the following matches is incorrect? (NEET 2014)
a) Aromatic amines – bladder cancer
b) Schistosomiasis – bladder cancer
c) Benzene – Leukemia
d) Nitrates – Skin cancer

54) Carcinoembryonic antigen is raised in which of the following nonneoplastic conditions? (NEET 2014)
a) Hepatitis
b) Pancreatitis
c) Hemolytic anemia
d) Ulcerative colitis

55) Paraneoplastic syndrome – Hypercalcemia of malignancy is produced due to ectopic production of which hormone? (NEET 2014)
a) PTHrP
b) 1, 25 dihydroxy Vitamin D
c) PGE2
d) Parathormone

56) Point mutation in which proto-oncogene is responsible for the development of gastrointestinal stromal tumor: (NEET 2014)
a) KIT b) ALK
c) RET d) FLT3

57) The phenomenon by which the cancer cells are able to sustain and proliferate under adverse conditions of hypoxia is: (NEET 2014)
a) Warburg
b) Wanton
c) Wormian
d) Wolf

58) True about primary gastric lymphoma is: (NEET 2014)
a) Affects young adults
b) Surgery is never indicated
c) T cell lymphoma
d) H. pylori infection increases the risk

59) Carcinoma due to inherited mutation of p53 proto-oncogene: (NEET 2014)
a) Li-Fraumeni syndrome
b) Familial adenomatous polyposis
c) Retinoblastoma
d) Osteosarcoma

60) **Grade of tumor denotes: (NEET 2014)**
a) Degree of differentiation
b) Degree of anaplasia
c) Stage of disease
d) Vascular invasion

61) **RB gene is located on: (NEET 2014)**
a) 13p b) 13q
c) 15p d) 15q

62) **K-ras mutation is seen in: (NEET 2014)**
a) Pancreatic carcinoma
b) Prostatic cancer
c) Gastric cancer
d) Hepatic cancer

63) **Excessive fibrosis in tumor is called: (NEET 2014)**
a) Anaplasia b) Metaplasia
c) Desmoplasia d) Dysplasia

64) **AFP is tumor marker for: (NEET 2014)**
a) Hepatocellular carcinoma
b) Prostate carcinoma
c) Renal cell carcinoma
d) Colon carcinoma

65) **Overgrowth of a skin structure at a localized region: (NEET 2013)**
a) Hamartoma b) Malignant tumor
c) Choriostoma d) Polyp

66) **Retinoblastoma is associated with: (NEET 2013)**
a) Osteosarcoma
b) Hepatocellular ca
c) SCC
d) Osteoclastoma

67) **MYC gene is: (NEET 2013)**
a) Protein kinase inhibitor
b) Growth factor inhibitor
c) GTPase
d) Transcription activator

68) **An example of a tumor suppressor gene is: (NEET 2013)**
a) Myc b) Fos
c) Ras d) RB

69) **Which of the following is DNA repair defect? (NEET 2013)**
a) Xeroderma-pigmentosum
b) Retinoblastoma
c) Neurofibromatosis
d) MEN-I

70) **Carcinoma of lung, best marker is: (NEET 2013)**
a) CEA
b) AFP
c) HCG
d) CA-15-3

71) **Telomerase: (NEET 2013)**
a) RNA polymerase
b) Causes carcinogenesis
c) Present in somatic cells
d) Absent in germ cells

72) **Marker for ovarian cancer in serum is: (NEET 2013)**
a) CA-125
b) Fibronectin
c) Acid phosphatase
d) PSA

73) **Cell growth can be stopped at some specific checkpoints in the cell cycle as depicted. Which stage of the cell cycle demonstrates the primary point in regulation of cell growth? (AIIMS Nov 2015)**

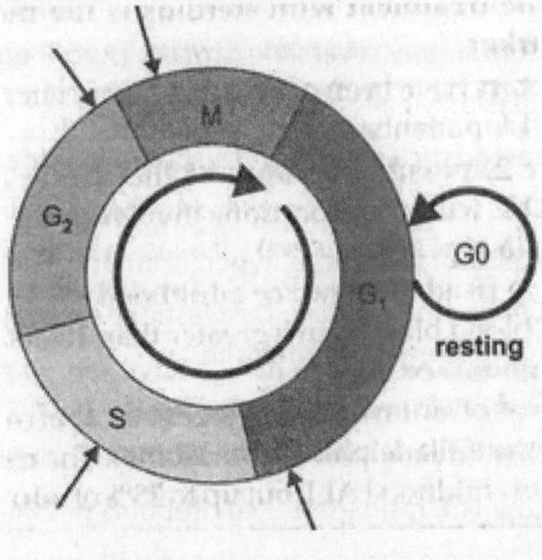

a) End of M b) End of G1
c) End of S d) End of G

74) **The tumor suppressor gene p 53 induces cell cycle arrest at: (NEET 2013)**
a) G2-M phase
b) S-G1 phase
c) G1 - S phase
d) G0 phase

CHAPTER 7: NEOPLASIA

Ans. 1) **A. Benign appearing mass composed of cells indigenous to the particular site (Ref: 8 ed. Robbins p.262-63, 9 ed. p. 267-69)**

Let's be familiar with following terminologies:

Hamartoma:

- Excessive and localized overgrowth of cells and tissues confined to the organ of its origin

Choristoma (heterotopia):

- Described as **heterotopic rest of cells** Q
- **Localized collection of cells** at a site other than **site of origin**
- **Example:** Pancreatic tissue may be found in the submucosa of the stomach, duodenum, or small intestine (most common)

Differentiation:

- Extent to which **the neoplastic parenchymal cells** resemble the corresponding normal parenchymal cells, both morphologically and functionally

Anaplasia:

- Lack of differentiation and is considered a hallmark of malignancy Q

Metaplasia:

- Defined as the replacement of one type of cell with another type

Ans. 2) **D. Completely reversible process (Ref: 8 ed. Robbins p.265, 9 ed. p. 270-71, f-7-10)**

Dysplasia: Means disordered growth

Characteristic Features of Dysplasia include:

- Loss in uniformity and architectural orientation Q of individual cells
- **Pleomorphic, large hyperchromatic nuclei** with **high nuclear to-cytoplasmic ratio**
- **Carcinoma in situ** Q: Dysplastic changes which involve the **entire thickness of the epithelium**, being confined to the **basement membrane**
- Does not necessarily progress to cancer
- Mild to moderate dysplastic changes and can revert back to normal

Ans. 3) **C. Low N:C ratio (Ref: 8 ed. Robbins p. 264-66, 9 ed. p. 269-70, f-7-8,9, t-7-2)**

Morphologic changes associated with malignancy:

- **Pleomorphism** Q — Variation in size and shape of cells
- **Abnormal nuclear morphology** – Nuclei contain abundant chromatin (**hyperchromatic**) and becomes **large in comparison to cytoplasm** of the cell
- **N:C ratio** may approach **1:1** instead of the normal 1:4 or 1:6
- **Mitoses** – Reflects **higher proliferative activity** but it can also be seen in **normal tissues** exhibiting rapid turnover, such as **bone marrow**
- **Loss of polarity** Q – **Tumor cell orientation of** is **markedly disturbed** (i.e. they lose normal polarity)
- Formation of **tumor giant cells** Q
- **Ischemic necrosis** Q

Ans. 4) **D. Shortening of cell cycle (Ref: 8 ed. Robbins p. 266, f-7-11)**

Factors that affect the **rate of growth of tumor** Q:

- **Doubling time** of **tumor cells**
- **Fraction of tumor cells** that are in the replicative pool

- **Rate at which cells are shed or die**

Note:

- **Dividing tumor cells** do not necessarily complete the cell cycle **more rapidly** than normal cells [Q]
- Hence, growth of the tumor is **not associated** with **shortening of cell-cycle** time [Q]

Ans. 5) **C. Tumor cells enter the cell cycle and become susceptible to drug therapy (Ref: 8 ed. Robbins p. 266-67, f-7-11)**

- **Susceptibility** to the **cancer chemotherapy** depends on the **growth fraction** of tumor cells [Q]
- Because, most of the **anticancer agents** act on **dividing cells** of cell cycle [Q]
- Tumor containing cells, which are in G_0 **phase**, will be **slow growing** and are **refractory to treatment** with drugs that **kill dividing cells** [Q]
- Treatment of tumors with **low growth fraction (e.g., cancer of colon and breast)** [Q] involves strategy in which tumor cells are made to shift from G_0 into the cell cycle
- This is done by **de-bulking** the tumor with **surgery** or **radiation** [Q]
- As a result, **tumor cells** enter the **cell cycle** and become **susceptible** to drug therapy
- This forms the **basis of combined modality treatment** [Q]

Ans. 6) **A. MDR 1(Multiple drug resistance-1) (Ref: 8 ed. Robbins p. 267, 9 ed. p. 305)**

- Cancer cells have **"stem-cell like" properties,** which are essential for **tumor persistence**
- **Cancer stem cells** have **high resistance** to **conventional therapies**, because of expression of factors, such as **multiple drug resistance-1 (MDR1)** [Q]
- **Tumor-initiating cells (T-ICs)** [Q] – Allow human tumor to grow and maintain itself indefinitely
- **T-ICs** have been identified in **breast carcinoma, Glioblastoma multiforme, colon cancer and AML**

Ans. 7) **B. When stem cell transforms into a different cell type (Ref: 8 ed. Robbins p. 267)**

- **Trans-differentiation** [Q]: When **mature cell/non stem cell** [Q] differentiate into **another cell**
- In **trans-differentiation**, only **mature cell/non-stem cell** is transformed into other cell type, while in **metaplasia**, either stem cell or non-stem cell transforms into other cell type
- Hence, all **trans-differentiation processes** are **metaplasia**, but **not all metaplasia** are **trans-differentiation** [Q]

Ans. 8) **B. Metastasis (Ref: 8 ed. Robbins p. 268-69, 9 ed. p. 271-73)**

- **Metastasis** [Q] is the most **reliable feature** which differentiates **malignant** from **benign tumors** followed by **invasiveness** [Q]
- Cancers evolve from a **pre-invasive stage** referred to as **carcinoma in situ**

Ans. 9) **B. Basal cell carcinoma (Ref: 8 ed. Robbins p. 269, 9 ed. p. 272)**

- **Invasiveness of cancers** permits them to penetrate into blood vessels, lymphatics and body cavities
- All **tumors** can metastasize except **gliomas** [Q] and **basal cell carcinomas** [Q]

Ans. 10) **B. Hematogenous spread is typical of carcinomas (Ref: 8 ed. Robbins p. 269-70, 9 ed. p. 273-74)**

- **Lymphatic spread** is the **most common pathway** [Q] for dissemination of carcinomas
- **Hematogenous spread** is typical of **sarcomas** [Q] but can also be seen with carcinomas

Sentinel Lymph Node [Q]**:**

- First node in a **regional lymphatic basin** that receives **lymph flow** from the primary tumor
- Used for detecting the spread of **breast cancers** [Q], **melanomas, colon cancers**

Points to Remember:

- **Breast carcinoma** preferentially spreads to **bone** [Q]
- **Bronchogenic carcinomas** tend to involve the **adrenals and brain** [Q]
- **Neuroblastomas** spread to the **liver** and **bones** [Q]

Ans. 11) B. Rhabdomyosarcoma

Neural invasion[Q] **is seen in:**

- **Adenoid cystic carcinoma** of salivary gland
- **Polymorphous low grade adenocarcinoma**
- **Prostatic adenocarcinoma**
- **Pancreatic adenocarcinoma**
- **Capillary hemangioma/Juvenile hemangioendothelioma**

Ans. 12) D. p 16/INK4a – Renal cell carcinoma (Ref: 8 ed. Robbins p. 274-76, t-7-4, 9 ed. p. 279-80)

Inherited cancer syndromes and the **genes** responsible for them include:

- **RB** - Retinoblastoma
- **p53** - Li-Fraumeni syndrome [Q]
- **P16/INK4A** - Melanoma [Q]
- **APC** - Familial adenomatous polyposis/colon cancer [Q]
- **NF1, NF2** - Neurofibromatosis 1 and 2
- **BRCA1, BRCA2** - Breast and ovarian tumors [Q]
- **MEN1, RET** - Multiple endocrine neoplasia 1 and 2 [Q]
- **MSH2, MLH1, MSH6** - Hereditary nonpolyposis colon cancer (HNPCC) [Q]
- **PTCH** - Nevoid basal cell carcinoma syndrome [Q]
- **PTEN** - Cowden syndrome (epithelial cancers)
- **LKB1** - Peutz-Jeghers syndrome (epithelial cancers)
- **VHL** - Renal cell carcinomas [Q]

Ans. 13) A. 3% (Ref: 8 ed. Robbins p. 275)

- **BRCA1** [Q] **and BRCA2** [Q] mutation are seen in **no more** than **3%** of **breast cancers**

Ans. 14) D. Angiosarcoma (Ref: 8 ed. Robbins p. 274, t-7-3)

Occupational cancers include:

- **Vinyl chloride – Angiosarcoma** [Q] and liver cancer
- **Arsenic and arsenic compounds** [Q] – Lung, skin, hemangiosarcoma
- **Asbestos** [Q] – Lung, mesothelioma, gastrointestinal tract
- **Benzene** [Q] – Leukemia, Hodgkin lymphoma
- **Beryllium and beryllium compounds** [Q] – Lung
- **Cadmium and cadmium compounds** [Q] – Prostate
- **Chromium compounds** [Q] – Lung
- **Nickel compounds** [Q] – Nose, lung

Ans. 15) D. Lung carcinoma (Ref: 8 ed. Robbins p. 276-77, t-7-5)

Cancers Associated with Infectious Agents:

Pathology	**Associated neoplasm**	**Etiological agent**
Opisthorchis, cholangitis	**Cholangiosarcoma** [Q], colon carcinoma	Liver fluke (Opisthorchis viverrini)
Chronic cholecystitis	Gallbladder cancer	Bacteria, Gall stones
Gastritis/ulcers	**Gastric adenocarcinoma** [Q], MALT	*Helicobacter pylori* [Q]
Hepatitis	Hepatocellular carcinoma	Hepatitis B and/or C virus
Mononucleosis	B-cell non-Hodgkin lymphoma and Hodgkin lymphoma	EBV [Q]

Cont.

Cont.

AIDS	**Non-Hodgkin lymphoma** Q, Squamous cell carcinoma, Kaposi sarcoma	HIV Q, HHV-8 Q
Osteomyelitis	Carcinoma in draining sinuses	Bacterial infection
Pelvic inflammatory disease, chronic cervicitis	Ovarian carcinoma, cervical/anal carcinoma	Gonorrhea, Chlamydia, HPV
Chronic cystitis	Bladder, liver, rectal carcinoma	Schistosomiasis

Ans. 16) C. Tumors are polyclonal (Ref: 8 ed. Robbins p. 276-78, 9 ed. p. 280-81, f-7-22)

Molecular Basis of Cancer Q:

A) **Nonlethal genetic damage** Q lies at the heart of carcinogenesis

B) **Tumor** is formed by **clonal expansion** of a **single precursor cell** that has incurred the genetic damage (i.e. **tumors are monoclonal**) Q

C) **Four classes** of **normal regulatory genes:**
- **Proto-oncogenes**
- **Tumor suppressor genes**
- Genes that regulate programmed cell death (**apoptosis**)
- Genes involved in **DNA repair**

Note: Regulatory genes are the **principal targets** of **genetic damage**

D) **Carcinogenesis** is a **multistep process** at the phenotypic and the genetic levels and occurs due to accumulation of **multiple mutations**

Ans. 17) D. ERBB-1 is associated breast cancer (Ref: 8 ed. Robbins p. 280-81, 9 ed. p. 282-86, t-7-5)

A) **RET proto-oncogene** Q:
- **Receptor tyrosine kinase**, expressed in **neuroendocrine cells,** such as **Para follicular C cells** of **thyroid** Q, **adrenal medulla** Q and **parathyroid cell precursors**
- **Point mutations** in **RET proto-oncogene** – associated with **MEN 2A** and **2B** Q and **familial medullary thyroid carcinoma** Q
- **MEN-2A** (**point mutation** in **RET extracellular domain** Q) leads to **medullary thyroid carcinomas** Q and **adrenal and parathyroid tumors**
- **MEN-2B** (**point mutation** in the **RET cytoplasmic catalytic domain** Q) leads to **thyroid** and **adrenal tumors without** involvement of **parathyroid**

B) **Epidermal growth factor (EGF) receptor:**
- **ERBB1** Q **(EGF receptor gene)** – Overexpressed in **squamous cell carcinomas of the lung** Q, **glioblastomas, head and neck tumors**
- **ERBB2 gene (also called HER-2/NEU)** Q – Amplified in **breast cancers** Q and **adenocarcinomas** of the **ovary, lung, stomach and salivary glands**
- Thus, **ERBB-2** Q is **associated** with breast cancer and **not ERBB-1**

Ans. 18) B. *SIS* (Ref: 8 ed. Robbins p. 280-81, 9 ed. p. 282-86, t-7-5)

Important oncogenes and associated human tumors (Asked repeatedly in entrance exams):

Category	Proto-oncogene	Associated Human Tumor
Growth Factors		
PDGF-β chain	*SIS* (official name PBGFB)	Astrocytoma, Osteosarcoma
Fibroblast growth factors	HST1 FGF3	Stomach cancer Bladder cancer, Breast cancer, Melanoma
TGF-α	TGFA	Astrocytoma, Hepatocellular carcinomas
HGF	HGF	Thyroid cancer

Cont.

Cont.

Growth factor receptors		
EGF-receptor family	ERBB1(EGFR) ERRB2	Squamous cell carcinoma of lung Breast cancer
FMS-like tyrosine kinase 3	FLT3	Breast and ovarian cancers
Receptor for neurotrophic factors	RET	Leukemia Multiple endocrine neoplasia 2A and B Familial medullary thyroid carcinomas
PDGF receptor	PDGFRB	Gliomas, leukemias
Receptor for KIT ligand	KIT	Gastrointestinal stromal tumors, seminomas, leukemias

Ans. 19) C. Bladder tumors (Ref: 8 ed. Robbins p. 281-82, 9 ed. p. 284, t-7-5)

Point mutation of the **RAS family** genes is the **single most common** abnormality of **proto-oncogenes** in human tumors. **Examples:**

- **Carcinomas** Q (particularly from **colon** and **pancreas**) have mutations of **KRAS** Q
- **Bladder and kidney tumors** Q have **HRAS** Q mutations
- **Hematopoietic tumors** and **melanomas** Q bear **NRAS** Q mutations

Ans. 20) A. GAP's (Ref: 8 ed. Robbins p. 281-82, 9 ed. p. 285-86, f-7-25)

Salient Features of RAS:

- Member of family of small **G proteins** that bind **guanosine nucleotides** (guanosine triphosphate, GTP and guanosine diphosphate, GDP)
- **Normally RAS proteins** flip back and forth between an excited **signal-transmitting state** and **quiescent state**
- In **inactive state** Q, **RAS proteins** bind to **GDP** Q
- Stimulation of cells by growth factors leads to **exchange of GDP for GTP** Q that generates active RAS
- **Activated RAS** Q stimulates **mitogen-activated protein (MAP) kinase cascade** Q, which signals **cell proliferation**
- **GTP hydrolysis**, converts the **GTP bound, active RAS** to the **GDP-bound, inactive form**
- **GTPase activating proteins (GAPs) increases the GTPase activity**, leading to **termination** of **signal transduction**
- GAPs function as **"brakes"** Q that prevent uncontrolled RAS activity
- Mutation in **Neurofibromin 1** Q, a **GAP**, is associated with **familial neurofibromatosis type 1**

Note:

- Mutations in **BRAF** have been **detected** in **melanomas** and **benign nevi** Q

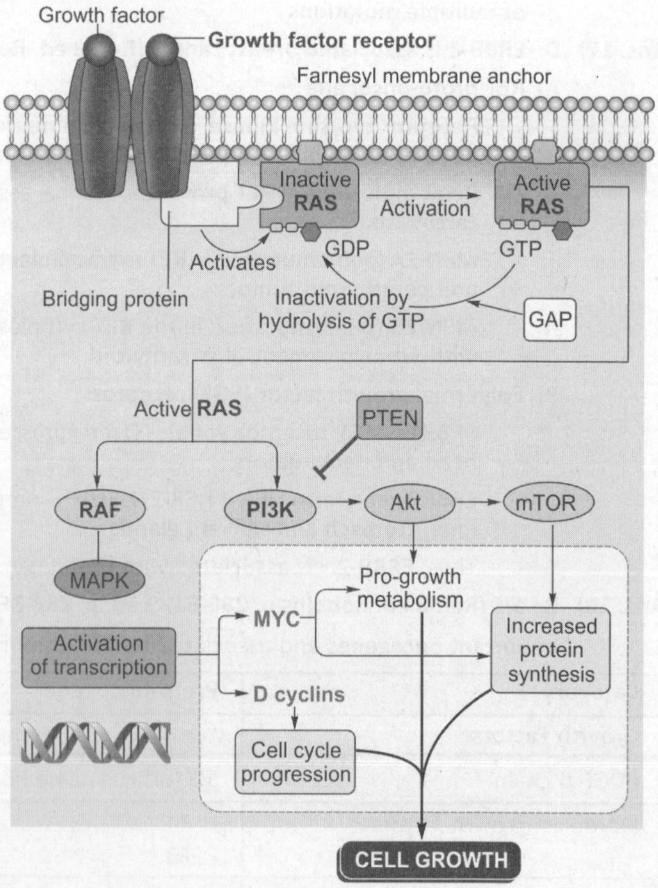

Growth factor signaling pathways in cancer

Ans. 21) C. C-MYC (Ref: 8 ed. Robbins p. 284-86, 9 ed. 292-93, f-7-29)

- Cell cycle goes through **G_0-G1-S-G_2-M phases**
- **Cell cycle regulators** include **Cyclins (Cyclin D, Cyclin E)** Q **and Cyclin dependent kinases** Q

Cyclin-Cyclin dependent kinase complex:

- **Cyclin D–CDK4, cyclin D–CDK6** and **cyclin E–CDK2** regulate the **G1-to-S transition** by phosphorylation of the **RB protein** Q
- **Cyclin A–CDK2** and **cyclin A–CDK1** are active in the **S phase** Q
- **Cyclin B–CDK1** is essential for **G2-to-M transition** Q

CDKIs (Cyclin dependent kinase inhibitors):

- **INK4 inhibitors** Q: Composed of **p16, p15, p18, p19** can block the activity of **cyclin D–CDK4** Q **and cyclin D–CDK6** Q
- **CIP/WAF** Q family of **CDKIs – p21, p27 and p57** can **inhibit all CDKs**

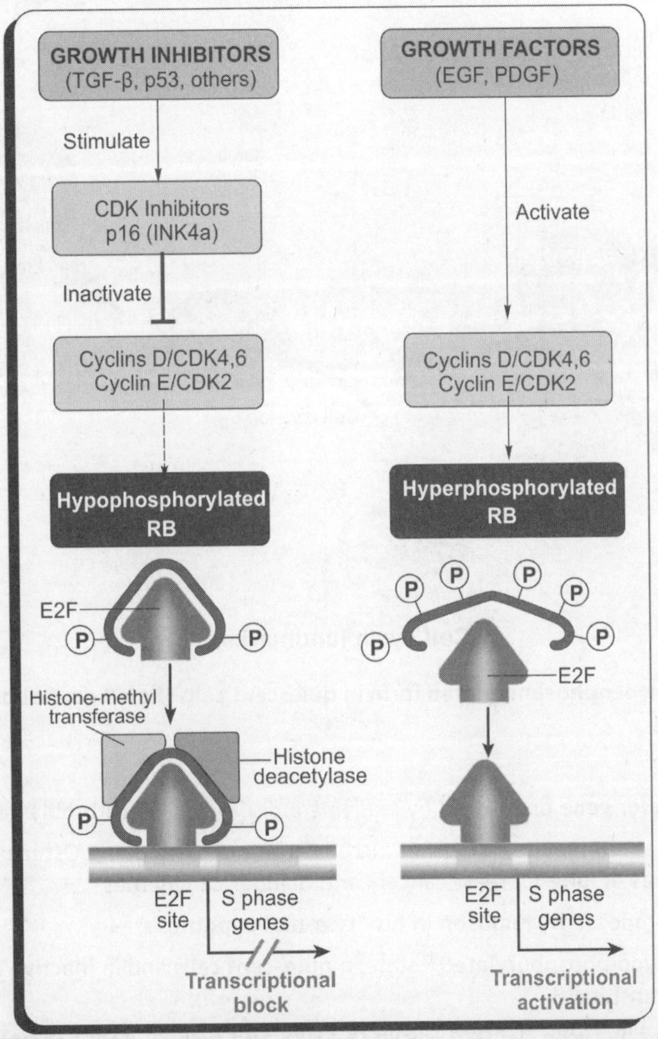

Role of RB in regulating the G1-S checkpoint of cell cycle

Ans. 22) C. Cells damaged by ionizing radiation activate G_1/S checkpoint (Ref: 8 ed. Robbins p. 285-86, 9 ed. p. 25-26, 292-293, f-1-17-18)

- **Two main cell cycle checkpoints: G_1/S transition** Q and **G_2/M** Q

G_1/S checkpoint Q:

- **Checks for DNA damage** Q and if damage is present, DNA-repair mechanisms arrest the cell cycle
- Prevents the replication of cells that have **defects in DNA** Q

G2/M checkpoint Q:

- **Monitors** the completion of **DNA replication** Q and checks whether the cell can safely initiate **mitosis** Q and **separate sister chromatids**
- Plays a role in cells exposed to **ionizing radiation** Q
- **Defects** in this checkpoint give rise to **chromosomal abnormalities** Q
- **p53** Q **(induces** the **cell cycle inhibitor p21** Q) is required for the **G1/S checkpoint** and also forms a **main component** of the **G2/M checkpoint**

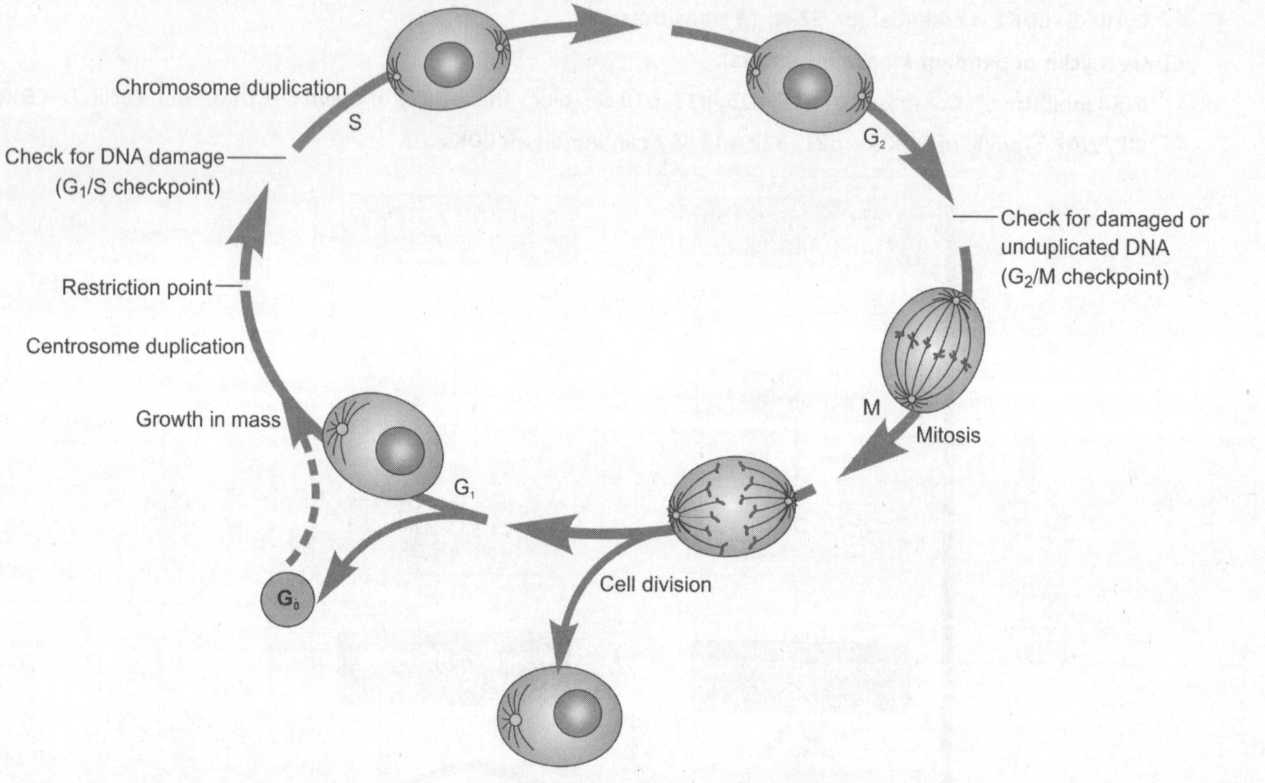

Cell cycle landmarks

Ans. 23) C. RB exists in active hyper phosphorylated form in quiescent cells (Ref: 8 ed. Robbins p. 286-90, 9 ed. p. 292-93, f-7-28-29, t-7-7)

RB:

- First **tumor suppressor gene** discovered by studying a disease called **retinoblastoma**
- Patients with familial retinoblastoma are at increased risk of developing **Osteosarcoma**Q, **Glioblastoma** Q and **Small cell carcinomas of lung** Q, breast cancers and bladder carcinomas
- Pathogenesis was proposed by **Knudson** in his **"two-hit"** hypothesis
- Exists in an **active hypo-phosphorylated** Q state in **quiescent cells** and in **inactive hyper phosphorylated** Q state in **G1/S cell cycle transition** Q
- **RB** is phosphorylated by **cyclin D–CDK4, cyclin D–CDK6 and cyclin E–CDK2 complexes** Q
- **Phosphorylation of RB** is **inhibited** by **CDKIs (p16/INK4a)** Q

Ans. 24) C. Activity in the cell decreases following UV radiation and stimulates the cell cycle (Ref: 8 ed. Robbins p. 290-92, 9 ed. p. 292-96, f-7-30, t-7-7)

p53 – guardian of genome Q ("molecular policeman")

- Located on chromosome **17p13.1** Q
- **Prevents** the propagation of **genetically damaged cells**
- **Levels of p53** are negatively regulated by **MDM2/MDMX** Q

- Has short half-life **(20 minutes)** Q
- Activity increases following **UV radiation** Q

p53 inhibits neoplastic transformation by:

a) Activation of temporary cell cycle arrest **(quiescence)**
b) Induction of permanent cell cycle arrest **(senescence)**
c) Triggering of programmed cell death **(apoptosis)**

p53 brings **cell cycle arrest** by:

- Activation of CDK inhibitor **CDKN1A (p21)** Q
- Inducing certain proteins, such as **GADD45 (growth arrest and DNA damage)** Q
- Activation of **BAX gene** Q which promotes **apoptosis**

Main tumor suppressor genes

Gene	Protein	Familial syndromes	Sporadic cancers
Inhibitors of Mitogenic Signaling Pathways			
APC	Adenomatous polyposis coliprotein	Familial colonic polyps and carcinomas	Carcinomas of stomach, colon, pancreas; melanoma
NF-1	Neurofibromin-1	Neurofibromatosis type 1	Neuroblastoma, juvenile myeloid leukemia
NF-2	Merlin	Neurofibromatosis type 2	Schwannoma, meningioma
PTCH	Patched	Gorlin syndrome	Basal cell carcinoma, Medulloblastoma
PTEN	Phosphatase and tensin homologue	Cowden syndrome	Carcinomas and lymphoid tumors
SMAD2, SMAD4	SMAD2, SMAD4	Juvenile polyposis	Colonic and Pancreatic carcinoma
Inhibitors of Cell Cycle Progression			
RB	Retinoblastoma (RB) protein	Familial retinoblastoma syndrome	Retinoblastoma; osteosarcoma, carcinomas of breast, colon, lung
CDKN2A	p16/INK4a and p14/ARF	Familial melanoma	Pancreatic, breast, esophageal carcinoma, melanoma, leukemias
Inhibitors of "Pro-growth" Programs of Metabolism and Angiogenesis			
VHL	Von Hippel Lindau (VHL) protein	Von Hippel Lindau syndrome (cerebellar hemangioblastoma, retinal angioma, renal cell carcinoma)	Renal cell carcinoma
STK11	Liver kinase B1 (LKB1) or STK11	Peutz-Jeghers syndrome (GI polyps, GI cancers, pancreatic carcinoma)	Diverse carcinomas
Inhibitors of Invasion and Metastasis			
CDH1	E-cadherin	Familial gastric cancer	Gastric carcinoma, lobular breast carcinoma

Cont.

Cont.

Enablers of Genomic Stability			
TP53	p53 protein	Li-Fraumeni syndrome	Most human cancers
DNA Repair Factors			
BRCA1, BRCA2	Breast cancer-1 and breast cancer-2 (BRCA1 and BRCA2)	Familial breast and ovarian carcinoma; carcinoma of male breast; chronic lymphocytic leukemia (BRCA-2)	Rare
MSH2, MLH1, MSH6	MSH1, MLH1, MSH6	Hereditary nonpolyposis colon carcinoma	Colonic and endometrial carcinoma
Unknown Mechanisms			
WT1	Wilms tumor-1 (WT1)	Familial Wilms tumor	Wilms tumor, certain leukemias
MEN1	Menin	Multiple endocrine neoplasia-1 (MEN1; pituitary, parathyroid, and pancreatic endocrine tumors)	Pituitary, parathyroid, and pancreatic endocrine tumors

Ans. 25) A. Resistant to chemotherapy (Ref: 8 ed. Robbins p. 292, 9 ed. p. 296)

- **Irradiation and chemotherapy**, used in cancer treatment, mediate their effects by **inducing DNA damage** and subsequent **apoptosis**
- Tumors with normal **p53 activity** responds well to treatment **(e.g. testicular teratocarcinomas and childhood acute lymphoblastic leukemia's)** Q
- Tumors that carry **p53 mutations (lung cancers and colorectal cancers)** Q are **resistant to chemotherapy and irradiation**

Ans. 26) D. Pathway is located in the nucleus of cell (Ref: 8 ed. Robbins p. 292-94, 9 ed. 296-97, f-7-31)

APC/β-Catenin Q**:**

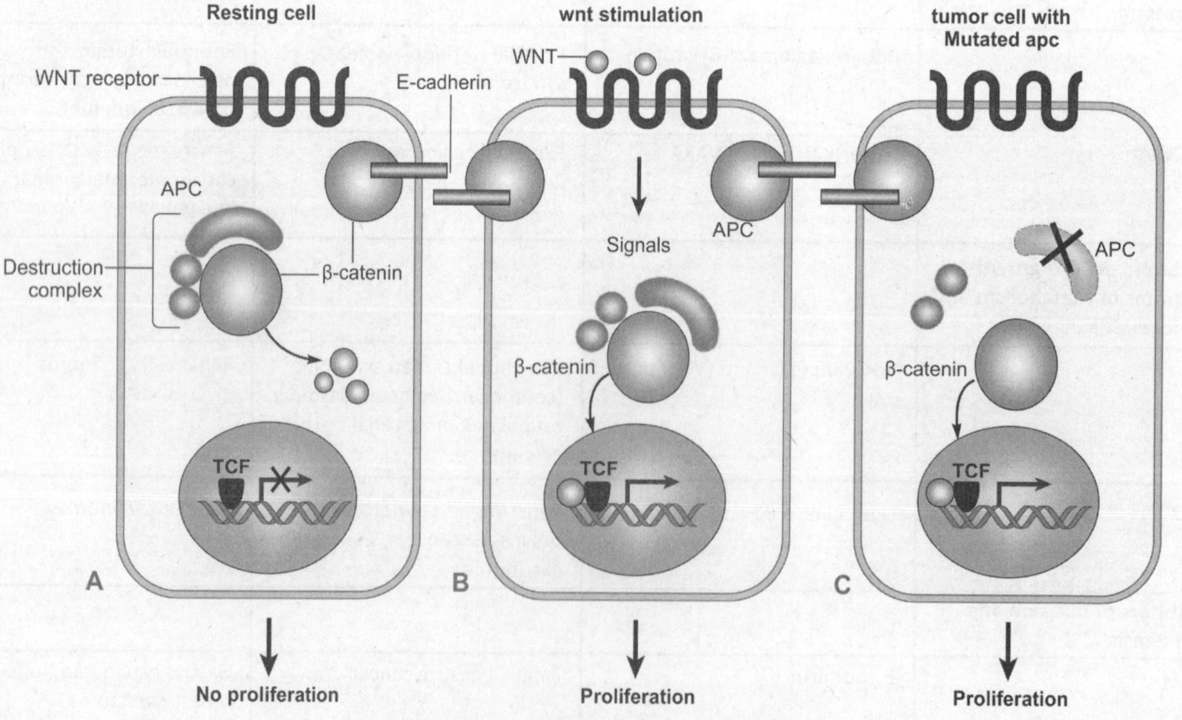

WNT- APC- β-catenin signalling pathway

- Gene is located in **cytosol** Q of the cell
- **Adenomatous polyposis coli** genes (APC) Q are example of **tumor suppressors** Q
- Germ-line mutations at the **APC (5q21)** loci are associated with **familial adenomatous polyposis** Q
- APC protein down-regulate **β-catenin** Q
- **Dysregulation** of **APC/β-catenin pathway** leads to **colon cancers**, **hepatoblastomas** and **hepatocellular carcinomas** Q

Ans. 27) D. Neurofibromin facilitates the conversion of the RAS from an inactive to active stage (Ref: 8 ed. Robbins p. 294-95, f-7-26, 9 ed. p. 298)

NF1 Q:

- **Tumor suppressor gene**, located in **inner aspect of plasma membrane**
- Encodes protein **Neurofibromin** Q, which is a **GAP (GTPase activating protein)**
- Located on **chromosome 17q11** Q and facilitates the conversion of RAS from an active to inactive stage
- **NF - 1 mutation** is associated with **optic nerve gliomas** Q, **neurofibromas** Q, **Lisch nodules** Q **and café-au-lait spots**

Ans. 28) D. All of the above (Ref: 8 ed. Robbins p. 292-94, 9 ed. p. 298)

NF-2 gene:

- Product of the **NF2 gene** is **neurofibromin 2** or **merlin** Q
- **Germline mutation** in **NF2 gene** predispose to the development of **neurofibromatosis type 2**
- **Mutation** predisposes to **bilateral acoustic nerve Schwannoma** Q, **meningiomas** Q and **ependymomas** Q

Ans. 29) A. Aerobic glycolysis (Ref: 8 ed. Robbins p. 303-04, 9 ed. p. 300-01)

Warburg effect/ Aerobic glycolysis Q:

- **Cancer cells shows** a cellular metabolism **characterized** by **high levels of glucose uptake** and **increased conversion of glucose** to **lactose** via the **glycolytic pathway** Q
- **Cancer cells** rely on **aerobic glycolysis** yielding only **2 ATP's** and not on oxidative phosphorylation which yields 36 ATP's. Why?

Answer:

- **Aerobic glycolysis** provides rapidly **dividing tumor cells** with **metabolic intermediates**, needed for synthesis of **cellular components** Q
- **Mitochondrial oxidative phosphorylation** does not provide **metabolic intermediates** Q

Ans. 30) D. In cancer cells telomerase activity is lost (Ref: 8 ed. Robbins p. 296-97, 9 ed. p. 303-04, f- 7-34)

- **Normal human cell** becomes **senescent** after **60 to 70 doublings**, which occurs due to **progressive shortening** of **telomeres** at the ends of chromosomes Q
- In tumor cells **telomerase activity** is **up-regulated** Q
- **Telomerase enzyme** is **absent** from **normal somatic cells** and thus they lead to progressive **loss of telomeres** Q
- **Telomerase activity** has been noted in more than **90%** of **human tumors**

Ans. 31) D. BCL2 overexpressing lymphocytes arise due to explosive cell proliferation (Ref: 8 ed. Robbins p. 296-97)

Follicular B-cell lymphomas:

- Shows a characteristic **t (14; 18)** Q **translocation**
- Results in overexpression of the **BCL2 protein** Q, which is an **anti-apoptotic** protein
- Leads to a steady accumulation of **B-lymphocytes**, resulting in **lymphadenopathy** and **marrow infiltration**
- **BCL2 overexpressing** lymphocytes arise from **reduced cell death** of lymphocytes rather than **explosive cell proliferation**
- Hence, **B-cell lymphomas** are **indolent (slow growing)** Q as compared to other lymphomas

Ans. 32) D. bFGF (Ref: 8 ed. Robbins p. 298, 9 ed. p. 305-06)

- Relative lack of oxygen stimulates **HIF1α**, which then activates variety of **pro-angiogenic** cytokines, such as **VEGF** Q and **bFGF** Q **(basic fibroblast growth factor)**
- **Potent angiogenesis inhibitors** Q include – **angiostatin**, **endostatin**, **thrombospondin-1** and **vasculostatin**

Ans. 33) A. CXCR4 (Ref: 8 ed. Robbins p. 300, 9 ed. p. 308)

Chemokines:

- Play an **important role** in determining the site (target tissue) for **metastasis**

Example:

- **Breast cancer cells** express the **chemokine receptors CXCR4** Q and **CCR7** Q
- **Chemokine receptors** are found in the tissues in which **breast cancers metastasize** Q
- Breast cancer metastasis to the **lymph nodes** and **lungs**, can be decreased by blocking the interaction between **CXCR4** and its **receptor** Q

Ans. 34) D. Any of the above (Ref: 9 ed. Robbins p. 308)

- Stage of **dormancy** i.e. prolonged survival of **micrometastases** Q without progression is described in **melanoma, breast cancer** and **prostate cancer** Q

Ans. 35) B. RANKL (Ref: 8 ed. Robbins p. 300, 9 ed. p. 309)

- **Breast carcinomas** metastasizing to the bone produces **osteolytic lesion** Q
- Breast cancer cells secrete **parathyroid hormone–related protein (PTHRP)** Q, which stimulates **osteoblasts** Q to make **RANK ligand (RANKL)** Q
- **RANKL activates osteoclasts**, which **leads to degradation** of bone matrix and release of the growth factors like **IGF** and **TGF-β**

Ans. 36) D. Lung is the most common site of metastasis (Ref: 8 ed. Robbins p. 269-70, 9 ed. p. 274-75)

- **Liver** Q is the **most common site** of **metastasis** and not lung

Ans. 37) D. miR 10b inhibits metastasis (Ref: 8 ed. Robbins p. 302, 9 ed. p. 309)

Micro-RNAs:

- **miR 335** and **miR 126 suppress** metastasis of **breast cancer**
- **miR 10b** Q **promote** metastasis

Note: SNAIL and **TWIST**, promote a **process** called **epithelial-to-mesenchymal transition (EMT)** in **breast cancers** Q

Epithelial Mesenchymal Transition Q:

- Carcinoma cells **down-regulate** certain epithelial markers (e.g., **E-cadherin**) Q
- Carcinoma cells **up-regulate** certain mesenchymal markers (e.g., **vimentin** and **smooth muscle actin**) Q
- **SNAIL and TWIST** down-regulate **E-cadherin expression**, a key event in EMT

Ans. 38) D. All of the above (Ref: 8 ed. Robbins p. 302, 9 ed. p. 301)

Autophagy:

- In situations of **oxygen** and **glucose deprivation**, cells arrest their growth and cannibalize their own organelles, proteins and membranes for energy production
- **PTEN** Q: **Tumor suppressor** gene, which **promote autophagy** in tumor cells
- In order for its survival, **tumor cells** use **autophagy** to become **"dormant"**, making themselves resistant to therapies that kill actively dividing cells

Ans. 39) D. t(14;18) – Burkitt lymphoma (Ref: 8 ed. Robbins p. 305-06, 9 ed. p. 316-17, t-7-8)

- In **Burkitt lymphoma** Q the most common form of translocation is **t (8:14)** Q
- In **CML** Q, **BCR-ABL fusion** Q protein has a **molecular weight** of **210kD** Q, whereas in **ALL** Q, **190-kD** Q protein is formed

Ans. 40) B. Osteosarcomas (Ref: 9 ed. Robbins p. 318-19)

- Genomic sequencing has brought **chromosome "catastrophes"** termed **chromothrypsis (chromosome shattering)** Q as a cause of **rearrangements**
- **Chromothrypsis** is seen in: **osteosarcomas** Q and **gliomas** Q

Ans. 41) A. miR-200 (Ref: 9 ed. Robbins p. 320)

Non-coding RNA's:

- **OncomiRs** – are important for **invasiveness** and **metastasis of tumor cells**. Examples – **miR-200** Q, **miR-155**

- **Tumor suppressive miRs – miR-15** and **miR-16** are **frequent genetic lesions** seen in **chronic lymphocytic leukemia**Q

Ans. 42) B. UV-B (Ref: 9 ed. Robbins p. 324)

- **UV rays** from solar system are divided into **three wavelength ranges: UVA (320-400 nm), UVB (280-320 nm) and UVC (200-280 nm)**
- **UVB** Q is believed to be responsible for the **induction of cutaneous cancers** Q
- **UVC**, a **potent mutagen**, is filtered out by the **ozone layer** surrounding the earth

Also know,

- **Most frequent cancers** due to **Ionizing radiation** are **myeloid neoplasms** Q

Ans. 43) D. Gag, pol, env plays a role in cancer development (Ref: 8 ed. Robbins p. 312-13, 9 ed. p. 325-26)

Human T-cell leukemia virus type 1 (HTLV-1) Q:

- Causative agent for cancer in humans
- Similar to the human immunodeficiency virus, **HTLV-1** has **tropism** for CD4+ T cells Q and also contains the ***gag, pol, env*** and long-terminal-repeat regions
- ***Tax*** Q – Another region, which plays an **important role** in **development of leukemia**
- **HTLV-1 infection** causes **cell proliferation** through **stimulatory effects of *Tax***, which leads to an **increased risk of mutations** and **genomic instability**

Ans. 44) A. Oncogenic RNA virus (Ref: 8 ed. Robbins p. 313-14, 9 ed. p. 326-27, f-7-45)

Human Papilloma Virus (HPV):

- **Oncogenic DNA virus** Q
- HPV subtypes (e.g., 1, 2, 4 and 7) cause **benign squamous papillomas (warts)** Q
- **High-risk HPVs** (e.g. **types 16 and 18**) Q have been **implicated** in **squamous cell carcinoma (SCC) of the cervix** Q and **anogenital region** Q
- **Genital warts** have **low malignant potential** and **are associated** with **low-risk HPVs**, predominantly **HPV-6** Q **and HPV-11** Q
- **Oncogenic potential** Q of HPV can be related to the products of two viral genes, **E6 and E7** Q

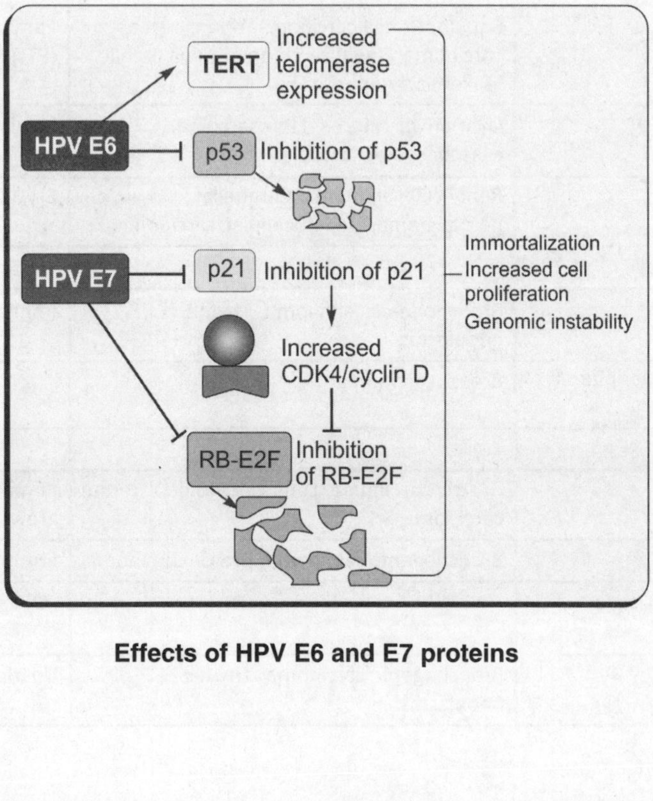

Effects of HPV E6 and E7 proteins

Ans. 45) A. LMP-1 (Ref: 8 ed. Robbins p. 314-15, 9 ed. p. 327, f-7-46)

Epstein - Barr virus (EBV) Q:

- Infects **B lymphocytes** Q using the **complement receptor CD21** Q
- Has **strong association** with **Burkitt Lymphoma** Q especially in **immunosuppressed patients**
- EBV gene, **latent membrane protein-1 (LMP-1)** Q, acts as an **oncogene** and induces **B-cell lymphomas** Q
- **Nasopharyngeal carcinoma** Q, **Hodgkin lymphoma** Q is also associated with EBV infection

Ans. 46) D. All of the above (Ref: 8 ed. Robbins p. 316, 9 ed. p. 329)

H. pylori infection Q:

- Leads to **chronic gastritis**
- Implicated in the development of **gastric adenocarcinomas** and **gastric lymphomas** Q
- ***Cytotoxin-associated A (CagA)*** gene is associated with **gastric adenocarcinoma**
- **Gastric lymphomas** are of **B-cell** Q origin and are called as **lymphomas of mucosa-associated lymphoid tissue, or MALTomas** Q

Ans. 47) D. Small-cell carcinoma of lung (Ref: 8 ed. Robbins p. 321-22, 9 ed. p. 330-31, t-7-11)

- **Endocrinopathies** are frequently encountered **Para-neoplastic syndromes**
- **Cushing syndrome** Q is most commonly seen in **small-cell carcinoma of lung** Q, which is due to excessive production of **corticotrophin** Q
- **Hypercalcemia** Q {due to **Parathyroid hormone–related protein (PTHRP)**} Q is seen in **SCC lung** Q, **Breast carcinoma** Q, **Renal cell carcinoma** Q, **Adult T-cell leukemia/lymphoma** Q

Paraneoplastic syndromes Q:

Clinical syndromes	**Major forms of underlying cancer**	**Causal mechanism**
Endocrinopathies Q		
Cushing syndrome	Small-cell carcinoma of lung, Pancreatic carcinoma, Neural tumors	ACTH or ACTH-like substance
Syndrome of inappropriate antidiuretic hormone secretion	Small-cell carcinoma of lung, Intracranial neoplasms	Antidiuretic hormone or atrial natriuretic hormones
Hypercalcemia	Squamous cell carcinoma of lung, Breast carcinoma, Renal carcinoma, Adult T-cell leukemia/lymphoma	Parathyroid hormone-related protein (PTHRP), TGF-α, TNF, IL-1
Hypoglycemia	Ovarian carcinoma, Fibrosarcoma, Mesenchymal sarcomas	Insulin or insulin-like substance
Polycythemia	Renal cell carcinoma, Cerebellar hemangioma, Hepatocellular carcinoma	Erythropoietin
Nerve and Muscle syndromes Q		
Myasthenia	Bronchogenic carcinoma, Thymic neoplasms	Immunologic
Disorders of the central and peripheral nervous system	Breast carcinoma	
Dermatologic Disorders Q		
Acanthosis nigricans	Gastric carcinoma, Lung carcinoma, Uterine carcinoma	Immunologic; secretion of epidermal growth factor
Dermatomyositis	Bronchogenic carcinoma, Breast carcinoma	Immunologic
Osseous, Articular and Soft Tissue Changes Q		
Hypertrophic osteoarthropathy and clubbing of the fingers	Bronchogenic carcinoma, Thymic neoplasms	Unknown

Contd.

Contd.

Vascular and Hematologic Changes [Q]		
Venous thrombosis (Trousseau phenomenon)	Pancreatic carcinoma, Bronchogenic carcinoma, Other cancers	Tumor products (mucins that activate clotting)
Disseminated intravascular coagulation	Acute promyelocytic leukemia, Prostatic carcinoma	Tumor products that activate clotting
Nonbacterial thrombotic endocarditis	Advanced cancers	Hypercoagulability
Red cell aplasia	Thymic neoplasms	Unknown
Others		
Nephrotic syndrome	Various cancers	Tumor antigens, immune complexes

Ans. 48) D. All of the above (Ref: 9 ed. Robbins p. 334)

Uses of Immunohistochemistry [Q]:

- Categorization of undifferentiated malignant tumors
- Determination of site of origin of metastatic tumors
- Detection of molecules that have prognostic or therapeutic significance

Ans. 49) A. DNA sequencing (Ref: 8 ed. Robbins p. 321-22, 9 ed. p. 330-31)

NextGen sequencing [Q]:

- **DNA sequencing methods** which rely massively on **parallel sequencing**
- **DNA sequencing**, is technically, **simpler** that RNA sequencing

Ans. 50) B. HCG – Seminoma (Ref: 8 ed. Robbins p. 326-27, 9 ed. p. 337-38, t-7-12)

- **AFP and HCG** [Q] levels are **elevated** in more than 80% of individuals with **NSGCT (Non Seminomatous germ cell tumor)** [Q]
- Only in 15% of **seminomas** have elevated HCG levels
- **CEA** [Q] – Increased in carcinomas of the colon, pancreas, stomach and breast
- **AFP** [Q] – Hepatocellular carcinomas [Q], yolk sac cancers, teratocarcinomas and embryonal cell carcinomas
- **CA-125** [Q] – Ovarian cancer [Q]
- **CA-19-9** [Q] – Colon cancer, pancreatic cancer [Q]
- **CA-15-3** [Q] – Breast cancer

Selected tumor markers	
Tumor markers [Q]	**Tumor types** [Q]
Hormones [Q]	
Human chorionic gonadotropin	Trophoblastic tumors, Nonseminomatous testicular tumors
Calcitonin	Medullary carcinoma of thyroid
Catecholamine and metabolites	Pheochromocytoma and related tumors
Oncofetal Antigens [Q]	
α-Fetoprotein	Liver cell cancer, Nonseminomatous germ cell tumors of testis
Carcinoembryonic antigen	Carcinomas of the colon, pancreas, lung, stomach and heart
Isoenzymes [Q]	
Prostatic acid phosphatase	Prostate cancer
Neuron-specific enolase	Small-cell cancer of lung, Neuroblastoma

Contd.

Contd.

Specific Proteins [Q]	
Immunoglobulins	Multiple myeloma and other gammopathies
Prostate-specific antigen and prostate-specific membrane antigen	Prostate cancer
Mucins and Other Glycoproteins [Q]	
CA-125	Ovarian cancer
CA-19-9	Colon cancer, Pancreatic cancer
CA-15-3	Breast cancer
Cell-Free DNA Markers [Q]	
TP53, APC, RAS mutants in stool and serum	Colon cancer
TP53, RAS mutants in stool and serum	Pancreatic cancer
TP53, RAS mutants in sputum and serum	Lung cancer
TP53 mutants in urine	Bladder cancer

Ans. 51) A. 25 U/ ml

- Normal value of CA-125 is less than 35 U/mL **Refer Q 50 for details**

Ans. 52) C. Metaplasia (Ref: 9th ed. Robbins p. 270-271) Refer Q 1 for details

Ans. 53) D. Nitrates - skin cancer (Ref: 8 ed. Robbins p. 274) Refer Q 14 and 15 for details

Ans. 54) B. Pancreatitis (Ref: 9 ed. Robbins p. 337) Refer Q 50 for details

Ans. 55) A. PTHrP (Ref: 9 ed. Robbins p. 330-31)

Paraneoplastic hypercalcemia of malignancy:

- Parathyroid hormone-related protein (PTHRP) is the most important hormone responsible for it
- Seen in carcinomas of the breast, lung, kidney and ovary

Ans. 56) A. KIT (Ref: 9 ed. Robbins p. 284) Refer Q 18 for details

Ans. 57) A. Warburg (Ref: 9 ed. Robbins p. 300) (Refer Q 29 for details)

Ans. 58) D. H. pylori infection increases the risk (Ref: 9 ed. Robbins p. 329) Refer Q 46 for details

Ans. 59) A. Li Fraumeni syndrome (Ref: 9 ed. Robbins p. 279-80) Refer Q 12 for details

Ans. 60) A. Degree of differentiation (Ref: 9 ed. Robbins p. 267-271)

Grading of tumor is based on the degree of differentiation of tumor cells and the number of mitosis within the tumor

Ans. 61) B. 13q (Ref: 9 ed. Robbins p. 291)

Ans. 62) A. Pancreatic carcinoma (Ref: 9 ed. Robbins p. 284)

Ans. 63) C. Desmoplasia (Ref: 9 ed. Robbins p 266)

Ans. 64) A. Hepatocellular carcinoma (Ref: 9 ed. Robbins p. 337) Refer Q 50 for details

Ans. 65) A. Hamartoma (Ref: 9 ed. Robbins p 267-69) Refer Q 1 for details

Ans. 66) A. Osteosarcoma (Ref: 9 ed. Robbins p. p. 292-93) Refer Q 23 for details

Ans. 67) D. Transcription activator (Ref: 9 ed. Robbins p. 292-93) Refer Q 21 for details

Ans. 68) D. RB (Ref: 9 ed. Robbins 292-93) Refer Q 23 for details

Ans. 69) A. Xeroderma Pigmentosum (Ref: 9 ed. Robbins p. 314)

- Xeroderma Pigmentosum – inherited disorder of DNA repair

Ans. 70) A. CEA (9 ed. Robbins p. 337-38) Refer Q 50 for details

Ans. 71) B. Causing carcinogenesis (Ref: 9 ed. Robbins p. 303-04) Refer Q 30 for details

Ans. 72) A. CA-125 (Ref: 9 ed. Robbins p. 337-38) Refer Q 50 for details

Ans. 73) B. End of G1 (Ref: 9 ed. Robbins p. 292-93) Refer Q 21 and 22 for details

Ans. 74) C. G1-S phase (Ref: 9 ed. Robbins p. 25-26, 292-93) Refer Q 22 for details

8 Infectious Diseases

How to go about this chapter?

- **Be thorough with the following topics:**
  - **Common viral infections and its histopathological features especially HSV, CMV and EBV**
  - **Mycobacterium tuberculosis**
  - **Mycobacterium avium-intracellulare complex**
  - **Mycobacterium leprae**
  - **Syphilis**
  - **Fungus – candida, aspergillus, zygomycosis, mucor, dimorphic fungi**
  - **Parasitic infections – Plasmodium vivax, falciparum, hydatid disease**
  - **Recent advances in infectious diseases**

TECHNIQUES FOR DIAGNOSING INFECTIOUS AGENTS

1) **Mucicarmine stain is used to diagnose:**
a) Mycobacteria b) Amebae
c) Fungi d) Cryptococci

VIRAL INFECTIONS

2) **Cell surface receptor(s) which bind to viral hemagglutinin protein in measles:**
a) CD46 b) SLAM
c) Nectin 4 d) All of the above

3) **Following is seen in measles:**
a) Osteoclastic giant cells
b) Langhans giant cells
c) Toutan's giant cells
d) Warthin-Finkeldey cells

4) **Most common extra-salivary gland complication of mumps:**
a) Orchitis b) Pancreatitis
c) Aseptic meningitis d) Encephalitis

5) **Cause for genital herpes:**
a) HSV-1 b) HSV-2
c) HHV-8 d) HHV-7

6) **Latency in EBV infection is seen due to following protein(s):**
a) EBNA-1 b) LMP-1
c) EBNA-2 d) Any of the above

7) **Atypical lymphocytes in EBV infection, seen in blood can be:**
a) CD8+- T-cells
b) CD4+-T-cells
c) Both of the above
d) None of the above

8) **All are TRUE about EBV infection EXCEPT:**
a) Atypical lymphocytes
b) Expansion of paracortical areas by T-cells
c) Intranuclear basophilic inclusions
d) Spleen is enlarged in most of cases

9) **Following is the most specific criteria for diagnosing infectious mononucleosis:**
a) Atypical lymphocytosis
b) Positive monospot test
c) Rising titer of EBV nuclear antigen
d) Hypogammaglobulinemia

BACTERIAL INFECTIONS

10) **A pregnant female on non-vegetarian diet, presents with fever and neck rigidity since one week. On admission, CSF analysis were performed and it shows presence of gram positive intracellular bacteria, which most likely would be:**
a) Listeria monocytogenes
b) Toxoplasmosis
c) Mycobacterium tuberculosis
d) Cryptococcus

11) All are TRUE about the tuberculosis EXCEPT:
a) Incidence is increasing due to HIV
b) Mantoux test detects the disease
c) Viable organisms may remain dormant for ages in lungs
d) Flourishes in poverty, crowding and debilitating diseases

12) Which of the following cell helps to restrict tuberculosis infection?
a) T_H1 b) T_H2
c) B cell d) Plasma cell

13) Genetic polymorphism in the following gene leads to ineffective immune response to T.B.:
a) LMP-1 b) EBNA-2
c) NRAMP-1 d) TLR2

14) All of the following are TRUE about secondary tuberculosis EXCEPT:
a) Arises in a previously sensitized host
b) Involves the apex of the upper lobes
c) Presents with lower and middle lobe consolidation
d) Reinfection plays an important role

15) All are the components of tubercular granuloma EXCEPT:
a) Caseous necrosis
b) Epithelioid histiocytes
c) Lymphocytes
d) Neutrophils

16) CD 4 cell count for developing the MAC infection:
a) <400 cells/mm^3 b) <300 cells/mm^3
c) <100 cells/mm^3 d) <60 cells/mm^3

17) All are TRUE about M. leprae EXCEPT:
a) Complete protection against infection through BCG
b) Favor cooler areas of skin
c) T_H1 response plays a role
d) Extremely slow course

18) Neuronal involvement dominates in:
a) Tuberculoid leprosy
b) Lepromatous leprosy
c) Both of the above
d) None of the above

19) All are TRUE about Lepromatous leprosy EXCEPT:
a) Affects CNS
b) Also called as multibacillary leprosy
c) Leonine facies is a distinctive feature
d) Associated with male sterility

20) All are TRUE about syphilis EXCEPT:
a) Spirochetes are abundant in the chancre
b) Secondary syphilis is characterized by skin lesions over trunk
c) Neurosyphilis manifests as tabes dorsalis and general paresis
d) Early congenital syphilis is manifested by nasal discharge and congestion

21) All are TRUE about syphilitic gumma EXCEPT:
a) Also called as benign tertiary syphilis
b) Resembles tubercles
c) Involves skin, subcutaneous tissue and bone
d) Treponemas are abundant in gummas

22) Saddle nose deformity is seen in:
a) Congenital Syphilis
b) Primary Syphilis
c) Secondary Syphilis
d) None of the above

FUNGAL INFECTIONS

23) All are TRUE about candidiasis EXCEPT:
a) *C. albicans* is the most frequent cause
b) Appears as yeast like forms in tissue sections
c) Septate hyphae are the most important diagnostic clue
d) Periodic acid–Schiff (PAS) is most commonly used to identify them

24) Following special stain is used to visualize fungus:
a) Gomori Methenamine-silver stain
b) Perl's stain
c) Prussian blue stain
d) Reticulin stain

25) Most common fungus responsible for endocarditis:
a) Candida b) Cryptococcus
c) Aspergillus d) Mucor

26) All are true about Cryptococcosis EXCEPT:
a) Has a yeast form
b) In lung it presents as a coin lesion
c) India ink preparation is used to visualize the pseudohyphae
d) Can cause disseminated disease

27) All are correctly matched regarding Aspergillus infection EXCEPT:
a) Aspergillus fumigatus – ABPA
b) Aspergilloma – target lesions
c) Invasive aspergillosis – neutropenia
d) Aspergillus – septate hyphae and fruiting bodies

28) All are TRUE about zygomycosis EXCEPT:
a) Includes Rhizopus, Mucor species
b) More common in immunocompromised individuals
c) Forms non septate hyphae with acute angle branching
d) Rhinocerebral mucormycosis is a mostly notable in diabetics

29) Dimorphic fungi include(s):
a) Blastomycosis

b) Histoplasma
c) Coccidioidomyces
d) All of the above

PARASITIC INFECTIONS

30) All are TRUE regarding Malaria infection EXCEPT:
a) Infectious stage is *sporozoite*
b) In hepatocytes, *merozoite* form is seen
c) First stage of parasite is *trophozoite*
d) *P. falciparum* forms latent *hypnozoites* in hepatocytes

31) *P. falciparum* causes more severe disease because:
a) It is able to infect red blood cells of any age
b) Causes infected red cells to clump together (rosette)
c) Stimulates production of high levels of cytokines
d) All of the above

32) All of the following confers resistance to malaria infection EXCEPT:
a) HbS b) HbC
c) HbD d) Duffy antigen

33) Dürck granulomas are seen in:
a) Liver b) Spleen
c) Brain d) Kidney

34) Maltese cross appearance is a characteristic feature of:
a) Trypanosomiasis
b) Plasmodium vivax
c) Plasmodium falciparum
d) Babesiosis

35) All of the following are correct about Hydatid disease EXCEPT:
a) Caused by *E. granulosus*
b) For *E. granulosus*, definitive hosts are dogs
c) Cysts are most commonly found in lung
d) Daughter cysts often develop into large mother cyst

36) Which of the following is the recently described infectious agent?
a) HIV b) KSHV
c) West-Nile fever d) SARS coronavirus

37) Obliterative endarteritis of the vasa vasorum of aorta is seen in: (NEET 2014)
a) Syphilis b) Wegener's
c) Churg Strauss d) Cold hemoglobinuria

38) Warthin-finkeldey cells are seen in: (NEET 2014)
a) Measles b) Mumps
c) Rubella d) Poliomyelitis

39) A man presents with maculopapular rash. He gives a history of previous painless rash. Infection is due to: (AIPGMEE 2012)
a) Treponema pallidum
b) Chlamydia
c) Haemophilus ducreyi
d) Granulomatous disease

40) Which of the following is a special stain used to diagnose fungal hyphae in tissues? (AIIMS May 2013)
a) Masson trichome
b) Silver methenamine
c) Congo Red
d) Alizarin Red

41) Phagocytosis of Mycobacterium Tuberculosis by macrophages is mainly mediated by: (AIIMS May 2014)
a) IL6 b) IL3
c) IL 12 d) IFN gamma

42) Lipogranulomatous condition is: (AIIMS May 2014)
a) TB b) Viral
c) Fungal d) Chalazion

43) A farmer presents with multiple discharging sinuses. HPE showed the following and confirms diagnosis of: (AIIMS Nov 2015)

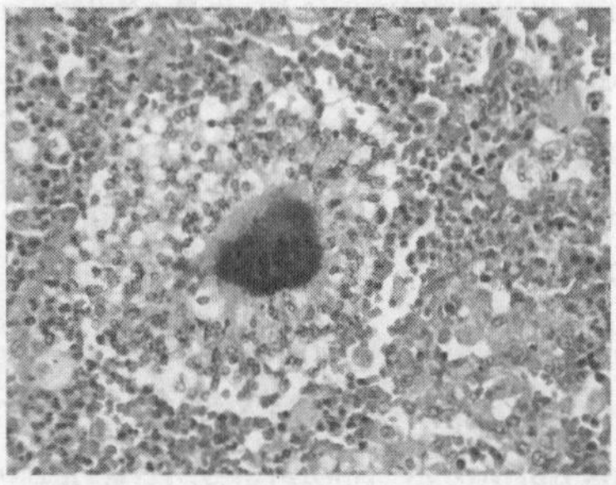

a) Actinomycosis b) Nocardiosis
c) Mycetoma d) Candida

44) Following malarial parasite is shown in the center of photomicrograph: (AIIMS Nov. 2015)

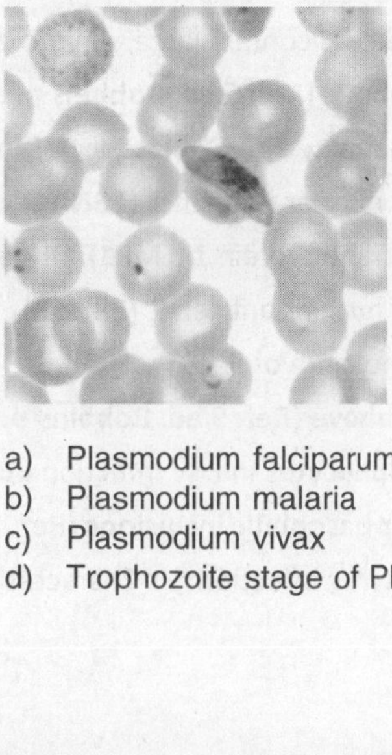

a) Plasmodium falciparum
b) Plasmodium malaria
c) Plasmodium vivax
d) Trophozoite stage of Plasmodium ovale

CHAPTER 8: INFECTIOUS DISEASES

Ans. 1) D. Cryptococci (Ref: 9 ed. Robbins p. 353-54)

Special Techniques for **Diagnosing Infectious Agents** Q:

Techniques	Infectious Agents
Gram stain	Most bacteria
Acid-fast stain	Mycobacteria, Nocardiae (modified)
Silver stains	Fungi, Legionellae, Pneumocystis
Periodic acid-schiff	Fungi, Amebae
Mucicarmine	Cryptococci
Giemsa	Campylobacter, Leishmaniae, Malaria parasites
Molecular diagnostic assays	Gonorrhea, chlamydial infection, tuberculosis and herpes encephalitis

Ans. 2) All of the above (Ref: 9 ed. Robbins p. 355)

Three cell-surface receptors have been identified for the **virus** Q:

- **CD46** (a complement regulatory protein that **inactivates C3 convertase**): Expressed on **all nucleated cells** Q
- **Signaling lymphocytic activation molecule (SLAM)**: Expressed on **cells of the immune system** Q
- **Nectin 4**: Expressed on **epithelial cells** Q

Ans. 3) D. Warthin-Finkeldey cells (Ref: 9 ed. Robbins p. 355, f-8-8)

Morphology of Lymphoid Organs in Measles:

- Marked follicular hyperplasia, large germinal centers
- **Warthin-Finkeldey cells** Q – **multinucleate giant cells**, which have **eosinophilic nuclear and cytoplasmic inclusion bodies**

Ans. 4) C. Aseptic meningitis (Ref: 9 ed. Robbins p. 356)

- **Aseptic meningitis** Q is the most **common extra-salivary gland** complication of **mumps infection**
- **Mumps parotitis** is bilateral in 70% of cases

Ans. 5) B. HSV-2 (Ref: 9 ed. Robbins p. 357-58, f-8-9)

- **Gingivostomatitis**, encountered in children is caused by **HSV-1** Q
- **Genital herpes** is most often caused by **HSV-2** Q
- **HSV-2** can be transmitted to **neonates** during the passage through the birth canal of infected mothers
- **Herpes viruses** are responsible for **latent infections** in **humans** Q
- HSV-infected cells contain large, pink to purple **(Cowdry type A) intranuclear inclusions** Q

Ans. 6) D. Any of the above (Ref: 9 ed. Robbins p. 360-61, f-8-13)

EBV proteins that play a role in **latency of infection** Q:

- Epstein-Barr nuclear antigen 1 **(EBNA1)**
- Latent membrane protein 1 **(LMP1)**: Drives B cell activation and proliferation by mimicking active form of **CD 40** Q
- Epstein-Barr nuclear antigen 2 **(EBNA2)**
- **vIL-10** – homologue of IL-10

Ans. 7) C. Both of the above (Ref: 9 ed. Robbins p. 361)

- **Atypical lymphocytes** in EBV infection includes **EBV-specific CD8+ cytotoxic T cells** Q and **CD16+ NK cells** Q

Ans. 8) C. Intra-nuclear basophilic inclusions (Ref: 8 ed. Robbins p. 354-57, 9 ed. p. 359-62, f-8-12-13)

- ***Cytomegalovirus* infection** Q – Characteristic feature is prominent **basophilic intra-nuclear inclusions**

- In **HSV** Q – **Glassy intra-nuclear** herpes simplex **inclusion bodies** Q are seen

Epstein Bar Virus Q:

- **Peripheral blood** – shows **absolute lymphocytosis** Q; composed of **atypical lymphocytes** Q
- **Lymph node morphology** – most striking feature is **expansion of Para cortical areas** by **activated T cells**
- **Splenomegaly** and **hepatomegaly** are **commonly seen**

Ans. 9) C. Rising titer of EBV nuclear antigen (Ref: 9 ed. Robbins p. 361-62)

Diagnosis of **Infectious mononucleosis** depends on the **following findings** in **increasing order of specificity** Q:

a) **Lymphocytosis** with characteristic **atypical lymphocytes** Q in the peripheral blood

b) **Positive heterophile antibody reaction (Monospot test)** Q

c) **Rising titer of specific antibodies for EBV antigens** Q (viral capsid antigens, early antigens, or **Epstein-Barr nuclear antigen**)

Ans. 10) A. Listeria monocytogenes (Ref: 9 ed. Robbins p. 366)

Listeria monocytogenes Q:

- **Gram-positive bacillus** that causes severe **food-borne infections** in vulnerable hosts
- Food products contaminated with bacteria includes **dairy products, chicken** and **hot dogs** Q
- **Pregnant women** Q, neonates, older adults and immunosuppressed persons are particularly **susceptible**
- Evokes an **exudative pattern of inflammation** Q with **numerous neutrophils**
- **Meningitis** Q is indistinguishable from other bacteria
- **CSF microscopy** – presence of **gram-positive**, mostly **intracellular bacilli** is **diagnostic** Q

Ans. 11) B. Mantoux test detects the disease (Ref: 8 ed. Robbins p. 366-67, 9 ed. p. 371)

Mycobacterium Tuberculosis Q:

- Is responsible for tuberculosis
- Infection with **HIV** makes people more susceptible
- Tuberculosis flourishes in poverty, crowding and chronic debilitating illness
- Increased risk in diabetes mellitus, Hodgkin lymphoma, chronic lung disease (e.g. silicosis), chronic renal failure, malnutrition, alcoholism and immunosuppression
- **Infection**: Presence of organisms, which may or may not cause clinically significant disease

Mantoux test Q:

- **Delayed hypersensitivity** to ***M. tuberculosis* antigens**
- **Intra-cutaneous injection** of **purified protein derivative (PPD)** of *M. tuberculosis* induces a visible and palpable induration that peaks in **48 to 72 hours** Q
- **Positive tuberculin test** signifies **T cell–mediated immunity** Q to **mycobacterial antigens** and **does not differentiate** between **infection** and **disease**
- **False-negative reactions** Q – Viral infections, sarcoidosis, malnutrition, Hodgkin lymphoma, immunosuppression and overwhelming active tuberculous disease
- **False-positive reactions** Q – Infection by **atypical mycobacteria** or **prior vaccination** with **BCG** (Bacillus Calmette-Guerin)

Ans. 12) A. T_H1 (Ref: 8 ed. Robbins p. 367-68, 9 ed. p. 371-72, f-8-24)

Mycobacterial antigens are displayed to T cells, which differentiates into **T_H1** cells

Mature T_H1 cells:

- Produces **IFN-γ** Q, which enables macrophages to contain *M. tuberculosis* infection
- Results in formation of **granulomas** Q and **caseous necrosis**
- Activated macrophages differentiate into **"epithelioid histiocytes"** Q that characterize **granulomatous response**

Ans. 13) C. NRAMP-1 (Ref: 8 ed. Robbins p. 368)

- **Polymorphisms** in the **NRAMP1 gene** Q leads to ineffective immune response to tuberculosis

Ans. 14) C. Presents with lower and middle lobe consolidation (Ref: 8 ed. Robbins p. 368-69, 9 ed. p. 373-74, f-8-25)

Progressive primary tuberculosis:

- Presents with **lower** and **middle lobe consolidation** Q, **hilar lymphadenopathy** and **pleural effusion**
- Rare cavitation
- **Lymphohematogenous dissemination** may result in development of **tuberculous meningitis** and **miliary tuberculosis**

Secondary tuberculosis:

- Arises in **previously sensitized host**
- Due to reactivation of a **latent infection/reinfection**
- **Reactivation** Q is **more common** in **low-prevalence** Q areas, while **reinfection** Q plays an important role in **highly contagious** Q regions
- Involves the **apex** Q of **upper lobes** Q of one or both lungs

Ans. 15) D. Neutrophils (Ref: 8 ed. Robbins p. 370-71, 9 ed. p. 374-76, f-8-27)

Let us get familiar with following terms:

- **Ghon's focus** – 1- to 1.5 cm area of gray-white inflammation with consolidation

Ghon complex:

- **Tubercle bacilli**, either free or within phagocytes, drain to the **regional nodes**, which often show **caseation**
- Combination of **parenchymal lung lesion** and **nodal involvement** is referred to as **Ghon complex**

Granulomatous inflammatory reaction Q:

- Granulomas are composed of **caseous necrosis** surrounded by **epithelioid histiocytes**; **lymphocytes** and **multinucleate giant cells**

Ans. 16) D. <60 cells/mm^3 (Ref: 8 ed. Robbins p. 372, 9 ed. p. 376-77)

***M. avium-intracellulare* complex**, or **MAC**:

- Caused by *Mycobacterium avium* and *M. intracellulare* species
- Commonly seen in **AIDS** patients, with low numbers of **CD4+ lymphocytes (<60 cells/mm^3)** Q
- Granulomas, lymphocytes and tissue destruction are **rare**
- **Hallmark** in HIV patients–abundant **acid-fast bacilli** Q within macrophages

Ans. 17) A. Complete protection against infection through BCG (Ref: 8 ed. Robbins p. 372-73, 9 ed. p. 377-78)

Leprosy or Hansen's disease Q:

- **Slowly progressive infection** caused by **Mycobacterium leprae** Q
- Virulence is based on the properties of its **cell wall**
- **Cell wall** is similar to that of **M. tuberculosis** and **immunization** with **BCG** Q confers partial protection against M. leprae infection
- Cooler areas of skin are more severely affected than warmer areas

Patterns of disease by M. leprae:

- **Tuberculoid leprosy**
- **Lepromatous leprosy**
- **Intermediate form** called **borderline leprosy**

Note:

Tuberculoid leprosy patients have **T_H1 response** Q **associated** with production of **IL-2** and **IFN-γ** Q

Ans. 18) A. Tuberculoid leprosy (Ref: 8 ed. Robbins p. 372-73, 9 ed. p. 377)

- **Neuronal involvement** dominates **tuberculoid leprosy** [Q]
- **Nerves** become enclosed within **granulomatous inflammatory reactions** and are **destroyed** [Q]

Ans. 19) A. Affects CNS (Ref: 8 ed. Robbins p. 373-74, 9 ed. p. 377)

Lepromatous leprosy or **multibacillary leprosy** [Q]:

- Involves skin, peripheral nerves, anterior chamber of the eye, upper airways, testes, hands and feet
- **Vital organs** and **CNS** are **rarely** affected as their **core temperature** is **too high**
- Lesions contain **large aggregates** of **lipid-laden macrophages** which are filled with **masses ("globi") of acid-fast bacilli**
- **Nodular lesions** coalesce to yield a distinctive **leonine facies**
- **Testes** are usually **extensively involved**, leading to **sterility**

Ans. 20) B. Secondary syphilis is characterized by skin lesions over trunk (Ref: 8 ed. Robbins p. 374-77, 9 ed. p. 380-81)

Primary Syphilis [Q]:

- Characterized by a **single firm, non-tender, raised, red lesion (chancre)** [Q] on the penis, cervix, vaginal wall, or anus
- Spirochetes are plentiful within the **chancre**

Secondary Syphilis [Q]:

- Occurs due to the **proliferation of spirochetes** within skin and mucocutaneous tissues
- Skin lesions frequently occur on the **palms or soles** [Q] of the feet

Tertiary Syphilis:

a) Cardiovascular syphilis **(syphilitic aortitis)**
b) **Neurosyphilis** – presents as **tabes dorsalis** [Q], general paresis
c) **CSF examination** – shows **pleocytosis** [Q] (increased numbers of inflammatory cells), elevated protein levels, or **decreased glucose**
d) **Benign tertiary syphilis** – characterized by formation of **gummas**

Congenital Syphilis:

- Presents as early (infantile) and late (tardive) syphilis
- **Early congenital syphilis** is manifested by **nasal discharge** and **congestion (snuffles)** [Q]
- Late manifestations of congenital syphilis include a triad of **interstitial keratitis, Hutchinson teeth** and **eighth-nerve deafness**

Jarisch-Herxheimer reaction [Q]:

- Seen during **antibiotic treatment** of **syphilis**
- Patients with **high bacterial load**, following antibiotic therapy, leads to massive release of endotoxins, resulting in a **cytokine storm**
- Manifests with high fever, rigors, hypotension and leukopenia
- Also seen in **Lyme disease** [Q]

Ans. 21) D. Treponemas are abundant in gummas (Ref: 8 ed. Robbins p. 374-77, 9 ed. p. 381, f-8-34, 36)

Benign tertiary syphilis:

- Characterized by the **formation of gummas** [Q]
- Gummas are **most commonly** seen in bone, skin and the mucous membranes of the upper airway and joints
- **Gummas** vary in size from **microscopic lesions** resembling **tubercles** to **large tumor-like masses**
- **Hepar lobatum** – scarring because of gummas in the liver
- **Treponemas** are **scant** [Q] in **gummas** and are difficult to identify

Ans. 22) A. Congenital Syphilis (Ref: 8 ed. Robbins p. 377)

Congenital Syphilis is characterized by:

- Diffuse rash
- **Syphilitic osteochondritis** and **periostitis** – causing the **destruction of the vomer** leading to **collapse of the bridge of the nose** and characteristic **saddle nose deformity** Q
- **Liver** – Diffuse fibrosis, gummas being **rarely found** in the liver
- Late manifestations include a **distinctive triad** of **interstitial keratitis, Hutchinson teeth** and **eighth-nerve deafness** Q

Ans. 23) **C. Septate hyphae are the most important diagnostic clue (Ref: 8 ed. Robbins p. 382-84, 9 ed. p. 386-87, f-8-42)**

- In tissue sections, ***C. albicans*** can appear as **yeast like forms**
- **Pseudo hyphae** Q are an important diagnostic clue and **true hyphae** (defined by the presence of septae) are rarely seen
- Organisms may be visible with routine **hematoxylin and eosin** stain Q
- Special "fungal" stains include **Gomori methenamine–silver** Q **and periodic acid–Schiff** Q

Ans. 24) **A. Gomori Methenamine-silver stain (Ref: 8 ed. Robbins p. 384, 9 ed. p. 386)**

- Special fungal stains used are **Gomori methenamine-silver** and **periodic acid-Schiff** Q

Ans. 25) **A. Candida (Ref: 8 ed. Robbins p. 385, 9 ed. p. 387)**

- **Candida endocarditis** is the most common **fungal endocarditis** Q
- **Predisposing condition**: **Prosthetic heart valves** or **intravenous drug abusers** Q

Ans. 26) **C. India ink preparation is used to visualize the pseudo-hyphae (Ref: 8 ed. Robbins p. 384, 9 ed. p. 387-88, f-8-43)**

- **Cryptococcus neoformans** grows as **encapsulated yeast** Q and presents as an **opportunistic infection**
- **Cryptococcal yeast** has **thick gelatinous capsule** Q that stains **intense red** with **periodic acid-Schiff** and **Mucicarmine** Q
- **India ink** Q **preparations** create a **negative image** Q (**thick capsule** is seen as a **clear halo** in a dark background)
- **Lung** is the **primary site of infection** and forms **solitary pulmonary granuloma** Q similar to the **circumscribed (coin) lesion** caused by **Histoplasma** Q
- **C. neoformans** primarily affects **CNS** Q
- Immunosuppressed individuals can show involvement of meninges or perivascular Virchow-Robin spaces, producing **soap-bubble lesions** Q

Ans. 27) **B. Aspergilloma – target lesions (Ref: 8 ed. Robbins p. 384-85, 9 ed. p. 388-89, f-8-44)**

- **Aspergillus** is a mold that causes **allergies** (**Allergic bronchopulmonary aspergillosis**), often seen in **asthmatic people** Q
- **Aspergillus fumigatus** produces severe **invasive infections** in **immunocompromised individuals**
- **Invasive aspergillosis** is an **opportunistic infection**, associated with **neutropenia** and in lung, it forms **target lesions** Q
- Aspergillus forms **fruiting bodies** (usually in **lung cavities**) and **septate filaments**, which shows **branching** at **acute angles** Q **(40 degrees)**
- Has a tendency to **invade blood vessels**
- **Colonizing aspergillosis/Aspergilloma** – **proliferating masses of hyphae** which form brownish **"fungal balls"** within **pulmonary cavities** Q

Hence, **aspergilloma** doesn't result in formation of **target lesions** (which are formed by invasive aspergillosis)

Ans. 28) **C. Forms non-septate hyphae with acute angle branching (Ref: 8 ed. Robbins p. 385-86, 9 ed. p. 389-90, f-8-45)**

- **Zygomycosis (mucormycosis, phycomycosis)** Q is an **opportunistic infection** and includes Mucor, Rhizopus, Absidia and Cunninghamella species
- **Predisposing factors** include neutropenia, corticosteroids, diabetes mellitus, iron overload and breakdown of the cutaneous barrier

- **Zygomycetes** form **non-septate, fungal hyphae** with **right-angle branching** Q
- In **diabetics, fungus** may spread from **nasal sinuses** to the orbit and brain, giving rise to **rhinocerebral mucormycosis** Q

Ans. 29) **D. All of the above (Ref: 8 ed. Robbins p. 386, 9 ed. p. 390)**

Dimorphic Fungi: Q

- Grows as a **yeast** in human tissue but as a **hyaline mold** under laboratory culture conditions, at room temperature Q
- Examples – Include **blastomyces, histoplasma** and **coccidioidomycosis** Q

Ans. 30) **D. *P. falciparum* forms latent hypnozoites in hepatocytes (Ref: 8 ed. Robbins p. 386-87, 9 ed. p. 390-91, f-8-46)**

Life cycle of *Plasmodium* parasite:

- Infectious stage of malaria is the **sporozoite** Q, which enters into hepatocyte and rapidly multiply, releasing **merozoites**
- **P. vivax** and **P. ovale** forms **latent hypnozoites** in **hepatocytes** Q, which is responsible for relapse of **malaria**
- In **RBC, trophozoite** Q is the **first stage** of the **parasite** followed by the **schizont**, each of which develops into a **merozoite**, which infects **additional RBC's**
- Few parasites in RBC's develop into *gametocytes* that infect the mosquito

Thus, **P. vivax** and **P. ovale** form **latent hypnozoites** Q and not *P. falciparum*.

Ans. 31) **D. All of the above (Ref: 8 ed. Robbins p. 387, 9 ed. p. 391, f-8-47)**

Factors responsible for **P. falciparum** pathogenicity:

- Infects RBC's of any age, as compared to other species which infect only young or old red cells
- Causes **infected red cells** to clump together and cause **endothelial cells sequestration**
- Stimulates the production of **high levels of cytokines,** including **TNF, IFN-γ and IL-1**

Ans. 32) **C. HbD (Ref: 8 ed. Robbins p. 387)**

Common mutations which confer resistance to **malaria**:

- Patients **heterozygous** for **sickle cell trait (HbS)** Q
- **HbC** Q **mutation, protects** against **severe malaria** by reducing parasite proliferation
- **P. vivax** enters **red cells** by binding to the **Duffy blood group antigen** Q, individuals who do not have the Duffy antigen are resistant to malaria

Ans. 33) **C. Brain (Ref: 8 ed. Robbins p. 388, 9 ed. p. 392, f-8-47)**

- **Dürck granulomas** Q are characteristic of **malignant cerebral malaria** Q
- **P. falciparum** causes **malignant cerebral malaria** and shows **brain vessels** containing **parasitized red cells**

Ans. 34) **D. Babesiosis (Ref: 8 ed. Robbins p. 388, 9 ed. p.392, f-8-48)**

Babesiosis Q:

- Organisms resemble **P. falciparum** Q ring forms, but **lack hemozoin pigment**
- **Peripheral smear** – erythrocytes with babesia have diagnostic **Maltese cross** Q **(tetrads) appearance**

Ans. 35) **C. Cysts are most commonly found in lung (Ref: 8 ed. Robbins p. 392-93, 9 ed. p.395-96)**

Hydatid disease: Q

- Caused by **ingestion of eggs** of **echinococcal species**
- **For Echinococcus granulosus** the **definitive hosts** are **dogs** and humans are accidental intermediate hosts
- **E. granulosus cysts** are **most commonly** found in **liver** Q, followed by lung, bone, brain or other organs

Microscopy: Q

- Enclosing an opalescent fluid, there is inner, nucleated, **germinative layer** Q and an outer, opaque, **non-nucleated layer** Q with innumerable delicate laminations
- **Daughter cysts** often develop within the **large mother cyst**
- **Hydatid sand** Q – Degenerating scolices of the worm produce a fine, sand like sediment within the hydatid fluid

Ans. 36) D. SARS coronavirus (Ref: 9 ed. Robbins p. 400-01)

Recently Recognized **Infectious Agents** and **Manifestations** [Q]:

Date Recognized	Infectious Agent	Manifestations
1977	Ebola virus Hantaan virus Legionella pneumophila Campylobacter jejuni	Epidemic Ebola hemorrhagic fever Hemorrhagic fever with renal syndrome Legionnaire disease Enteritis
1980	HTLV-I	T-cell lymphoma or leukemia, HTLV-associated myelopathy
1981	Staphylococcus aureus	Toxic shock syndrome
1982	Escherichia coli O157:H7 Borrelia burgdorferi	Hemorrhagic colitis, hemolytic uremic syndrome Lyme disease
1983	HIV Helicobacter pylori	AIDS Gastric ulcers
1988	Hepatitis E	Enterically transmitted hepatitis
1995	KSHV (HHV-8)	Kaposi sarcoma in AIDS
1999	West Nile virus	West Nile fever, neuroinvasive disease
2003	SARS coronavirus	Severe acute respiratory syndrome

Ans. 37) A. Syphilis (Ref: 9 ed. Robbins p. 379, 501-505)

- Syphilitic aortitis is caused by endarteritis of the vasa vasorum of the proximal aorta

Ans. 38) A. Measles (Ref: 9 ed. Robbins p. 355) Refer Q 3 for details

Ans. 39) A. Treponema pallidum (Ref: 9 ed. Robbins p. 380-81) Refer Q 21, 22 & 23 for details

Ans. 40) B. Silver methenamine (Ref: 9 ed. Robbins p. 386-87) Refer Q 23 for details

Ans. 41) D. IFN gamma (Ref: 9 ed. Robbins, p. 493-494)

- Tuberculosis is a communicable chronic granulomatous disease caused by Mycobacterium tuberculosis
- Mycobacteria are slender rods that are acid-fast

Pathogenesis:

- Pathologic features include caseating granulomas and cavitation
- Processed mycobacterial antigens reach the draining lymph nodes and are presented to CD4 T cells by dendritic cells and macrophages
- Macrophage secretes IL-12; which leads to the activation of CD4+ T cells (TH1 subset) which secretes IFN-γ
- IFN-γ released by CD4+ T cells of the TH1 subset leads to further activation of macrophages, which in turn leads to stimulation of:
  a) **TNF – recruits monocytes, which undergo differentiation into "epithelioid histiocytes"**
  b) **Nitric oxide – has excellent antibacterial activity**
  c) **Reactive oxygen species: Antibacterial activity**
- **Hence, defects in TH1 response results in poorly formed granulomas, absence of resistance and disease progression**

Ans. 42) D Chalazion (Ref: http://www.images.Illissionforvisionusa.org/anatomy/2007/01/chalazion-or-lipogranulomatous.html)

Chalazion or Lipogranulomatous Inflammation:

Definition – Localized lipogranulomatous inflammatory condition that involves sebaceous glands of the eyelid presumably due to duct obstruction

Etiology:

- Duct obstruction
- Non-infectious causes – neoplastic conditions especially sebaceous carcinoma
- Infections, particularly staphylococcus infection of the meibomian glands

Histopathology:

- Lipogranulomatous inflammation
- In paraffin sections, clear circular empty spaces (presumably represent lipid) are surrounded by nodular collections of epithelioid histiocytes

Ans. 43) A. Actinomycosis (Ref: Internet)

- Causative agent in humans is Actinomyces israelii (gram-positive bacterium)
- Gomori methenamine-silver stain is used to demonstrate these oranisms

Note:

- Nocardia organisms are acid fast bacilli

Ans. 44) A. Plasmodium Falciparum (Ref: 9 ed. Robbins p. 390-91) Refer Q 30 & 31 for details

Note: Gametocyte stage of Plasmodium falciparum appears banana shaped, as shown in the micro-photograph

9 Environmental and Nutritional Diseases

How to go about this chapter?

- **Be thorough with the following topics:**
  - **Environmental pollution**
  - **Occupational health hazards**
  - **Effects of alcohol**
  - **Drug abuse**
  - **Nutritional diseases**

ENVIRONMENTAL POLLUTION

1) **Particulate matter of which size are most dangerous?**
   a) <10 μm b) <20 μm
   c) <30 μm d) <40 μm

2) **All of the following are blood and marrow findings in lead poisoning EXCEPT:**
   a) Ringed sideroblasts
   b) Basophilic stippling
   c) Microcytic hypochromic RBC's
   d) Macrocytic RBC's

OCCUPATIONAL HEALTH RISKS: INDUSTRIAL AND AGRICULTURAL EXPOSURES

3) **All are TRUE regarding smoking EXCEPT:**
   a) Associated with increased risk of multiple cancers and lung diseases
   b) Associated with increased risk of Myocardial Infarction and atherosclerosis
   c) Maternal smoking increases the risk of spontaneous abortions
   d) Passive smoking inhalation in non-smokers can be estimated by measuring the blood levels of nicotine

EFFECTS OF ALCOHOL

4) **In potentiating the effect of the anti-depressant drugs in alcoholics which enzyme plays a major role:**
   a) CYP2E1
   b) ADH
   c) ALDH
   d) Catalase

INJURY BY THERAPEUTIC DRUGS AND DRUGS OF ABUSE

5) **Thrombocytopenia can be caused by:**
   a) Methyldopa
   b) Penicillin
   c) Quinidine
   d) Any of the above

6) **All are TRUE about oral contraceptive pills (OCP) EXCEPT:**
   a) OCP's increase the risk of breast cancer
   b) OCP's protect against endometrial cancer
   c) OCP's increases the risk of thromboembolism
   d) OCP's do not increase the risk of cardiovascular disease in young women

7) **Product of acetaminophen responsible for hepatocellular injury:**
   a) CYP2E1 b) GSH
   c) NAPQI d) None of the above

INJURY BY PHYSICAL AGENTS

8) **Effects of radiation on hemato-lymphoid system includes all EXCEPT:**
   a) Shrinkage of lymph node and spleen
   b) Lymphocytosis is seen
   c) Bone marrow aplasia
   d) Granulocyte count begins to fall at end of first week

9) **Radiation induced cancer include:**
   a) Papillary thyroid carcinoma
   b) Follicular carcinoma of thyroid
   c) Lymphoma
   d) Seminoma

NUTRITIONAL DISEASES

10) Retinoids are useful for treatment of:
a) Severe acne
b) Psoriasis
c) Promyelocytic leukemia
d) Any of above

11) All are TRUE about leptin EXCEPT:
a) Stimulated by abundant fat stores
b) Leptin mutation results in obesity
c) Can function as anti-inflammatory cytokine
d) Stimulates physical activity, energy expenditure

12) Gut hormones include all EXCEPT:
a) Gherlin
b) Leptin
c) PYY
d) Amylin

13) Radiation exposure during infancy has been linked to which one of the following carcinoma? (NEET 2013)
a) Breast
b) Melanoma
c) Thyroid
d) Lung

14) Lead causes following EXCEPT: (NEET 2013)
a) Uroporphyrinuria
b) Sideroblastic anemia
c) Basophilic stippling
d) Macrocytic anemia

15) UV radiation: (NEET 2013)
a) Prevents formation of Pyrimidine dimers
b) Stimulates formation of pyrimidine dimers
c) Purine dimers
d) None

16) Indoor air pollution doesn't lead to: (AIIMS Nov 2013)
a) Chronic lung disease
b) Impaired neurological development
c) Adverse pregnancy outcome
d) Pneumonia in child

CHAPTER 9: ENVIRONMENTAL AND NUTRITIONAL DISEASES

Ans. 1) **A. <10 μm (Ref: 8 ed. Robbins p. 405, 9 ed. p. 409)**

Particulate matter ("soot"):

- Particles that are **less than 10 μm** [Q] in diameter are **most harmful**
- Because the particles, greater than **10 μm** in **diameter** [Q] are removed in nose, or trapped by mucociliary epithelium of the airways

Ans. 2) **D. Macrocytic RBC's (Ref: 8 ed. Robbins p. 406-07, 9 ed. p. 410-12, f-9-5-7)**

- Lead **inhibits** the activity of **two enzymes** involved in heme synthesis, **δ-aminolevulinic acid dehydratase** [Q] and **ferrochelatase** [Q]

Features in blood and marrow include:

- **Ringed sideroblasts** [Q] – red cell precursors with **iron-laden mitochondria** [Q], detected with **Prussian blue stain** [Q]
- **Microcytic, hypochromic** anemia, accompanied by mild **hemolysis** [Q]
- **Punctate basophilic stippling** [Q] of RBC's

Ans. 3) **D. Passive smoking inhalation in non-smokers can be estimated by measuring the blood levels of nicotine (Ref: 8 ed. Robbins p. 410-12, 9 ed. p. 414-17, f-9-8-11, t-9-4)**

Adverse effects of smoking:

- **Lung** [Q] – emphysema, chronic bronchitis, chronic obstructive pulmonary disease and lung cancer
- **Heart** – increased risk of Atherosclerosis, myocardial infarcts
- **Cancers** – carcinoma of the oral cavity, esophagus, pancreas and bladder [Q]
- **Pregnancy – Maternal smoking** increases the risk of **spontaneous abortions** and **preterm births** and results in **intrauterine growth retardation**

Note:

- **Passive smoke inhalation** in **nonsmokers** can be estimated by measuring the blood levels of **cotinine** [Q], a metabolite of nicotine

Ans. 4) **CYP2E1 (Ref: 8 ed. Robbins p. 412-14, 9 ed. p. 417-19, f-9-12)**

Alcohol in the **blood** is **bio-transformed** to **acetaldehyde** in the liver by:

- Alcohol dehydrogenase **(ADH),** Microsomal ethanol-oxidizing system **(MEOS)** and Catalase

Note:

- Microsomal oxidation system involves **CYP2E1** [Q]
- When alcohol is present at **high concentrations** in blood, it competes with other **CYP2E1 substrates** and **delays drug catabolism**
- Hence, alcohol potentiates the **depressant effect** of **narcotic**, **sedatives** and **psychoactive drugs** in central nervous system

Ans. 5) **D. Any of the above (Ref: 8 ed. Robbins p. 416, 9 ed. p. 420, t-9-5)**

Common Adverse Drug Reactions and Their Agents [Q]:

Reaction	Major Offenders
Bone Marrow And Blood Cells	
Granulocytopenia, aplastic anemia, pancytopenia	Antineoplastic agents, immunosuppressives, chloramphenicol
Hemolytic anemia, thrombocytopenia	Penicillin, methyldopa, quinidine, heparin
Cutaneous	
Urticaria, macules, papules, vesicles, petechiae, exfoliative dermatitis, fixed drug eruptions, abnormal pigmentation	Antineoplastic agents, sulfonamides, hydantoins, antibiotics
Cardiac	
Arrhythmias	Theophylline, hydantoins, digoxin
Cardiomyopathy	Doxorubicin, daunorubicin

Cont.

Cont.

Renal	
Glomerulonephritis	Penicillamine
Acute tubular necrosis	Aminoglycoside antibiotics, cyclosporin, amphotericin B
Tubulointerstitial disease with papillary necrosis	Phenacetin, salicylates
Pulmonary	
Asthma	Salicylates
Acute pneumonitis	Nitrofurantoin
Interstitial fibrosis	Busulfan, nitrofurantoin, bleomycin
Hepatic	
Fatty change	Tetracycline
Diffuse hepatocellular damage	Halothane, isoniazid, acetaminophen
Cholestasis	Chlorpromazine, estrogens, contraceptive agents
Systemic	
Anaphylaxis	Penicillin
Lupus erythematosus syndrome (drug-induced lupus)	Hydralazine, procainamide
Bleeding	Warfarin, dabigatran
Central Nervous System	
Tinnitus and dizziness	Salicylates
Acute dystonic reactions and parkinsonian syndrome	Phenothiazine
Respiratory depression	Sedatives

Ans. 6) **A. OCP's increase the risk of breast cancer (Ref: 8 ed. Robbins p. 415, 9 ed. p. 421-22)**

OCP's are **protective against** or **does not increase the risk** Q of:
- Breast cancer
- Endometrial cancer and ovarian cancers
- Coronary artery disease in women younger than 30 years and non-smokers

OCP's increase the risk Q of:
- **Cervical carcinomas** (with prior infection with HPV)
- Venous thrombosis and pulmonary thromboembolism
- Coronary artery disease in women older than 35 years and who smoke
- **Hepatic adenoma** in older women

Ans. 7) **C. NAPQI (Ref: 8 ed. Robbins p. 416-17, 9 ed. p. 422, f-9-14)**
- **95%** of **acetaminophen** undergoes **detoxification** in the liver and is excreted in the urine as glucuronate or sulfate conjugates
- **5%** is metabolized by the activity of **CYP2E** to **NAPQI** (**N-acetyl- p-benzoquinoneimine**) Q (a highly reactive metabolite)
- **NAPQI** Q is normally conjugated with **glutathione (GSH)**
- In large doses, **unconjugated NAPQI** accumulates and causes hepatocellular injury leading to **centrilobular necrosis** Q and **liver failure**

Note:
- At early stages, **acetaminophen overdose** can be **treated** (within **12 hours**) by administration of **N-acetyl cysteine**Q, which restores **GSH**

Ans. 8) **B. Lymphocytosis is seen (Ref: 8 ed. Robbins p. 425, 9 ed. p.430)**

Effects of irradiation on **Hematopoietic** and **Lymphoid Systems** Q:
- **RBC counts** fall and **anemia** appears after **2 to 3 weeks**

- Severe **lymphopenia** (appear within **hours of irradiation**)
- **Leucopenia** (at the end of the first week)
- Shrinkage of the lymph nodes and spleen
- Very high doses of radiation induces **aplastic anemia**

Ans. 9) **A. Papillary thyroid carcinoma (Ref: 8 ed. Robbins p. 426, 9 ed. p. 432-33)**

- **Examples of Radiation induced cancer:** carcinoma of breast, lung, **Thyroid (Papillary Carcinoma)**[Q], leukemia, squamous cell carcinoma

Ans. 10) **D. All of the above (Ref: 8 ed. Robbins p. 421, 9 ed. p. 437)**

Retinoids are useful for[Q]:

- Severe acne
- Psoriasis
- Treatment of acute promyelocytic leukemia (by using **all-trans-retinoic acid**)

Ans. 11) **C. Can function as anti-inflammatory cytokine (Ref: 8 ed. Robbins p. 439-440, 9 ed. p. 444-45, f-9-30)**

Functions of Leptin[Q]:

- Hormone is synthesized by **fat cells** and secretion is **stimulated** when fat stores are **abundant**
- When there are **inadequate stores** of **body fat, leptin secretion** is diminished and food intake is increased and vice versa
- Stimulates **POMC/CART neurons**[Q] **(hypothalamus)** that produces **anorexigenic neuropeptides**
- **Leptin abundance** stimulates physical activity, heat production, and energy expenditure
- Acts as **pro-inflammatory cytokine**[Q] and participates in the regulation of hematopoiesis and lymphopoiesis

Ans. 12) **B. Leptin (Ref: 8 ed. Robbins p. 441-42, 9 ed. p. 444-48, f-9-30,31)**

- Gut hormones include **ghrelin, PYY, pancreatic polypeptide, insulin, and amylin**[Q]
- **Ghrelin**[Q] – produced in stomach and hypothalamus – **increases food intake** (orexigenic effect)
- **PYY** – secreted from endocrine cells in **ileum** and **colon**, their levels are low during fasting, leading to **hyperphagia and obesity** and **levels increase** shortly after food intake
- **Amylin – reduces food intake and weight gain** and is evaluated for the treatment of obesity and diabetes

Ans. 13) C. Thyroid (Ref: 9ed. Robbins p. 432-33) Refer Q9 for details

Ans. 14) D. Macrocytic anemia (Ref: 9 ed. Robbins p. 410-12) Refer Q 2 for details

Ans. 15) B. Stimulates formation of pyrimidine dimmers (Ref: 9 ed. Robbins p. 324)

- **UV rays cause DNA damage by forming pyrimidine dimmers which prevents replication**

Ans. 16) A. Impaired neurological development (Ref: Robbins 8th p. 403-405)

Indoor Air Pollution:

1. **Most common pollutant is tobacco smoke**
2. **Additional offenders are CO, nitrogen dioxide, asbestos**
3. **Volatile substances containing polycyclic aromatic hydrocarbons generated by cooking oils and coal burning are important indoor pollutants**
4. **Wood smoke, containing various oxides of nitrogen and carbon particulates, may not only be an irritant but also predisposes to lung infections and may contain far more dangerous carcinogenic polycyclic hydrocarbons**
5. **Bio-aerosols can cause Legionnaire's disease, viral pneumonia, common cold**
6. **Radon (radioactive gas derived from uranium) is widely present in soil and in homes, can predispose to lung cancer**
7. **Exposure to formaldehyde causes breathing difficulties and a burning sensation in the eyes and throat, and can trigger asthma attacks**

10 Diseases of Infancy and Childhood

How to go about this chapter?

- **Following topics, one should be thorough with:**
  - **Hyaline membrane disease**
  - **Necrotizing enterocolitis**
  - **Immune hydrops**
  - **ABO incompatibility**
  - **Cystic fibrosis**
  - **Childhood teratoma and small round blue cell tumors**
  - **Neuroblastoma**
  - **Wilm's tumor**

PREMATURITY AND FETAL GROWTH RESTRICTION

1) **All are TRUE about respiratory distress syndrome (RDS) EXCEPT:**
a) Due to deficiency of pulmonary surfactant
b) Incidence of RDS is inversely proportion to gestational age
c) Glucocorticoids play an important role
d) Cesarean section helps to reduce its risk

2) **Complications associated with pre-term birth:**
a) Necrotizing enterocolitis
b) Intraventricular hemorrhage
c) Patent ductus arteriosus
d) Any of the above

3) **Most important mediator responsible in pathogenesis of *Necrotizing Enterocolitis*:**
a) Platelet Activating Factor (PAF)
b) Epidermal Growth Factor (EGF)
c) Fibroblastic Growth Factor (FGF)
d) Vascular Endothelial Growth Factor (VEGF)

FETAL HYDROPS

4) **All are TRUE about immune hydrops EXCEPT:**
a) D antigen is major cause of Rh incompatibility
b) Concurrent ABO incompatibility protects the mother against Rh immunization
c) Initial exposure to Rh antigens evokes the formation of IgG antibodies
d) Antibody response depends on the dose of immunizing antigen

5) **Incidence of Rh incompatibility decreases when immunization is given:**
a) At 28 weeks of gestation
b) Within 72 hours of delivery
c) At the time of abortion
d) Any of the above

6) **ABO incompatibility all are TRUE EXCEPT:**
a) Anti-A and Anti-B antibodies are of IgM type
b) Many cells other than red cells express A and B antigens
c) Occurs in approximately 20-25% of pregnancies
d) There is effective protection against ABO reactions

7) **Levels of bilirubin responsible for neural damage in erythroblastosis fetalis:**
a) > 5 mg% b) >10 mg%
c) >15 mg% d) >20 mg%

INBORN ERRORS OF METABOLISM AND OTHER GENETIC DISORDERS

8) **Phenylketonuria (PKU) occurs due to deficiency of:**
a) Phenylalanine hydroxylase
b) Dihydropteridine reductase
c) Tetrahydrobiopterin
d) Tyrosinase

9) **Galactosemia occurs due to deficiency of:**
a) Galactokinase
b) Galactose-1-phosphate uridyl transferase
c) Galacticol
d) Galactose

10) All are TRUE about Cystic Fibrosis EXCEPT:
a) Autosomal recessive inheritance
b) Mutation in CFTR gene
c) Affects the sweat glands
d) Meconium ileus can be seen

11) Most common cause of death in Cystic fibrosis is:
a) Meconium ileus
b) Exocrine Pancreatic insufficiency
c) Diabetes
d) Cardiorespiratory complications

TUMORS AND TUMOR-LIKE LESIONS OF INFANCY AND CHILDHOOD

12) Most common tumors of infancy:
a) Hemangiomas
b) Lymphangiomas
c) Teratomas
d) Fibrous tumors

13) Following fusion transcript is seen In congenital fibrosarcoma:
a) ETV6-TRKC
b) PI3K/AKT
c) N-Myc
d) Any of the above

14) All are TRUE about childhood teratomas EXCEPT:
a) Sacrococcygeal teratoma are most common in childhood
b) Associated with congenital anomalies
c) 75% of these tumors are immature teratomas
d) Malignant potential correlates with the amount of immature tissue

15) Differential diagnosis of small round cell tumors includes all EXCEPT:
a) Medulloblastoma
b) Hepatoblastoma
c) Pheochromocytoma
d) Wilm's tumor

16) All are TRUE about Neuroblastoma EXCEPT:
a) Is the most common extra-cranial solid tumor of childhood
b) Can show spontaneous tumor regression
c) ALK gene mutation is noted in familial cases
d) Children younger than 1 year has worse prognosis

17) Most common site of neuroblastoma:
a) Adrenals
b) Sympathetic chain
c) Kidney
d) Posterior mediastinum

18) All of the following are TRUE about Neuroblastoma EXCEPT:
a) Range in size from nodules to large masses
b) Homer-Wright psudorosettes can be found
c) Schwannian stroma is associated with worse prognosis
d) Metastasis involves liver, lung, bone marrow

19) Following are associated with good prognosis in Neuroblastoma EXCEPT:
a) Stage 4S
b) Age < 18 months
c) N - Myc amplification
d) TRKA expression

20) All are TRUE about Wilm's tumor EXCEPT:
a) Most common primary pediatric renal tumor
b) Presents between 2-5 years of age
c) 90% tumors occurs bilaterally
d) Indicates a relationship between malformation and neoplasia

21) Associated malformation(s) in Wilms tumor include(s):
a) WAGR syndrome
b) Denys-Drash Syndrome
c) Beckwith-Wiedemann Syndrome
d) All of the above

22) All of the following are TRUE about Wilms tumor EXCEPT:
a) Large, solitary, well-circumscribed mass
b) Classically shows tri-phasic pattern
c) Most of tumors reveal anaplasia
d) Anaplasia correlates with p53 mutations

23) TRUE about nephrogenic rests:
a) Precursor lesions of Wilms
b) Seen in renal parenchyma adjacent to Wilms tumor
c) Frequency increases to 100% in bilateral Wilms tumor
d) All of the above

24) Most common type of class II mutation in cystic fibrosis is: (NEET 2014)
a) Missense mutation
b) Frame-shift
c) Non sense
d) Deletion

25) Most common known causes of congenital anomalies in humans are: (NEET 2014)
a) Chromosomal aberrations
b) Maternal infections
c) Drugs
d) Irradiation

26) Wilm's tumor associated with all EXCEPT: (NEET 2014)
a) WAGR
b) Beckwith-Wiedemann
c) Denys-Drash
d) DiGeorge syndrome

27) Most important prognostic factor of Wilms tumour: (NEET 2013)

a) Histopathology
b) Ploidy of cells
c) Age < 1 yr
d) Mutation of 1p gene

28) Cystic fibrosis is associated with all except: (NEET 2013)

a) Infertility
b) Azoospermia
c) Nasal polyps
d) Renal failure

29) Gene for Wilm's tumor is located on: (NEET 2013)

a) Chromosome 1
b) Chromosome 10
c) Chromosome 11
d) Chromosome 12

CHAPTER 10 – DISEASES OF INFANCY AND CHILDHOOD

Ans. 1) **D. Cesarean section helps to reduce its risk (Ref: 8 ed. Robbins p. 456-58, 9 ed. 457-59, f-10-6, 7)**

RDS/Hyaline membrane disease:

- Seen in **preterm infants**
- Associated with male gender, maternal diabetes, cesarean section [Q]
- **Chest X-ray** reveals **ground-glass picture** [Q]
- **Predisposing factor – lung immaturity** [Q]
- Incidence of RDS is inversely proportional to **gestational age** [Q]
- Fundamental defect in RDS is **deficiency of pulmonary surfactant** [Q]
- **Surfactant synthesis** is **increased** by cortisol, insulin, prolactin, thyroxine, **TGF-β**[Q] and is suppressed by **insulin** [Q]
- **Labor** [Q] increases **surfactant synthesis**
- **Cesarean section** before onset of labor may increase the risk of RDS
- Microscopically, **eosinophilic hyaline membranes** [Q] line the **respiratory bronchioles**, alveolar ducts and alveoli

Complications in treatment of RDS:

- **High concentration** and **prolonged oxygen administration** leads to **retrolental fibroplasia** (also called **retinopathy of prematurity**) [Q] and **bronchopulmonary dysplasia** [Q]

Ans. 2) **D. Any of the above (Ref: 9 ed. Robbins p. 459)**

Most common complications associated with **preterm birth**[Q]:

- Patent ductus arteriosus
- Intraventricular hemorrhage
- Necrotizing enterocolitis

Ans. 3) **A. Platelet Activating Factor (PAF) (Ref: 8 ed. Robbins p. 458, 9 ed. p. 459)**

Pathogenesis of NEC:

- **Immaturity of lungs/Prematurity** (defined by **gestational age** less than **37 weeks**) is the most important predisposing factor
- Most cases are associated with **enteral feeding**[Q]
- **Platelet activating factor (PAF)** [Q] brings **apoptosis** of **enterocytes**, thus increasing **mucosal permeability**

Ans. 4) **C. Initial exposure to Rh antigens evokes the formation of IgG antibodies (Ref: 8 ed. Robbins p. 460-62, 9 ed. p. 461-62, f-10-10)**

Immune hydrops:

- Develops when **fetal red cells** reach **maternal circulation** and results in **antibody response** (more than 1 mL of Rh-positive fetal red cells is required)
- **D antigen** [Q] is a major cause of **Rh incompatibility**
- Initial exposure to Rh antigen evokes the formation of **IgM antibodies** [Q]
- **Rh disease** is uncommon after **first pregnancy**
- However, during **subsequent pregnancy** (due to **IgG antibody** response) the risk of **immune hydrops** is increased

  Concurrent **ABO incompatibility** protects the mother against Rh immunization??

- Because, fetal red cells are removed from the maternal circulation by **anti-A** or **anti-B IgM antibodies**, which **does not cross the placenta**

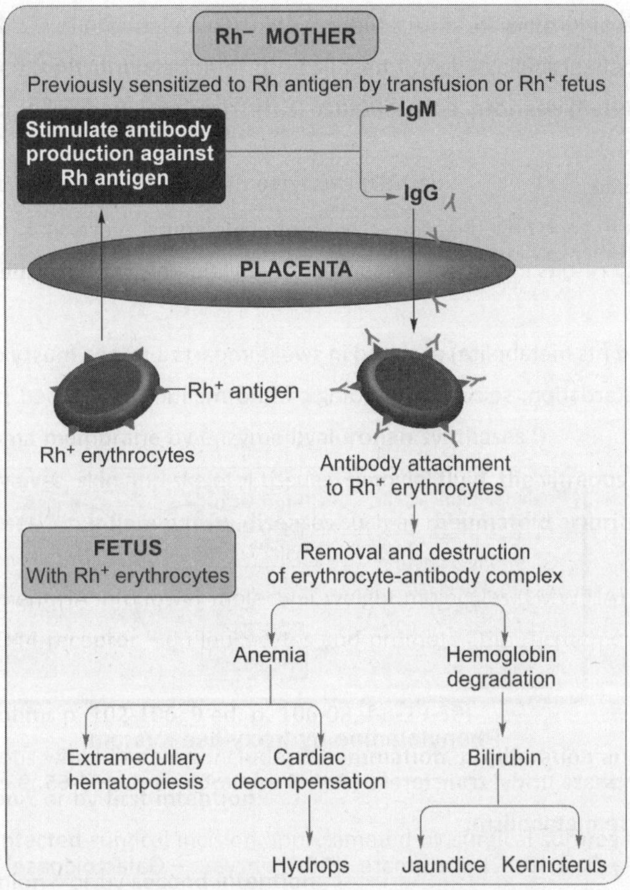

Pathogenesis of immune hydrops fetalis

Ans. 5) **D. Any of the above (Ref: 8 ed. Robbins p. 460-62, 9 ed. p. 462)**

- Incidence of **maternal Rh iso-immunization** has decreased significantly due to use of **Rhesus immune globulin (RhIg)** containing **anti-D antibodies** Q
- **Administration of RhIg** at **28 weeks** Q of **pregnancy** and **within 72 hours** Q **of delivery** is **beneficial**
- Immunization to **Rh negative mothers** decreases the risk for **hemolytic disease** in **Rh-positive neonates** in subsequent pregnancies
- **RhIg** is also administered following abortions Q

Ans. 6) **D. There is effective protection against ABO reactions (Ref: 8 ed. Robbins p. 460-62, 9 ed. p. 462)**

ABO incompatibility

- Occurs in **20% to 25% of pregnancies** Q
- **Anti-A** and **anti-B antibodies** are of the **IgM type** Q, which **do not** cross the placenta
- **Neonatal red cells** express **blood group antigens** A and B poorly
- Cells, other than red cells, express A and B antigens and thus absorb some of the transferred antibody
- **ABO hemolytic disease** occurs in infants of **group A or B,** who are born of group O mothers
- Disease is always **milder** than **Rh incompatibility**; but there is **no effective protection** against **ABO reactions**

Ans. 7) **D. >20 mg% (Ref: 8 ed. Robbins p. 462, 9 ed. p. 463, f-10-13)**

"Kernicterus" [Q]**:**

- Most serious **CNS complication** in **fetal hydrops**
- There is **yellow discoloration of basal ganglia** [Q], thalamus, cerebellum, cerebral gray matter and spinal cord
- Blood bilirubin levels greater than **20 mg%** [Q] in term infants induces **neural damage**

Ans. 8) **A. Phenylalanine hydroxylase (Ref: 8 ed. Robbins p. 462-64, 9 ed. p. 464-65, f-10-14)**

Phenylketonuria (PKU) [Q]**:**

- **Autosomal recessive**
- Due to mutations in gene encoding the enzyme **phenylalanine hydroxylase (PAH)** [Q]
- Enzyme deficiency results in inability to convert **phenylalanine** into **tyrosine**

Clinical Features:

- **Phenyl-acetic acid** (its metabolite) excreted in sweat imparts a strong **musty or mousy odor** [Q] to affected infants
- Severe mental retardation, seizures, neurologic abnormalities, decreased pigmentation of hair and skin and eczema

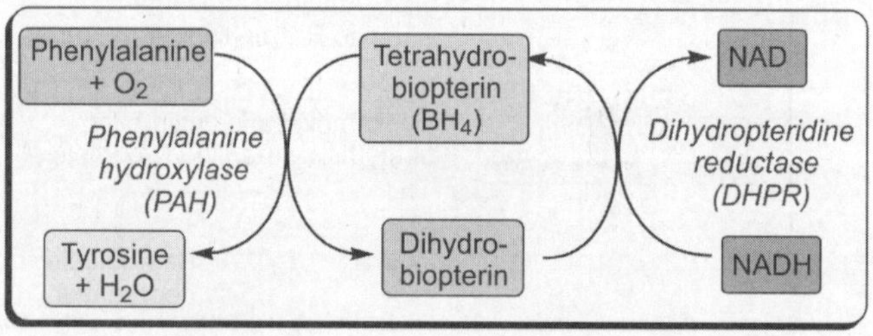

Phenylalanine hydroxylase system

Ans. 9) **B. Galactose-1-phosphate uridyl transferase (Ref: 8 ed. Robbins p. 464-65, 9 ed. p.465-66, f-10-16)**

Pathways of galactose metabolism:

a. Galactose + ATP → Galactose-1-phosphate + ADP (enzyme – **Galactokinase)**

b. Galactose-1-phosphate → UDP-galactose+glucose-1-phosphate (enzyme – **galactose-1-phosphate uridyl transferase)** [Q]

c. UDP-galactose → UDP glucose (enzyme – **UDP-galactose-4-epimerase)**

Galactosemia: [Q]

- Autosomal recessive disorder
- **Most common cause** – lack of **galactose-1-phosphate uridyl transferase (also known as GALT)** [Q]
- Galactose-1-phosphate accumulates in liver, spleen, lens of the eye, kidneys, heart muscle, cerebral cortex and erythrocytes

Diagnosis:

- Demonstration of **reducing sugar** (other than glucose), in the urine
- Deficiency of **GALT** in **leukocytes** and **erythrocytes** are reliable parameters

Ans. 10) **C. Affects the sweat glands (Ref: 8 ed. Robbins p. 465-70, 9 ed. p. 466-71, f- 10-17)**

Cystic Fibrosis:

- Disorder of **ion transport** in **epithelial cells**
- Affects **fluid secretion** in **exocrine glands** and epithelial lining of the respiratory, gastrointestinal and reproductive tracts
- **Results** from **abnormal function** of **epithelial chloride channel protein** encoded by **cystic fibrosis trans-membrane conductance regulator (CFTR)** gene

- **CFTR gene** is located on **chromosome 7q31.2**[Q]
- **Pulmonary manifestations** are associated with mutation of **mannose-binding lectin 2 (MBL2)** [Q] and **transforming growth factor β1 (TGFB1)** [Q]

Morphology:

- **Pancreas** – atrophy of the exocrine glands and progressive fibrosis
- **Small-bowel** – obstruction due to **meconium ileus**
- **Liver** – Bile canaliculi are plugged by mucinous material, ductular proliferation, portal inflammation, hepatic steatosis and focal biliary cirrhosis
- **Azoospermia, infertility**, congenital bilateral absence of the **vas deferens** are found in 95% of the males

Pulmonary Manifestations:

- Chronic bronchitis, bronchiectasis, lung abscesses
- **Staphylococcus aureus, Haemophilus influenzae** and **Pseudomonas aeruginosa** are **most common organisms** for **lung infections**
- **Burkholderia cenocepacia** [Q] is the **most common opportunistic infection** [Q]

Note:

- **Sweat glands** are **morphologically unaffected** [Q]

Ans. 11) D. Cardiorespiratory complications (Ref: 8 ed. Robbins p. 470-71, 9 ed. p.471)

- **Cardiorespiratory complications** are the **most common cause** of **death**
- **Exocrine pancreatic insufficiency** occurs in **85% to 90%** of patients with cystic fibrosis and is associated with **"severe" CFTR mutations** on both alleles

Diagnosis [Q]**:**

- **Persistently elevated** sweat electrolyte concentrations [Q]
- In patients with at least one **"mild" CFTR mutation** and with a normal sweat test **(<60 mM/L)**, measurement of **nasal trans-epithelial potential difference** [Q] is a useful adjunct test
- **Cystic fibrosis** patients demonstrate significantly **more negative baseline nasal potential difference** [Q] than **controls**
- **CFTR gene sequencing** [Q] is the **"gold standard"** for diagnosis of **cystic fibrosis**

Ans. 12) A. Hemangiomas (Ref: 8 ed. Robbins p. 473, 9 ed. p.474, f-10-22)

- **Hemangiomas** are the **most common tumors of infancy** [Q]

Ans. 13) A. ETV6-TRKC (Ref: 8 & 9 ed. Robbins p. 474)

- In **congenital-infantile fibro-sarcomas, t(12;15) (p13;q25)** results in generation of **ETV6-NTRK3/TRKC fusion transcript** [Q]
- **ETV6-NTRK3 fusion transcript** is a useful **diagnostic marker** [Q]

Ans. 14) C. 75% of these tumors are immature teratomas (Ref: 8 ed. Robbins p. 474, 9 ed. p. 474-75, f-10-23)

Childhood Teratomas [Q]**:**

- **Sacrococcygeal teratomas** [Q] are the **most common** teratomas of childhood
- **Age group** – exhibits two peaks: first at 2 years of age and the second in late adolescence or early adulthood
- **75%** are **mature teratomas** [Q]
- Malignant potential correlates with **the amount of immature tissue** [Q] (particularly immature **neuroepithelial element)**
- **Sites** [Q] – testis, ovaries, mediastinum, retro-peritoneum and head and neck

Ans. 15) C. Pheochromocytoma (Ref: 8 ed. Robbins p. 475, 9 ed. p. 475, t-10-7)

Differential diagnosis of **small round blue cell tumors** [Q]**:**

- Neuroblastoma, Wilms tumor, Lymphoma (ALL), Rhabdomyosarcoma, Ewing sarcoma/primitive Neuroectodermal tumor, Medulloblastoma and Retinoblastoma

Common Malignant Neoplasms of Infancy and Childhood

0-4 years	5-9 years	10-14 years
Leukemia	Leukemia	
Retinoblastoma	Retinoblastoma	
Neuroblastoma	Neuroblastoma	
Wilms tumor		
Hepatoblastoma	Hepatocellular carcinoma	Hepatocellular carcinoma
Rhabdomyosarcoma Teratomas	Soft tissue sarcoma	Soft-tissue sarcoma
Central nervous system tumors	Central nervous system tumors, Ewing sarcoma Lymphoma	Osteogenic sarcoma, Thyroid carcinoma, Hodgkin disease

Ans. 16) D. Children younger than 1 year has worse prognosis (Ref: 8 ed. Robbins p.475-76, 9 ed. p. 477, t-10-8)

Characteristic Features of **Neuroblastic Tumors:**

- Differentiation into **mature elements** (spontaneous or therapy-induced) and **spontaneous tumor regression** [Q] is seen
- **Neuroblastoma** [Q] is the most common **extra-cranial solid tumor of childhood** [Q]
- **Germline mutations** in ***anaplastic lymphoma kinase (ALK)*** [Q] gene have been identified as a **major cause** of familial predisposition to **neuroblastoma**
- Children **younger than 18 months** [Q] of age have **better prognosis**

Note: Refer answer 19

Ans. 17) A. Adrenals (Ref: 8 ed. Robbins p.476, 9 ed. p. 476, f-10-24)

- 40% of neuroblastomas arise in **adrenal medulla** [Q]
- Other sites: **Along the sympathetic chain**, i.e. paravertebral region of the abdomen (25%) and posterior mediastinum(15%)

Ans. 18) C. Schwannian stroma is associated with worse prognosis (Ref: 8 & 9 ed. Robbins p.476-77, f-10-26)

Neuroblastomas:

- Range in size from **minute nodules to large masses** and may **spontaneously regress**

Histologically [Q]**:**

- Composed of small, primitive-appearing cells with dark nuclei, scant cytoplasm, growing in solid sheet
- Background demonstrates **neuropil** (faintly eosinophilic fibrillary material)
- **Homer-Wright pseudo rosettes** [Q] – tumor cells are concentrically arranged about a central space filled with **neuropil**
- **Ganglioneuroblastoma:** Composed of **ganglion cells** (cells with abundant cytoplasm, large vesicular nuclei and prominent nucleolus) admixed with primitive **neuroblasts**
- **Ganglioneuromas**: **Better differentiated lesions**, with many more **mature ganglion** cells and few **neuroblasts**
- **Maturation of neuroblasts** into **ganglion cells** is accompanied by the **appearance of Schwann cells** [Q]
- Presence of **schwannian stroma** is associated with a **favorable outcome**
- **Metastasis** can be seen in liver, lungs, bone marrow and bones

Ans. 19) C. N-Myc amplification (Ref: 8 & 9 ed. Robbins p.477-79, t-10-8)

Most important **prognostic factors** in **neuroblastomas** include [Q]:

Variable	Favorable	Unfavorable
Stage	Stage 1, 2A, 2B, 4S	Stage 3, 4
Age Q	<18 months	>18 months
Evidence of schwannian stroma and gangliocytic differentiation Q	Present	Absent
DNA ploidy	Hyperdiploid or neartriploid	Near-diploid
N-MYCQ	Not amplified	Amplified
Chromosome 17q gain	Absent	Present
Chromosome 1p loss	Absent	Present
Chromosome 11q loss	Absent	Present
TRKA expression Q	Present	Absent
TRKB expression	Absent	Present
Telomerase expression Q	Low or absent	Highly expressed

- **N-MYC amplification** Q – **most important genetic abnormality** used for the prognosis of **neuroblastic tumors** Q

Ans. 20) C. 90% tumors occurs bilaterally (Ref: 8 ed. Robbins p.479)

Wilms tumor:

- Most common **primary childhood renal tumor** Q
- Peak incidence is between **2 and 5 years** and 95% occur before age of 10 years Q
- **5% to 10%** of Wilms tumor involves both kidneys Q

Ans. 21) D. All of the above (Ref: 8 & 9 ed. Robbins p.479-80)

Associations with **Wilm's tumor** include:

A) ***WAGR syndrome*** Q:

- Characterized by Wilms, aniridia, genital anomalies and mental retardation
- Demonstrates Wilms tumor–associated gene, ***WT1*** Q and autosomal dominant gene for aniridia (***PAX6***) Q, both located on **chromosome 11p13** Q

B) ***Denys-Drash syndrome*** Q:

- Characterized by **gonadal dysgenesis (male pseudo-hermaphroditism)** and **diffuse mesangial sclerosis**
- Patients demonstrate **germline abnormalities** in **WT1**Q
- **Increased risk** for developing **germ cell tumors – gonadoblastomas** Q
- **WT1 protein** is critical for **normal renal** and **gonadal development**

C) ***Beckwith-Wiedemann syndrome (BWS)*** Q:

- Characterized by **organomegaly, macroglossia, hemi hypertrophy, omphalocele** and abnormal large cells in the **adrenal cortex (adrenal cytomegaly)** Q

- Shows **genomic imprinting** Q
- Chromosomal region is localized to **11p15.5 ("WT2")** Q
- Patients are at increased risk for **Wilms tumor, hepatoblastoma, pancreatoblastoma, adrenocortical tumors** and **rhabdomyosarcoma** Q

Note:

Nephrogenic rests Q are precursor lesions of **Wilms tumors**

Ans. 22) C. Most of tumors reveal anaplasia (Ref: 8 & 9 ed. Robbins p.480-81, f-10-28,29)

Morphology of Wilms tumor:

Grossly:

- Presents as a large, **solitary, well-circumscribed mass** Q

- Cut section – tumor is soft, **homogeneous** and tan to gray with occasional foci of hemorrhage, cyst formation and necrosis

Microscopically Q**:**

Tri-phasic pattern consisting of **blastemal**, **stromal** and **epithelial cell types**

- **Blastemal** component Q – sheets of **small blue cells**
- **Epithelial** component Q – in form of **abortive tubules** or **glomeruli**
- **Stromal cells** are usually **fibrocytic** or **myxoid** in nature

Points to Remember:

- **5%** of tumors reveal **anaplasia** Q (defined by the presence of cells with large, hyperchromatic, pleomorphic nuclei and abnormal mitoses)
- **Presence of anaplasia** correlates with **p53 mutation** Q
- **Adverse prognostic** factors – **loss of genetic material** on **chromosomes 11q and 16q** and **gain of chromosome 1q** in the **tumor cells**

Ans. 23) D. All of the above (Ref: 8 & 9 ed. Robbins p.480)

Nephrogenic Rests Q**:**

- **Precursor lesions of Wilms tumors** Q
- **Frequency** – seen in adjacent **renal parenchyma** in **25% to 40%** of **unilateral tumors** and in **100%** cases of **bilateral Wilms tumors** Q

Ans. 24) D. Deletion (Ref: 9 ed. Robbins p. 468)

- Most common class II mutation is deletion of three nucleotides coding for phenylalanine at amino acid position 508 (ÄF508)

Ans. 25) A. Chromosomal aberrations (Ref: 9 ed. Robbins p. 454)

Ans. 26) D. DiGeorge syndrome (Ref: 9 ed. Robbins p. 479-480) Refer Q 21 for details

Ans. 27) A. Histopathology (Ref: 9 ed. Robbins p.480-81) Refer Q 22 for details

- **Anaplastic histology remains a critical determinant of adverse prognosis**

Ans. 28) D. Renal failure (Ref: 9 ed. Robbins p. 466-71) Refer Q10 & 11 for details

Ans. 29) C. Chromosome 11 (Ref: 9 ed. Robbins p.479-80) Refer Q 21 for details

11 Blood Vessels

How to go about this chapter?

- **Following topics are asked repeatedly in PG entrance exams and one should be thorough with:**
  - **Endothelial cell dysfunction**
  - **Vascular pathology in hypertension**
  - **Atherosclerosis**
  - **Aneurysms**
  - **Vasculitis – small, medium, large**
  - **Vascular tumors – Glomus tumor, Kaposi sarcoma, Bacillary angiomatosis, Angiosarcoma**

VASCULAR STRUCTURE AND FUNCTION

1) All are TRUE about the blood vessels EXCEPT:
a) Tunica media is the thickest layer
b) Internal elastic lamina is present between intima and media
c) Inner portion of media derives nutrition through vasa vasorum
d) External elastic lamina is present on outer aspect of media

2) All are responsible for endothelial dysfunction EXCEPT:
a) Laminar flow
b) Hypertension
c) Cytokines
d) Cigarette smoke

3) TRUE about endothelial cells:
a) Contains *Webel-Palade* bodies
b) They can be recognized immunohistochemically
c) Intimal thickening is a response to vascular injury
d) All of the above

HYPERTENSIVE HEART DISEASE

4) Liddle syndrome is caused by mutation in:
a) Aldosterone synthase
b) 11β-hydroxylase
c) Na^+ channel protein
d) 17α-hydroxylase

5) Features of vascular pathology in hypertension is/are:
a) Hyaline arteriosclerosis
b) Hyperplastic arteriosclerosis
c) Necrotizing arteriolitis
d) All of the above

ATHEROSCLEROSIS

6) TRUE about atherosclerosis is/are:
a) Characterized by intimal lesions called atheroma
b) Increased LDL is associated with increased risk for MI
c) Non-modifiable and modifiable risk factors
d) All of the above

7) TRUE about pathogenesis of atherosclerosis:
a) Endothelial injury
b) Accumulation of lipoproteins
c) Hemodynamic disturbances
d) All of the above

8) All are TRUE about morphology of atherosclerosis EXCEPT:
a) Fatty streaks are the earliest lesion
b) Atherosclerotic lesions appear eccentric
c) Coronary arteries are involved to a greater degree followed by abdominal aorta
d) Vessels of the upper extremities are spared

9) Major consequence/s of atherosclerosis include(s):
a) Myocardial infarction
b) Cerebral infarction
c) Aortic aneurysms
d) All of the above

ANEURYSMS AND DISSECTION

10) All are TRUE about aneurysm EXCEPT:
a) Can be saccular or fusiform

b) Decreased MMP contributes to aneurysm formation
c) Hypertension is associated with aneurysms of ascending aorta
d) Mycotic aneurysms occurs due to septic embolus

11) All are TRUE about Aortic dissection EXCEPT:
a) Associated with Hypertension
b) Seen in patients with connective tissue abnormalities
c) Common in atherosclerosis patients
d) Most commonly seen in ascending aorta

VASCULITIS

12) All are the examples of small vessel vasculitis EXCEPT:
a) Wegener's Granulomatosis
b) Churg-Strauss syndrome
c) Microscopic Polyangiitis
d) Polyarteritis Nodosa

13) PR-3 ANCA is specific for:
a) Granulomatosis with Polyangiitis
b) Microscopic Polyangiitis
c) Polyarteritis Nodosa
d) Churg-Strauss Syndrome

14) All are TRUE about Giant cell Arteritis EXCEPT:
a) Granulomatous inflammation of large sized artery
b) Occurs in younger individuals
c) Segmental involvement of artery
d) Corticosteroids are effective in treatment

15) All are TRUE about Takayasu Arteritis EXCEPT:
a) Involves Aortic arch
b) Also known as pulseless disease
c) Doesn't involve the pulmonary artery
d) Characterized by transmural inflammation

16) All are TRUE about Polyarteritis Nodosa (PAN) EXCEPT:
a) Involves the pulmonary circulation
b) Association with Hepatitis B
c) All stages of activity coexist in different vessels
d) Renal involvement is the most common cause of death

17) TRUE about Kawasaki disease:
a) Predilection for coronary arteries
b) Endothelial cell autoantibodies
c) Also known as mucocutaneous lymph node syndrome
d) All of the above

18) All are TRUE about Microscopic Polyangiitis EXCEPT:
a) Also called as Leukocytoclastic vasculitis
b) All lesions tend to be of the same age
c) Pulmonary capillaries are commonly involved
d) Associated with PR-3 ANCA

19) All are TRUE about Churg-Strauss Syndrome EXCEPT:
a) Characterized by eosinophilia, asthma and granulomas
b) MPO-ANCA positivity is seen
c) Myocardial involvement is common
d) Affects medium size vessels

20) Granulomatosis with polyangiitis is characterized by:
a) Necrotizing granulomas
b) Affects the small vessels
c) Renal disease is commonly seen
d) All of the above

21) TRUE about Thromboangiitis Obliterans (Buerger Disease):
a) Involves large arteries
b) Associated with PR3-ANCA
c) Heavy cigarette smokers are at risk
d) Seen in older individuals

VEINS AND LYMPHATICS

22) All of the following causes Superior Vena Caval syndrome EXCEPT:
a) Bronchiogenic carcinoma
b) Mediastinal Lymphoma
c) High grade Renal Cell Cancer
d) None of the above

23) All of the following are associated with secondary lymphedema EXCEPT:
a) Post irradiation fibrosis
b) Filariasis
c) Following surgical procedures
d) Milroy disease

VASCULAR TUMORS

24) Distinction between benign and malignant vascular tumors can be done best by:
a) Cytological atypia
b) Mitotic figures
c) Obvious vascular channel formation
d) CD31 positivity

25) All are TRUE about Capillary Hemangioma EXCEPT:
a) Can occur on salivary gland
b) Regresses by seventh week of life
c) Also called strawberry Hemangioma
d) Also called as juvenile Hemangioendothelioma

26) All are TRUE regarding Cavernous hemangiomas EXCEPT:
a) Association with VHL disease
b) Regresses spontaneously

c) Vulnerable to traumatic ulceration and bleeding
d) None of the above

27) All are TRUE regarding Pyogenic granuloma EXCEPT:
a) Commonly seen in oral cavity and fingers
b) Associated with history of trauma
c) Recurrence is common
d) Capillary lobule formation indicates benign process

28) All are TRUE about Glomus tumors EXCEPT:
a) Painful lesions
b) Subungual region is the most common site
c) >2 cms in size
d) Numerous mast cells can be seen

29) Causal organism of Bacillary Angiomatosis is:
a) Mycobacterium tuberculosis
b) Mycobacterium leprae
c) Helicobacter pylori
d) Bartonella Henselae

30) All are TRUE about Kaposi Sarcoma (KS) EXCEPT:
a) Is common in AIDS patients
b) Caused by HHV-8
c) Four forms of the disease are recognized
d) Classic form of KS is associated with HIV

31) All are TRUE about Angiosarcoma EXCEPT:
a) Chemical carcinogenesis play a role
b) Older individuals are commonly affected
c) Radical mastectomy is a risk factor
d) CD34 is used to demonstrate endothelial cell of origin

32) All are TRUE about Hemangiopericytoma EXCEPT:
a) Tumor derived from pericytes
b) Most common in lower extremity
c) Endothelial cell markers positivity on IHC
d) Can metastasize

33) C-ANCA is associated with: (NEET 2014)
a) Wegener's granulomatosis
b) Microscopic polyangiitis
c) Churg Strauss syndrome
d) Goodpasture syndrome

34) Tumor(s) associated with tuberous sclerosis is/are: (NEET 2014)
a) Renal angiomyoma
b) Subependymal giant cell astrocytoma
c) Rhabdomyoma heart
d) All of the above

35) Hepatitis B is associated with: (NEET 2014)
a) Wegener's granulomatosis
b) Systemic lupus erythematosus
c) Polyarteritis nodosa
d) Sjögren syndrome

36) Patient with chronic hypertension will show following changes on histology of kidney: (NEET 2014)
a) Hyaline arteriosclerosis
b) Hyperplastic arteriosclerosis
c) Onion skin lesions
d) Vessel lumen dilatation

37) Most common site of glomus tumor is: (NEET 2014)
a) Under fingernails b) Under toenails
c) Neck d) Axilla

38) Which of the following is not a large vessel vasculitis? (NEET 2014)
a) Takayasu arteritis
b) Cogan syndrome
c) Churg Strauss syndrome
d) Giant cell arteritis

39) HLA B51 is associated with: (NEET 2014)
a) Behcet's disease
b) Churg Strauss syndrome
c) Microscopic polyangiitis
d) Polyarteritis nodosa

40) p ANCA associated vasculitis is: (NEET 2014)
a) Temporal arteritis
b) Microscopic polyangiitis
c) Takayasu arteritis
d) Polyarteritis nodosa

41) Histologic finding in hyperplastic arteriosclerosis: (NEET 2014)
a) Concentric layer onion skin lesion
b) Mucinous intimal thickening
c) Fibrinoid atherosclerosis
d) All of the above

42) Libman sack's endocarditis is seen in: (NEET 2014)
a) SLE
b) Systemic sclerosis
c) Dermatomyositis
d) Inclusion body myositis

43) Irreversible injury to myocardial cell occurs in: (NEET 2014)
a) 20 - 40 min b) 40 - 60 min
c) 60 - 80 min d) 80 -100 min

44) Marker of Angiosarcoma is: (NEET 2014)
a) CD 31 b) Cytokeratin
c) Vimentin d) CD 55

45) Which is associated with vasculitis of medium size vessels? (NEET 2013)
a) Temporal arteritis
b) Wegeners granulomatosis
c) Polyarteritis nodosa
d) Tuberous sclerosis

46) Which is not a characteristic feature of Wegener Granulomatosis: (NEET 2013)
a) Granuloma in vessel wall
b) Focal necrotizing glomerulonephritis
c) Positive for c ANCA
d) Involves large vessels

47) Atherosclerosis is seen with which bacteria: (NEET 2013)
a) Staph aureus
b) Streptococcus pneumonia
c) Chlamydia
d) Mycobacteria

48) Most common histological finding in benign hypertension is: (NEET 2013)
a) Proliferating endarteritis
b) Necrotizing arteriolitis
c) Hyaline arteriosclerosis
d) Cystic medial necrosis

49) Glomus tumor is seen in: (NEET 2013)
a) Retro peritoneum
b) Soft tissue
c) Distal portion of digits
d) Proximal portion of digits

50) All is TRUE about Giant cell arteritis EXCEPT: (NEET 2013)
a) Involves large to small sized arteries
b) Granulomatous inflammation
c) Most commonly involved artery is abdominal aorta
d) Segmental nature of the involvement

51) Most common cause of dissecting hematoma is: (NEET 2013)
a) Hypertension b) Marfan's
c) Latrogenic d) Kawasaki

52) Pyogenic granuloma all are true except: (NEET 2013)
a) Bacterial infection b) Bleeding
c) Benign tumor d) Capillary hemangioma

53) In PAN, cysts are seen in all EXCEPT: (NEET 2013)
a) Lung b) Pancreas
c) Liver d) Heart

54) Atheromatous changes of blood vessels affects early in: (NEET 2013)
a) Kidney b) Heart
c) Liver d) Spleen

55) Kaposi sarcoma is seen with: (NEET 2013)
a) HCV b) HPV
c) HSV d) HHV

56) Most common cause of aortic aneurysm is: (NEET 2013)
a) Syphilis b) Marfan's syndrome
c) Atherosclerosis d) Congenital

57) Which of the following is abdominal angiitis? (NEET 2013)
a) Giant cell arteritis
b) Takayasu arteritis
c) Kawasaki disease
d) Polyarteritis Nodosa

58) Medial calcification is seen in: (NEET 2013)
a) Atherosclerosis
b) Arteriosclerosis
c) Monckeberg's sclerosis
d) Dissecting aneurysm

59) Sturge Weber syndrome is associated with: (NEET 2013)
a) Port wine stain
b) Cavernous hemangioma
c) Lymphangioma
d) Hemangiosarcama

60) The following change in the vessel is seen initially in Raynaud's phenomenon: (NEET 2013)
a) No change (Fibrinoid necrosis, thrombosis)
b) Thrombosis
c) Fibrinoid necrosis
d) Hyaline sclerosis

61) All of the following conditions are associated with granulomatous pathology, EXCEPT: (AIPGMEE 2010)
a) Wegner's granulomatosis
b) Takayasu Arteritis
c) Polyarteritis Nodosa
d) Giant cell arteritis

62) Not a predisposing factor for atherosclerotic plaque formation: (AIPGMEE 2011)
a) Apo E
b) Alpha 2-macroglobulin
c) Oxidized LDL
d) Increased homocystiene

63) What does "cardiac polyp" means? (AIIMS MAY 2011)
a) Acute infarct
b) Cardiac aneurysm
c) Benign tumour
d) Fibrinous clot

64) In a specimen of kidney, fibrinoid necrosis is seen and onion peel appearance is also present. Most probable pathology is: (AIIMS May 2011)
a) Hyaline degeneration
b) Hyperplastic arteriosclerosis
c) Glomerulosclerosis
d) Fibrillary glomerulonephritis

CHAPTER 11: BLOOD VESSELS

Ans. 1) C. Inner portion of media derives nutrition through vasa vasorum (Ref: 8 ed. Robbins p. 488-89, 9 ed. p. 483-84)

- **Three concentric layers** of blood vessels include **intima, media and adventitia** Q
- **Intima** is separated from the media by a dense elastic membrane called **internal elastic lamina** Q
- **Inner aspect of the media** receives oxygen and nutrients from the **vessel lumen**
- However, the **outer portions of the media** Q are nourished by **vasa vasorum** Q
- Outer limit of the media of **most arteries** has well-defined **external elastic lamina** Q

Ans. 2) A. Laminar flow (Ref: 8 ed. Robbins p. 490-91, 9 ed. p. 485-86, f-11-2)

Causes of endothelial dysfunction include:

- **Hypertension** Q, cytokines, complement, bacterial products, lipid products, **Advanced Glycation End products (in Diabetes)** Q, hypoxia and viruses
- **Turbulent flow** Q is responsible for endothelial dysfunction and not laminar flow

Ans. 3) D. All of the above (Ref: 8 ed. Robbins p.490-93, f-11-2,3)

Points to Remember Regarding endothelial cells:

- For maintaining **vessel wall homeostasis** and **circulatory function**
- Contains **Weibel-Palade bodies** Q, the organelles for **von Willebrand's factor** Q
- **Immunohistochemical markers** – Antibodies to **von Willebrand's factor** and/or platelet-endothelial cell adhesion molecule-1 **(PECAM-1 or CD31)** Q
- **Endothelial dysfunction** Q induces **thrombogenic** surface and leads to initiation of thrombus formation, **atherosclerosis** and vascular lesions of **hypertension** Q
- **Vascular injury**— Results in the formation of a **neo-intima** Q

Ans. 4) C. Na+ channel protein (Ref: 8 ed. Robbins p. 493, 9 ed. p. 490)

Single gene disorders Q which plays a role in **essential hypertension**:

- Disorders affecting the enzymes involved in aldosterone metabolism (e.g., **aldosterone synthase, 11β-hydroxylase, 17α-hydroxylase**) Q
- Mutations that affect **sodium reabsorption**. E.g. **Liddle syndrome** Q, caused by mutations in epithelial **Na + channel protein** Q

Ans. 5) D. All of the above (Ref: 8 ed. Robbins p.495-96, 9 ed. p. 490-91, f-11-6)

Vascular pathology in **hypertension:**

Hyaline arteriosclerosis Q**:**

- Seen in **diabetic microangiography** Q and **hypertension** Q
- Due to **plasma protein leakage** across injured endothelial cells
- **Arteriolar wall** is **thickened** with **increased protein deposition (hyalinized)** and markedly narrowed lumen

Hyperplastic Arteriolosclerosis Q**:**

- Seen in **severe (malignant) hypertension** Q
- Vessels exhibit **onion-skin lesions** Q, characterized by **concentric, laminated thickening** of the walls and luminal narrowing
- **Necrotizing arteriolitis** – kidney shows **fibrinoid deposits** and vessel wall necrosis Q

Ans. 6) D. All of the above (Ref: 8 ed. Robbins p. 496-98, 9 ed. p. 491-94, f-11-7, t-11-2)

Atherosclerosis:

- Characterized by **intimal lesions** called **atheromas** Q, which consists of a raised lesion with a **soft, yellow, grumous core of lipid** covered by a **white fibrous cap**

Non modifiable risk factors Q**:**

- Increasing age, Male gender, Family history, Genetic abnormalities

Modifiable Risk Factors Q –

- Hyperlipidemia, Hypertension, Cigarette smoking, Diabetes, C-reactive protein

Points to Remember:

- **Low-density lipoprotein (LDL) cholesterol** Q **("bad cholesterol")** is associated with increased risk
- **Higher levels of HDL correlate** with **reduced risk**
- **Inflammation** Q – is associated with **atherosclerotic plaque** formation
- **C-reactive protein (CRP)** Q (synthesized by liver Q) predicts the risk of **myocardial infarction, stroke, peripheral arterial disease and sudden cardiac death** Q
- **Hyperhomocystinemia** Q, **Metabolic syndrome** Q, **Lipoprotein (a)** Q **levels** are associated with **increased risk** of coronary and cerebrovascular disease risk

Ans. 7) D. All of the above (Ref: 8 ed. Robbins p. 496-98, 9 ed. p. 494-96, f-11-10, 11)

Pathogenesis of **Atherosclerosis:**

A) Endothelial injury Q:

- Due to hypertension, hyperlipidemia, toxins from cigarette smoke, homocysteine, inflammatory cytokines (e.g. tumor necrosis factor [TNF])

B) Hemodynamic disturbances Q:

- Leads to **plaque formation** at the areas of disturbed flow patterns i.e. at **ostia** of exiting vessels, branch points and along the **posterior wall of the abdominal aorta** Q

C) Dyslipoproteinemias Q:

- **Lipoproteins** within **intima** are ingested by **macrophages** Q, leading to formation of **foam cells** Q

D) Inflammation Q:

- At injured vessel, **endothelial cells** bind to monocytes and T cells
- Monocytes transform into **macrophages**

E) Infection Q:

- **Herpes-virus, cytomegalovirus** and **Chlamydia pneumoniae** are commonly seen

F) Smooth Muscle Proliferation Q:

- Due to growth factors like **PDGF, FGF and TGF-α**
- Intimal smooth muscle cell proliferation Q and ECM deposition Q (collagen) convert a **fatty streak** Q (the **earliest lesion**) into **mature atheroma**

Atheroma: consists of dysfunctional endothelial cells, proliferating smooth muscle cells and admixed lymphocytes and macrophages

Ans. 8) C. Coronary arteries are involved to a greater degree followed by abdominal aorta (Ref: 8 ed. Robbins p.502-504, 9 ed. p. 496-99, f-11-12-15)

Morphology of Atherosclerosis Q:

Fatty streaks Q:

- **Earliest lesion** to appear
- Begins as multiple **flat yellow spots**, which coalesce into elongated streaks **1 cm or more in length**

Atherosclerotic Plaque Q: Appears white to yellow and superimposed **thrombus** over ulcerated plaque is **red brown**

Vessels involved in **descending order:**

- **Lower abdominal aorta** Q
- **Coronary arteries** Q
- Popliteal arteries, internal carotid arteries and the vessels of the circle of Willis

Note: Vessels of the upper extremities are usually **spared** Q

Complications of Atherosclerotic Plaques [Q]**:**

- **Rupture, ulceration, or erosion** which induces **thrombosis** [Q]
- Hemorrhage into a plaque
- Athero-embolism
- Aneurysm formation
- Vasoconstriction

Ans. 9) D. All of the above (Ref: 8 ed. Robbins p.504, 9 ed. p. 499-500)

Major consequences of **atherosclerosis** [Q]:

- Myocardial infarction
- Cerebral infarction (stroke)
- Aortic aneurysms
- Peripheral vascular disease (gangrene of the legs)

Ans. 10) B. Decreased MMP contributes to aneurysm formation (Ref: 8 ed. Robbins p.506-07, 9 ed. p. 501-02, f-11-18)

- **Aneurysm** is a **localized abnormal dilation** of a blood vessel

True aneurysm [Q]

- Involves an **intact** attenuated **arterial wall** or **thinned ventricular wall** of the heart
- **Types** – Saccular aneurysm and fusiform aneurysm

False aneurysm [Q]**:**

- Defect in the **vascular wall** leads to **extravascular hematoma** which communicates with intravascular space **(pulsating hematoma)**

Pathogenesis:

- Defect in the connective tissue of vascular wall e.g. **Marfan syndrome**, Ehlers-Danlos syndrome
- **Increased MMP (Matrix Metalloproteinase) production** [Q], which brings about degradation of **Extra Cellular Matrix (ECM)** in arterial wall
- **Decreased tissue inhibitor of metalloproteinase (TIMP)** [Q] expression can also contribute to ECM degradation
- **Histologically, cystic medial degeneration** [Q] of the vessels is seen

Causes of aortic aneurysms:

- **Atherosclerosis** – leading to **abdominal aortic aneurysms** [Q]
- **Hypertension** – associated with **aneurysms of ascending aorta** [Q]
- **Mycotic aneurysms** [Q] – occurs due to
  a) Embolization of **septic embolus** [Q] from **infective endocarditis**
  b) Extension of adjacent **suppurative process** [Q]
  c) Organisms directly infecting the **arterial wall**

Ans. 11) C. Common in atherosclerosis patients (Ref: 8 ed. Robbins p.508-10, 9 ed. p. 504-05, f-11-21-22)

Predisposing factors [Q]**:**

- **Aortic dissection** occurs in **hypertensive patients** [Q]
- **Inherited or acquired connective tissue** disorders (e.g., Marfan syndrome, Ehlers- Danlos syndrome, Vitamin C deficiency, copper metabolic defects) [Q]

Morphology [Q]**:**

- Most frequent histologically detectable lesion is **cystic medial degeneration** [Q]

DeBakey classification – two types:

- **Type A dissection (proximal), (types I and II)** – involving either both the ascending and descending aorta or just the ascending aorta

- **Type B dissections or DeBakey type III (distal)** – distal to origin of subclavian artery
- Serious complications predominantly occur in **type A dissections** Q

Note:

- Dissection is **unusual** in the presence of **atherosclerosis** Q
- In **spontaneous dissections**, tear is found in the **ascending aorta** Q, usually within **10 cm** of the aortic valve

Ans. 12) D. Polyarteritis Nodosa (Ref: 8 ed. Robbins p.511, 9 ed. p. 505-06, t-11-3, f-11-23)

Classification of Immune Mediated Vasculitis Q:

a) Large Vessel Vasculitis Q – Giant-cell (temporal) arteritis, Takayasu arteritis

b) Medium Vessel Vasculitis Q – Polyarteritis nodosa, Kawasaki disease

c) Small Vessel Vasculitis Q:

- **ANCA associated** – Granulomatosis with Polyangiitis (Wegener granulomatosis), Churg-Strauss syndrome, Microscopic polyangiitis
- **Immune complex mediated** – SLE, Henoch- Schönlein purpua, Cryoglobin vasculitis, Goodpasture disease

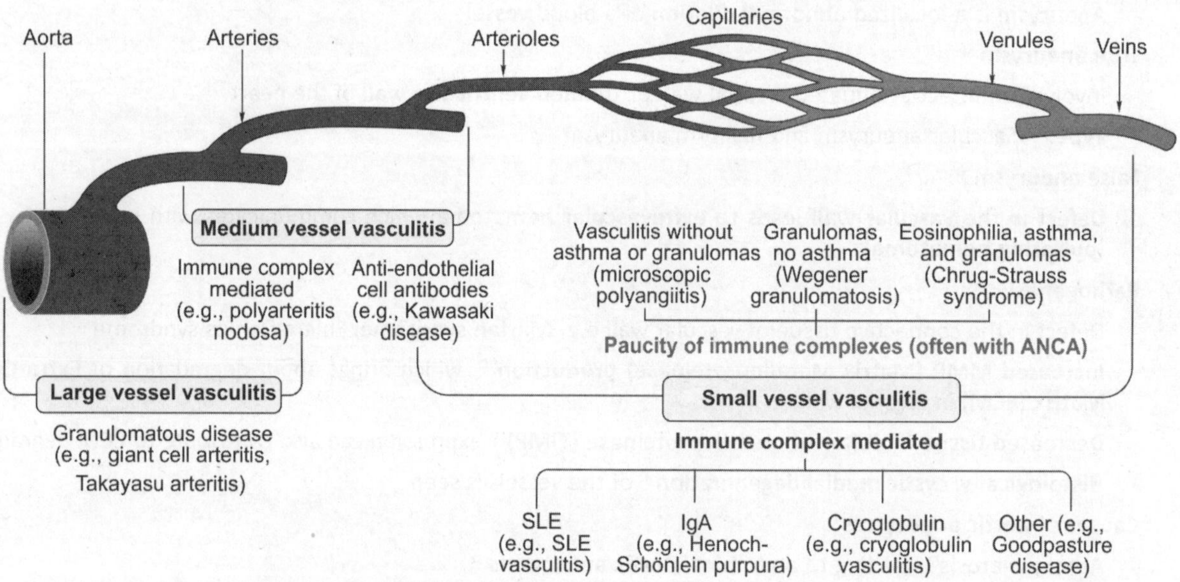

Different types of vasculitis according to the sites involved

Ans. 13) A. Granulomatosis with Polyangiitis (Ref: 8 ed. Robbins p.511, 9 ed. p. 507, t-11-3)

- **Anti-neutrophil Cytoplasmic Antibodies** Q – Previously classified into cytoplasmic (c-ANCA) or perinuclear (p-ANCA)
- **Anti-proteinase-3 (PR3-ANCA) or c-ANCA** Q– seen in **Granulomatosis with Polyangiitis** (Wegener granulomatosis) Q
- **Anti-myeloperoxidase (MPO-ANCA) or p-ANCA** Q – seen in **Microscopic polyangiitis** and **Churg-Strauss syndrome** Q

Ans. 14) B. Occurs in younger individuals (Ref: 8 ed. Robbins p.512-13, 9 ed. p. 507-08, f-11-24)

Giant-cell (temporal) arteritis Q:

- Most common form of vasculitis among **elderly individuals** Q
- **Characterized** by **granulomatous inflammation** Q of large to small-sized arteries
- Most commonly involves **temporal** Q, **ophthalmic** and **vertebral artery**

Morphology Q:

- **Nodular vessel wall thickening**
- **Tunica media** shows **granulomatous inflammation**, composed of T cells, macrophages and multinucleated giant cells

Diagnosis [Q]:

- Depends on **biopsy** [Q] and **histologic confirmation**
- **Giant-cell arteritis** is extremely **segmental**, adequate biopsy requires **2- to 3-cm** [Q] **length of artery**

Treatment – Corticosteroids, anti-TNF therapy

Ans. 15) C. Doesn't involve the pulmonary artery (Ref: 8 ed. Robbins p.513-14, 9 ed. p. 508-09, f-11-25)

Takayasu Arteritis:

- **Granulomatous vasculitis** [Q] of medium and larger arteries characterized by weakening of the pulses in the upper extremities (**pulseless disease**)
- Characterized by **trans-mural fibrous thickening** of the **aorta**
- **<50 years** – Takayasu Arteritis, **>50 years** – Giant cell arteritis

Morphology:

- Involves **aortic arch** [Q], **pulmonary artery** [Q]
- **Microscopically**, there is **destruction of arterial media** by **mononuclear inflammatory cells** with **giant cells**

Ans. 16) A. Involves the pulmonary circulation (Ref: 8 ed. Robbins p.514-15, 9 ed. p. 509-10, f-11-26)

Polyarteritis Nodosa (PAN) [Q]:

- **Systemic vasculitis** of small or medium-sized muscular arteries
- Involves renal and visceral vessels but **spares the pulmonary circulation** [Q]
- 30% of patients have **chronic hepatitis B** infection with **HBsAg-HbsAb complexes** [Q]

Morphology [Q]:

- **Acute phase** is **characterized** by **segmental trans-mural necrotizing inflammation** [Q] of small to medium-sized arteries, accompanied by **fibrinoid necrosis** [Q]
- In **chronic phase**, there is **fibrous thickening** of the vessel wall
- **All stages of activity (acute and late stage)** [Q] coexist in different vessels or even within the same vessel
- **Renal arterial involvement** is often **prominent** and a **major cause of death** [Q]

Ans. 17) D. All of the above (Ref: 8 ed. Robbins p.515, 9 ed. p. 510)

Kawasaki disease (mucocutaneous lymph node syndrome) [Q]:

- **Acute febrile, self-limited illness** of **infancy** and **childhood**
- **Arteritis** affecting **large** to **medium-sized** vessels
- Predilection for **coronary artery involvement** [Q]
- Formation of **autoantibodies** to **endothelial cells** [Q] and **smooth muscle cells**

Ans. 18) D. Associated with PR-3 ANCA (Ref: 8 ed. Robbins p.515, 9 ed. p. 510-11, f-11-27)

Microscopic Polyangiitis:

- **Necrotizing vasculitis** which affects **capillaries**, **arterioles** and **venules**
- Also known as **hypersensitivity vasculitis** or **leukocytoclastic vasculitis** [Q]
- In **contrast to PAN**, all lesions of **microscopic polyangiitis** tend to be of the **same age**
- **Necrotizing glomerulonephritis (90%)** and **pulmonary capillaritis** [Q] are common
- **MPO-ANCAs** [Q] are causally implicated

Morphology:

- Segmental **fibrinoid necrosis** [Q] of the **tunica media**
- **Leukocytoclastic vasculitis** [Q] – infiltration and fragmentation of neutrophils is seen in and around blood vessels

Ans. 19) D. Affects medium size vessels (Ref: 8 ed. Robbins p.516, 9 ed. p. 511, f-11-27)

Churg-Strauss syndrome [Q]:

- **Small-vessel necrotizing vasculitis** [Q]

- Characterized by **asthma** Q, allergic rhinitis, lung infiltrates, **peripheral hyper eosinophilia** Q and **necrotizing granulomas** Q
- Shows **MPO-ANCA** Q **positivity**
- **Myocardial involvement** may give rise to **cardiomyopathy** and is the **most common** cause of death
- **Myocardium shows eosinophilic infiltrates** Q

Ans. 20) A. All of the above (Ref: 8 ed. Robbins p.516-17, 9 ed. p. 511-12, f-11-27)

Granulomatosis with Polyangiitis (Wegener granulomatosis) is characterized by:

a) **Acute necrotizing granulomas** Q of **upper respiratory tract** or **lower respiratory tract** or both
b) **Necrotizing or granulomatous vasculitis** Q of small to medium-sized vessels
c) **Renal disease** in the form of focal and segmental necrotizing glomerulonephritis (early stage) and **crescentic glomerulonephritis** Q (later stage)

Other Features:

- **PR3-ANCAs** Q (c-ANCA) is present in up to **95%** of cases

Ans. 21) C. Heavy cigarette smokers are at risk (Ref: 8 ed. Robbins p.517, 9 ed. p. 512, f-11-28)

Thromboangiitis Obliterans/Buerger Disease Q:

- Seen exclusively in **heavy cigarette smokers** Q, usually before the age of 35 years Q

Microscopically Q:

- **Acute** and **chronic vasculitis** of **medium-sized and small arteries** Q of extremities
- Thrombus contains **small micro-abscesses** Q composed of **neutrophils** surrounded by **granulomatous inflammation**
- Characteristic feature is **instep claudication** Q
- Symptoms are relieved dramatically by **abstinence of cigarette smoking** Q

Ans. 22) C. High Grade Renal Cell Cancer (Ref: 8 ed. Robbins p.519, 9 ed. p. 515)

Superior vena caval syndrome Q:

- Caused by neoplasms that compress or invade superior vena cava
- **E.g. – Bronchogenic carcinoma** Q or **Mediastinal lymphoma** Q

Inferior vena caval syndrome Q:

- Caused by neoplasms that compress or invade the inferior vena cava
- **E.g. – Hepatocellular carcinoma** Q and **renal cell carcinoma** Q

Ans. 23) D. Milroy disease (Ref: 8 ed. Robbins p.520, 9 ed. p. 515)

Milroy disease Q **(heredofamilial congenital lymphedema** Q**):**

- Characterized by lymphatic agenesis or hypoplasia

Secondary or obstructive lymphedema Q:

Causes: Malignant tumors Q, Surgical procedures (axillary lymph nodes in radical mastectomy Q), Post-irradiation fibrosis, Filariasis

Ans. 24) C. Obvious vascular channel formation (Ref: 8 ed. Robbins p.520, 9 ed. p. 515-16, t-11-4)

Classification of vascular tumors:

Benign Neoplasms:

- Hemangioma – Capillary Hemangioma, Cavernous Hemangioma, Pyogenic granuloma
- Lymphangioma – Simple (capillary) lymphangioma, Cavernous lymphangioma (cystic hygroma)
- Glomus tumor
- Vascular ectasias – Nevus flammeus, Spider telangiectasia (arterial spider), hereditary hemorrhagic telangiectasis (Osler-Weber-Rendu disease)
- Reactive vascular proliferations – Bacillary angiomatosis

Intermediate grade neoplasms:

- Kaposi sarcoma
- Hemangioendothelioma

Malignant neoplasms:

- Angiosarcoma
- Hemangiopericytoma

Benign tumors:

- Produce **obvious vascular channels** Q filled with blood cells, lined by a layer of normal-appearing endothelial cells

Malignant tumors:

- More cellular, shows cytologic atypia, mitotic figures; but **do not form well-organized vessels** Q
- **Endothelial derivation** of neoplasms can be confirmed by immunohistochemical demonstration of **CD31** Q or **von Willebrand's factor** Q

Ans. 25) B. Regresses by seventh week of life (Ref: 8 ed. Robbins p. 520-21, 9 ed. p. 516, f-11-30, Ackerman 10 ed. p. 2152)

Capillary Hemangioma:

- Also called as **"strawberry" or juvenile Hemangioma** Q
- Grows **rapidly** in the **first few months**, fades at 1 to 3 years of age and **completely regresses by 7** Q years of **age** in 90% of cases
- **Sites** – Skin, subcutaneous tissues and **oral cavity, lips** Q, liver, spleen and kidneys, salivary glands, breast
- **Microscopically** Q – **Un-encapsulated aggregates** of closely packed, thin-walled capillaries, lined by flattened endothelium

Ans. 26) B. Regresses spontaneously (Ref: 8 ed. Robbins p.520-21, 9 ed. p. 516, f-11-30, Ackerman 10 ed. p.2152)

Features of Cavernous Hemangioma Q:

- Frequently involve deep structures and can be **locally destructive** Q
- Has **no spontaneous tendency to regress** Q and may require **surgery**
- Forms a component of **von Hippel-Lindau disease** Q, with **cavernous hemangiomas** arising within the **cerebellum, brain stem**, or **retina**

Microscopy Q:

- **Un-encapsulated** lesion, composed of **large, cavernous blood-filled vascular spaces**, separated by a modest connective tissue stroma
- Intravascular thrombosis with **dystrophic calcification** is common

Ans. 27) C. Recurrence is common (Ref: 8 ed. Robbins p.521, 9 ed. p. 516-17, f-11-30. Ackerman 10 ed. p.184-86)

Pyogenic Granuloma Q:

- Presents clinically as rapidly growing **polypoidal red mass**
- **Sites – oral cavity** Q, mucosa, fingers
- One third of the lesions develop after **trauma** Q
- Lesions can **spontaneously regress** Q
- Recurrence is rare Q

Microscopy Q:

- Epidermis shows ulceration and is lined by **granulation tissue** epithelium Q
- **Capillary lobule formation** Q with central branching vessel **(feeder vessel)**, surrounding which endothelial cell proliferation is seen

Note:

- Capillary lobule formation indicates a **benign process** [Q]
- Curettage and cautery is usually curative

Ans. 28) C. >2 cms in size (Ref: 8 ed. Robbins p.522, 9 ed. p. 517, Ackerman 10 ed. p.2153-54)

Glomus Tumors:

- Benign, **painful tumors** [Q] arising from smooth muscle cells of the glomus body
- **Most commonly found** in the digits, especially under the **fingernails** [Q]

Morphology:

- Lesions are round, slightly elevated, red-blue, firm nodules, usually **<1 cm in diameter** [Q]

Histologically [Q]:

- Aggregates, nests and masses of specialized glomus cells with branching vascular channels
- Individual tumor cells are **small**, **uniform** and **round or cuboidal**, with scant cytoplasm
- **Mast cells** [Q] are frequently seen accompanying the tumor cells
- **IHC** [Q] – Desmin, Actin, Vimentin positivity

Ans. 29) D. Bartonella Henselae (Ref: 8 ed. Robbins p.522-23, 9 ed. p. 517-18, f-11-31)

Bacillary Angiomatosis:

- **Opportunistic infection** in immune-compromised individuals e.g. **AIDS**
- **Sites** – skin, bone, brain and other organs

Causative agents:

- **Gram-negative** bacilli e.g. **Bartonella henselae** [Q], (organism responsible for **cat-scratch disease**[Q]) and **B. quintana**[Q], causative agent of **"trench fever"**
- Bacteria are demonstrated by molecular methods such as **polymerase chain reaction, Warthin Starry stain** [Q]
- **Vascular proliferation** is induced by **HIF-1α** [Q] by the bacteria; which in turn drives **VEGF production** [Q]

Ans. 30) D. Classic form of KS is associated with HIV (Ref: 8 ed. Robbins p.523-24, 9 ed. p. 518-19, f-11-32)

Kaposi Sarcoma (KS) [Q]:

- Common in patients with AIDS

Four forms [Q]:

*a) **Chronic KS (classic or European KS)***:
  - Not associated with human immunodeficiency virus (HIV) [Q]
  - Tumors are asymptomatic and remain localized to the skin and subcutaneous tissue

*b) **Lymphadenopathic KS (African or endemic KS)***:
  - Not associated with HIV [Q]
  - Patients presents with lymphadenopathy

*c) **Transplant-associated KS***:
  - Occurs in patients with solid-organ transplantation and those on long-term immunosuppression
  - **An aggressive (fatal) tumor** with nodal, mucosal and visceral involvement

*d) **AIDS-associated (epidemic) KS***:
  - Seen in a third of AIDS patients, particularly male homosexuals

Pathogenesis [Q]:

- 95% of lesions show association with **Human herpesvirus-8 (HHV-8)** [Q] or **KS associated herpes virus (KSHV)** [Q]
- Transmitted by sexual route
- **KSHV** induces a **lytic** as well as **latent infection** in **endothelial cells**, which proliferate

Morphology [Q]:

3 stages are recognized:

Patch stage – red to purple macules confined to distal lower extremities

Plaque stage – presents as raised plaques

Nodule stage – composed of sheets of plump, proliferating spindle cells seen mostly in dermis or subcutaneous tissues

Ans. 31) D. CD34 is used to demonstrate endothelial cell of origin (Ref: 8 ed. Robbins p.524-25, 9 ed. p. 519-20, f-11-33)

Angiosarcomas [Q]:

- Malignant endothelial neoplasm that affects older adults
- **Sites** [Q] – Most commonly skin, soft, tissue, breast and liver
- **Hepatic angiosarcomas** [Q] are associated with exposure of **Arsenic** [Q], **Thorotrast** [Q] and **Polyvinyl chloride** [Q]
- Can arise in the setting of **lymphedema**, after **radical mastectomy** [Q] for breast cancer
- **Endothelial cell origin** can be demonstrated by staining for **CD31** [Q] or **von Willebrand factor** [Q]

Thus CD31 and not CD 34, is used for demonstration of endothelial cells on IHC

Ans. 32) C. Endothelial cell markers positivity on IHC (Ref: Ackerman 10 ed. 2155-56, f-25-123)

Hemangiopericytoma:

- Arise from **pericytes** [Q] (myofibroblast-like cells that are normally arranged around capillaries and venules)
- **Special stains** confirm that **pericytes** are outside the **endothelial cell basement membrane**
- **Sites** [Q] – Lower extremities (especially the **thigh**), retro-peritoneum
- Metastasis can be seen hematogenously to lungs, bone or liver

Also Know:

Tumors with Hemangiopericytomatous like pattern [Q]:

- Solitary fibrous tumor, Synovial sarcoma, MPNST, Mesenchymal chondrosarcoma, Phosphaturic mesenchymal tumor, Infantile fibro sarcoma and Thymoma

Ans. 33) A. Wegener's granulomatosis (Ref: Robbins 9 ed. p.1122) Refer Q 13 for details

Ans. 34) D. All of the above (Ref: Robbins 9th ed. p. 1316-1317)

Ans. 35) C. Polyarteritis nodosa (Ref: 9ed Robbins, p. 509-10) Refer Q 16 for details

Ans. 36) A. Hyaline arteriosclerosis (Ref: 9th ed. Robbins p. 490) Refer to Q 5 for details

Ans. 37) A. Under fingernails (Ref: 9 ed. Robbins p. 517) Refer Q 28 for details

Ans. 38) C. Churg-Strauss syndrome (Ref: 9 ed. Robbins p. 511) Refer Q 19 for details

Ans. 39) A. Behcet's disease (Ref: 9ed. Robbins p. 511)

- HLA-B51 is associated with Behcet's disease

Ans. 40) B. Microscopic polyangiitis (Ref: 9 ed. Robbins p. 510-11)

Ans. 41) D. All of the above (Ref: Robbins p. 490-91) Refer Q 5 for details

Ans. 42) A. SLE (Ref: 9 ed. Robbins p. 562)

Ans. 43) A. 20-40 min (Ref: 9 ed. Robbins p. 541)

Ans. 44) A. CD 31 (Ref: 9 ed. Robbins p. 519) Refer Q 31 for details

Ans. 45) C. Polyarteritis nodosa (Ref: 9 ed. Robins p. 505-06) Refer Q 12 for details

Ans. 46) D. Involves large vessels (Ref: 9 ed. Robbins p. 511-12) Refer Q 20 for details

Ans. 47) C. Chlamydia (Ref: 9 ed. Robbins p. 494-96) Refer Q 7 for details

Ans. 48) C. Hyaline arteriosclerosis

Ans. 49) C. Distal portion of digits (Ref: 9 ed. Robbins p. p. 517) Refer Q 28 for details

Ans. 50) C. Most commonly involved artery is abdominal aorta (Ref: 9 ed. Robbins p. 507-08) Refer Q 14 for details

Ans. 51) A. Hypertension (Ref: 9 ed. Robbins p. 504-05) Refer Q 11 for details

Ans. 52) A. Bacterial infection (Ref: 9 ed. Robbins p. 516-17) Refer Q 27 for details

Ans. 53) A. Lung (Ref: 9 ed. Robbins p. 509-10) Refer Q 16 for details

Ans. 54) B. Heart (Ref: 9 ed. Robbins p. 496-99) Refer Q 8 to Q 10 for details

Ans. 55) D. HHV (Ref: 9 ed. Robbins p. 9 ed. p. 518-19) Refer Q 30 for details

Ans. 56) C. Atherosclerosis (Ref: 9 ed. Robbins p. 501-02) Refer Q 10 for details

Ans. 57) B. Takayasu arteritis (Ref: 9 ed. Robbins p. 508-09) Refer Q 12 & 15 for details

Abdominal aorta involvement can lead to abdominal pain

Ans. 58) C. Monckeberg's sclerosis (Ref: 9 ed. Robbins p. 491)

- Mönckeberg medial sclerosis is characterized by calcification of the walls of muscular arteries and involved the internal elastic membrane

Ans. 59) A. Port wine/stain (Ref: 9 ed. Robbins p. 516)

Sturge-Weber syndrome:

- Unilateral facial nevus (port-wine stain)
- Ipsilateral venous angiomas in cortical leptomeninges, mental retardation, seizures, hemiplegia and skull radio-opacities

Ans. 60) A. No change (Fibrinoid necrosis, thrombosis)

Ans. 61) C. Polyarteritis Nodosa (Ref: 9 ed. Robbins p. 509-10) Refer Q 13 to Q 16 for details

Ans. 62) B. Alpha 2-macroglobulin (Ref: 9 ed. Robbins p. 491-94) Refer Q 6 for details

Ans. 63) D. Fibrinous clot

- **Postmortem fibrinous clot in the heart is called cardiac polyp**

Ans. 64) B. Hyperplastic arteriosclerosis Ref: 9 ed. Robbins p. 490-91) Refer Q 5 for details

12

The Heart

How to go about this chapter?

- **One should be thorough with the following repeatedly asked topics:**
  - **Normal anatomy of the heart**
  - **Right and left sided heart failure**
  - **Congenital heart diseases – Atrial Septal Defect, Ventricular Septal Defect, Coarctation of Aorta, Tetralogy of Fallot**
  - **Ischemic heart disease**
  - **Valvular heart diseases – Rheumatic Heart Disease, Mitral Valve Prolapse, Infective endocarditis, Nonbacterial Thrombotic Endocarditis, Libman-Sacks endocarditis**
  - **Carcinoid heart disease**
  - **Dilated cardiomyopathy, Hypertrophic Cardiomyopathy**
  - **Myocarditis and pericarditis**
  - **Atrial myxomas**

EFFECTS OF AGING ON THE HEART

1) **Features of aging heart includes:**
a) Valvular thickening
b) Lambl excrescences
c) Lipofuscin deposits
d) All of the above

HEART FAILURE

2) **All are TRUE regarding cardiac hypertrophy EXCEPT:**
a) Pressure overload leads to concentric increase in wall thickness
b) Volume overload is characterized by ventricular dilation
c) Fetal cardiac genes can be expressed in adults
d) Left Ventricular thickness becomes 1.3-1.5cms in hypertrophy

3) **All are the features of Left sided Heart failure EXCEPT:**
a) Pulmonary congestion and edema
b) Heart failure cells
c) Kerly B lines
d) Ascites

4) **TRUE about Right sided heart failure:**
a) Most commonly it occurs due to left sided heart failure
b) Cor pulmonale occurs due to parenchymal lung diseases
c) Right atrial dilation
d) All of the above

CONGENITAL HEART DISEASE

5) **In cardiac development, cells derived from second heart field gives rise to all EXCEPT:**
a) Outflow tract
b) Atria
c) Right ventricle
d) Left ventricle

6) **TRUE about etiopathogenesis of Congenital heart disease:**
a) Single gene mutations
b) Chromosomal deletions
c) Trisomy and monosomy
d) All of the above

7) **All are TRUE about right to left shunt EXCEPT:**
a) Cyanosis
b) Paradoxical embolism
c) Hypertrophy osteoarthropathy
d) Eisenmenger syndrome

8) **Most common type of Atrial Septal Defect (ASD) is:**
a) Secundum ASD
b) Primum ASD
c) Sinus venosus
d) None of the above

9) **All are TRUE about Ventricular septal defect EXCEPT:**
a) Most common form of congenital cardiac anomaly
b) Associated with Tetralogy of Fallot
c) Most common type is infundibular VSD
d) 50% of VSD close spontaneously

10) **Preservation of ductal patency is done by:**
a) Prostaglandin F b) Prostaglandin G
c) Prostaglandin E d) Prostaglandin D

11) **All are TRUE about Tetralogy of Fallot EXCEPT:**
a) Cyanosis at birth
b) Degree of cyanosis depends upon the degree of pulmonary stenosis
c) Right ventricular failure is commonly seen
d) Right Aortic arch is seen in 25% of patients

12) **All of the following are TRUE about Coarctation of Aorta (COA) EXCEPT:**
a) Males are affected twice as females
b) Associated with Bicuspid Aortic Valve
c) COA with Patent ductus arteriosus (PDA) manifests in late adult life
d) Infantile forms produces cyanosis in lower half of body

ISCHEMIC HEART DISEASE

13) **All are TRUE about Pre-infarction Angina EXCEPT:**
a) Also called as Prinzmetal variant angina
b) Pattern of increasingly frequent pain
c) Can occur at rest
d) Warning sign of Myocardial Infarction (MI)

14) **Mechanism/s responsible for pathogenesis of MI:**
a) Coronary artery occlusion
b) Vasospasm
c) Emboli from left atrium
d) All of the above

15) **All are TRUE about myocardial injury in MI EXCEPT:**
a) Onset of ATP depletion occurs within seconds
b) Reperfusion therapy can make the infarction reversible within 6 hours
c) Permanent damage occurs after 2-4 hours
d) Ischemia is more pronounced in sub-endocardial zone

16) **All are TRUE about sub-endocardial infarction EXCEPT:**
a) Ischemic necrosis limited to 1/3 - 1/2 of ventricular wall
b) Sub-endocardial zone is least perfused region
c) Can occur due to severe reduction of blood pressure
d) Also referred to as 'ST elevation' infarcts

17) **Right coronary artery infarct involves all of the following EXCEPT:**
a) Posterior wall of the left ventricle
b) Posterior portion of the ventricular system
c) Anterior portion of the ventricular system
d) Posterior right ventricular free wall

18) **In the area of infarcted myocardium, well established granulation tissue appears after:**
a) 4-12 hours b) 3-7 days
c) 10-14 days d) 2-8 weeks

19) **Most sensitive and specific biomarkers of myocardial damage:**
a) Troponins
b) Creatine kinase MM
c) Lactate dehydrogenase
d) Myoglobin

20) **Complication/s following acute MI include(s):**
a) Arrhythmias
b) Myocardial rupture
c) Pericarditis
d) All of the above

21) **Electrical abnormalities of heart that predispose to sudden cardiac death (SCD) include:**
a) Long QT syndrome
b) Brugada syndrome
c) Short QT syndrome
d) Any of the above

HYPERTENSIVE HEART DISEASE

22) **All are the features of left ventricular hypertrophy on microscopy EXCEPT:**
a) Increased transverse diameter of myocytes
b) Interstitial fibrosis
c) Left ventricular cellular and nuclear enlargement
d) Fat in the ventricular wall disappears

VALVULAR HEART DISEASE

23) **All are TRUE about non-rheumatic aortic stenosis EXCEPT:**
a) Valve area 0.5-1cm^2
b) Heaped up calcified masses
c) Commissural fusion
d) Normal Mitral valve

24) **TRUE about Bicuspid Aortic valve:**
a) Rare congenital cardiovascular malformation
b) Mitral valve involvement is always seen
c) Larger cusp has a midline raphe
d) Rarely associated with Aortic stenosis

25) **All are TRUE about Mitral valve prolapse EXCEPT:**
a) Myxomatous degeneration is the key histologic change

b) Associated with Marfan syndrome
c) TGF-β deficiency causes Myxomatous change
d) Rarely leads to complications

26) All are TRUE about Rheumatic heart disease (RHD) EXCEPT:
a) Most common cause of Mitral stenosis
b) Aschoff bodies are seen
c) Antischkow cells are pathognomic
d) Mac Callam plaques are seen in right atrium

27) All are TRUE about Rheumatic heart disease EXCEPT:
a) Pancarditis is common
b) Vegetations along the line of closure
c) Mac Callam plaques commonly seen in Left Atrium
d) Tricuspid valve involvement is frequent

28) Complications of chronic RHD are:
a) Atrial fibrillation
b) Thromboembolism
c) Infective endocarditis
d) All of the above

29) Major offender/s of infective endocarditis in intravenous drug abusers is/are:
a) Streptococcus viridans
b) Staphylococcus aureus
c) Haemophilus
d) Any of the above

30) Prosthetic valve endocarditis is caused by:
a) Staphylococcus aureus
b) Staphylococcus epidermidis
c) Streptococcus viridans
d) Haemophilus

31) Vegetations characteristic of Infective endocarditis:
a) Small warty projections
b) Friable, bulky, destructive
c) Small, bland
d) None of the above

32) Most commonly Infective endocarditis vegetations affect/s:
a) Mitral valve
b) Aortic valve
c) Mitral and Aortic valve
d) Pulmonary valve

33) Non Bacterial Thrombotic endocarditis is associated with:
a) Squamous cell carcinoma
b) Small cell carcinoma
c) Mucinous adenocarcinoma
d) Papillary carcinoma

34) Most frequent valve involved in SLE:
a) Mitral b) Aortic
c) Pulmonary d) Tricuspid

35) All are TRUE about Carcinoid heart disease EXCEPT:
a) Associated with carcinoid syndrome
b) Plaque like endocardial thickening
c) Involves left sided heart valves
d) Gastrointestinal carcinoids don't induce carcinoid heart disease

36) Complications of Artificial valves include/s:
a) Thrombosis
b) Infective endocarditis
c) Intravascular hemolysis
d) All of the above

CARDIOMYOPATHIES

37) Investigation of choice for cardiomyopathies include:
a) ECG
b) TMT
c) Echocardiography
d) Endomyocardial biopsy

38) All are TRUE about Dilated cardiomyopathy (DCM) EXCEPT:
a) Heart is enlarged, flabby
b) Causes diastolic dysfunction
c) Dilatation of all chambers of heart
d) Interstitial and endocardial fibrosis is seen

39) Genetic influences in DCM involve(s):
a) Dystrophin
b) Desmin
c) Laminin A
d) All of the above

40) All are TRUE about Hypertrophic Cardiomyopathy (HCM) EXCEPT:
a) Most common heart disorder caused by a single gene mutation
b) Abnormal diastolic filling
c) Intermittent ventricular outflow obstruction
d) Ventricular dilatation is commonly seen

41) Region most commonly involved in HCM:
a) Sub-aortic b) Aortic
c) Mitral d) Pulmonary

42) Following mutations are noted in HCM EXCEPT:
a) β-myosin heavy chain (β-MHC)
b) Cardiac TnT
c) α-tropomyosin
d) Desmin

43) Toxic product(s) implied in the pathology of Loeffler endomyocarditis:
a) IL-1
b) Major basic protein
c) Chemotaxin
d) All of the above

44) **Causative agent(s) of myocarditis include(s):**
a) Cox-sackie virus A
b) Cytomegalovirus
c) Trichinosis
d) All of the above

45) **Normal pericardial sac contains ...... of fluid.**
a) <50 ml b) <30 ml
c) <20 ml d) <10 ml

PRIMARY CARDIAC TUMORS

46) **Most frequent type of pericarditis:**
a) Serous pericarditis
b) Purulent pericarditis
c) Fibrinous pericarditis
d) Hemorrhagic pericarditis

47) **All are TRUE about cardiac myxomas EXCEPT:**
a) Most common primary tumor of heart
b) Involves right atrium
c) Mobile tumors exert wrecking ball effect
d) Fever and malaise are commonly associated features

48) **TSC1 mutation is associated with the following cardiac tumors:**
a) Cardiac myxoma
b) Papillary fibroelastoma
c) Rhabdomyoma
d) Lipoma

49) **Ladder tears are: (NEET 2014)**
a) Spiral tears of aortic intima
b) Vertical tears of aortic intima
c) Horizontal tears of aortic intima
d) Oblique tears of aortic intima

50) **Antischkow cells are: (NEET 2014)**
a) Modified macrophages
b) Modified neutrophils
c) Modified B cells
d) Modified RBCs

51) **Site of carcinoid in heart: (NEET 2014)**
a) Tricuspid valve b) Aortic valve
c) Mitral valve d) Left atrium

52) **Which worm causes myocarditis? (NEET 2014)**
a) Trichuris
b) Trichinella
c) Enterobius
d) Strogyloides

53) **Which isoenzyme of LDH is seen in heart? (NEET 2014)**
a) LDH1 b) LDH2
c) LDH3 d) LDH4

54) **Burkitts lymphoma is caused by: (NEET 2014)**
a) EBV b) HPV
c) HSV d) RSV

55) **Most common benign heart tumor is: (NEET 2013)**
a) Rhabdomyoma
b) Hemangioma
c) Lipoma
d) Myxoma

56) **7-day-old MI the most sensitive biochemical marker: (NEET 2013)**
a) Troponin-T b) CPK MB
c) IDH d) Myoglobin

57) **Vegetations in Libman sac endocarditis are: (NEET 2013)**
a) Large and fragile
b) Small warty along the line of closure of valve
c) Small or medium sized on either or both sides of valve
d) Small bland vegetations

58) **Most common site of artery of atherosclerosis: (NEET 2013)**
a) LAD
b) RCA
c) LCX
d) Diagonal branch of LAD

59) **Post MI day 10 which enzyme is raised? (NEET 2013)**
a) LDH b) CPK
c) Troponin d) Myoglobin

60) **Cells seen after 72 hours in the infarcted area in MI are: (NEET 2013)**
a) Neutrophils
b) Lymphocytes
c) Macrophages
d) Monocytes

61) **Mc Callums patch is diagnostic of: (NEET 2013)**
a) Infective endocarditis
b) Rheumatic endocarditis
c) Myocardial infarction
d) Tetralogy of Fallot

62) **Heart failure cells are seen in: (NEET 2013)**
a) Kidney b) Heart
c) Lungs d) Brain

63) **A young female patient came for routine examination. On examination a mid-systolic click was found. There is no history of RHD. The histopathological examination is most likely to show: (AIIMS May 2012)**
a) Myxomatous degeneration and prolapse of the mitral valve
b) Fibrinous deposition on the tip of papillary muscle
c) Rupture of chordae tendinae
d) Aschoff nodule on the mitral valve

64) Tigered effect in myocardium is due to: (NEET 2013)
a) Malignant change
b) Fat deposition
c) Seen in rheumatic fever
d) Associated with myocarditis

65) A 45-year-old male had severe chest pain and was admitted to the hospital with a diagnosis of acute myocardial infarction. Four days later he died and autopsy showed transmural coagulative necrosis. Which of the following microscopic features will be seen on further examination? (AIIMS MAY 2011)
a) Fibroblasts and collagen
b) Granulation tissue
c) Neutrophilic infiltration surrounding coagulative necrosis
d) Granulomatous inflammation

66) Which of the following have most friable vegetation? (AIPGMEE 2010)
a) Infective endocarditis
b) Libman Sack's endocarditis
c) Rheumatic heart disease
d) SLE

67) Characteristic pathological finding in carcinoid heart disease is: (AIPGMEE 2010)
a) Fibrous endocardial thickening of right ventricle, tricuspid valve and pulmonary valve
b) Endocardial thickening of tricuspid valve with severe tricuspid stenosis
c) Collagen rich, elastic deposits in endocardium of right ventricle and pulmonary valve
d) Calcification of tricuspid and pulmonary valve

68) Athlete died sudden cardiac death. Following histopathology slide confirms the diagnosis, and is: (AIIMS Nov 2015)

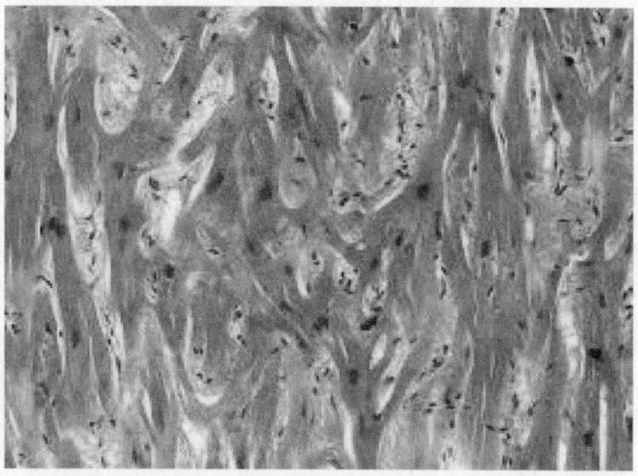

a) Hypertrophic obstructive cardiomyopathy
b) Rheumatic heart disease
c) Heart block
d) Dilated cardiomyopathy

69) Most common site of artery of atherosclerosis: (NEET 2013)
a) LAD
b) RCA
c) LCX
d) Diagonal branch of LAD

CHAPTER 12 – THE HEART

Ans. 1) **D. All of the above (Ref: 8 ed. Robbins p. 532, 9 ed. p. 525-26, t-12-1)**

Features of the aging heart:

- Valvular aging – include calcification of the mitral annulus and aortic valve
- **Lambl excrescences** Q – small filiform processes on the closure lines of aortic and mitral valves
- Deposition of **amyloid, lipofuscin** Q
- **Brown atrophy** Q – extensive lipofuscin deposition in a small, atrophied heart, seen in cachexic patients

Ans. 2) **D. Left Ventricular thickness becomes 1.3-1.5 cms in hypertrophy (Ref: 8 ed. Robbins p. 533-35, 9 ed. p. 527-29, f-12-1, 2)**

Cardiac hypertrophy:

- **Pressure-overload hypertrophy** Q – seen in **hypertension** or **aortic stenosis** Q, with concentric increase in wall thickness of ventricles
- **Volume-overload hypertrophy** – characterized by ventricular dilation
- **Fetal cardiac development genes** (e.g. β-myosin heavy chain, **natriuretic peptides** Q and collagen) can be seen in adults
- **Atrial Natriuretic Factor/peptide (ANF/ANP)** Q – used to assess the function of heart in CHF patients
- Normal **right ventricle thickness** is **0.3 - 0.5 cm** Q and **left ventricle** thickness is **1.3-1.5 cm** Q. Hence, in hypertrophy, thickness increases much more than normal

Ans. 3) **D. Ascites (Ref: 8 ed. Robbins p.535-36, 9 ed. p. 529-30)**

Left-sided heart failure Q:

- **Causes** – Ischemic heart disease, hypertension, aortic and mitral valvular diseases, myocardial diseases
- Impaired **left ventricular function** usually causes dilation of the **left atrium** Q and increases the risk of **atrial fibrillation**
- **Risk factors – Hypertension** Q **(most common)**, diabetes mellitus, obesity and bilateral renal artery stenosis

Lungs:

- **Pulmonary congestion and edema** Q – responsible for characteristic **Kerley B lines** Q on **chest X-Ray**
- **Hemosiderin-laden macrophages/Heart failure cells** Q – Red cells which extravasate into the edema fluid and are phagocytosed by macrophages

Ans. 4) **D. All of the above (Ref: 8 ed. Robbins p.536-37, 9 ed. p. 530-31)**

Right heart failure:

- Most common cause is **left-sided heart failure** Q
- **Cor pulmonale** Q is **most commonly** associated with **parenchymal diseases of the lung**
- Minimal pulmonary congestion

Morphology Q:

- **Heart** Q – Dilatation and hypertrophy of right atrium and ventricle
- Pleural, pericardial and peritoneal spaces – effusion can develop leading to **ascites**
- Subcutaneous tissues – Peripheral edema, anasarca

Liver and **portal system** Q:

- **Congestive hepatomegaly** Q due to **passive congestion**
- **Nutmeg liver** Q – **Congested red-brown** areas around the central vein and **normal colored** tan periportal regions
- **Centrilobular necrosis** Q
- **Cardiac sclerosis and cirrhosis** Q (long standing cases)
- **Spleen** – Congestive splenomegaly

Ans. 5) **D. Left ventricle (Ref: 8 ed. Robbins p.537-38, 9 ed. p. 531-32, f-12-3)**

Heart develops from **two heart fields** [Q] in which:

- Cells derived from the **first heart field** [Q] give rise to the **left ventricle**
- Cells derived from the **second heart field** [Q] give rise to the **outflow tract**, **right ventricle** and most of the **atria** [Q]

Ans. 6) **D. All of the above (Ref: 8 ed. Robbins p.538-39, 9 ed. p. 532-33, t-12-3)**

Causes of Congenital Heart Disease:

- Single gene mutations, small chromosomal deletions, trisomy and Monosomy

Examples include:

- **GATA4**, **TBX5** and **NKX2-5** genes are **mutated** in patients with **atrial and ventricular septal defects** [Q]
- **GATA4** [Q] and **TBX20** are mutated in adult-onset cardiomyopathy
- **NOTCH1** [Q] – associated with bicuspid aortic valve
- **JAG1 and NOTCH2** [Q] – Tetralogy of Fallot, Alagille Syndrome
- **Fibrillin** [Q] – Marfan Syndrome
- **Chromosome 22q11.2 deletion** [Q] – DiGeorge syndrome
- **Trisomy 21 (Down syndrome)** [Q] – **Most common** genetic cause of congenital heart disease. **Endocardial cushion defects** [Q] are most commonly seen

Ans. 7) **D. Eisenmenger syndrome (Ref: 8 ed. Robbins p.539-40, 9 ed. p. 533, f-12-4)**

- **Shunt** is an **abnormal communication** between chambers or blood vessels

Salient Features of right to left shunt [Q]:

- **Hypoxemia and cyanosis** [Q] – occurs due to admixture of poorly oxygenated venous blood with systemic arterial blood (called **cyanotic congenital heart disease**) [Q]
- Emboli from the peripheral veins can bypass the lungs and directly enter the systemic circulation (**paradoxical embolism**) [Q]
- **Hypertrophic osteoarthropathy** [Q] – Clubbing of tips of the fingers and toes
- **Examples** [Q] – Tetralogy of Fallot, Transposition of the great arteries, Persistent truncus arteriosus, Tricuspid atresia, Total anomalous pulmonary venous connection

Salient Features of Left to right shunt [Q] :

- **Right ventricular hypertrophy** [Q] – due to the increased pulmonary blood flow
- When **pulmonary vascular resistance** [Q] approaches **systemic levels**, a new **right-to-left shunt** [Q] can develop, leading to development of **Eisenmenger syndrome** [Q]
- **Examples** include – Atrial septal defect, Ventricular Septal Defect, patent ductus arteriosus and atrioventricular septal defects

Ans. 8) **A. Secundum ASD (Ref: 8 ed. Robbins p.540-41, 9 ed. p. 534-35, f-12-4)**

Three major types of ASDs:

- Secundum ASD (**90%** of all ASDs)
- Primum ASD
- Sinus venosus

Thus, **Secundum ASD** [Q] are most commonly found

Ans. 9) **C. Most common type is infundibular VSD (Ref: 8 ed. Robbins p.541, 9 ed. p. 535, f-12-4,5)**

Ventricular Septal Defect:

- **Most common form** [Q] of **congenital cardiac anomaly**
- Commonly seen in association with **Tetralogy of Fallot** [Q]
- 50% of small muscular VSDs **close spontaneously** [Q]

- **Treatment – Surgical or Catheter-based closure** of asymptomatic VSDs is delayed beyond **infancy** Q

Morphology Q **– Two types:**

- **Membranous VSD** Q **– 90%** involve the region of the **membranous interventricular septum (most common type)**
- **Infundibular VSD** Q – Defect lies below the pulmonary valve

Ans. 10) C. Prostaglandin E (Ref: 8 ed. Robbins p.542, 9 ed. p. 535)

- **Patent duct** is useful in infants with **congenital malformations** which obstruct the pulmonary or systemic outflow tract. E.g. **Aortic valve atresia** Q
- Preservation of ductal patency is done by administering **Prostaglandin E** Q

Ans. 11) C. Right ventricular failure is commonly seen (Ref: 8 ed. Robbins p.542-43, 9 ed. p. 535-36, f-12-6)

Four cardinal features of **Tetralogy of Fallot (TOF)** Q:

1) Ventricular Septal Defect
2) Obstruction of the right ventricular outflow tract (sub-pulmonary stenosis)
3) An aorta that overrides the Ventricular Septal Defect
4) Right ventricular hypertrophy

Morphology: Q

- Heart is **boot-shaped** Q due to **right ventricular hypertrophy**
- **Sub pulmonic stenosis** Q: leading to **right ventricular outflow tract obstruction**
- **Right aortic arch** Q is present in about 25% of cases

Clinical Features Q:

- Clinical consequences depends on the severity of **sub-pulmonary stenosis** Q
- If **sub-pulmonary stenosis** is mild, the shunt may be **left-to-right** Q, without cyanosis (so-called **pink tetralogy**) Q
- When the obstruction increases in severity, **right-to-left** Q shunting develops, producing cyanosis (**classic TOF**)
- **Right ventricular failure** is rare Q

Ans. 12) C. COA with Patent ductus arteriosus (PDA) manifests in late adult life (Ref: 8 ed. Robbins p.544, 9 ed. p. 537, f-12-8)

Coarctation of the Aorta (COA) Q

- Males are affected twice as often as females, except females with **Turner syndrome**
- Associated with **bicuspid aortic valve** Q in 50% of cases

Two classic forms:

A) Infantile form (COA with a patent ductus arteriosus) Q:

- Presents with **tubular hypoplasia** of **aortic arch** proximal to **patent ductus arteriosus (PDA)**
- Symptomatic in **early childhood** Q and presents with cyanosis localized to the lower half of the body Q

B) Adult form (COA without a patent ductus arteriosus) Q:

- Presence of a ridge like in-folding of the aorta, opposite the closed ductus arteriosus **(ligamentum arteriosum)**
- Asymptomatic till adult life and presents with **hypertension in upper extremities** and **weak pulses and hypotension** in the lower extremities
- Associated with claudication and coldness Q

Ans. 13) A. Also called as Prinzmetal variant angina (Ref: 8 ed. Robbins p.546-47, 9 ed. p. 539-40, f-12-9)

Angina Pectoris:

- Characterized by paroxysmal and recurrent attacks of sub-sternal or precordial chest discomfort
- Three overlapping patterns —1) **stable or typical angina** 2) **Prinzmetal variant angina** and 3) **unstable or crescendo angina**

1) Stable angina/Typical angina pectoris [Q]**:**
- Most common form, produced by **increased cardiac workload**
- **Relieved by rest** or administering **nitroglycerin**

2) Prinzmetal variant angina [Q]**:**
- Caused by **coronary artery spasm** [Q]
- Angina attacks are unrelated to physical activity, heart rate, or blood pressure
- Responds promptly to **nitroglycerin** [Q] and calcium channel blockers

3) Unstable or crescendo/pre-infarction angina [Q]**:**
- Pattern of **increasingly frequent pain** [Q] and of prolonged duration
- Can be precipitated even by lower levels of physical activity or at rest [Q]
- Occurs due to the **disruption of an atherosclerotic plaque** with superimposed **partial (mural) thrombosis** and possibly **embolization** or **vasospasm (or both)**
- Serves as a **warning sign for acute MI** [Q]

Point to Remember:

Silent ischemia – Ischemic events are not perceived by patients. Seen most commonly in Diabetics

Ans. 14) D. All of the above (Ref: 8 ed. Robbins p.547, 9 ed. p. 540)

Pathogenesis of **myocardial ischemia**:

1) Coronary Arterial Occlusion [Q] **(90%** of cases):
- Coronary angiography, within **4 hours** of onset of MI shows thrombosed coronary artery in **90%** of cases

2) Vasospasm [Q] with or without coronary atherosclerosis

3) Emboli from left atrium [Q] caused by **atrial fibrillation**, **mural thrombus**, vegetations of infective endocarditis, or paradoxical emboli

4) Ischemia [Q] of **small intramural coronary vessels** caused by **vasculitis**, disorders due to **sickle cell disease**, amyloid deposition

Ans. 15) B. Reperfusion therapy can make the infarction reversible within 6 hours (Ref: 8 ed. Robbins p.547-49, 9 ed. p. 540-43, f-12-10,11,12, t-12-4)

Myocardial changes seen after myocardial infarction:

Early changes:
- **Loss of adenosine triphosphate (ATP)** [Q] and **accumulation of lactate** [Q]
- **Myocardial injury** is **reversible** [Q] for approximately **30 minutes** [Q]
- Benefits of reperfusion is maximum in first **30 minutes** [Q]
- Severe ischemia lasting **20 to 30 minutes** or longer leads to **irreversible damage (necrosis)** of cardiac myocytes

Late changes:
- **Permanent damage** occurs when **perfusion of the myocardium** is severely reduced for **2 to 4 hours** [Q]
- **Ischemia** is most pronounced in the **sub-endocardium** [Q]
- **Necrosis** occurs within **6 hours** [Q] of the onset of severe MI

Ans. 16) D. Also referred to as 'ST elevation' infarcts (Ref: 8 ed. Robbins p.550, 9 ed. p. 543, f-12-12, 13)

Transmural infarcts [Q]**:**
- **Most myocardial infarcts** are **transmural** [Q]
- **Ischemic necrosis** involves full thickness of the **ventricular wall**
- Results due to the **combination** of chronic coronary atherosclerosis, acute plaque change and superimposed thrombosis
- Also known as **"ST elevation infarcts"** [Q]

Sub-endocardial infarct/non-ST elevation infarcts [Q]:

- **Sub-endocardial zone** is the **least perfused region** [Q] and is **most vulnerable**
- Occurs due to **prolonged, severe reduction** in **systemic blood pressure**

Ans. 17) C. Anterior portion of the ventricular system (Ref: 8 ed. Robbins p.550-51, 9 ed. p. 544, f-12-13,14,15,16)

Coronary arteries and the **areas involved** by their infarction:

- **Left anterior descending coronary artery** [Q]: **Anterior wall** of the **left ventricle** near the apex; anterior portion of ventricular septum; and apex circumferentially
- **Right coronary artery** [Q]: Inferior/posterior wall of left ventricle; posterior portion of ventricular septum; and inferior/posterior right ventricular free wall
- **Left circumflex coronary artery** [Q]: Lateral wall of left ventricle except at the apex

Ans. 18) C. 10-14 days (Ref: 8 ed. Robbins p.550-53, 9 ed. p. 543-46, t-12-5)

Evolution of morphological changes in **Myocardial Infarction** [Q]:

Reversible Injury

Time	Gross features	Microscopy
0 - ½hour	None	None

Irreversible Injury [Q]

½ – 4 hour	None	Waviness of fibers
4 – 12 hourSS	Dark mottling (occasional)	Coagulation necrosis; edema; hemorrhage
12 – 24 hourS	**Dark mottling**	Ongoing coagulation necrosis, early infiltration by neutrophils
1 – 3 days	Mottling with yellow tan infarct at the center	Coagulation necrosis, **brisk interstitial infiltrate of neutrophils**
3 – 7 days	Hyperemic border; central yellow-tan softening	Disintegration of dead myofibers, early phagocytosis of dead cells by macrophages at infarct border
7 – 10 days	Maximally yellow-tan and soft, with depressed red-tan margins	**Well-developed phagocytosis of dead cells**; early granulation tissue at margins
10 – 14 days	Red-gray depressed infarct borders	**Well-established granulation tissue** with collagen deposition
2 – 8 weeks	**Gray-white scar**	Increased collagen deposition, with decreased cellularity
>2 months	Scarring complete	Dense collagenous scar

Points to Remember:

Triphenyltetrazolium chloride [Q]:

- Highlights the area of necrosis
- Imparts a **brick-red color** [Q] to **non-infarcted myocardium** due to preserved dehydrogenase activity
- As **dehydrogenase leak out** [Q] through the damaged membranes of a dead cell, an **infarct** appears as an unstained **pale zone** [Q]

Note:

- **"Silent" MIs** are particularly common in **elderly** and in **diabetes mellitus** [Q] patients

Ans. 19) A. Troponins (Ref: 8 ed. Robbins p.555-56, 9 ed. p. 547, f-12-17)

Laboratory evaluation of MI [Q]:

- Based on measuring the blood levels of myoglobin, cardiac **troponins T and I**, MB fraction of **Creatine kinase (CK-MB)**, lactate dehydrogenase

A) **Troponins I and T** Q:

- **Most sensitive** and **specific** biomarker
- **Troponins I and T** levels begins to rise at **2 to 4 hours** of the onset of MI, peaks at **48 hours** and persist for approximately **7 to 10 days** Q

B) **CK-MB**:

- **Sensitive** but not specific and is also elevated when **skeletal muscle is injured**
- **CK-MB** begins to rise **within 2 to 4 hours** of the onset of MI, peaks at 24 hours and returns to the normal within approximately **72 hours** Q

Note: Unchanged levels of CK-MB and troponin over a period of **2 days** excludes the diagnosis of MI

Ans. 20) D. All of the above (Ref: 8 ed. Robbins p. 556-57, 9 ed. p. 547-49, f-12-18, 19)

Complications following Acute MI Q:

- **Contractile dysfunction** Q – leads to left ventricular failure, cardiogenic shock
- **Arrhythmias** Q – sinus bradycardia, heart block (asystole), tachycardia, ventricular premature contractions or ventricular tachycardia and ventricular fibrillation
- **Myocardial rupture – anterolateral ventricular free wall (most common)** Q, **ventricular septum** (less common) and **papillary muscle** (least common)
- **Pericarditis** Q – fibrinohemorrhagic pericarditis **(Dressler syndrome)**

Important Points to Remember:

- **Anterior transmural infarcts** Q can lead to **free-wall rupture, mural thrombi** and **aneurysm**
- **Posterior transmural infarcts** Q can be complicated by **conduction blocks, right ventricular involvement**

Ans. 21) D. Any of the above (Ref: 8 ed. Robbins p.558-59, 9 ed. p. 551-52)

Sudden Cardiac Death (SCD):

- As a consequence of **lethal arrhythmia** (e.g., asystole, ventricular fibrillation)
- **Acute myocardial ischemia** Q – **most common** trigger for **fatal arrhythmias**

Electrical abnormalities Q that predispose to **SCD** Q:

- **Long QT syndrome** Q, **Brugada syndrome, short QT syndrome, polymorphic ventricular tachycardia**, Wolff-Parkinson-White syndrome, congenital sick sinus syndrome and isolated cardiac conduction disease
- **Long QT syndrome** can predispose to **malignant ventricular arrhythmias** Q, which occurs due to the mutation in **gene** encoding **KCNQ1** Q

Ans. 22) D. Fat in the ventricular wall disappears (Ref: 8 ed. Robbins p. 559-60, 9 ed. p. 552-53, f-12-20)

- Ventricular wall fat **disappears** in **right ventricular hypertrophy** Q

Left side (Systemic) Hypertensive heart disease:

- Left ventricular wall thickness may exceed **2.0 cm** Q

Microscopy:

- **Earliest change** Q - Increase in the **transverse diameter of myocytes** Q
- **Cellular and nuclear enlargement** Q with **interstitial fibrosis** Q in advanced stage

Cor pulmonale Q

- **Acute cor pulmonale** can follow **massive pulmonary embolism** Q
- **Chronic cor pulmonale** Q results from **right ventricular hypertrophy** secondary to **chronic lung diseases** Q
- In **chronic cor pulmonale** Q, right ventricular wall thickens up to **1.0 cm**

Microscopy:

- Normally, the **myocytes** of right ventricle are **haphazardly arranged** Q and the wall contains **transmural fat** Q
- In right ventricular hypertrophy, **fat in the wall disappears** Q and the myocytes are aligned **circumferentially** Q

Ans. 23) C. Commissural fusion (Ref: 8 ed. Robbins p.561-62, 9 ed. p. 554-55, f-12-21)

In Valvular Heart Disease:

- **Stenosis** is the failure of a valve to open completely
- **In-sufficiency**, results from failure of a valve to close completely, thus allowing reverse flow

Morphology of **calcific aortic stenosis**:

- **Hallmark** of **non-rheumatic, calcific aortic stenosis** is **heaped-up calcified masses** Q within the aortic cusps
- **Functional valve area** is **decreased** leading to outflow obstruction
- Commissural fusion is **not** seen Q
- Mitral valve is generally **normal** Q
- **Rheumatic aortic stenosis** – Patients have **commissural fusion** and structural **abnormalities of the mitral valve** Q
- Normal **aortic valve** area is **4 cm^2**, however in severe **aortic stenosis**, the valve area is reduced to **0.5 to 1 cm^2**

Ans. 24) C. Larger cusp has a midline raphe (Ref: 8 ed. Robbins p.562-63, 9 ed. p. 555-56, f-12-21)

Bicuspid Aortic Valve (BAV):

- Most frequent **congenital cardiovascular malformation** Q
- Only **two functional cusps** Q are seen in **bicuspid aortic valve** Q
- Larger cusp shows fusion at its center, called as **midline raphe** Q and is a major site of calcific deposits
- **Complications** include **aortic stenosis** Q or **regurgitation** Q, **infective endocarditis** Q and **aortic dilation** Q and/or **dissection** Q
- **Mitral valve** is **normal** in these patients

Ans. 25) C. TGF-β deficiency causes Myxomatous change (Ref: 8 ed. Robbins p.563-64, 9 ed. p. 556-57, f-12-22)

Mitral Valve Prolapse (MVP):

- One or both mitral valve leaflets are **"floppy" and prolapse** and projects into the left atrium during systole Q
- **Myxomatous degeneration** Q is the key histologic change
- Associated with **Marfan syndrome**, due to mutation in **fibrillin-1 (FBN-1)** Q
- **Increased TGF-β** Q levels, leads to **valvular myxomatous change,** which can be **prevented** by **TGF-β inhibitors** Q
- Physical examination reveals a **mid-systolic click** Q
- Diagnosis is confirmed by **echocardiography**

Ans. 26) D. Mac Callam plaques are seen in right atrium (Ref: 8 ed. Robbins p.565-66, 9 ed. p. 557-59, f-12-23, 24)

Rheumatic Fever (RF):

- Occurs few weeks following an episode of **group A streptococcal pharyngitis** Q
- **Acute rheumatic carditis** Q is a frequent manifestation during the **active phase**
- **RF** is the most common cause of **mitral stenosis** Q

Morphology:

Heart:

- **Aschoff bodies**–Focal inflammatory lesions Q, which consists of lymphocytes, plasma cells and plump activated macrophages called **Anitschkow cells (pathognomonic for RF)** Q
- Antischkow cells have abundant cytoplasm and round-to ovoid nuclei in which the chromatin is disposed in a central, slender, wavy ribbon **("caterpillar cells")**
- Aschoff bodies are seen in any of the three layers of heart **(Pancarditis)**
- **Vegetations (verrucae)** Q, along the lines of closure of valves
- **MacCallum plaques – Sub-endocardial lesions (irregular thickenings)**, seen in **left atrium** Q

Ans. 27) D. Tricuspid valve involvement is frequent (Ref: 8 ed. Robbins p. 565-66, 9 ed. p. 557-59, f-12-23, 24)

- **Mitral valve** Q – **Most commonly** affected followed by the aortic valve and results in **"fish mouth"** or **"buttonhole" stenosis**

- **Tricuspid valve** is rarely involved

Pathogenesis:

- **Acute rheumatic fever** results from **immune responses** to **group A streptococci**
- **Antibodies** directed against the **M proteins of streptococci** [Q] have been shown to cross-react with **self-antigens in the heart**

Clinical Features [Q]**:**

- **Major manifestations:**
  a) **Migratory polyarthritis** of the large joints b) **Pancarditis**, c) Subcutaneous nodules d) Erythema marginatum of the skin e) Sydenham chorea (a neurologic disorder with involuntary rapid, purposeless movements)
- **Minor manifestations:** Fever, arthralgia, or elevated blood levels of acute-phase reactants

Note:

Diagnosis is **established** by **Jones criteria** [Q]:

- Evidence of preceding group A streptococcal infection
- Presence of two of the major manifestations or one major and two minor manifestations.

Ans. 28) D. All of the above (Ref: 8 ed. Robbins p.565-66, 9 ed. p. f-12-23, 24)

Salient Features of Rheumatic Fever (RF):

- **Acute RF** appears **10 days to 6 weeks** [Q] after an episode of pharyngitis caused by **group A streptococci** [Q]
- **Age group – 5 and 15** years
- Antibodies to **one** or **more streptococcal enzymes, streptolysin O** and **DNase B**, can be detected in the sera of patients

Complications in chronic RHD patients [Q]:

- **Arrhythmias (atrial fibrillation)**, thromboembolism, infective endocarditis, cardiac murmurs, cardiac hypertrophy and dilation and heart failure

Ans. 29) B. Staphylococcus aureus (Ref: 8 ed. Robbins p.566-68, 9 ed. p. 559-61, f-12-24, 25)

Infective Endocarditis (IE) [Q]:

- Microbial infection of **heart valves** or **endocardium** leading to formation of **vegetations**
- **Vegetations** [Q] are composed of **thrombotic debris** and **organisms**

Two types:

a) **Acute infective endocarditis** – Caused by infection of previously normal heart valve by a **highly virulent organism**
b) **Sub-acute IE** – Insidious infection of deformed valves, by organisms of lower virulence

Etiology and Pathogenesis [Q]:

- **Predisposing conditions** [Q] – rheumatic heart disease (in past), mitral valve prolapse, degenerative calcific valvular stenosis, bicuspid aortic valve, artificial valves
- **Streptococcus viridans** [Q] – **common** agent responsible for **endocarditis** of native but previously damaged valves
- **Staphylococcus aureus** [Q] **(S. aureus)** is the major offender in IE among **intravenous drug abusers**
- **Prosthetic valve endocarditis** is **most commonly** caused by coagulase negative **S. epidermidis** [Q]

Ans. 30) B. Staphylococcus epidermidis (Ref: 8 ed. Robbins p. 567, 9 ed. p. 559-60, 563)

- **Prosthetic valve endocarditis** is caused most commonly by **coagulase-negative staphylococci** (e.g. **S. epidermidis)** [Q]

Ans. 31) B. Friable, bulky, destructive (Ref: 8 ed. Robbins p. 566-68, 9 ed. p. 560, f-12-24)

Morphology [Q]:

- **Hallmark of IE** is presence of a **friable, bulky, potentially destructive vegetations** [Q]
- **Aortic and mitral valves** [Q] – **most common** sites of infection
- **Right heart valves** may also be involved, particularly in **intravenous drug abusers** [Q]

- Vegetations may erode into the underlying myocardium and produce **ring abscess**
- Embolic fragments may contain large numbers of **virulent organisms**
- **Abscesses** often develop at the sites where the emboli lodge, leading to **septic infarcts or mycotic aneurysms**

Ans. 32) C. Mitral and Aortic valve (Ref: 8 ed. Robbins p. 566-68, 9 ed. p. 560, f-12-25,26)

Refer to question 31

Ans. 33) C. Mucinous adenocarcinoma (Ref: 8 ed. Robbins p. 568-69, 9 ed. p. 561-62, f-12-26)

Nonbacterial Thrombotic Endocarditis (NBTE) Q:

- Characterized by **small sterile thrombi**, measuring **1-5 mm** in size
- Occur singly or multiply **along the line of closure of the leaflets or cusps** Q
- Vegetations **do not elicit** Q any **inflammatory reaction**

Predisposing Conditions Q:

- Seen in **cancer or sepsis patients** (so previously called as ***Marantic endocarditis*** Q)
- Associated with **mucinous adenocarcinomas** Q and the **pro-coagulant effects** are due to tumor-derived **mucin** or **tissue factor** Q
- As a part of **Trousseau syndrome** in **migratory thrombophlebitis** Q
- **Endocardial trauma**, due to an indwelling catheter

Ans. 34) A. Mitral (Ref: 8 ed. Robbins p. 569, 9 ed. p. 562, f-12-24)

- **Libman-Sacks endocarditis**, is occasionally encountered in **SLE** Q
- **Mitral** Q and **tricuspid valves** are **most commonly** involved
- Vegetations are **small (1–4 mm in diameter)** Q, single or multiple, **sterile** Q, have a **warty (verrucous) appearance** on either or both sides of **valves**
- **Histologically,** vegetations may contain **hematoxylin bodies** Q (homogeneous remnants of nuclei damaged by anti-nuclear antigen bodies)

Ans. 35) C. Involves left sided heart valves (Ref: 8 ed. Robbins p. 569-70, 9 ed. p. 562, f-12-27)

Carcinoid Heart Disease Q:

- **Most common cardiac manifestation** is **tricuspid insufficiency** Q followed by pulmonary valve insufficiency

How the cardiac lesions are brought about?

- Due to the elaboration of **serotonin (5-hydroxytryptamine)**, kallikrein, bradykinin, histamine, prostaglandins and tachykinins

Why gastrointestinal carcinoids do not usually induce carcinoid heart disease?

- Because the **key bioactive mediators** released into the **portal circulation** by **gut carcinoid tumors** are readily **metabolized by the liver** Q and do not reach the heart

Why predominantly right heart is involved?

- Due to the inactivation of both **serotonin and bradykinin** during passage **through the lungs** Q by **monoamine oxidase** present in **pulmonary vascular endothelium**

Morphology:

- **Intimal plaque like thickenings** of the **endocardial surfaces** of the cardiac chambers and valve leaflets

Ans. 36) D. All of the above (Ref: 8 ed. Robbins p. 570-71, 9 ed. p. 563, f-12-28, t-12-10)

Complications of cardiac valve prostheses include Q:

- Thromboembolism
- Infective endocarditis
- Structural deterioration
- Intravascular hemolysis due to high shear forces

Ans. 37) D. Endomyocardial biopsy (Ref: 8 ed. Robbins p. 572)

- **Endomyocardial biopsies** Q are used in **diagnosis and management** Q of individuals with myocardial disease

Ans. 38) B. It causes diastolic dysfunction (Ref: 8 ed. Robbins p. 573-75, 9 ed. p. 565-68, t-12-11, f-12-29-32)

Dilated Cardiomyopathy (DCM) Q:

- Characterized by progressive **cardiac dilation** and **contractile (systolic) dysfunction** Q

Morphology Q:

- Heart is **enlarged**, **heavy** and **flabby**, due to dilation of all chambers Q
- **Mural thrombi** Q are common and are a source of **thromboemboli**

Histology:

- Most of muscle cells are **hypertrophied** with **enlarged nuclei** Q
- **Interstitial and endocardial fibrosis** is present Q

Pattern	Left Ventricular Ejection Fraction	Causes
Dilated (systolic dysfunction)	<40%	Genetic; alcohol; peripartum; myocarditis; hemochromatosis; chronic anemia; doxorubicin (Adriamycin) toxicity; sarcoidosis; idiopathic
Hypertrophic (diastolic dysfunction)	50% to 80%	Genetic; Friedreich ataxia; storage diseases; infants of diabetic mother
Restrictive (diastolic dysfunction)	45% to 90%	Amyloidosis; radiation-induced fibrosis; idiopathic

Ans. 39) D. All of the above (Ref: 8 ed. Robbins p.573-75, 9 ed. p. 565-68, f-12-30,31)

Pathogenesis of DCM:

a) **Genetic influences** Q:
   - **AD** inheritance is the **predominant pattern** Q
   - Also seen are **X-linked**, **autosomal-recessive** and **mitochondrial inheritance** patterns
   - **Mutations in the following genes** are noted: **Dystrophin** Q (X-linked cardiomyopathy), **cardiac α-actin, Desmin** and **lamin A and lamin C**

b) **Myocarditis** Q:
   - Viral nucleic acids from **Coxsackievirus B** Q and other **Enteroviruses** have been detected in the myocardium of patients with DCM

c) **Alcohol and other toxins** Q:
   - **Alcohol abuse** and chemotherapeutic agents, including **doxorubicin** (Adriamycin)

d) **Childbirth**:
   - **Peripartum cardiomyopathy**, which occurs **late in pregnancy** or several weeks to months **postpartum** Q

Ans. 40) D. Ventricular dilatation is commonly seen (Ref: 8 ed. Robbins p.575-77, 9 ed. p. 569-70, f-12-31,34)

Hypertrophic Cardiomyopathy (HCM):

- Characterized by myocardial hypertrophy, **abnormal diastolic filling** Q, intermittent ventricular outflow obstruction
- Caused by **mutations** in genes encoding **sarcomeric proteins** Q
- **Most common** cardiovascular disorder caused by **single gene mutations** Q
- Heart is thick-walled, heavy, **hyper-contracting** Q, in striking contrast to the flabby, **hypo-contracting** heart of DCM
- Causes **diastolic dysfunction** Q
- One of the most common causes of **sudden death** in young athletes Q
- Has to be distinguished from **deposition diseases** (e.g., amyloidosis, Fabry disease) Q and **hypertensive heart disease**

Ans. 41) **A. Sub-aortic (Ref: 8 ed. Robbins p.575-77, 9 ed. p. 569, f-12-34)**

Morphology of HCM:

- **Asymmetric septal hypertrophy** Q: Characterized by disproportionate thickening of the ventricular septum
- On **cross-section**, ventricular cavity is compressed into a **"banana-like" configuration** Q
- Marked hypertrophy is **most prominent** in the **sub-aortic region** Q

Histologic Features:

- Extensive **myocyte hypertrophy** Q, with transverse myocyte diameters > than **40 μm** (normal=15 μm)
- **Myofiber disarray** Q
- Interstitial fibrosis

Ans. 42) **D. Desmin (Ref: 8 ed. Robbins p.575-77, 9 ed. p. 566, 569, f-12-30)**

Mutations causing HCM are found in:

- Genes encoding β-**myosin heavy chain (β-MHC)** Q **– most common**
- Genes for **cardiac TnT**, **α-tropomyosin** and **myosin-binding protein C (MYBP-C)** Q

Ans. 43) **B. Major basic protein (Ref: 8 ed. Robbins p.577, 9 ed. p. 570)**

Restrictive cardiomyopathies include:

- Endomyocardial fibrosis
- Loeffler endomyocarditis
- Endocardial fibroelastosis

Loeffler endomyocarditis Q

- Associated with **peripheral eosinophilia** Q and eosinophilic infiltrates in other organs
- **Major basic protein** Q, from eosinophils, initiates **Endomyocardial necrosis**
- Associated with **myeloproliferative disorder** (with chromosomal rearrangements involving either the **PDGFRα or PDGFRβ genes)**

Salient Features Q of restrictive cardiomyopathy –

- Decrease in ventricular compliance which results in impaired ventricular filling during **diastole**

Causes:

- **Idiopathic** or
- Associated with **radiation fibrosis, amyloidosis, sarcoidosis, metastatic tumors, inborn errors of metabolism** Q

Ans. 44) **D. All of the above (Ref: 8 ed. Robbins p. 578, 9 ed. p. 57-71, t-12-13, f-12-35)**

Major Causes of Myocarditis:

a) Infections:

- Viruses – **Coxsackievirus** Q, ECHO, influenza, **HIV**, **cytomegalovirus** Q
- Chlamydia – C. psittaci
- Rickettsiae – R. typhi, typhus fever
- Bacteria – **Corynebacterium diphtheriae** Q, Neisseria meningococcus, Borrelia (Lyme disease)
- Fungi – Candida
- Protozoa – **Trypanosoma cruzi (Chagas disease)** Q, toxoplasmosis
- Helminths – **Trichinosis** Q

b) Immune mediated:

- Post-viral
- Post-streptococcal (rheumatic fever)
- Systemic lupus erythematosus
- Drug hypersensitivity (e.g., methyldopa, sulfonamides)

- Transplant rejection

c) Unknown – Sarcoidosis, Giant cell myocarditis

Ans. 45) A. < 50 ml (Ref: 8 ed. Robbins p. 581, 9 ed. p. 573)

- **Pericardial sac** contains **less than 50 mL** of thin, clear, straw-colored fluid
- Effusions of **less than 500 mL** Q produces a **characteristic globular enlargement** of heart shadow on **chest radiographs**
- Rapidly developing fluid collection of **200 to 300 mL** fluid produce fatal **cardiac tamponade** Q

Ans. 46) C. Fibrinous pericarditis (Ref: 8 ed. Robbins p. 581-82, 9 ed. p. 573-74)

Serous Pericarditis:

- Produced by Noninfectious, inflammatory diseases
- **Examples –** Rheumatic fever, SLE and scleroderma, tumors and uremia

Fibrinous and **serofibrinous pericarditis**:

- **Most frequent type** of **pericarditis**

Causes:

- **Acute MI, Post-infarction (Dressler) syndrome, uremia, chest radiation**, rheumatic fever, SLE and trauma

Purulent or suppurative pericarditis:

- **Cause** – Direct extension from neighboring infections, seedling from blood, lymphatic extension

Hemorrhagic Pericarditis:

- **Most common** cause is spread of a **malignant neoplasm** to the **pericardial space**
- Also, seen in **bacterial infections**, patients with underlying bleeding diathesis and tuberculosis

Caseous Pericarditis: e.g. Tuberculosis

Ans. 47) B. Involves right atrium (Ref: 8 ed. Robbins p.583-84, 9 ed. p. 575-76, f-12-38)

Atrial myxomas:

- **Most common primary tumor** Q of the heart in adults
- 90% are located in the **left atria** Q

Morphology:

- **Site: Fossa ovalis** Q in the **atrial septum, sessile or pedunculated** lesions
- Range in size from 1 cm to 10 cm
- **Pedunculated form** exert a **"wrecking-ball" effect**, causing damage to **valve leaflets**
- **Histologically** Q – composed of **stellate** or **globular myxoma cells** embedded in abundant **amorphous extracellular matrix**

Clinical Features:

- **Fever and malaise** Q, due to the elaboration of the **cytokine IL-6** Q
- **Carney complex** Q (seen in 10% of cases) – **Autosomal-dominant** transmission, multiple cardiac and often **extra cardiac** (e.g., skin) **myxomas** Q, **pigmented skin lesions** Q and **endocrine over activity** Q
- **PRKAR1 mutation** Q is noted in **Carney complex patients**

Ans. 48) C. Rhabdomyoma (Ref: 8 ed. Robbins p.583-84, 9 ed. p. 576)

Rhabdomyoma Q:

- **Most frequent primary tumor** of the **heart** in infants and children
- Often associated with **tuberous sclerosis** Q, caused by **defects** in **TSC1 or TSC2** Q **tumor suppressor genes**

Ans. 49) C. Horizontal tears of aortic intima (Ref: Textbook of forensic medicine and toxicology: Principles and practice p. 385)

- Ladder tears are the horizontal tears of intima

Ans. 50) A. Modified macrophages (Ref: 9 ed. Robbin's p. 558) Refer Q 26 for details

Ans. 51) A. Tricuspid valve (Ref: 9 ed. Robbin's p. 562) Refer Q 35 for details

Ans. 52) B. Trichinella (Ref: 9 ed. Robbins p. 571, t-12-13) Refer Q 44 for details

Ans. 53) A. LDH1

LDH-1 is seen in heart and red blood cells and in brain

Ans. 54) A. EBV (Ref: 9 ed. Robbins p. 597-598) Refer Q 44 for details

Ans. 55) D. Myxoma (Ref: 9 ed. Robbins p. 575-76) Refer Q 47 and 48 for details

Ans. 56) A. Troponin T (Ref: 9 ed. Robbins p. 547) Refer Q 19 for details

Ans. 57) C. Small or medium sized on either or both sides of valve (Ref: 9ed. Robbins p. 562) Refer Q 34 for details

Ans. 58) A. LAD (Ref: 9 ed. Robbins p. 544) Refer Q 17 for details

Ans. 59) A. LDH (Ref: 9 ed. Robbins 9 ed. p. 547, f-12-17) Refer Q 19 for details

Lactate Dehydrogenase

- Seen at 24 hrs post MI
- Peaks at 4-5 days
- Returns to normal at 10 days

Ans. 60) C. Macrophages (Ref: 9 ed. Robbins p. 543-46) Refer Q 18 for details

Ans. 61) B. Rheumatic endocarditis (Ref: 9 ed. Robbins p. 557-59) Refer Q 26 for details

Ans. 62) C. Lungs (Ref: 9 ed. Robbins p. 529-30) Refer Q 3 for details

Ans. 63) A. Myxomatous degeneration and prolapse of the mitral valve (Ref: 9 ed. Robbins p. 556-57) Refer Q 25 for details

Ans. 64) B. Fat deposition

Tigered effect: Grossly apparent bands of yellowed myocardium (containing fat) alternating with bands of darker, red-brown, uninvolved heart

Ans. 65) C. Neutrophilic infiltration surrounding coagulative necrosis (Ref: 9 ed. Robbins p. 543-46) Refer Q 18 for details

Ans. 66) A. Infective endocarditis (Ref: 9ed. Robbins p. 560) Refer Q 31, 33 and 34 for details

Ans. 67) A. Fibrous endocardial thickening of right ventricle, tricuspid valve and pulmonary valve (Ref: 9 ed. Robbins p. 562) Refer Q 35 for details

Also know:

- Intimal plaque like thickenings of the endocardial surfaces of the right side cardiac chambers and valve leaflets are characteristically seen

Ans. 68) A. Hypertrophic obstructive cardiomyopathy (Ref: 9 ed. Robbins p. 569) Refer Q 40 and 41 for details

Ans. 69) A. Left Anterior descending artery (Ref: 9 ed. Robbins p. 544) Refer Q 17 for details

- Left anterior descending – most common artery involved in MI

13 The Lung

How to go about this chapter?

- **One should be thorough with the following repeatedly asked topics:**
  - **Atelectasis**
  - **ARDS**
  - **Emphysema**
  - **Chronic bronchitis**
  - **Asthma**
  - **Bronchiectasis**
  - **Interstitial pneumonia**
  - **Anthracosis**
  - **Silicosis**
  - **Asbestosis**
  - **Sarcoidosis**
  - **Pulmonary infections**
  - **Bronchopneumonia**
  - **Histoplasmosis**
  - **Pulmonary squamous cell carcinoma, adenocarcinoma, bronchioloalveolar carcinoma, small cell carcinoma, carcinoid tumors**
  - **Paraneoplastic syndromes**
  - **Mesothelioma**

INTRODUCTION

1) **All are TRUE about development of lung EXCEPT:**
a) Bronchioles divide into terminal bronchioles
b) Terminal bronchioles are devoid of cartilage and sub-mucus glands
c) Bronchioles are lined by stratified squamous epithelium
d) Distal to terminal bronchiole is acinus

CONGENITAL ANOMALIES

2) **Most common foregut cyst include:**
a) Bronchogenic cyst
b) Esophageal cyst
c) Enteric cyst
d) Hilar cyst

ATELECTASIS

3) **All are TRUE about atelectasis EXCEPT:**
a) Resorption atelectasis is seen in bronchiectasis
b) Compression atelectasis occurs in pleural cavity filled by fluid/air
c) Contraction atelectasis occurs in fibrosis of lung
d) Atelectasis is an irreversible disorder

ACUTE LUNG INJURY AND ACUTE RESPIRATORY DISTRESS SYNDROME

4) **TRUE about Acute Lung Injury/ARDS:**
a) Associated with sepsis
b) Alveolar walls are lined by hyaline membranes
c) Comprises both alveolar epithelial and endothelial injury
d) All of the above

OBSTRUCTIVE LUNG DISEASES

5) **Most common type of emphysema is:**
a) Centriacinar
b) Panacinar
c) Paraseptal
d) Irregular

6) Centriacinar emphysema affects most commonly:
a) Upper lobe
b) Lower lobe
c) Middle lobe
d) None of the above

7) Most severely affected region of lung in Panacinar emphysema is:
a) Upper lobe
b) Middle lobe
c) Basal/lower lobe
d) None of the above

8) Emphysema associated with alpha -1- antitrypsin deficiency:
a) Centriacinar emphysema
b) Panacinar emphysema
c) Paraseptal emphysema
d) Irregular emphysema

9) Spontaneous pneumothorax in young adults is associated with:
a) Centriacinar emphysema
b) Panacinar emphysema
c) Paraseptal/Distal airway emphysema
d) Irregular emphysema

10) Apical blebs/ bullae formation occurs in:
a) Centriacinar emphysema
b) Panacinar emphysema
c) Paraseptal emphysema
d) Irregular emphysema

11) All are TRUE regarding pathogenesis of Emphysema EXCEPT:
a) Destruction of alveolar wall is by protease–antiprotease mechanism
b) Alpha-1- antitrypsin deficiency leads to increase neutrophil elastase
c) Alpha-1- antitrypsin deficiency is inherited as autosomal recessive disorder
d) Occurs due to increase protease activity and low antiprotease activity

12) Smoking leads to emphysematous damage in following ways EXCEPT:
a) Neutrophils and macrophage accumulate in alveoli
b) Leads to increase ROS, which depletes antioxidants
c) Leads to functional Alpha-1- antitrypsin deficiency
d) Lung parenchyma destruction stops after cessation of smoking

13) All are seen in patients with emphysema EXCEPT:
a) Dyspnea
b) Expiratory airflow limitation
c) Blue bloaters
d) Weight loss

14) TRUE about chronic bronchitis:
a) Hyper-secretion of mucus
b) Tobacco smoke is a risk factor
c) Increase in goblet cell hyperplasia
d) All of the above

15) Reid index in chronic bronchitis is:
a) Increased
b) Decreased
c) Both of the above
d) None of the above

ASTHMA

16) All of following cytokines mediate early phase of asthma EXCEPT:
a) IL-1 b) IL-5
c) IL-13 d) IL-4

17) Following cytokine(s) are involved in late phase reaction of asthma:
a) Acetylcholine b) Histamine
c) Leukotrienes d) All of the above

18) Following is/are implicated in genetics of asthma:
a) Chromosome 5q
b) ADAM33
c) IL-4 polymorphisms
d) All of the above

19) TRUE about morphology of Asthma:
a) Occlusion of bronchi by mucus plugs
b) Curschmann spirals
c) Charcot-Leyden crystals
d) All of the above

20) Bronchiectasis is associated with:
a) Cystic fibrosis
b) Post-infectious conditions
c) Bronchial obstruction
d) All of the above

21) All are TRUE about the morphology of Bronchiectasis EXCEPT:
a) Affects bilateral upper lobes
b) Dilation of airways
c) Bronchioles can be followed up to pleural surfaces
d) Pseudo stratification of the columnar cells can be seen

CHRONIC DIFFUSE INTERSTITIAL (RESTRICTIVE) DISEASES

22) All are the Fibrosing types of Interstitial Lung Disease EXCEPT:
a) Idiopathic Pulmonary Fibrosis
b) Cryptogenic Organizing Pneumonia
c) Desquamative Interstitial Pneumonia
d) Pneumoconiosis

23) All are TRUE about the pathogenesis of Idiopathic pulmonary fibrosis (IPF) EXCEPT:
a) Increased telomerase activity
b) Increased TGF-β1 activity
c) Decreased Caveolin-1 activity
d) Increased myofibroblasts

24) IPF most commonly involves:
a) Upper lobe
b) Bilateral basal lobes
c) Sub-pleural region
d) Middle lobe of right lung

25) All are TRUE about Cryptogenic Organizing Pneumonia EXCEPT:
a) Also known as Bronchiolitis Obliterans organizing pneumonia
b) Histologically it shows Masson bodies
c) Interstitial fibrosis and honey combing is seen
d) Good prognosis

26) Following connective tissue disease(s) is/are associated with Interstitial lung disease:
a) Rheumatoid arthritis
b) Systemic sclerosis
c) Lupus erythematosus
d) All of the above

27) Particle size which predisposes to pneumoconiosis:
a) 1 to 5 μ b) 5 to 10 μ
c) 10-15 μ d) 15-20 μ

28) All are TRUE about Anthracosis EXCEPT:
a) Also known as coal workers pneumoconiosis (CWP)
b) Lower lobes are most commonly involved in simple CWP
c) Complicated CWP leads to massive fibrosis
d) Coal dust does not increase the susceptibility to tuberculosis

29) All are TRUE about silicosis EXCEPT:
a) Crystalline forms are more fibrogenic
b) TNF plays an important role
c) Produces nodules in upper zone of lungs
d) Doesn't increase the susceptibility to tuberculosis

30) Occupational exposure of Asbestos is associated with:
a) Localized fibrous plaques
b) Pleural effusions
c) Parenchymal interstitial fibrosis
d) All of the above

31) All are TRUE about pathogenesis of Asbestosis EXCEPT:
a) Serpentine chrysotile form of asbestos is most prevalent
b) Amphiboles are more pathogenic
c) Serpentine chrysotile form leads to mesothelioma
d) Serpentine forms are flexible and in lungs can be removed by mucociliary elevator

32) All are TRUE about the morphology of asbestosis EXCEPT:
a) Pleural plaques are the most common manifestation of asbestos exposure
b) Diffuse pulmonary interstitial fibrosis
c) Concomitant cigarette smoking leads to increase risk of mesothelioma
d) Asbestos body is a characteristic feature

33) Granulomatous diseases include(s):
a) Sarcoidosis
b) Mycobacterial infections
c) Fungal infections
d) All of the above

34) TRUE about morphology of Sarcoidosis:
a) Non caseating granulomas
b) Schaumann bodies and asteroid bodies
c) Lungs are the most common site of involvement
d) All of the above

35) Hypersensitivity Pneumonitis include(s):
a) Farmer's Lung
b) Pigeon breeders lung
c) Humidifier lung
d) All of the above

36) Mutation which leads to Acquired Pulmonary Alveolar Proteinosis is:
a) SP-A b) SP-C
c) GM-CSF d) ABCA-3

37) Most frequent mutated gene in Surfactant Dysfunction Disorders:
a) ABCA3 b) SP-A
c) SP-B d) SP-C

38) Pulmonary embolus can be differentiated from postmortem clot by:
a) Red brown in color
b) Lines of Zahn
c) Presence of neutrophils
d) None of the above

39) Pulmonary hypertension is due to mutation in following gene receptor:
a) TGF- β
b) Bone morphogenetic protein (BMP)
c) Activin
d) Inhibin

40) All are TRUE about Goodpasture syndrome EXCEPT:
a) Autoantibodies against NC4A3
b) Lungs are spared
c) Linear deposits on Immunofluorescence
d) Most common cause of death is uremia

PULMONARY INFECTIONS

41) Most common cause of community acquired bacterial pneumonia:
a) Streptococcus pneumoniae
b) Haemophilus influenza
c) Pseudomonas aeruginosa
d) Staphylococcus aureus

42) Most common cause of meningitis in young children, before the advent of vaccine:
a) H. Influenza
b) Streptococcus
c) Staphylococcus
d) Moraxella catarrhalis

43) Following is responsible for pneumonia in intravenous drug abusers:
a) Staphylococcus aureus
b) Moraxella catarrhalis
c) Klebsiella pneumonia
d) Pseudomonas aeruginosa

44) TRUE about Pseudomonas infection:
a) Commonly causes hospital acquired infections
b) Occurs in cystic fibrosis patients
c) Extra pulmonary spread is seen
d) All of the above

45) Organism found in aquatic environments which leads to pneumonia is:
a) Pseudomonas b) Legionella
c) Staphylococcus d) Moraxella

46) Patchy consolidation is a characteristic feature in:
a) Bronchopneumonia
b) Lobar pneumonia
c) Any of the above
d) None of the above

47) Most common agent causing Community Acquired Atypical Pneumonia:
a) Mycoplasma
b) Adenovirus
c) Influenza virus
d) Respiratory syncytial virus

48) Cause of Primary cryptogenic lung abscess:
a) Hematogenous seedling by pyogenic organisms
b) Traumatic penetration of lungs
c) Aspiration
d) No cause found

49) All are TRUE about Histoplasmosis EXCEPT:
a) Clinical and morphological resemblance to tuberculosis
b) Dimorphic fungi
c) Tree bark appearance
d) Immunocompromised hosts show well-formed granulomas

50) Differential diagnosis of Solitary Pulmonary nodule include/s:
a) Tuberculosis
b) Sarcoidosis
c) Coccidioidomycosis
d) All of the above

51) TRUE about pulmonary disease in HIV infection:
a) Tubercular infections occur when CD4+ counts >200 cells/mm^3
b) Pneumocystis pneumonia occurs when CD4+ counts are less than 200 cells/mm^3
c) Mycobacterium avium complex infections occurs when CD4+ counts are less than 50 cells/mm^3
d) All of the above

TUMORS

52) Cancer associated genes involved in small cell carcinoma of lung include(s):
a) C-KIT
b) p53
c) 3p
d) All of the above

53) Precursor stage(s) seen in carcinoma lung include(s):
a) Squamous dysplasia
b) Carcinoma in situ
c) Adenocarcinoma in situ
d) All of the above

54) Most common site where lung carcinoma metastasize:
a) Adrenals b) Liver
c) Brain d) Bone

55) TRUE about Adenocarcinoma lung:
a) Located peripherally in lung
b) Most commonly seen in smokers
c) Doesn't metastasize
d) More frequently associated with history of smoking

56) Following pattern of growth is noted in Bronchioloalveolar carcinomas:
a) Glandular b) Sheets
c) Singly d) Lepidic

57) All are TRUE about molecular genetics of Squamous cell carcinomas EXCEPT:
a) P53 mutation
b) Loss of RB1 gene expression
c) P16/INK4A inactivation
d) EGFR mutation

58) Azzopardi effect is noted in:
a) Squamous cell carcinomas
b) Small cell carcinomas
c) Adenocarcinomas
d) Bronchioloalveolar carcinoma

59) **Paraneoplastic Syndrome in lung carcinomas occurs due to:**
a) ADH b) ACTH
c) Parathormone d) All of the above

60) **Carcinoma of lung is associated with:**
a) Leukemoid reactions
b) Peripheral neuropathy
c) Lambert-Eaton myasthenic syndrome
d) All of the above

61) **TRUE about Neuroendocrine tumors of lung:**
a) Diffuse Idiopathic Pulmonary Neuroendocrine Cell Hyperplasia is a precursor lesion
b) Typical and Atypical carcinoids are associated with MEN-1
c) Neuroendocrine differentiation is confirmed by Immunohistochemistry
d) All of the above

62) **All are TRUE about Carcinoid tumor EXCEPT:**
a) Grow as spherical polypoidal mass
b) Typical carcinoid have 2-10 mitosis/10 hpf
c) Atypical Carcinoids can show a foci of necrosis
d) Classical Carcinoid Syndrome is rare

63) **Normal pleural fluid quantity is:**
a) <5 ml b) <10 ml
c) <15 ml d) <20 ml

64) **Mesotheliomas are differentiated from Adenocarcinomas in following ways EXCEPT:**
a) Positive staining for acid mucopolysaccharide
b) CEA positivity
c) Positive staining for Calretinin
d) Positive staining for cytokeratin 5/6

65) **What is the characteristic histological finding of chronic radiation pneumonitis? (NEET 2014)**
a) Foam cells in vessel wall
b) Fibroblasts in lumen
c) Epithelial cell hyperplasia
d) Presence of giant cells in vessel wall

66) **Most common malignancy in lung is: (NEET 2014)**
a) Small cell carcinoma
b) Squamous cell carcinoma
c) Adenocarcinoma
d) Lymphoma

67) **Reid index in increased in: (NEET 2014)**
a) Chronic bronchitis
b) Emphysema
c) Bronchiectasis
d) ARDS

68) **Which is the most common site for extra-thoracic metastases in patients with lung carcinoma? (NEET 2014)**
a) Kidneys b) Liver
c) Vertebral body d) Adrenal glands

69) **Mesothelioma is positive for which intermediate filament? (NEET 2014)**
a) Vimentin b) Cytokeratin
c) GFAP d) Desmin

70) **Keratinization and pearl formation is characteristic of: (NEET 2014)**
a) Squamous cell carcinoma
b) Basal cell carcinoma
c) Melanoma
d) Lymphoma

71) **TRUE about Kartagener syndrome is all EXCEPT: (NEET 2014)**
a) Dextrocardia
b) Infertility
c) Bronchiectasis
d) Mental retardation

72) **Calretinin is used in: (NEET 2014)**
a) Mesothelioma b) Hamartoma
c) Choristoma d) Chordoma

73) **Alpha 1 antitrypsin deficiency seen in: (NEET 2014)**
a) Emphysema
b) Bronchitis
c) ARDS
d) Bronchiectasis

74) **Creola bodies are seen in: (NEET 2013)**
a) Bronchial asthma
b) Chronic bronchitis
c) Emphysema
d) Bronchiectasis

75) **Bronchogenic sequestration is seen in which lobe? (NEET 2013)**
a) Left lower lobe
b) Right upper lobe
c) Left middle lobe
d) Left upper lobe

76) **Which one of the following sets of components of cigarette smoke is a causal agent of coronary artery disease? (NEET 2013)**
a) Tar and nicotine
b) Nicotine and carbon monoxide and tar
c) Carbon monoxide and tar
d) Carbon dioxide

77) **In which of the following location, carcinoid tumor is most common? (NEET 2013)**
a) Esophagus b) Lung
c) Stomach d) Appendix

78) **Sequestrated lobe of lung is commonly supplied by: (NEET 2013)**
a) Pulmunory artery
b) Intercoastal artery
c) Descending aorta
d) Bronchial artery

79) Carcinoid tumor develops from: (NEET 2013)
a) Hematopoietic cells
b) Kulschitsky cells
c) Neuroglial cells
d) None of the baove

80) Marker of small cell cancer of lung is: (NEET 2013)
a) Chromogranin b) Cytokeratin
c) Desmin d) Vimentin

81) Most common mediastinal tumor is: (NEET 2013)
a) Neurogenic tumor
b) Pericardial cyst
c) Hernia
d) Teratoma

82) Collapse of lung is called: (NEET 2013)
a) Emphysema b) Bronchiectasis
c) Atelectasis d) Bronchitis

83) A female presents with history of progressive breathlessness. Histology shows heterogenous patchy fibrosis with several fibroblastic foci. The most likely diagnosis is: (AIPGMEE 2010)
a) Cryptogenic organizing pneumonia
b) Nonspecific interstitial pneumonia
c) Usual interstitial pneumonia
d) Desquamative interstitial pneumonia

84) In a 70-year-old man who was working in an asbestos factory for 10-15 years, on routine X-Ray a mass was seen in right apical region of the lung. Biopsy was taken from the mass. Which of the following is seen on electron microscopic examination? (AIIMS Nov 2013)
a) Numerous long, slender microvilli
b) Melanosomes
c) Desmosomes
d) Neurosecretory granules in cytoplasm

85) A 65-year-old chronic smoker presented with a central lung mass with distal bronchiectasis and recurrent pneumonia. A grayish white tumor was resected. Which of the following histopathological finding is most likely to be seen? (AIIMS Nov 2014)
a) Small cells with scant cytoplasm, ill-defined cell borders and hyperchromatic nuclei with nuclear moulding
b) Derivatives of all three germ layers are seen
c) Tall columnar cells with cytoplasmic and intra alveolar mucin
d) Palisading or rosette-like arrangements of cells separated by abundant fibro-vascular stroma

CHAPTER 13 – THE LUNG

Ans. 1) C. Bronchioles are lined by stratified squamous epithelium (Ref: 8 ed. Robbins p. 678-79, 9 ed. p. 669-70, f-15-1)

Development of Lung Q:

- Midline trachea develops two lung buds
- **Right lung bud** Q divides into **three** lobar bronchi and the **left** Q into **two** lobar bronchi, thus giving rise to **three lobes on the right** and **two on the left**
- **Right main stem bronchus** is **more vertical** Q and more directly in line with the trachea
- **Progressive branching** of the bronchi forms **bronchioles** Q
- Bronchioles **lack cartilage** and **sub-mucosal glands** within their walls
- Further branching of bronchioles leads to **terminal bronchioles**
- Part of the lung distal to the terminal bronchiole is called **acinus** Q
- An acinus is composed of **terminal bronchioles, alveolar ducts** and **alveolar sacs** and are the site of **gas exchange**
- **Pulmonary lobule** Q: Cluster of **three to five terminal bronchioles**, each with its **acinus** Q
- Entire respiratory tree, including **larynx, trachea and bronchioles**, is lined by **pseudo-stratified, tall, columnar, ciliated epithelial cells**, except for vocal cords, which are lined by **stratified squamous epithelium** Q
- Alveolar epithelium consists of: **Type I pneumocytes** covering **95%** of alveolar surface and rounded **type II pneumocytes**
- **Type II cells** synthesize **surfactant** Q
- Alveolar walls are **perforated** by numerous **pores of Kohn** Q, which permit the passage of bacteria and exudate between adjacent alveoli

Ans. 2) A. Bronchogenic cyst (Ref: 8 ed. Robbins p.679, 9 ed. p. 670)

Foregut Cysts Q

- Arise from primitive foregut and are most often located in the **hilum** or **middle mediastinum** Q
- Cysts are classified as **bronchogenic (most common)** Q, esophageal, or enteric

Ans. 3) D. Atelectasis is an irreversible disorder (Ref: 8 ed. Robbins p. 679-80, 9 ed. p. 670-71, f-15-2)

Atelectasis: Incomplete expansion of lungs (neonatal atelectasis) or **collapse** of the previously inflated lung

Acquired Atelectasis can be of **3 types:**

A) Resorption atelectasis Q**:**

- Consequence of **complete obstruction** of an airway
- Mediastinum **shifts toward** the atelectatic lung
- Most commonly found in **bronchial asthma** Q, **chronic bronchitis, bronchiectasis** Q, postoperative states, aspiration of foreign bodies

B) Compression atelectasis Q**:**

- Occurs when the **pleural cavity** is partially or completely filled by **fluid exudate, tumor, blood or air (pneumothorax)** Q
- Mediastinum shifts away from the **affected lung**

C) Contraction atelectasis Q**:**

- Occurs when local or generalized **fibrotic changes** in lung or pleura prevent full expansion
- Because, the collapsed lung parenchyma can be re-expanded, **atelectasis is a reversible disorder** Q (except contraction type)

Ans. 4) D. All of the above (Ref: 8 ed. Robbins p. 680-82, 9 ed. p. 672-73, t-15-2, f-15-3,4)

Acute respiratory distress syndrome (ARDS)/Acute Lung Injury (Non-cardiogenic pulmonary edema) Q**:**

- Characterized by abrupt onset of hypoxemia and **bilateral pulmonary infiltrates**
- Due to **inflammation** associated increase in pulmonary vascular permeability and **epithelial** and **endothelial cell death** [Q]
- **Common causes** [Q] – Sepsis, pulmonary infections (viral, mycoplasma, pneumocystis), gastric aspiration and mechanical trauma

Pathogenesis [Q]**:**

- **Endothelial activation** – Due to **increased TNF expression** [Q]
- **Adhesion** and **extravasation of neutrophils**
- Accumulation of **intra-alveolar fluid** and formation of **hyaline membranes** [Q]

Morphology [Q]**:**

- Histologic manifestation is **diffuse alveolar damage (DAD)** [Q]
- **Alveolar walls** are lined with **hyaline membranes** [Q]

Ans. 5) **A. Centriacinar (Ref: 8 ed. Robbins p. 684-87, 9 ed. p. 674-75, f-15-6-8)**

Emphysema:

- Characterized by **irreversible enlargement of airspaces** distal to the **terminal bronchioles** [Q], with **destruction of their walls**, without fibrosis
- **Four major types** [Q]: (1) Centriacinar (2) Panacinar (3) Paraseptal and (4) Irregular
- **Centriacinar emphysema** is the **most common form** [Q]

Ans. 6) **A. Upper lobe (Ref: 8 ed. Robbins p. 684-87, 9 ed. p. 675, f-15-6-8)**

Centriacinar Emphysema:

- **Central or proximal parts** [Q] of **acini**, formed by **respiratory bronchioles** [Q], are affected, whereas distal alveoli are **spared**
- Lesions are more common and severe in **upper lobes** [Q]
- Occurs predominantly in **heavy smokers** [Q] and in association with chronic bronchitis

Ans. 7) **C. Basal/lower lobe (Ref: 8 ed. Robbins p. 684-87, 9 ed. p. 675, f-15-6)**

Panacinar Emphysema [Q]**:**

- Acini are enlarged from the level of **respiratory bronchiole** to the terminal blind alveoli
- Most common in **lower zones** [Q] and most severe at the **bases** [Q]

Ans. 8) **B. Panacinar emphysema (Ref: 8 ed. Robbins p. 684-87, 9 ed. p. 675)**

- **Panacinar emphysema** is associated with **α1-antitrypsin (α1- AT) deficiency** [Q]

Ans. 9) **C. Paraseptal/Distal airway emphysema (Ref: 8 ed. Robbins p. 684-87, 9 ed. p. 675-76, f-15-6-8)**

Distal Acinar (Paraseptal) Emphysema [Q]**:**

- **Proximal portion** of the **acinus** is **normal** and **distal part** [Q] is predominantly involved
- Severe in **upper half** of the **lungs** [Q]
- Characteristic finding – **multiple, continuous, enlarged airspaces** ranging from **0.5 cm** to **2.0 cm** in diameter, forming **cyst like structures**
- Associated with **spontaneous pneumothorax** [Q] in young adults

Ans. 10) **D. Irregular emphysema (Ref: 8 ed. Robbins p.684-87, 9 ed. p. 677)**

- **Large apical blebs or bullae** are **more characteristic** [Q] of **irregular emphysema** secondary to scarring

Ans. 11) **C. Alpha-1- antitrypsin deficiency is inherited as autosomal recessive disorder (Ref: 8 ed. Robbins p. 684-87, 9 ed. p. 676-77, f-15-8)**

Pathogenesis of Emphysema [Q]**:**

A) Inflammatory mediators and leukocytes:

- **Leukotriene B4, IL-8, TNF** [Q]

B) Protease-antiprotease imbalance:

- Deficiency of protective **anti-proteases** [Q] is seen in **emphysema** patients
- Patients with **α1-antitrypsin** [Q] deficiency, are at increased risk for emphysema
- **α1-antitrypsin**, secreted by neutrophils, is a major **inhibitor of proteases (elastase)**
- **α1-antitrypsin** is encoded by **co-dominantly** [Q] **expressed genes** on the proteinase inhibitor (Pi) locus on **chromosome 14** [Q]

C) Role of smoking in emphysema:

- Leads to **accumulation of neutrophils and macrophages** in alveoli
- **Nicotine** activate **NF-κB** [Q], which increases **TNF** and **IL-8** levels
- **Enhances elastase** [Q] activity in **macrophages**
- **Tobacco smoke** contains **abundant reactive oxygen species** [Q], which leads to inactivation of anti-proteases **("functional" α1-antitrypsin deficiency)** [Q]

Morphology [Q]:

- **Voluminous lungs**, often overlapping the heart
- **Cut surface** – large, dilated alveoli
- **Microscopically** – abnormally large alveoli are separated by thin septa with focal centrilobular fibrosis

Ans. 12) D. Lung parenchyma destruction stops after cessation of smoking (Ref: 8 ed. Robbins p. 684-87, 9 ed. p. 676-77)

- Refer to answer number 11

Ans. 13) C. Blue bloaters (Ref: 8 ed. Robbins p. 684-87, 9 ed. p. 677)

Clinical Features of Emphysema [Q]:

- Patients with severe emphysema, **over-ventilate** and remain well oxygenated and are designated as **pink puffers** [Q]
- **Dyspnea** is the **first symptom**, with **cough or wheezing** and weight loss
- Barrel shaped chest
- **Spirometry** (key to diagnosis) shows **expiratory airflow limitation** [Q]
- **Death** in **most patients with emphysema occurs due to** 1) Respiratory acidosis and coma 2) Right-sided heart failure 3) Pneumothorax

Ans. 14) D. All of the above (Ref: 8 ed. Robbins p. 687-88, 9 ed. p. 678-79)

Chronic Bronchitis [Q]:

Definition: Persistent cough with **sputum production** for at least **3 months** in at least **2 consecutive years**, in the absence of any other identifiable cause

Pathogenesis [Q]:

A) Primary or initiating factor seems to be **tobacco smoke** [Q]

B) Hyper-secretion of mucus (earliest feature) occurs due to:

- **Hypertrophy of sub-mucosal glands** and **goblet cells** of small airways
- Proteases released from neutrophils, such as **neutrophil elastase** [Q] and **cathepsin**

C) Inflammation

D) Infection

Ans. 15) A. Increased (Ref: 8 ed. Robbins p. 687-88, 9 ed. p. 679)

- **Reid index** [Q] is ratio of the **thickness of mucous gland layer** to the **thickness of the wall between the epithelium and cartilage**
- **Reid index (normally 0.4)** is **increased** [Q] in **chronic bronchitis**
- Patient presents with **mild cyanosis ("blue bloaters")** [Q]

Complication – Obliteration of the lumen due to fibrosis (**Bronchiolitis Obliterans**)

Morphology of **Chronic Bronchitis** ᵠ

- **Chronic inflammation (lymphocytes)** of the airways and enlargement of the **mucus-secreting glands** ᵠ of the trachea and bronchi

	Predominant Bronchitis ᵠ	Predominant Emphysema ᵠ
Age (years)	40–45	50–75
Dyspnea	Mild; late	Severe; early
Cough	Early; copious sputum	Late; scanty sputum
Infections	Common	Occasional
Respiratory insufficiency	Repeated	Terminal
Cor pulmonale	Common	Rare; terminal
Airway resistance	Increased	Normal or slightly increased
Elastic recoil	Normal	Low
Chest radiograph	Prominent vessels; large heart	Hyperinflation; small heart
Appearance	Blue bloater	Pink puffer

Ans. 16) A. IL-1 (Ref: 8 ed. Robbins p.689-90, 9 ed. p. 679-81, f-15-10)

Cytokines involved in **early phase of asthma**:

- **IL-4** stimulates **B-cells** and leads to production of **IgE** ᵠ
- **IL-5** recruits **eosinophils** ᵠ
- **IL-13** stimulates **mucus secretion** ᵠ from bronchial submucosal glands

Early-phase (immediate hypersensitivity) reaction ᵠ:

- Dominated by bronchoconstriction, increased mucus production and vasodilation with increased vascular permeability

Ans. 17) D. All of the above (Ref: 8 ed. Robbins p. 689-90, 9 ed. p. 679-81, f-15-10)

Mediators involved in **late phase of asthma** ᵠ:

- **Eotaxin** ᵠ – potent **chemo-attractant** and activator of **eosinophils** ᵠ
- **Major basic protein** ᵠ **(eosinophils)** causes **epithelial damage** and airway constriction
- **Leukotrienes C4, D4 and E4, acetylcholine** leads to **bronchospasm** ᵠ
- **Histamine, Prostaglandin D2** are potent **broncho-constrictors**
- **IL-1, TNF** and **IL-6** also play an important role

Ans. 18) D. All of the above (Ref: 8 ed. Robbins p. 691, 9 ed. p. 681-82)

Genes reported in Asthma include:

- **Chromosome 5q**, encoding the **cytokines** IL-3, IL-4, IL-5, IL-9 and IL-13 and the IL-4 receptor
- **Polymorphisms** in the **IL13** gene has strongest association with asthma or allergic disease
- **Polymorphism** in gene encoding **ADAM-33** results in proliferation of bronchial smooth muscle cells and fibroblasts
- **β2-adrenergic** receptor gene
- **IL-4 receptor** gene variants are associated with atopy, elevated total serum IgE and asthma

Ans. 19) D. All of the above (Ref: 8 ed. Robbins p. 691-92, 9 ed. p. 682-83, f-15-10, 11)

Morphology of Asthma ᵠ:

- Occlusion of bronchi and bronchioles by **thick, tenacious mucus plugs** ᵠ
- **Curschmann spirals** ᵠ **– spiral shaped mucus plugs** containing whorls of **shed epithelium**
- **Charcot-Leyden crystals** ᵠ are composed of eosinophil protein crystalloid **galectin – 10**

Ans. 20) D. All of the above (Ref: 8 ed. Robbins p. 692-93, 9 ed. p. 683)

Bronchiectasis Q

- Characterized by **permanent dilation** of **bronchi** and **bronchioles** Q
- Caused by **destruction of muscle and elastic tissue**, due to chronic necrotizing infections

Associated with:

- **Congenital/ hereditary conditions: Cystic fibrosis** Q, immunodeficiency states, **primary ciliary dyskinesia** Q, **Kartagener syndrome (bronchiectasis, sinusitis and situs inversus)** Q
- **Infections –** Necrotizing pneumonia due to bacterial, viral or **fungal** infections **(Allergic bronchopulmonary aspergillosis)** Q
- **Bronchial obstruction**, due to tumor, foreign bodies
- **Other conditions** – Rheumatoid arthritis, systemic lupus erythematosus, inflammatory bowel disease, COPD and post-transplantation
- Idiopathic

Ans. 21) A. Affects bilateral upper lobes (Ref: 8 ed. Robbins p. 692-93, 9 ed. p. 683-84, f-15-12)

Morphology Q**:**

- **Bronchiectasis** usually affects the **lower lobes bilaterally** Q

Gross:

- Bronchi and bronchioles are **dilated** and can be **followed** up to the **pleural surfaces**
- In normal lung, the bronchioles **cannot be followed** beyond **2 to 3 cm** from the pleural surfaces Q
- **Cut surface** Q – dilated bronchi show cysts filled with mucopurulent secretions

Microscopy Q**:**

- **Acute and chronic inflammatory infiltrate** within the walls of the bronchi and bronchioles
- **Desquamation** of the lining epithelium and extensive areas of necrotizing ulceration
- **Fibrosis** Q of bronchial and bronchiolar walls develops in **chronic cases**

Ans. 22) C. Desquamative Interstitial Pneumonia (Ref: 8 ed. Robbins p. 694, 9 ed. p. 684-85, t-15-5)

Major Categories of Chronic Interstitial Lung Disease:

a) Fibrosing Q**:**

- Usual interstitial pneumonia (idiopathic pulmonary fibrosis)
- Nonspecific interstitial pneumonia
- Cryptogenic organizing pneumonia
- Associated with connective tissue diseases
- Pneumoconiosis
- Drug reactions
- Radiation pneumonitis

b) Granulomatous – Sarcoidosis, Hypersensitivity pneumonitis

c) Eosinophilic

d) Smoking Related Q**:**

- Desquamative interstitial pneumonia
- Respiratory bronchiolitis-associated interstitial lung disease

e) Other – Pulmonary alveolar proteinases

Ans. 23) A. Increased telomerase activity (Ref: 8 ed. Robbins p. 694-95, 9 ed. p. 685-86, f-15-13)

Pathogenesis of Idiopathic Pulmonary Fibrosis (IPF) Q

- Caused by repeated cycles of **epithelial activation/injury** Q, which gives rise to exuberant **fibroblastic/ myofibroblastic** proliferation

Implicated factors [Q]**:**

Environmental factors:

- Smoking, occupational exposure, other irritants, toxins, viral infection

Genetic factors:

- Telomerase mutations (**germline loss-of-function mutations** in **TERT** and **TERC genes**, which encode components of **telomerase**)
- Mutation in the gene encoding **surfactant**

Role of Increased TGF-β1 in IPF [Q]:

- Fibrogenic and favors the transformation of **fibroblasts into myofibroblasts** [Q]
- Negatively regulates **telomerase activity** [Q]
- Inhibits **Caveolin-1** [Q], leading to **increased TGF** production

Note:

New therapies – **neutralizing TGF-β1, enhancing telomerase activity**, or **augmenting caveolin-1** may lead to future treatments in IPF patients

Ans. 24) C. Sub-pleural (Ref: 8 ed. Robbins p. 694-95, 9 ed. p. 686, f-15-14,15)

Morphology of IPF:

- **Histological pattern** of fibrosis is referred to as **usual interstitial pneumonia (UIP)**

Grossly:

- **Pleural surfaces** of the lung are **cobblestoned**
- **Cut surface – Fibrosis of the lung parenchyma**, seen in **sub-pleural regions** [Q]

Microscopically:

- **Hallmark of UIP** is **patchy interstitial fibrosis** [Q]
- **Earliest lesion** – Lung shows **fibroblastic foci,** however in **late stages** it shows **honeycomb fibrosis** [Q]

Clinical course – presents as dyspnea on exertion and dry cough. Hypoxemia, cyanosis and clubbing occur later on in disease

Ans. 25) C. Interstitial fibrosis and honey combing is seen (Ref: 8 ed. Robbins p. 696, 9 ed. p. 687, f-15-16)

Cryptogenic organizing pneumonia or **Bronchiolitis Obliterans organizing pneumonia:**

- Unknown etiology
- Patients present with **cough and dyspnea**

Histologically:

- **Masson bodies** [Q] **(polypoidal plugs** of loose organizing connective tissue) are seen within alveolar ducts, alveoli and often bronchioles
- **Interstitial fibrosis or honeycomb lung** [Q] is not seen
- **Good prognosis**

Ans. 26) D. All of the above (Ref: 8 ed. Robbins p. 696, 9 ed. p. 687)

Pulmonary Involvement in Autoimmune Diseases [Q]:

- **Rheumatoid arthritis** – Chronic pleuritis, diffuse interstitial pneumonitis and fibrosis, intrapulmonary rheumatoid nodules, pulmonary hypertension
- **Systemic sclerosis (scleroderma)** – Diffuse interstitial fibrosis
- **Lupus erythematosus** – parenchymal infiltrates

Ans. 27) A. 1 to 5μ (Ref: 8 ed. Robbins p. 696-97, 9 ed. p. 688)

- **Particles** which range from **1 to** 5μ [Q] in diameter are most dangerous
- Particles reach **terminal small airways** and **settle** in their linings
- **Smaller the particle**, the more rapidly it causes **acute lung injury** [Q]

Ans. 28) B. Lower lobes are most commonly involved in simple CWP (Ref: 8 ed. Robbins p.697-98, 9 ed. p. 689-90, f-15-17)

Anthracosis:

- **Coal-induced pulmonary lesion** in coal miners
- Classified into three types: a) Asymptomatic Anthracosis b) Simple CWP c) Complicated CWP, or progressive massive fibrosis (PMF)

Simple CWP Q:

- Characterized by **coal macules** (1 to 2 mm in diameter) and **coal nodules**
- **Upper lobes** and **upper zones of the lower lobes** Q are commonly involved
- Can predispose to **centrilobular emphysema** Q

Complicated CWP Q **(progressive massive fibrosis)**

- Characterized by multiple blackened **scars, > 1 cm** and **< 10 cm** in greatest diameter

Ans. 29) D. Doesn't increase the susceptibility to tuberculosis (Ref: 8 ed. Robbins p. 698-99, 9 ed. p. 690, f-15-18,19)

Silicosis:

- **Most prevalent** Q chronic occupational disease in the world
- Silica occurs in both **crystalline** Q and **amorphous forms** Q
- **Crystalline forms** Q (including **quartz**, crystobalite and tridymite) are much more fibrogenic **(especially quartz)**
- Silica causes activation and **release of mediators** (IL-1, **TNF**, fibronectin, lipid mediators, oxygen-derived free radicals and fibrogenic cytokines)
- Patients with silicosis have **increased susceptibility to tuberculosis** Q

Morphology

Grossly:

- Nodules in the **upper zones of the lungs** Q and these nodules may coalesce into **hard, collagenous scars**
- **Calcification** of lymph nodes are seen radiographically as **eggshell calcification** Q
- Coalescence of lesions produces **progressive massive fibrosis**

Microscopy

- Hallmark lesion is characterized by a central area of whorled collagen fibers with peripheral zone of dust-laden macrophages
- **Polarized microscopy** – Nodules reveals **birefringent silicate particles** (silica is weakly birefringent)

Ans. 30) D. All of the above (Ref: 8 ed. Robbins p. 699, 9 ed. p. 690-91, f-15-20,21)

Occupational exposure to **asbestos** Q is associated with:

- **Localized fibrous plaques** Q/diffuse pleural fibrosis
- Pleural effusion
- Parenchymal interstitial fibrosis **(asbestosis)** Q
- Lung carcinoma
- **Mesotheliomas** Q
- Laryngeal and other extrapulmonary neoplasms, including **colon carcinomas**

Ans. 31) C. Serpentine chrysotile form leads to mesothelioma (Ref: 8 ed. Robbins p.699-701, 9 ed. p. 691-92, f-15-20,21)

Pathogenesis of Asbestosis Q

- **Two distinct forms** Q of asbestos: serpentine and amphibole
- **Serpentine chrysotile** Q accounts for most of the asbestos used in industry
- **Amphiboles** are **more pathogenic** and can lead to **mesothelioma** Q
- **Chrysotiles** are more **flexible** and get impacted in the **upper respiratory passages** Q and are removed by the **mucociliary elevator**

- In contrast, **the straight, stiff amphiboles** can penetrate deeper into the lungs
- Both amphiboles and serpentines are **fibrogenic** Q
- **Tobacco smoke** increases the oncogenicity of the fibers Q

Ans. 32) C. Concomitant cigarette smoking leads to increase risk of mesothelioma (Ref: 8 ed. Robbins p.699-701, 9 ed. p. 691-92, f-15-20,21)

Morphological features of **asbestosis** includes:

- Asbestosis begins in the **lower lobes** Q and **sub-pleurally**
- Diffuse pulmonary interstitial fibrosis, with presence of multiple **asbestos bodies** Q
- **Asbestos bodies** appear as **golden brown, fusiform or beaded rods** with a translucent center
- **Pleural plaques** Q **(most common** manifestation of **asbestos exposure)** – seen on parietal pleura and domes of diaphragm
- Both **lung carcinoma** Q and **mesothelioma** Q (pleural and peritoneal) can develop
- **Concomitant cigarette smoking** Q greatly **increases the risk of lung carcinoma** Q but not of mesothelioma

Ans. 33) E. All of the above (Ref: 8 ed. Robbins p.701, 9 ed. p. 693-94)

- **Non-caseating granulomas** Q – seen in Sarcoidosis, Mycobacterial and fungal infections, Berylliosis

Note:

- **Immunological abnormalities** in sarcoid granulomas include **intra-alveolar** and **interstitial accumulation** of CD4+ T cells
- Resulting in increased **CD4/CD8 T-cell ratio** Q

Ans. 34) D. All of the above (Ref: 8 ed. Robbins p.702-03, 9 ed. p. 693-94)

Histology of Sarcoidosis:

- Non-caseating granulomas composed of aggregates of **epithelioid macrophages** and **giant cells**
- **Schaumann bodies** Q **– Laminated concretions** composed of calcium and proteins
- **Asteroid bodies** Q **– Stellate inclusions** in **giant cells**

Sites of involvement:

- **Lungs** Q are the **most common site** of **involvement**
- Occasionally the heart, kidneys, central nervous system and endocrine glands (pituitary) involvement can occur

Ans. 35) D. All of the above (Ref: 8 ed. Robbins p.703-04, 9 ed. p. 694-95)

Examples of **Hypersensitivity Pneumonitis** include:

- **Farmer's lung** Q results from exposure to dusts generated from humid, warm, newly harvested **hay** (permits the **rapid proliferation** of **spores** of thermophilic actinomycetes)
- **Pigeon breeder's lung** Q (bird fancier's disease) is provoked by proteins from serum, excreta, or feathers of birds
- **Humidifier or air-conditioner lung** is caused by thermophilic bacteria in heated water reservoir

Ans. 36) C. GM-CSF (Ref: 8 ed. Robbins p.705-06, f-15-25, 9 ed. p. 696-97)

Pulmonary Alveolar Proteinosis (PAP) Q

- Accumulation of **acellular surfactant** in the intra-alveolar and bronchiolar spaces
- Three distinct classes of the disease—acquired, congenital and secondary PAP

Pathogenesis of PAP Q:

- **Autoimmune PAP – anti–GM-CSF antibody** is found in the serum and bronchial fluid
- **Secondary PAP –** uncommon, seen in malignancies, hematopoietic disorders, immunodeficiency disorders
- **Hereditary PAP** – occurs in **neonates** and occurs due to the **mutations** that **disrupt genes** involved in **GM-CSF signaling** Q

Morphology:

- Lungs show **homogeneous, granular precipitate** within alveoli

- Alveolar precipitate is **periodic acid–Schiff positive** [Q]

Ans. 37) A. ABCA3 (Ref: 9 ed. Robbins p. 696-97)

Mutated genes involved in **Surfactant Dysfunction Disorders:**

a) ATP-binding cassette protein member 3 (**ABCA3**) [Q] – Most frequently mutated gene
   - **Ultra structurally – Small lamellar bodies** with **electron dense cores** are **diagnostic**

b) **Surfactant protein C** is the **second** most commonly **mutated gene**

c) **Surfactant protein B** is the **least commonly** mutated gene

Ans. 38) B. Lines of Zahn (Ref: 8 ed. Robbins p.706-07, 9 ed. p. 698)

- **Pulmonary embolus** can be distinguished from a **postmortem clot** by the presence of the **lines of Zahn** [Q] in the thrombus

Ans. 39) B. Bone morphogenetic protein (BMP) (Ref: 8 ed. Robbins p.708-09, 9 ed. p. 699-700, f-15-29, 30)

- **Familial Pulmonary Hypertension** occurs due to the mutations in the **bone morphogenetic protein receptor type 2 (BMPR2)** [Q] signaling pathway
- **BMPR2 mutation** causes **increased smooth muscle** survival and proliferation
- **BMPR2** belongs to **TGF-β receptor family**, which binds to variety of cytokines, including **TGF-β, bone morphogenetic protein (BMP), activin** and **inhibin**

Ans. 40) B. Lungs are spared (Ref: 8 ed. Robbins p.709-10, 9 ed. p. 701)

Goodpasture Syndrome [Q]

- Autoimmune disease involving **kidneys** and **lungs**
- Occurs due to circulating autoantibodies against the **noncollagenous domain of the α3 chain of collagen IV** [Q]
- Most common associated lesions – **Rapidly progressive glomerulonephritis** [Q] and **necrotizing hemorrhagic interstitial pneumonitis** [Q]
- **Immunofluorescence** [Q] – **Linear deposits** [Q] of **immunoglobulin's** along the **glomerular basement membrane**
- Most common cause of death is **uremia** [Q]
- HLA associations : **HLA-DRB1*1501 and *1502**

Ans. 41) A. Streptococcus pneumoniae (Ref: 8 ed. Robbins p.711, 9 ed. p.702)

- **Streptococcus pneumoniae**, or **pneumococcus**, is the **most common** cause of **community-acquired acute pneumonia** [Q]

Ans. 42) A. H. Influenza (Ref: 8 ed. Robbins p.711-12, 9 ed. p.703)

Points to Remember about ***Haemophilus influenzae*** [Q]

- **Gram-negative organism**, a major cause of life-threatening acute **lower respiratory tract infections** and **meningitis** in **young children**
- Before the advent of vaccine, **H. Influenza** was a common cause of **meningitis** [Q] in young children (<5 years of age)
- **Most common** bacterial cause of **acute exacerbation of COPD**

Ans. 43) A. Staphylococcus Aureus (Ref: 8 ed. Robbins p. 712, 9 ed. p. 703)

- **Intravenous drug abusers** [Q] are at **high risk** of developing **staphylococcal pneumonia** and **endocarditis**
- **Lung abscess** and **empyema** are associated complications

Ans. 44) D. All of the above (Ref: 8 ed. Robbins p. 712, 9 ed. p. 703)

Pseudomonas Aeruginosa

- Most common cause of **hospital-acquired infections** [Q]
- Seen in **neutropenic** [Q] patients and those with **cystic fibrosis** [Q]
- Can invade blood vessels with consequent extra pulmonary spread

Ans. 45) **B. Legionella (Ref: 8 ed. Robbins p. 712, 9 ed. p. 703-04)**

Legionella pneumophila [Q]

- Causes **Legionnaires' disease** and **Pontiac fever**
- Organism is seen in **artificial aquatic environments** [Q], such as **water-cooling towers**
- **Mode of transmission** [Q] – Inhalation of **aerosolized organisms** or aspiration of contaminated drinking water
- **Predisposing factors** [Q] include cardiac, renal, immunological, hematologic disease and organ transplant recipients

Ans. 46) **A. Bronchopneumonia (Ref: 8 ed. Robbins p. 712-14, 9 ed. p. 704, f-15-32-33)**

Morphology of Pneumonia [Q]:

Divided into two types:

Lobar pneumonia – Fibrinosuppurative consolidation of an **entire lobe**

Bronchopneumonia – Patchy consolidation of the lung

Lobar pneumonia:

- **Four stages** [Q] have been described: **Congestion**, **Red hepatization**, **Gray hepatization** and **Resolution**
- **Gross examination** – Affected lobe appears to have liver-like consistency, hence the term **hepatization** [Q]

Bronchopneumonia [Q]:

- Consolidation may be patchy and frequently bilateral and basal

Complications of Pneumonia [Q]

- **Abscess formation** (particularly common with **type 3 pneumococci** or **Klebsiella infections**)
- **Empyema**
- **Bacteremic dissemination** to the heart valves, pericardium, brain, kidneys, spleen or joints

Ans. 47) **A. Mycoplasma (Ref: 8 ed. Robbins p. 714-15, 9 ed. p. 704-05)**

Primary Atypical Pneumonia [Q]

- Characterized by **moderate amount of sputum** and elevated white cell count
- Absence of consolidation and lack of alveolar exudate
- **Most common** causative agent – ***Mycoplasma pneumoniae*** [Q]
- Other causative agents – Influenza virus types A and B, respiratory syncytial virus, adenovirus, rhinoviruses, rubeola and varicella; *Chlamydia pneumoniae*; *Coxiella burnetii* (Q-fever)

Ans. 48) **D. No cause found (Ref: 8 ed. Robbins p.716-17, 9 ed. p. 708-09, f-15-36)**

- **Lung abscess – Local suppurative process** that produces **necrosis** of **lung tissue**
- **Primary cryptogenic lung abscesses** [Q] – When **no causative agent** is identified

Causative Organisms of **Lung Abscess** [Q]:

- Staphylococcus aureus
- Anaerobic organisms – Bacteroides, Fusobacterium and Peptococcus species

Morphology: [Q]

- **Pulmonary abscesses** due to aspiration are more common on the **right** [Q] side (as right main bronchus is **more vertical)**
- Continued infection leads to **gangrene of lung**
- **Cardinal histologic change** [Q] is **suppurative destruction** of lung parenchyma within the **central area of cavitation**

Ans. 49) **D. Immunocompromised hosts show well-formed granulomas (Ref: 8 ed. Robbins p.717-18, 9 ed. p. 708-09)**

Clinical presentation of **Histoplasmosis** resembles **tuberculosis** [Q] and includes:

- **Coin lesions** [Q] on chest radiography
- Lung disease, involving **lung apices**

- **Extra pulmonary sites** include mediastinum, adrenals, liver or meninges, which show localized lesions
- **Widely disseminated disease** in **Immunocompromised patients**

Morphology:

- **Dimorphic fungus** Q
- In lung, infection produces **epithelioid cell granulomas** Q, which are not found in **immunosuppressed individuals** Q
- Lesions undergo fibrosis and concentric calcification **(tree-bark appearance)** Q

Differential Diagnosis – Tuberculosis, sarcoidosis and coccidioidomycosis

Ans. 50) D. All of the above (Ref: 8 ed. Robbins p.717-19, 9 ed. p. 709-10)

D/D of coin lesions Q in lungs include:

- Tuberculosis, Sarcoidosis, Histoplasmosis, Blastomycosis, Coccidioidomycosis,
- Miliary tuberculosis, Metastasis, Pulmonary hamartoma
- So called sclerosing Hemangioma, Inflammatory myofibroblastic tumor, Carcinoid

Ans. 51) D. All of the above (Ref: 9 ed. Robbins p. 709-10)

Pulmonary Disease in **Human Immunodeficiency Virus Infection:**

- Bacterial and tubercular infections occur at **higher CD4+ counts (>200 cells/mm^3)** Q
- **Pneumocystis pneumonia** occurs at CD4+ counts **less than 200 cells/mm^3** Q
- **Cytomegalovirus**, fungal and Mycobacterium avium complex infections occurs at CD4+ counts less than **50 cells/mm^3** Q

Ans. 52) D. All of the above (Ref: 8 ed. Robbins p.722-23, 9 ed. p. 713-14)

Lung cancers can be divided into two clinical subgroups: Small cell carcinoma and non-small cell carcinoma

- In **small cell lung carcinoma** Q, cancer associated genes include: C-KIT, MYCN, p53, 3p, RB and BCL2
- Genes most commonly affected in **non-small cell lung carcinoma** Q include: EGFR, KRAS, p53, p16 INK4a

Ans. 53) D. All of the above (Ref: 8 ed. Robbins p. 723-24, 9 ed. p. 714-15, f-15-41-42)

Precursor (Pre-invasive) Lesions of **carcinoma lung includes:**

a) **Squamous dysplasia** and **carcinoma in situ** Q
b) **Atypical adenomatous hyperplasia** Q
c) **Adenocarcinoma in situ** (formerly called as **Bronchioloalveolar carcinoma**)
d) Diffuse idiopathic pulmonary neuroendocrine cell hyperplasia (DIPNECH)

Ans. 54) A. Adrenals (Ref: 8 ed. Robbins p. 723)

- Distant spread of lung carcinoma occurs through both lymphatic and hematogenous pathway
- **Adrenals** Q are most commonly involved, followed by the liver, brain and bone

Ans. 55) A. Located peripherally in lung (Ref: 8 ed. Robbins p. 724-25, 9 ed. p. 715-16, f-15-44)

Salient Features of Adenocarcinomas Q:

- Malignant epithelial tumor with glandular differentiation or mucin production
- Most common type of **lung cancer** in women and **nonsmokers**
- Lesions are more **peripherally located** Q and are smaller
- Pattern of growth includes **acinar, papillary, bronchioloalveolar** and **solid**
- Tumor shows positivity for **thyroid transcription factor-1 (TTF-1)** Q
- Grows more slowly than squamous cell carcinoma but tend to metastasize widely
- **KRAS** and **epidermal growth factor receptor gene (EGFR) mutations** Q are seen

Ans. 56) D. Lepidic (Ref: 8 ed. Robbins p. 725-27, 9 ed. p. 715, f-15-42)

Note: 9 ed. Robbins mentions that **Adenocarcinoma in situ** is the new name given to **bronchioloalveolar carcinoma**

Bronchioloalveolar Carcinoma Q

- **Macroscopically**, the tumor occurs in the **peripheral portions** of the lung and are less than **3 cms**
- **Histologically**, the key feature is **Lepidic** Q growth pattern – neoplastic cells resembles **butterflies** sitting on a **fence**
- Composed of **dysplastic cells** which grow along **preexisting alveolar septae**
- Two subtypes: **nonmucinous** and **mucinous**

Ans. 57) D. EGFR mutation (Ref: 8 ed. Robbins p. 726, 9 ed. p. 713-14)

Following **gene abnormalities** are noted in **Squamous cell carcinoma of lung** Q:

- p53 mutation
- Loss of protein expression of tumor suppressor gene **RB1**
- Inactivation of **p16 (INK4a)**
- **HER-2/NEU** is **highly expressed** in **cancers**
- **Amplification of FGFR1** (gene encoding **fibroblast growth factor receptor tyrosine kinase** has been recently described)
- **EGFR overexpression** has been noted and not mutation

Ans. 58) B. Small cell carcinomas (Ref: 8 ed. Robbins p.726-27, 9 ed. p. 717, f-15-43)

Azzopardi effect Q:

- **Basophilic staining** of vascular walls, which occurs due to encrustation by DNA from necrotic tumor cells
- Seen in **small cell carcinomas**Q, which on immunohistochemistry shows positivity of **chromogranin, synaptophysin** and **CD57**

Ans. 59) D. All of the above (Ref: 8 ed. Robbins p.728-29, 9 ed. p. 718-19)

Paraneoplastic syndromes Q – occurs due to the hormones or hormone-like factors which include:

- Antidiuretic hormone **(ADH)**, leading to hyponatremia due to SIADH
- Adrenocorticotropic hormone **(ACTH)**, producing Cushing syndrome
- **Parathormone**, parathyroid hormone-related peptide, prostaglandin E, leading to **hypercalcemia**
- **Calcitonin**, causing hypocalcemia
- **Gonadotropins**, causing gynecomastia
- **Serotonin** and **bradykinin**, associated with the carcinoid syndrome

Note:

- **Small cell carcinomas** Q – produce **Cushing syndrome (ACTH)** and **SIADH (ADH)**
- **Squamous cell carcinomas** – produce **hypercalcemia** Q

Ans. 60) D. All of the above (Ref: 8 ed. Robbins p.729, 9 ed. p. 718-19)

Systemic manifestations Q of **lung carcinoma** includes:

- Lambert-Eaton myasthenic syndrome
- Peripheral neuropathy
- Acanthosis nigricans
- Leukemoid reactions
- Hypertrophic pulmonary osteoarthropathy

Pancoast Tumors Q:

- **Lung cancers** located in **superior pulmonary sulcus** can invade **cervical sympathetic plexus**, leading to **Horner syndrome** Q (enophthalmos, ptosis, miosis and anhidrosis)

Ans. 61) D. All of the above (Ref: 8 ed. Robbins p.729-30, 9 ed. p. 719-20, f-15-47)

Points to Remember about **Neuroendocrine cell tumors (NET) of lung:**

- **Diffuse idiopathic pulmonary neuroendocrine cell hyperplasia (DIPNECH)** Q is the **precursor** lesion
- NET's include – **Benign tumorlets**, **carcinoids** and highly aggressive **small cell carcinoma** and **large cell neuroendocrine carcinoma of the lung** Q
- **Atypical carcinoids** can show **p53 mutations** and abnormalities of ***BCL2* and *BAX* expression**

Ans. 62) B. Typical carcinoid have 2-10 mitosis/10 hpf (Ref: 8 ed. Robbins p.729-30, 9 ed. p. 719-20, f-15-47)

Carcinoid Tumors Q:

Grossly

- Most tumors grow as **spherical polypoid masses**
- Can present as **intraluminal mass** that penetrate the **bronchial wall** and extends into the peribronchial tissue, producing **collar-button lesion** Q

Histologically Q

- Tumor is composed of **organoid**, **trabecular**, **palisading**, or **rosette-like arrangements** of cells separated by a **delicate fibro vascular stroma**
- Tumor cells are **regular** and have **uniform round nuclei** and moderate amount of **eosinophilic cytoplasm**
- **Typical carcinoids** Q have **< 2 mitoses/10 hpf** and lack necrosis
- **Atypical carcinoids** Q have **2-10 mitoses/hpf** and/or foci of necrosis

Clinical Features:

- Presents as **classic carcinoid syndrome**, with intermittent attacks of diarrhea, flushing and cyanosis
- **Bronchial carcinoids** can **metastasize**

Ans. 63) C. <15 ml (Ref: 8 ed. Robbins p.731, 9 ed. p. 721)

- Normally, no more than **15 mL** Q of serous, acellular, clear fluid lubricates the pleural surface

Ans. 64) B. CEA positivity (Ref: 8 ed. Robbins p.733-34, 9 ed. p. 723-24, f-15-52)

Mesotheliomas microscopically are classified into:

a) **Epithelioid**

b) **Sarcomatoid** or

c) **Mixed types**

Differentiation of mesotheliomas from Adenocarcinomas is done by a panel of special stains.

Features that favor mesothelioma include:

- Positive staining for **acid mucopolysaccharide**
- **Lack of staining for carcinoembryonic antigen (CEA)** Q
- Positive staining for **Calretinin, Wilms tumor 1 (WT-1), cytokeratin 5/6** Q
- **Electron microscopy** – Presence of long microvilli and abundant tonofilaments

Ans. 65) A. Foam cells in vessel wall (Ref: Robbins 9th ed. p. 692-93)

Morphologic Changes in Radiation-Induced Lung Diseases:

- Diffuse alveolar damage
- Severe atypia of hyperplastic type II cells and fibroblasts
- Epithelial cell atypia and foam cells within vessel walls

Ans. 66) C. Adenocarcinoma (Ref: 9 ed. Robbins p. 715)

- Adenocarcinoma is now the most common form of lung cancer in women and, in many studies, men as well

Ans. 67) A. Chronic bronchitis (Ref: 9 ed. Robbins p. 679) Refer Q 15 for details

Ans. 68) D. Adrenal glands (Ref: 9 ed. Robbins p. 717) Refer Q 54 for details

Ans. 69) B. Cytokeratin (Ref: 9 ed. Robbins p. 724) Refer Q 64 for details

Ans. 70) A. Squamous cell carcinoma (Ref: 9 ed. Robbins p. 716-17)

Ans. 71) A. Dextrocardia (Ref: 9 ed. Robbins p. 683) Refer Q 20 for details

Ans. 72) A. Mesothelioma (Ref: 9 ed. Robbins p. 724) Refer Q 64 for details

Ans. 73) A. Emphysema (Ref: 9 ed. Robbins p. 675-678) Refer Q 11 for details

Ans. 74) A. Bronchial asthma (Ref: 9 ed. Robbins p. 682-83) Refer Q 19 for details

Ans. 75) A. Left lower lobe (Ref: 9 ed. Robbins p. 670)

Bronchogenic Sequestration:

- Refers to the presence of a discrete mass of lung tissue without any normal connection to the airway system

Ans. 76) B. Nicotine and carbon monoxide and tar

Ans. 77) B. Lung

Most common site for carcinoid tumor—Intestine or GIT as a whole followed by Bronchus (2nd most common site)

Ans. 78) C. Descending Aorta (Ref: 9 ed. Robbins p. 670)

Pulmonary sequestration:

- Refers to a discrete area of lung tissue that lacks any connection to the airway system
- Has abnormal blood supply arising from the aorta or its branches

Ans. 79) B. Kulschitsky cells

- Carcinoid tumours are neuroendocrine tumours arising from enterochromaffin cells (Kulschitsky cells of crypts of lieberkuhn)

Ans. 80) A. Chromogranin (Ref: 9 ed. Robbins p. 717) Refer Q 58 for details

Ans. 81) A. Neurogenic tumor (Ref: 9 ed. Robbins p. 626)

Ans. 82) C. Atelectasis (Ref: 9 ed. Robbins p. 670-71) Refer Q 3 for details

Ans. 83) C. Usual Interstitial Pneumonia (Ref: 9 ed. Robbins p. 686) Refer Q 21 to 25 for details

Ans. 84) A. Numerous long, slender microvilli (Ref: Robbins 8 ed. 700, 733) Refer Q 64 for details

- Most likely diagnosis on the basis of description is malignant mesothelioma

Mesothelioma:

a. Most specific neoplasm associated with asbestosis

b. Occurs after 1-2 years of exposure but incidence peaks at 20-35 years of exposure

c. Diagnosis:

- History of asbestos exposure
- Clinical signs and symptoms
- Radiographic findings
- Histopathological features
- Immunohistochemical and ultra-structural studies

d. Electron microscopy (ultra structural examination):

- Accepted as a gold standard
- Characterized by markedly elongated surface microvilli in the absence of secretory cytoplasmic granules

e. Features which differentiate mesothelioma from adenocarcinoma include:

1. Positive staining for acid mucopolysaccharide
2. Lack of staining for CEA and other epithelial glycoprotein antigens
3. Strong staining for keratin proteins
4. Positive staining for Calretinin, Wilms tumor1 (WT-1), Cytokeratin 5/6 and D2-40
5. On, electron microscopy, presence of long microvilli and abundant tonofilaments but absent micro villous rootlets and lamellar bodies

Ans. 85) A. Small cells with scant cytoplasm, ill-defined cell borders and hyperchromatic nuclei with nuclear moulding (Ref: 9ed. Robbins p. 717)

14 Head and Neck

How to go about this chapter?

- **One should be thorough with the following repeatedly asked topics:**
  - **Herpes simplex virus infection, Oral candidiasis, Rhinosporidiosis**
  - **Leukoplakia, Erythroplakia**
  - **Sinonasal (Schneiderian) Papilloma**
  - **Nasopharyngeal angiofibroma**
  - **Olfactory neuroblastoma**
  - **Nasopharyngeal carcinoma**
  - **Paraganglioma**
  - **Pleomorphic Adenoma, Warthin Tumor, Mucoepidermoid carcinoma, Adenoid cystic carcinoma, Acinic cell carcinoma**

INFLAMMATORY/ REACTIVE LESIONS

1) **Following is/are the fibrous tumors of the gingiva:**
   a) Irritation fibroma
   b) Pyogenic granuloma
   c) Peripheral ossifying fibroma
   d) All of the above

INFECTIONS

2) **All are TRUE about oro-facial Herpes simplex virus infections EXCEPT:**
   a) HSV-1 is the most common cause
   b) HSV-2 incidence is rising
   c) Intra-cytoplasmic inclusions are characteristic
   d) Tzanck test is used for diagnosis

3) **Most common type of oral candidiasis is:**
   a) Pseudomembranous
   b) Erythematous
   c) Hyperplastic
   d) None of the above

4) **TRUE about Rhinosporidiosis:**
   a) Causative agent is Klebsiella
   b) Microscopically, Mikulicz cells are characteristic
   c) Numerous globular cysts
   d) Bacterial disease

PRECANCEROUS AND CANCEROUS LESIONS

5) **All are TRUE about precancerous lesions of head and neck EXCEPT:**
   a) Leukoplakia presents as white patch
   b) Erythroplakia presents as red velvety patch
   c) Leukoplakia has a higher risk of malignant transformation
   d) Erythroplakia has a higher risk of malignant transformation

6) **Most common cancers of head and neck include:**
   a) Squamous cell carcinoma (SCC)
   b) Adenocarcinomas
   c) Melanomas
   d) Metastasis

7) **Genetic alterations in SCC include(s):**
   a) 3p and 9p21 deletions
   b) Inactivation of p16 gene
   c) P53 mutation
   d) All of the above

TUMORS OF NOSE, SINUSES AND NASOPHARYNX

8) **Agent responsible for Sinonasal Papilloma:**
   a) RSV
   b) CMV
   c) EBV
   d) HPV

9) All are TRUE regarding Nasopharyngeal Angiofibroma EXCEPT:
a) Occurs in older age group
b) Located in posterolateral wall of nose
c) Bleeds on biopsy
d) May regress after puberty

10) Olfactory neuroblastomas, sometimes may be associated with:
a) t(9;22) b) t(11;22)
c) t(15;17) d) Trisomy 8

11) All are TRUE about Nasopharyngeal carcinomas EXCEPT:
a) Bimodal age group
b) EBNA-1 (EBV genome) can be identified in tumor epithelial cells
c) Keratinizing SCC is most radiosensitive
d) Undifferentiated carcinoma is most radiosensitive

LARYNX

12) Potentially lethal laryngoepiglottitis in infants and young children is/are caused by:
a) RSV
b) H. Influenza
c) Beta-hemolytic streptococci
d) All of the above

13) Most common type of laryngeal cancer is:
a) Squamous cell carcinoma
b) Basaloid carcinoma
c) Spindle cell carcinoma
d) Verrucous carcinoma

14) Highest incidence of lymph nodes metastasis is seen in which type of laryngeal carcinoma?
a) Glottic
b) Supra-glottic
c) Sub-glottic
d) Trans-glottic

NECK

15) All are TRUE about Paraganglioma EXCEPT:
a) Most common site is adrenal medulla
b) Most common extra-nodal site is head and neck
c) Carotid body tumor is prototype of sympathetic paraganglioma
d) May metastasize to regional lymph nodes

SALIVARY GLANDS

16) All are TRUE about salivary gland tumors EXCEPT:
a) 65-80% arise in parotid gland
b) 15-30% tumors in parotid are malignant
c) Malignancy in salivary gland tumor is directly proportional to the size of gland
d) Warthin tumor occur more common in males

17) All are TRUE about Pleomorphic adenoma EXCEPT:
a) Also called as benign mixed tumor
b) Contains epithelial and mesenchymal components
c) Radiation exposure increases the risk
d) Doesn't undergo malignant transformation

18) TRUE about Warthin tumor:
a) Also called as Papillary Cystadenoma Lymphomatosum
b) Occurs exclusively in parotid gland
c) Increased risk in smokers and males
d) All of the above

19) Myoepitheliomas are of the following type(s):
a) Spindle cell
b) Clear cell
c) Hyaline (Plasmacytoid) cell
d) Any of the above

20) TRUE about Mucoepidermoid carcinoma:
a) Most commonly occur in parotid
b) Can be seen in minor salivary glands
c) Most common form of primary malignant tumor of salivary glands
d) All of the above

21) TRUE about Adenoid cystic carcinoma:
a) Most commonly involves parotid gland
b) Well encapsulated tumor
c) Tendency to invade perineural spaces
d) Doesn't metastasize

22) Acinic cell carcinoma rarely involves:
a) Parotid gland
b) Submandibular gland
c) Minor salivary glands
d) None of the above

23) Warthin's tumor is: (NEET 2014)
a) Multifocal and bilateral
b) Multifocal and unilateral
c) Unifocal and bilateral
d) Unifocal and unilateral

24) Most common malignant tumor of salivary glands: (NEET 2014)
a) Pleomorphic adenoma
b) Mucoepidermoid carcinoma
c) Warthin tumor
d) Acinar cell tumor

25) Following are TRUE about pleomorphic adenoma EXCEPT: (NEET 2014)
a) It is also called mixed tumor
b) It most commonly involves the parotid gland
c) Does not involve the submandibular gland
d) It is the most common neoplasm of the salivary glands

26) Which among the following is most common malignancy of salivary gland? (NEET 2013)
a) Pleomorphic adenoma
b) Adenocystic carcinoma
c) Mucoepidermoid carcinoma
d) Mixed tumour

27) Glomus cells are found in: (NEET 2013)
a) Carotid body
b) Thyroid carcinoma
c) Liver carcinoma
d) None

28) Which of the following is the most characteristic ultra-structural feature of paraganglioma on electron microscopy? (AIPGMEE 2010)
a) Shrunken mitochondria
b) Large Golgi apparatus
c) Frequent mitoses
d) Dense core neuroendocrine granules

CHAPTER 14: HEAD AND NECK

Ans. 1) **D. All of the above (Ref: 8 ed. Robbins p.741-42, 9 ed. p. 728-29, f-16-2,3)**

Fibrous proliferative lesions affecting **gingiva** includes:

a) **Irritation fibroma** – occurs in the buccal mucosa or at the gingivodental margin

b) **Pyogenic granuloma** [Q]:
- Pedunculated lesion
- Occurs in the gingiva of children, young adults and pregnant women
- Surface of the lesion is ulcerated and red to purple in color
- **Histologically** – It shows high vascular proliferation, similar to **granulation tissue**
- Considered to be a form of **Capillary Hemangioma** [Q]

c) **Peripheral ossifying fibroma** – Red, ulcerated and nodular lesions, can be mistaken clinically for pyogenic granulomas

d) **Peripheral giant cell granuloma** – composed of multinucleate, foreign body–like giant cells separated by a fibroangiomatous stroma

Ans. 2) **C. Intra-cytoplasmic inclusions are characteristic (Ref: 8 ed. Robbins p. 742-43, 9 ed. p. 729)**

Herpes Simplex Virus Type 1 (HSV-1) [Q]:
- Most common offending agent of oro-facial herpetic infection
- **Age group** – 2 to 4 years, results in abrupt onset of vesicles and ulcerations throughout the oral cavity, especially in **gingiva**

Morphology [Q]:
- Vesicles range from few millimeters to large bullae

Microscopy:
- Intracellular and intercellular edema
- **Epidermal cells** showing **eosinophilic intra-nuclear viral inclusions** [Q] and cells may fuse to produce **giant cells**
- **Tzanck test** [Q] is used as a **diagnostic test**, based on the **microscopic examination** of the vesicle fluid

Ans. 3) **A. Pseudomembranous (Ref: 8 ed. Robbins p.743, 9 ed. p. 729-30)**
- Three major clinical forms of oral candidiasis – **pseudo-membranous (thrush), erythematous and hyperplastic**

Pseudo-membranous candidiasis ("thrush") [Q]:
- Most common type affecting oral cavity, which presents as superficial, curdy and gray to white inflammatory membrane
- **Pseudomembrane** – Composed of **organisms** in a **fibrinosuppurative exudate** and can be readily scraped off
- **Predisposing factors** [Q] – Diabetes mellitus, organ or bone marrow transplant recipients, neutropenia, chemotherapy-induced immunosuppression, AIDS

Ans. 4) **C. Numerous globular cysts (Ref: 10 ed. Ackerman p.293)**

Rhinosporidiosis:
- Causative agent – **Rhinosporidium seeberi** [Q] (now thought a fish parasite)
- **Microscopy** [Q] shows **numerous globular cysts** [Q], each of which represents **thick-walled sporangium** containing numerous spores

Rhinoscleroma:
- Caused by an organism of the **Klebsiella** [Q] group
- **Microscopically**, the predominant cells are **foamy macrophages (Mikulicz cells)** and **plasma cells**
- Organisms can be identified using **periodic acid–Schiff (PAS)**

Ans. 5) **C. Leukoplakia has higher risk of malignant transformation (Ref: 8 ed. Robbins p.744-45, 9 ed. p. 731, f-16-4, 5)**

Leukoplakia

- **White patch** or plaque that **cannot be scraped off** [Q]
- **Grossly** – Appears as single or multiple white patches or plaques
- May show markedly **dysplastic changes** of the lining epithelium
- All leukoplakias must be considered **pre-cancerous** [Q]

Erythroplakia

- Presents as a **red, velvety** [Q] eroded area within the oral cavity
- Has a **higher risk** of **malignant transformation** [Q] than that seen with leukoplakia

Microscopy [Q]:

- **Superficial erosions** with **dysplasia, carcinoma in situ**, or **minimally invasive carcinoma** with **sub-epithelium** showing intense **inflammatory reaction**
- **Predisposing Factors** [Q]: Tobacco (cigarettes, pipes, cigars and chewing tobacco)

Ans. 6) **A. Squamous cell carcinoma (Ref: 8 ed. Robbins p.745-48, 9 ed. p. 731, f-16-7)**

- 95% of cancers of the head and neck are **squamous cell carcinomas** [Q], arising most commonly in the **oral cavity**

Predisposing Factors [Q]:

- Smoking tobacco and alcohol
- **Human Papilloma virus** infection
- Actinic radiation (sunlight) and pipe smoking (for cancer of the lower lip)
- Betel quid and paan chewing

Most common sites [Q] (in order of frequency) – **Ventral surface of the tongue**, floor of the mouth, lower lip, soft palate and gingiva

Ans. 7) **D. All of the above (Ref: 8 ed. Robbins p.745-48, 9 ed. p. 732-33, f-16-6)**

Genetic Alterations in SCC [Q]:

- **Loss of heterozygosity (LOH)** of **3p and 9p21**, results in **inactivation** of **p16 gene** (inhibitor of cyclin-dependent kinase)
- LOH at **17p** with mutation of the **p53 tumor suppressor gene** is associated with progression to **dysplasia**
- Amplification and **overexpression of cyclin D1 gene** (located on chromosome 11q13) activates **cell cycle progression**

Ans. 8) **D. HPV (Ref: 8 ed. Robbins p.751, 9 ed. p. 737, f-16-9)**

Sinonasal (Schneiderian) Papilloma [Q]:

- **HPV types 6 and 11** [Q] have been identified
- Three forms: **exophytic** (most common), **inverted** (most important biologically) and **cylindrical**
- **Nasal septum** [Q] – most common site of **exophytic type**
- **Lateral wall of nose** [Q] – most common site of **inverted type**
- Microscopically – proliferations of squamous or columnar epithelium are seen

Ans. 9) **A. Occurs in older age group (Ref: 10 ed. Ackerman p.305-06, 9 ed. p. 737)**

Nasopharyngeal Angiofibroma

- Occurs in males between **10 and 25 years** [Q] of age
- Arises from fibrovascular stroma located in the **posterolateral wall of the roof of the nose** [Q]
- Presents as a polypoid mass that bleeds severely on manipulation
- **Sites** [Q] – Protrude below the free edge of the soft palate, extend into the antrum, external orifice of the nose, posteriorly into the nasopharynx, or even into the orbit and cranial cavity

- **Differential Diagnosis** ᵠ – Lobular capillary hemangioma
- **Treatment** ᵠ – Usually regress after puberty. Surgical resection for early lesions and chemotherapy for advanced and aggressive lesions

Ans. 10) B. Trisomy 8 (Ref: 8 ed. Robbins p.751, 9 ed. p. 737)

Olfactory Neuroblastoma (Esthesioneuroblastoma) ᵠ:

- Composed of malignant **small round cells** ᵠ, resembling **neuroblasts**
- **Differential diagnosis** ᵠ – Small-cell tumors, such as lymphoma, Ewing sarcoma and Embryonal Rhabdomyosarcoma
- **Lacks 11;22 translocation** ᵠ, typical of Ewing sarcoma of bone
- Some of these tumors reveal **trisomy 8** ᵠ
- **Immunohistochemistry** ᵠ shows positivity for neuron-specific enolase, synaptophysin, CD56 and chromogranin

Ans. 11) C. Keratinizing SCC is most radiosensitive (Ref: 8 ed. Robbins p.751-52, 9 ed. p. 737-38, f-16-10)

Nasopharyngeal Carcinomas:

- **Bimodal age group** ᵠ (15-25 years and 60-69 years)
- 3 patterns: **Keratinizing squamous cell carcinomas, non-keratinizing squamous cell carcinomas** and **undifferentiated carcinomas (lymphoepithelioma)** ᵠ
- Undifferentiated and Non-keratinizing squamous cell nasopharyngeal carcinomas demonstrate components of EBV genome i.e. **EBNA-1** ᵠ

Treatment:

- **Radiotherapy** ᵠ is the standard modality of treatment
- **Undifferentiated carcinoma** is most **radiosensitive** ᵠ and **keratinizing squamous cell carcinoma** is **least** ᵠ radiosensitive

Ans. 12) D. All of the above (Ref: 8 ed. Robbins p.752, 9 ed. p. 738-39)

Laryngoepiglottitis:

- In **infants** and **young children – Respiratory Syncitial Virus (RSV), Haemophilus influenzae, or β-hemolytic streptococci** ᵠ are the causative agents

Ans. 13) A. Squamous cell carcinoma (Ref: 8 ed. Robbins p.753, 9 ed. p. 739-40)

- 95% of laryngeal carcinomas are typical **squamous cell carcinomas** ᵠ
- Four types of laryngeal cancer includes – **glottis, supra-glottic, subglottic, trans-glottic**

Ans. 14) D. Trans-glottic (Ref: 10 ed. Ackerman p.325)

- **Trans-glottic cancers** have highest risk of **lymph node metastasis** ᵠ

Ans. 15) C. Carotid body tumor is prototype of sympathetic paraganglioma (Ref: 8 ed. Robbins p.755-56, 9 ed. p. 741-42, f-16-13)

- **Paraganglia** – Clusters of neuroendocrine cells associated with sympathetic and parasympathetic nervous system
- **Most commonly** located in the **adrenal medulla** ᵠ, where they give rise to **pheochromocytomas** ᵠ
- 70% of **extra-adrenal paragangliomas** occur in the **head and neck** ᵠ region

Paragangliomas typically develop in **two locations**:

a) **Paravertebral Paraganglia** ᵠ (e.g. organs of Zuckerkandl) – Innervated by **sympathetic nervous system** ᵠ and are **chromaffin-positive**

b) Paraganglia related to the **great vessels** of the **head and neck** ᵠ (aorticopulmonary chain): e.g.

- **Carotid bodies (most common)** ᵠ; aortic bodies; jugulotympanic ganglia – and are innervated by the **parasympathetic** ᵠ nervous system

Carotid Body Tumor ᵠ

- Prototype of **parasympathetic paraganglioma,** arises at the **bifurcation of the common carotid artery**

Microscopy:

- **Composed of nests (Zellballen)** Q of **round to oval chief cells**, surrounded by delicate vascular septae
- **Chief cells** stain strongly for **chromogranin, synaptophysin, neuron-specific enolase, CD56 and CD57** Q
- **Sustentacular cells** (spindle-shaped stromal cells) are positive for **S-100 protein** Q

Ans. 16) C. Malignancy in salivary gland tumor is directly proportional to the size of gland (Ref: 8 ed. Robbins p.757, 9 ed. p. 744, t-16-4)

Overview of Salivary Gland Neoplasms:

- **65%-80%** arise within the **parotid**, 10% in the **submandibular gland** and the remainder in the minor salivary glands and sublingual glands
- Approximately, **15% to 30%** of tumors in parotid glands are malignant
- Ratio of salivary gland tumor being malignant is **inversely proportional to the size of the gland** Q
- **Warthin tumor** occurs more often in **males** than in females Q

Ans. 17) D. Doesn't undergo malignant transformation (Ref: 8 ed. Robbins p.757-59, 9 ed. p. 744-45, f-16-15,16)

Pleomorphic Adenoma:

- Also called as **mixed tumors** Q
- Consist of a mixture of **ductal (epithelial)** and **myoepithelial cells** and shows both **epithelial and mesenchymal differentiation** Q
- Radiation exposure **increases the risk** Q

Morphology Q:

Grossly Q – Presents as **rounded, encapsulated, well-demarcated masses**

Microscopy Q:

- **Epithelial elements** are arranged in acini, irregular tubules, strands, or sheets of cells
- **Epithelial cells** forming **well-developed ducts** are lined by cuboidal to columnar cells with an underlying layer of small **myoepithelial cells**
- Background **shows loose myxoid tissue** with islands of cartilage and rarely bone
- Carcinoma arising in a **pleomorphic adenoma** is referred to as a **carcinoma ex pleomorphic adenoma** Q or a **malignant mixed tumor** Q

Treatment Q – **Parotidectomy** is the treatment of choice

Ans. 18) D. All of the above (Ref: 8 ed. Robbins p.759, 9 ed. p. 745, f-16-17)

Warthin Tumor (Papillary Cystadenoma Lymphomatosum) Q

- Arises almost exclusively in the **parotid gland** Q
- Occurs more commonly in **males** Q, in fifth to seventh decades of life
- 10% are multifocal and 10% are bilateral
- **Smokers** Q are at increased risk of developing these tumors

Morphology Q:

Gross Q – Tumors are **round to oval, encapsulated masses**, 2 to 5 cm in diameter

Cut surface – Shows **multicystic spaces** filled with a mucinous or serous secretion

Microscopy Q:

- **Cystic spaces** are lined by a **double layer of neoplastic epithelial cells** resting on a **dense lymphoid stroma** with prominent germinal centers
- **Double layer** – Upper layer consists of columnar cells with abundant, finely granular, eosinophilic cytoplasm while lower layer is composed of cuboidal to polygonal cells

Ans. 19) D. Any of the above (Ref: 10 ed. Ackerman p. 829-830)

- Myoepitheliomas can be of **three types – Spindle cell type clear cell type** and **hyaline (plasmacytoid) type** Q

Ans. 20) D. All of the above (Ref: 8 ed. Robbins p.759-60, 9 ed. p. 745-46, f-16-18)

Mucoepidermoid Carcinomas:

- Most common form of **primary malignant tumor** Q of the salivary glands
- Most commonly occurs in the **parotid gland** Q
- Also seen in the **minor salivary glands** Q
- Associated with **t(11;19) chromosomal translocation**

Morphology:

- **Gross** Q –**circumscribed**, but **lack well-defined capsule**
- **Cut surface** – pale, gray-white, solid and frequently contain **small, mucin-containing cysts**

Microscopy Q:

- Tumor grows in nests, sheets and cords
- Tumor cells are composed of variable mixtures of **squamous cells, mucus-secreting cells and intermediate cells**
- Small to large **mucus-filled vacuoles** can be seen, which can be highlighted with mucin stains

Ans. 21) C. Tendency to invade perineural spaces (Ref: 8 ed. Robbins p.760-61, 9 ed. p. 746-47, f-16-19)

Adenoid Cystic Carcinoma Q

- Also called as **cylindroma** Q
- Most common site – **Minor salivary glands** Q (palate)
- Most common locations in major salivary glands: **Parotid** and **submandibular**
- Can show invasion into **perineural spaces** Q

Gross Q – Small, poorly encapsulated, infiltrative, gray-pink lesions

Microscopy Q:

- Cells are arranged in **tubular, solid, or cribriform patterns** Q
- Composed of small cells having dark, compact nuclei and scant cytoplasm
- Spaces between the tumor cells are filled with **hyaline material**
- Shows positivity with **CD117(cKIT)** Q

Ans. 22) C. Minor salivary glands (Ref: 9 ed. Robbins p. 747)

Acinic Cell Carcinoma:

- Most common site is **parotid** Q followed by **submandibular glands**
- **Rarely** involves **minor salivary glands** (which have **scant number** of **serous cells)**

Ans. 23) A. Multifocal and bilateral (Ref: 9 ed. Robbins p. 745)

- 10% are multifocal and 10% are bilateral
- Most Common benign Salivary gland tumor – Pleomorphic adenoma (mixed tumor)
- Most Common malignant tumor of salivary gland – Mucoepidermoid Carcinoma
- Most Common site of pleomorphic adenoma – Parotid gland
- Most Common site of Mucoepidermoid Carcinoma – Parotid gland
- Most Common site for Acinic cell carcinoma – Parotid gland
- Most Common site for Adenoid Cystic Carcinoma – Minor salivary glands
- Multifocal and bilateral Salivary gland tumor – Warthin tumor and Acinic cell tumor
- Salivary gland tumor with tendency to invade perineural space – Adenoid cystic carcinoma

Ans. 24) B. Mucoepidermoid carcinoma (Ref: 9 ed. Robbins 746) Refer Q 20 for details

Ans. 25) C. Does not involve the submandibular gland (Ref: 9 ed. p. 744-45) Refer Q 16 and 17 for details

Ans. 26) C. Mucoepidermoid Carcinoma (Ref: 9 ed. Robbins p. 745-46) Refer Q 20 for details

Ans. 27) A. Carotid body (Ref: 8 ed. Robbins p.755-56, 9 ed. p. 741-42, 517)

Ans. 28) D. Dense core neuroendocrine granules (Ref: 9 ed. Robbins p. 741-42) Refer Q 15 for details

Electron microscopy: Shows well-demarcated neuroendocrine granules (paravertebral tumors)

15 The Gastrointestinal Tract

How to go about this chapter?

- **One should be thorough with following topics:**
  - **Meckel diverticulum, Hirschsprung Disease, Barrett esophagus**
  - **Esophageal adenocarcinoma, Curling ulcers, Cushing ulcer**
  - ***H. pylori* gastritis, Autoimmune gastritis, Menetrier disease**
  - **Gastrinomas, Gastric adenomas, Gastric cancer, Gastric lymphomas**
  - **Carcinoid tumor, Gastrointestinal Stromal Tumor, Volvulus**
  - **Ischemic bowel disease, Celiac disease, Pseudomembranous colitis**
  - **Whipple disease, Amebiasis, Inflammatory bowel disease**
  - **Small intestinal polyps and associated syndromes, Familial adenomatous polyposis**
  - **Hereditary non-polyposis colorectal cancer (HNPCC)**
  - **Microsatellite instability**

CONGENITAL ABNORMALITIES

1) **All are TRUE about Meckel Diverticulum EXCEPT:**
   a) True diverticulum
   b) Can present as occult bleeding
   c) Most common site is sigmoid colon
   d) Most often symptomatic by age of 2 years

2) **All are TRUE about Congenital Hypertrophic Pyloric stenosis EXCEPT:**
   a) More common in males
   b) Presents in 2nd week of life
   c) Associated with Trisomy 21
   d) Monozygotic twins have high rate of concordance

3) **All of the following are TRUE about Hirschsprung disease EXCEPT:**
   a) Associated with Down Syndrome
   b) Also called as Congenital aganglionic megacolon
   c) Dilation of colon distal to affected segment
   d) Associated with RET mutations

4) **Causes of Acquired Megacolon include all EXCEPT:**
   a) Chagas disease
   b) Ulcerative colitis
   c) Hirschsprung disease
   d) Inflammatory stricture/neoplasm obstruction

ESOPHAGUS

5) **Patterson Brown Kelly syndrome includes all EXCEPT:**
   a) Iron deficiency anemia
   b) Glossitis
   c) Cheilosis
   d) Lower esophageal webs

6) **Achalasia is characterized by:**
   a) Increased LES tone
   b) Incomplete LES relaxation
   c) Aperistalisis of esophagus
   d) All of the above

7) **Mallory Weiss tear most commonly occurs in:**
   a) Esophagus b) Gastric mucosa
   c) Small Intestine d) Large Intestine

8) **Boerhaave Syndrome is characterized by rupture in:**
   a) Upper esophagus
   b) Mid-esophagus
   c) Distal esophagus
   d) Gastrointestinal junction

9) **Desquamative skin diseases affecting esophagus include(s):**
   a) Bullous Pemphigoid
   b) Epidermolysis Bullosa
   c) Both a + b
   d) Pemphigus Vulgaris

10) Herpetic infection in esophagus leads to:
a) Pseudo membrane formation
b) Punched out ulcers
c) Nuclear and cytoplasmic inclusions
d) Any of the above

11) Barret esophagus is characterized by all EXCEPT:
a) Intestinal metaplasia
b) Increased risk of esophageal carcinoma
c) Goblet cells are necessary for diagnosis
d) Features of dysplastic epithelium are absent

12) Epithelial dysplasia is noted in...... patients of Barret esophagus.
a) 0.2-2% b) 2-4%
c) 3-5% d) 5-10%

13) Intramucosal carcinoma is characterized by:
a) Invasion of neoplastic epithelial cells into lamina propria
b) Invasion of neoplastic epithelial cells into muscularis propria
c) Any of the above
d) None of the above

14) Risk factors for adenocarcinoma esophagus includes all EXCEPT:
a) Long standing GERD
b) Tobacco use
c) *H. pylori* infection
d) Prior radiation therapy

15) Progression of Barret esophagus to adenocarcinoma occurs through following genetic change(s):
a) p53 mutation
b) C-ERB-B2 amplification
c) Rb gene mutation
d) All of the above

16) Esophageal adenocarcinoma occurs in:
a) Proximal portion of esophagus
b) Middle third of esophagus
c) Distal third of esophagus
d) None of the above

17) Risk factors for Squamous cell carcinoma esophagus includes all EXCEPT:
a) Tobacco use
b) Alcohol
c) Plummer Vinson Syndrome
d) GERD

18) Squamous cell carcinoma esophagus occurs in:
a) Proximal 1/3 of esophagus
b) Middle 1/3 of esophagus
c) Distal 1/3 of esophagus
d) Any of the above

19) Most common benign tumor of esophagus:
a) Fibroma b) Leiomyoma
c) Lipoma d) Neurofibroma

STOMACH

20) G-cells which release gastrin are present in:
a) Cardiac glands b) Fundal glands
c) Antral glands d) Any of the above

21) Defense forces which protects gastric mucosal injury include(s):
a) Mucin secreted by surface foveolar cells
b) Elaboration of prostaglandins
c) Rich vascular supply
d) All of the above

22) An erosion is a defect in?
a) Mucosa
b) Sub mucosa
c) Muscularis
d) None of the above

23) All are TRUE about Curling ulcers EXCEPT:
a) Occurs in severe burns
b) Also seen in trauma patients
c) Affects distal duodenum
d) None of the above

24) Cushing ulcers are seen in patients with:
a) Intracranial disease
b) Severe burns
c) Trauma
d) Any of the above

25) Dieulafoy lesion is most commonly seen in:
a) Lesser curvature of stomach
b) Greater curvature of stomach
c) Antrum
d) Pylorus

26) Watermelon stomach is seen in:
a) Dieulafoy lesion
b) GAVE
c) *H. pylori* gastritis
d) Stress ulcers

27) All are TRUE about *H. pylori* organisms EXCEPT:
a) Spiral shaped organisms
b) Discovered by Warren and Marshall
c) Associated with duodenal ulcers
d) No association with gastric cancer

28) All are TRUE about pathogenesis of *H. pylori* gastritis EXCEPT:
a) Presents as antral gastritis
b) Can be associated with gastric atrophy
c) Cag A plays a role in gastritis
d) Infection results in decreased acid production

29) Special stains to demonstrate *H. pylori* includes all EXCEPT:
a) Warthin Starry
b) Giemsa
c) PAS
d) Silver stain

30) *H. pylori* can be found in following regions of gastric epithelium EXCEPT:
a) Superficial mucus overlying epithelial cells
b) Foveolar cells
c) Gastric pits
d) Areas showing intestinal metaplasia

31) Which biopsy is best used to diagnose *H. pylori*?
a) Antral b) Fundal
c) Cardiac d) Any of the above

32) Characteristic features of *H. pylori* gastritis in biopsy specimens:
a) Intraepithelial neutrophils
b) Sub-epithelial plasma cells
c) A+B
d) Lymphoid aggregates

33) *H. pylori* can be diagnosed by:
a) Rapid urease test
b) DNA detection by PCR
c) Bacterial culture
d) All of the above

34) Features of Autoimmune gastritis include(s):
a) Loss of parietal cells
b) Hypergastrinemia
c) Vitamin B12 deficiency
d) All of the above

35) Differentiating features between *H. pylori* gastritis and autoimmune gastritis includes all EXCEPT:
a) Sites of gastric mucosa involved
b) Gastrin levels
c) Its sequelae
d) Vitamin B 12 levels

36) Associated with Autoimmune gastritis include(s):
a) Hashimoto's thyroiditis
b) Addison's disease
c) Type 1 diabetes mellitus
d) All of the above

37) Most common cause of granulomatous gastritis in developed world includes:
a) Crohn disease b) Sarcoidosis
c) Mycobacteria d) CMV

38) Most common site for Peptic ulcer disease:
a) Duodenum b) Ileum
c) Jejunum d) Colon

39) Most common site for gastric peptic ulcer:
a) Greater curvature
b) Lesser curvature
c) A+B
d) None of the above

40) All are the gross features of Peptic Ulcer Disease EXCEPT:
a) Punched out defect
b) Heaped up margin
c) Mucosal margin may overhang base
d) Malignant transformation does not occur

41) All are TRUE about Menetrier disease EXCEPT:
a) Irregular enlargement of gastric rugae
b) In children, disease is self-limited
c) Increased risk of adenocarcinoma
d) Antrum is most commonly affected

42) All are TRUE about Gastrinomas EXCEPT:
a) Leads to Zollinger-Ellison Syndrome (ZES)
b) In stomach, it leads to increased parietal cells
c) Most commonly occurs in stomach
d) Has an association with MEN-1

43) In ZES, the predominant cell type is:
a) Mucous cell b) Parietal cell
c) Chief cell d) Endocrine cell

44) All are TRUE about fundic gland polyps EXCEPT:
a) Associated with Familial Adenomatosis polyposis syndrome
b) Increased risk in patients on PPI's
c) More common in women
d) Associated with adenocarcinoma

45) Increased risk of gastric adenocarcinoma is seen with:
a) Inflammatory gastric polyp
b) Gastritis cystica
c) Fundic gland polyp
d) Gastric adenomas

46) All are TRUE about epidemiology of gastric cancer EXCEPT:
a) Early gastric cancer is limited to mucosa and submucosa
b) Benzopyrene and N-nitroso compounds consumption leads to increased risk
c) Vitamin C, E intake is associated with reduced risk
d) Cancer of gastric antrum is on rise

47) Most common mutation seen in diffuse gastric cancer is:
a) CDH1 b) Beta catenin
c) P53 d) APC

48) All are TRUE about morphology of gastric cancers EXCEPT:
a) Intestinal type tumors form bulky masses
b) Diffuse tumors produces linitis plastica
c) Most commonly, it involves greater curvature
d) None of the above

49) All are TRUE about gastric cancer EXCEPT:
a) Intestinal type cancer has precursor lesions
b) Diffuse type cancer has reduced incidence
c) Depth of invasion is most important prognostic factor
d) Can metastasize to supraclavicular lymph node

50) Metastasis from gastric cancer can involve:
a) Virchow node
b) Sister-Mary Joseph nodule
c) Blumer shelf
d) All of the above

51) Most common site of extra nodal lymphoma:
a) Lung b) Liver
c) GIT d) Skin

52) Translocation(s) seen in gastric MALomas include(s):
a) t(11;18)
b) t(1;14)
c) t(14;18)
d) Any of the above

53) MALTomas express all of the markers EXCEPT:
a) CD5 b) CD19
c) CD20 d) CD43

54) All are TRUE about Carcinoid tumors EXCEPT:
a) Better known as well differentiated neuro-endocrine carcinoma
b) Most common site is tracheobronchial tree and lungs
c) In GIT, most commonly occurs in small intestine
d) Arise from the endocrine cells of the gut

55) Most common site of carcinoid tumor in GIT:
a) Proximal duodenum
b) Jejunum and ileum
c) Appendix
d) Colon

56) TRUE about the sites involved in gut carcinoid:
a) In appendix, it most commonly affects tip
b) In jejunum and ileum it can be seen throughout the mucosa
c) Rectum is more commonly involved than cecum
d) Any of the above

57) All are TRUE about carcinoid syndrome EXCEPT:
a) Strongly suggests metastatic disease
b) Mid-gut carcinoids are most commonly associated
c) Cutaneous flushing, bronchospasm, abdominal pain are manifestations
d) Occurs when tumors are confined to intestine

58) Most aggressive carcinoids is/are:
a) Foregut carcinoid
b) Mid-gut carcinoid
c) Hindgut carcinoid
d) Any of the above

59) Most common mesenchymal tumor affecting stomach is:
a) Gastrointestinal Stromal Tumor (GIST)
b) Leiomyoma
c) Schwannoma
d) None of the above

60) GIST arises from the following:
a) Smooth muscle
b) Nerve cells
c) Interstitial cells of Cajal
d) Vascular endothelium

61) TRUE about morphology of GIST include(s):
a) Solitary, well circumscribed mass
b) Metastasis can occur
c) C-KIT can be seen immunohistochemically
d) All of the above

62) All are TRUE about prognostic factors in GIST EXCEPT:
a) Tumor size <5 cms rarely metastasize
b) Small intestinal GIST are less aggressive than gastric GIST
c) >10 cm and >5 mitosis/50 hpf indicates high grade
d) None of the above

63) Carney's triad includes all EXCEPT:
a) Gastric GIST
b) Paraganglioma
c) Pulmonary chondroma
d) Neurofibromatosis

SMALL INTESTINE AND COLON

64) All are TRUE about intestinal obstruction EXCEPT:
a) Hernias, adhesions, volvulus account for 80% of mechanical obstruction
b) Tumors lead to 10-15% of obstructions
c) Pain and vomiting are presenting features
d) Sigmoid colon is most common site

65) Most common site of volvulus:
a) Sigmoid colon b) Cecum
c) Small bowel d) Stomach

66) Water shed zones include(s):
a) Splenic flexure
b) Recto sigmoid colon
c) Both A and B
d) None of the above

67) Surface epithelial atrophy and hyper proliferative crypts are features of:
a) Crohn disease
b) Ulcerative colitis
c) Ischemic bowel disease
d) Any of the above

68) Most common site of Angiodysplasia include(s):
a) Cecum b) Ileum
c) Jejunum d) Any of the above

69) All of the following predisposes to celiac disease EXCEPT:
a) Rye b) Wheat
c) Barley d) Maize

70) Most commonly associated with celiac disease:
a) HLA-DQ8 b) HLA-DQ4
c) HLA-DR4 d) Any of the above

71) TRUE about celiac disease are all EXCEPT:
a) In adults it presents with features of malabsorption
b) In infants the symptoms develop soon after birth
c) Has an association with dermatitis herpetiformis
d) Only treatment available is gluten free diet

72) TRUE about Abetalipoproteinemia:
a) X-linked disease
b) Associated with IPEX syndrome
c) Due to mutation in MTP
d) Mutation in FOXP3 gene

73) TRUE about Campylobacter enterocolitis:
a) Important cause of traveler's diarrhea
b) Association with Guillain Barre Syndrome
c) Can lead to reactive arthritis
d) All of the above

74) Reiter's syndrome is a complication of following infection:
a) Campylobacter b) E. coli
c) Shigella d) Salmonella

75) Features suggesting salmonella typhi infection includes all EXCEPT:
a) Payer patches hyperplasia
b) Oval ulcers along axis of ileum
c) Typhoid nodules
d) Non caseating granulomas

76) Which one of the following infection can be confused with Crohn disease?
a) E. coli b) Salmonella
c) Klebsiella d) Yersinia

77) Most common cause for traveler's diarrhea:
a) Enterotoxigenic E. Coli
b) Enterohemorrhagic E. Coli
c) Enteroinvasive E. Coli
d) Enteroaggregative E. Coli

78) TRUE about pseudomembranous enterocolitis:
a) Due to *clostridium difficile*
b) Due to third generation cephalosporins
c) Immunosuppression is a risk factor
d) All of the above

79) All are TRUE about Whipple disease EXCEPT:
a) Caused by *Tropheryma whippelli*
b) Gram positive actinomycete
c) Distended, foamy macrophages in small intestine
d) Cannot differentiate histologically from tuberculosis

80) Amebiasis most commonly affects:
a) Cecum b) Stomach
c) Duodenum d) Sigmoid colon

81) TRUE about Entamoeba histolytica:
a) Colonizes the colon and release trophozoites
b) Results in a flask shaped ulcer
c) Can lead to amebic liver abscess
d) All of the above

INFLAMMATORY BOWEL DISEASE

82) All of the following leads to increased susceptibility of Crohn disease EXCEPT:
a) NOD2 b) ATG16L1
c) IRGM d) IL23

83) Granulomas are a characteristic feature of:
a) Crohn disease
b) Ulcerative colitis
c) Both A and B
d) None of the above

84) Most common sites of Crohn disease includes all EXCEPT:
a) Terminal ileum b) Ileocecal valve
c) Cecum d) Rectum

85) Earliest Crohn disease lesion:
a) Aphthous ulcer
b) Fissure
c) Stricture
d) Cobblestone appearance

86) Extra intestinal manifestations of Crohn disease include(s):
a) Uveitis
b) Migratory polyarthritis
c) Pericholangitis
d) All of the above

87) All are morphological features of Ulcerative colitis EXCEPT:
a) Pan-colitis
b) Transmural
c) Normal serosal surface
d) Mucosal involvement

88) Serological investigation of choice for Crohn disease include:
a) P-ANCA
b) Anti-Saccharomyces cerevisiae antibody
c) C-ANCA
d) None of the above

89) All are TRUE about lymphocytic colitis EXCEPT:
a) Type of microscopic colitis
b) Increased intraepithelial lymphocytes
c) Dense sub-epithelial collagen layer
d) Associated with celiac disease

90) Non neoplastic polyps includes all EXCEPT:
a) Adenoma
b) Inflammatory
c) Hamartomatous
d) Hyperplastic

91) Solitary rectal ulcer syndrome is an example of:
a) Inflammatory polyp
b) Hamartomatous polyp
c) Hyperplastic polyp
d) Neoplastic polyp

92) All are TRUE about Juvenile polyps EXCEPT:
a) Associated with SMAD4 mutation
b) Most commonly occur in children less than 5 years of age
c) Most commonly seen in rectum
d) Dysplasia is not seen

93) All are TRUE about Peutz-Jeghers syndrome EXCEPT:
a) Multiple polyps, mucocutaneous hyperpigmentation
b) Also called as arborizing polyps
c) Mutation in the gene LKB1/STK11
d) Hamartomatous lesion leads to increased risk of carcinomas

94) Cowden syndrome patients are at increased risk for all EXCEPT:
a) Breast cancer
b) Gastrointestinal cancer
c) Endometrial cancer
d) Follicular carcinoma of thyroid

95) Hyperplastic polyp can be misinterpreted as:
a) Sessile serrated adenoma
b) Inflammatory polyp
c) Non-inflammatory polyp
d) None of the above

96) Polyps seen in Tuberous Sclerosis patients:
a) Inflammatory polyp
b) Hamartomatous polyp
c) Neoplastic polyp
d) Any of the above

97) TRUE about neoplastic polyps:
a) Most common neoplastic polyp is colonic adenoma
b) Precursor lesions to adenocarcinomas
c) Colorectal adenomas are characterized by epithelial dysplasia
d) All of the above

98) All are TRUE about sessile serrated adenoma EXCEPT:
a) Most common in right colon
b) Lack cytological features of dysplasia
c) Serrated surface confined to the surface
d) They have malignant potential

99) TRUE about Intramucosal carcinoma:
a) Have malignant potential
b) Invasion of lamina propria or muscularis propria is seen
c) Requires colectomy
d) All of the above

100) Familial Adenomatosis polyposis is characterized by all EXCEPT:
a) Develops more than 100 colonic adenomas
b) Associated with congenital hypertrophy of retinal pigment
c) 100% patients have mutations in APC gene
d) Colonic adenocarcinoma develops before age of 30 years

101) Gardner syndrome is characterized by all EXCEPT:
a) Osteomas of mandible
b) Epidermal cysts
c) Desmoid tumors
d) CNS tumors

102) TRUE about Lynch syndrome are all EXCEPT:
a) Autosomal Dominant disorder
b) Inherited mutations in mismatch repair genes
c) Cancer arises in left colon
d) Occurs in younger age group

103) TRUE about epidemiology of Colon cancer:
a) Low intake of dietary fibres
b) High intake of fat
c) Deficiency of Vitamin A, C, E
d) Any of the above

104) Following gene is/are involved in adenoma carcinoma sequence of colon cancer:
a) APC
b) K-RAS
c) SMAD-2
d) p 53
e) All of the above

105) All are TRUE about mismatch repair gene deficiency in colon cancer EXCEPT:
a) Mutations accumulate in microsatellite repeats
b) Silent mutations
c) K-RAS and p 53 mutation is commonly involved
d) Uncontrolled cell growth occurs due to TGF-β receptor mutation

106) Most commonly microsatellite mutation leads to carcinoma of:
a) Right colon
b) Left colon
c) Any of the above
d) Transverse colon

107) All are TRUE about adenocarcinoma colon EXCEPT:
a) Tumors of the right side causes napkin like constriction
b) Tumors of the proximal colon grow as polypoidal, exophytic masses
c) Tumors of the left colon can lead to obstruction
d) Tumors of the right colon rarely causes obstruction

108) TRUE about clinical features of colon cancers:
a) Right sided colon cancer presents with fatigue and weakness
b) Left side colon cancer presents with occult bleeding
c) Both of the above
d) None of the above

109) Ormond disease is:
a) Idiopathic
b) E. coli
c) S. pneumonia
d) Staphylococcus aureus

110) Tumors involving the peritoneum includes:
a) Metastasis
b) Mesothelioma
c) Desmoplastic small round blue cell tumors
d) All of the above

111) Which of the following gastric polyps has a malignant potential? (NEET 2014)
a) Adenomatous b) Hyperplastic
c) Fundic gland d) None of the above

112) Most common site for diverticulosis is: (NEET 2014)
a) Sigmoid colon b) Ascending colon
c) Transverse colon d) Splenic flexure

113) Gene responsible for Wilson disease is situated on which chromosome: (NEET 2014)
a) Chromosome 11 b) Chromosome 12
c) Chromosome 13 d) Chromosome 14

114) H pylori is associated with all of the following EXCEPT: (NEET 2014)
a) Increased risk of peptic ulcer disease
b) Increased risk of gastric lymphoma
c) Increased risk of antral gastric carcinoma
d) Increased risk of adenocarcinoma of esophagus

115) Majority of patients with HNPCC have mutations in: (NEET 2014)
a) MSH1 b) MSH2
c) MSH3 d) MSH4

116) Which of the following is not true about GIST? (NEET 2014)
a) Stomach is the most common site
b) High propensity of malignant change
c) Associated with c-KIT mutation
d) Histology shows spindle shaped cells

117) What is TRUE about ulcerative colitis? (NEET 2014)
a) Involves rectum and then whole colon backwards
b) Involves only colon
c) Skip lesions seen
d) Ileum not involved

118) MALToma is located in which layer of gastrointestinal tract? (NEET 2014)
a) Lamina Propria
b) Submucosa
c) Muscularis propria
d) Serosa

119) Most common site of tuberculosis in gastrointestinal tract is: (NEET 2014)
a) Stomach b) Small intestine
c) Rectum d) Ileocecal junction

120) Zollinger Ellison syndrome is caused by: (NEET 2014)
a) Gastrin secreting tumor
b) Somatostatin secreting tumor
c) CCK secreting tumor
d) Adrenalin secreting tumor

121) Most common site for colon cancer is: (NEET 2014)
a) Caecum
b) Transverse colon
c) Rectosigmoid
d) Ascending colon

122) H. pylori causes all EXCEPT: (NEET 2014)
a) Antral gastritis b) Gastric carcinoma
c) Atrophic gastritis d) GIST

123) Most common site of gastrointestinal carcinoid is: (NEET 2014)
a) Duodenum b) Appendix
c) Ileo-Jejunum d) Stomach

124) E- cadherin gene deficiency is seen in: (NEET 2013)
a) Gastric carcinoma
b) Intestinal carcinoma
c) Thyroid carcinoma
d) Pancreatic carcinoma

125) Gluten sensitive enteropathy is most strongly associated with: (AIIMS Nov 2014)
a) HLA-DR4 b) HLA-DQ2
c) HLA-DQ3D d) Blood group B

126) Skip areas are pathognomic of: (AIIMS Nov 2014)
a) Ulcerative colitis
b) Crohn disease
c) Intestinal obstruction
d) Ischemic bowel disease

127) Most common site of GIST is: (NEET 2013)
a) Ileum
b) Esophagus
c) Colon
d) Stomach

128) True about Ulcerative colitis is all EXCEPT: (NEET 2013)
a) Rectum involved
b) Pseudo polyps
c) Pan colitis
d) Non-caseating granuloma

129) Inheritance of Gardner syndrome is: (NEET 2013)
a) Autosomal recessive
b) Autosomal dominant
c) X-linked
d) None of the above

130) Toxic megacolon is seen in: (NEET 2013)
a) Chronic nonspecific ulcerative colitis
b) Crohn's disease
c) Colonic diverticulosis
d) Hamartomatous polyp

131) Osteomas, adenomatous polyps of intestine and periampullary carcinomas are seen in: (NEET 2013)
a) Cowden syndrome
b) Peutz Jeghers syndrome
c) FAP
d) Gardener syndrome

132) Diverticulum most common site is: (NEET 2013)
a) Sigmoid colon
b) Ileum
c) Ascending colon
d) Transverse colon

133) Achalasia cardia: (NEET 2013)
a) Absence of nerves
b) Absence of muscles
c) Hypertrophy of nerves
d) None

134) Which of the following markers is specific for Gastrointestinal stromal tumors (GIST)? (AIPGMEE 2010)
a) CD 117 b) CD 34
c) CD 23 d) S – 1000

135) TRUE about gastric carcinoma is: (AIPGMEE 2012)
a) Occult bleeding in stool is not common
b) Associated with achlorhydria/ hypochlorhydria
c) Always Squamous cell carcinoma
d) Radiosensitive

136) Most common mechanism of GERD: (AIIMS May 2012)
a) Transient decrease in pressure at LES
b) Hypotension at lower esophageal sphincter
c) Hiatus Hernia
d) Gastritis

137) In Barrett's Esophagus following is seen: (AIIMS May 2012, Nov 2014)
a) Intestinal Metaplasia
b) Intestinal Dysplasia
c) Gastric Dysplasia
d) Squamous Metaplasia

138) Due to popularity of refrigeration reducing the need to preserve food, which cancer's incidence has dramatically declined? (AIIMS May 2013)
a) Esophagus b) Stomach
c) Colon d) Nasopharynx

139) About gastrointestinal stromal tumour (GIST) all are TRUE EXCEPT: (AIIMS Nov 2014)
a) Most common site is stomach
b) Originates from interstitial cells of Cajal
c) Size plays a role in prognosis
d) ALK mutation is seen in most cases

140) 17-year-old boy had intussusception. The excised intestinal segment showed multiple polyps whose histopathology is shown in figure. Identify the pathology: (AIIMS Nov. 2015)

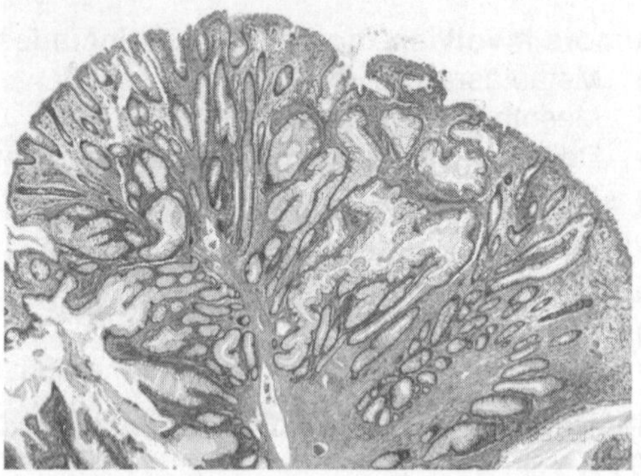

a) Hamartomatous polyp
b) Tubulovillous polyp
c) Juvenile polyp
d) Adenocarcinoma

141) A 30-year-old male patient presents with a history of heartburn. An upper GI endoscopy was done and a biopsy from a suspicious lesion showed the following picture. What does this show? Which special stain will you do for confirmation and what will you look for? (AIIMS Nov 2015)

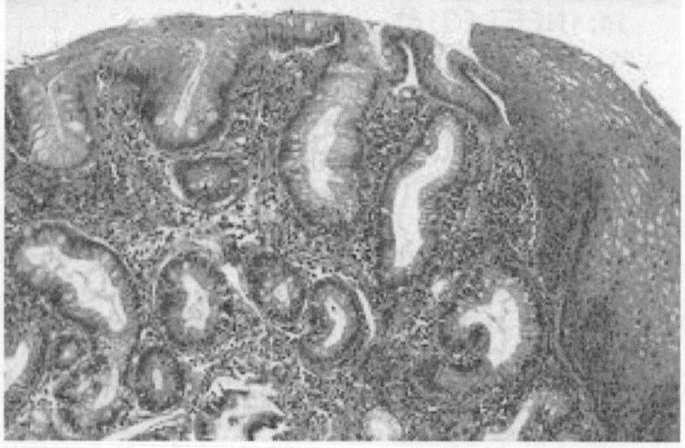

a) H. pylori infection, Silver stain, Gram-negative cocco-bacilli
b) Adenocarcinoma esophagus, mucin stain, mitotic figures
c) Squamous cell carcinoma, keratin stain
d) Barrett's esophagus, mucin stain, dysplasia

CHAPTER 15 – THE GASTROINTESTINAL TRACT

Ans. 1) C. Most common site is sigmoid colon (Ref: 8 ed. Robbins p.765-66, 9 ed. p. 751, f-17-2)

Meckel Diverticulum:

- Due to failed involution of the **vitelline duct**
- Most common site – **ileum** Q
- Can have **ectopic pancreatic** or **gastric tissue**, which may result in peptic ulceration and **occult bleeding** Q or abdominal pain
- A **true diverticulum** Q which includes mucosa, submucosa and muscularis propria

"Rule of 2s" Q **in Meckel Diverticulae:**

- Occurs in approximately **2%** of the population
- Present within **2 feet (85 cm)** of the **ileocecal valve**
- Approximately **2 inches (5 cm) long**
- Twice as common in males as in females and are most often symptomatic by age 2

Ans. 2) C. Associated with Trisomy 21 (Ref: 8 ed. Robbins p.766, 9 ed. p. 751)

Congenital hypertrophic pyloric stenosis:

- **Three to four times** more common in **males** Q
- **Monozygotic twins** have a high rate of **concordance**
- **Turner syndrome** Q and **trisomy 18** Q are also associated with the disease
- Presents in the **second or third week** of life
- Presents with persistent, projectile, non-bilious vomiting
- There is **hyperplasia** of the **muscularis propria** Q of **pylorus**
- Surgical splitting of the muscularis (**myotomy**) Q is curative

Ans. 3) C. Dilation of colon distal to affected segment (Ref: 8 ed. Robbins p.766-67, 9 ed. p. 751-52, f-17-3)

Hirschsprung Disease Q**:**

- 10% of cases occur in children with **Down syndrome** Q
- Also known as **congenital aganglionic megacolon** Q, in which ganglion cells undergo premature death
- Distal intestinal segment Q lacks **Meissner** sub-mucosal and Aurebach myentric plexus Q
- **Dilation of the colon proximal to the affected segment** Q
- **Loss-of-function mutations** in **receptor tyrosine kinase RET** Q is seen in familial cases

Morphology Q

- **Absence of ganglion cells** Q within the **affected segment**
- **Rectum** Q is **most commonly** affected
- **Aganglionic region** appears **normal grossly** and the normal innervated **proximal colon** may undergo **progressive dilation** Q, leading to **megacolon**

Ans. 4) C. Hirschsprung disease (Ref: 8 ed. Robbins p.766-67, 9 ed. p. 752)

Causes of Acquired megacolon Q

- Chagas disease
- Obstruction by a neoplasm or inflammatory stricture
- Toxic megacolon complicating ulcerative colitis
- Visceral myopathy

Ans. 5) D. Lower esophageal webs (Ref: 8 ed. Robbins p.767, 9 ed. p. 753)

Paterson-Brown-Kelly or Plummer-Vinson syndrome Q:

- Characterized by **upper esophageal webs** accompanied by **iron-deficiency anemia, glossitis** and **cheilosis** Q
- **Esophageal webs** are **most common** in **upper esophagus** and are **semi-circumferential** Q

Ans. 6) D. All of the above (Ref: 8 ed. Robbins p.767, 9 ed. p. 753-54)

Achalasia:

- Characterized by the **triad of incomplete LES relaxation, increased LES tone** and **aperistalsis of the esophagus** Q

Primary achalasia is **idiopathic** Q

Secondary achalasia Q is seen in:

- **Chagas disease**; **diabetic autonomic neuropathy**; infiltrative disorders such as **malignancy, amyloidosis, or sarcoidosis**; and lesions of **dorsal motor nuclei**

Ans. 7) A. Esophagus (Ref: 8 ed. Robbins p.768)

Mallory-Weiss Tear Q:

- **Linear lacerations** that are longitudinally **oriented** in the **esophagus** Q near the **gastro esophageal junction**
- Most often associated with **severe retching** or **vomiting** secondary to acute alcohol intoxication

Ans. 8) C. Distal esophagus (Ref: 8 ed. Robbins p.768, 9 ed. p. 754)

- **Boerhaave syndrome** Q is characterized by **distal esophageal rupture** and **mediastinitis**

Ans. 9) C. Both a + b (Ref: 8 ed. Robbins p.768, 9 ed. p. 754)

- **Desquamative skin diseases** which may affect esophagus includes **Bullous Pemphigoid** Q, **Epidermolysis bullosa** Q and, rarely **Crohn disease**

Ans. 10) B. Punched out ulcers (Ref: 8 ed. Robbins p.768-69, 9 ed. p. 755, f-17-4)

- **Candidiasis** leads to **pseudo membrane** Q formation
- **Herpes viruses** leads to **punched-out ulcers** Q and biopsy specimens demonstrate **nuclear viral inclusions** Q
- **CMV** causes **shallower ulcerations** Q and **biopsy** specimens demonstrate **nuclear and cytoplasmic inclusions** Q

Ans. 11) D. Features of dysplastic epithelium are absent (Ref: 8 ed. Robbins p.770-71, 9 ed. p. 757-58, f-17-7,8)

Barrett esophagus Q

- Complication of **chronic GERD** and is characterized by **intestinal metaplasia** Q within the **esophageal squamous mucosa**
- Leads to **epithelial dysplasia** Q **(pre-invasive lesion)** and **increased risk of esophageal adenocarcinoma** Q

Morphology Q

- Classified as **long segment**, in which **3 cm or more** of esophagus is involved, or **short segment**, in which **less than 3 cm** is involved

Microscopy Q

- **Goblet cells** Q which have distinct mucous vacuoles and are seen in **intestinal metaplasia** Q, are necessary for diagnosis
- **Low grade dysplasia and high-grade dysplasia** Q can be seen

Complication:

- May lead to **Intramucosal carcinoma** Q which is characterized by **invasion of neoplastic epithelial cells** Q into the lamina propria

Ans. 12) A. 0.2-2% (Ref: 8 ed. Robbins p.770, 9 ed. p. 757, f-17-7)

- **Epithelial dysplasia** Q, is detected in **0.2% to 2.0%** Q of patients with **Barrett esophagus** each year

Ans. 13) A. Invasion of neoplastic epithelial cells into lamina propria (Ref: 8 ed. Robbins p.771, 9 ed. p. 757)

- **Intramucosal carcinoma** Q is characterized by **invasion of neoplastic epithelial cells** into the **lamina propria** Q

Ans. 14) C. *H. pylori* infection (Ref: 8 ed. Robbins p.772, 9 ed. p. 758, f-17-9)

Risk factors for Adenocarcinoma of the Esophagus Q

- Barrett esophagus
- Long-standing GERD
- Tobacco use, obesity and prior radiation therapy

Reduced risk by diets rich in **fresh fruits** and **vegetables** and also with certain ***Helicobacter pylori*** Q serotypes

Ans. 15) D. All of the above (Ref: 8 ed. Robbins p.772, 9 ed. p. 758)

Following **genetic abnormalities** Q are noted in **adenocarcinoma of esophagus:**

- **p53 mutations** and **down regulation** of **cyclin dependent kinase inhibitor CDKN2A (p16/INK4a)** in early stages of esophageal adenocarcinoma
- **Amplification** of **c-ERB-B2, Cyclin D1** and **Cyclin E gene**
- **Mutation** of the **retinoblastoma tumor suppressor gene**

Ans. 16) C. Distal third of esophagus (Ref: 8 ed. Robbins p.772, 9 ed. p. 758, f-17-9,10)

Morphology:

- **Esophageal adenocarcinoma** usually occurs in the **distal third of the esophagus** Q

Grossly Q**:**

- Appears as a **flat** or **raised patch** which may reach up to **5 cm** or **more** in diameter and may infiltrate or ulcerate or invade deeply

Microscopically Q:

- Tumors most commonly produce **mucin** and **form glands** and are commonly seen in association with **Barrett esophagus** Q
- Tumors may show **tumor cells** composed of diffusely infiltrative **signet-ring cells** Q

Ans. 17) D. GERD (Ref: 8 ed. Robbins p.773-74, 9 ed. p. 759-60, f-17-9)

Risk Factors for SCC esophagus Q includes:

- **Alcohol** and **tobacco use**, poverty, caustic esophageal injury, achalasia, tylosis
- **Plummer-Vinson syndrome**, frequent consumption of very hot beverages, nutritional deficiencies, polycyclic hydrocarbons, nitrosamines
- Fungus-contaminated foods and **Human papillomavirus (HPV) infection** Q

Ans. 18) B. Middle 1/3 of esophagus (Ref: 8 ed. Robbins p.773-74, 9 ed. p. 759-60, f-17-9,10)

Morphology Q:

- Most common site of **squamous cell carcinomas** is **middle third of the esophagus** Q
- Begins as an **in situ lesion** Q termed as **squamous dysplasia**

Gross Q:

- Early lesions appear as **small, gray-white, plaque-like** thickenings
- **Polypoidal** or **exophytic** tumor masses, which may **protrude** and **obstruct** the lumen
- Appear as **ulcerated** or **diffusely infiltrative** lesion that spread within the esophageal wall and cause thickening, rigidity and luminal narrowing

Microscopy Q:

- Most squamous cell carcinomas are **moderately** to **well-differentiated** Q
- Histological variants include **verrucous squamous cell carcinoma, spindle cell carcinoma** and **Basaloid squamous cell carcinoma**

Lymph node metastases Q:

- Cancers in **upper third** of the **esophagus** metastasize to cervical lymph nodes
- Cancers in **middle third** favor Mediastinal, Para-tracheal and tracheobronchial nodes
- Cancers in the **lower third** spread to gastric and celiac nodes

Ans. 19) B. Leiomyoma (Ref: 8 ed. Robbins p.774)

- **Benign tumors of esophagus** are mostly **mesenchymal** in origin and most common are tumors of **smooth muscle origin** i.e. **Leiomyoma** Q.

Ans. 20) C. Antral glands (Ref: 8 ed. Robbins p.774, 9 ed. p. 760)

- Stomach is divided into **four major anatomic regions**: cardia, fundus, body and antrum
- **Antral glands** contain **G cells** Q, that release **gastrin** Q, which stimulate **parietal cells** Q leading to **luminal acid secretion**

Ans. 21) D. All of the above (Ref: 8 ed. Robbins p.774-75, 9 ed. p. 760-61, f-17-11)

- Gastric lumen is **strongly acidic** which helps in digestion, but can also lead to gastric mucosal damage

Mechanisms that protect the gastric mucosa Q:

- Mucin secreted by surface foveolar cells
- Mucus layer has a **neutral pH** because of **bicarbonate ion secretion** by surface epithelial cells
- **Rich vascular supply** delivers oxygen, bicarbonate and nutrients while washing away acid
- Elaboration of **Prostaglandin** and epithelial regenerative capacity

Any disruption in these protective mechanisms, may lead to acute or chronic gastritis

Ans. 22) A. Mucosa (Ref: 8 ed. Robbins p.775, 9 ed. p. 761, f-17-11)

- **Erosion** implies loss of **superficial epithelium**, leading to a **defect in the mucosa** that is limited to the lamina propria Q
- Accompanied by **neutrophilic infiltrate** within the mucosa

Ans. 23) C. Affects proximal duodenum (Ref: 8 ed. Robbins p.775, 9 ed. p. 762)

- **Curling ulcers** Q – Ulcers occurring in the **proximal duodenum** and are associated with **severe burns** or **trauma**
- **Stress ulcers** Q– Most common in individuals with **shock**, sepsis, or severe trauma

Ans. 24) A. Intracranial disease (Ref: 8 ed. Robbins p.775, 9 ed. p. 762)

Cushing ulcers Q:

- Gastric, duodenal and esophageal ulcers in persons with **intracranial disease** Q and have a high incidence of **perforation**

Ans. 25) A. Lesser curvature of stomach (Ref: 9 ed. Robbins p.762)

Dieulafoy Lesion Q:

- Caused by **submucosal artery** Q that does not branch properly within the wall of the stomach
- The diameter of **mucosal artery** becomes **3 mm**
- Most commonly found along the **lesser curvature** Q
- Erosion of the overlying epithelium can cause **gastric bleeding**

Ans. 26) GAVE (Ref: 9 ed. Robbins p. 762)

Gastric Antral Vascular Ectasia (GAVE) Q

- Responsible for non-variceal **upper gastrointestinal bleeding** Q
- **Endoscopy** – shows **longitudinal stripes** of edematous erythematous mucosa Q with alternating paler mucosa
- Sometimes referred to as **watermelon** Q **stomach**

Ans. 27) D. No association with gastric cancer (Ref: 8 ed. Robbins p.776-78, 9 ed. p. 763-64, f-17-12)

H. pylori Q

- Discovered by **Warren and Marshall** Q
- Spiral-shaped or curved bacilli
- Seen in patients with **duodenal ulcers** Q and **gastric ulcers** Q or **chronic gastritis** Q
- Most commonly affects the **antrum** Q
- Confers increased risk of **gastric cancer** Q

Ans. 28) D. Infection results in decreased acid production (Ref: 8 ed. Robbins p.776-78, 9 ed. p. 763-64, f-17-12)

H. pylori infection:

- Results in **increased acid production** and **disruption** of **normal gastric** and **duodenal protective mechanisms**
- Results in **antral gastritis** Q with **high acid production** Q, despite hypogastrinemia

Ans. 29) C. PAS (Ref: 8 ed. Robbins p.776-78, 9 ed. p. 763-64, f-17-12)

Special stains Q to demonstrate ***H. pylori* organisms**:

- **Giemsa**
- **Diff-Quik stains**
- **'Triple stain'** which includes Hematoxylin and Eosin, Alcian Blue (AB) (pH-2.5) and Warthin-Starry silver stain

Alcian Blue (pH – 2.5)/Periodic acid-Schiff (PAS) – demonstrates **intestinal metaplasia** Q

Ans. 30) D. Areas showing intestinal metaplasia (Ref: 8 ed. Robbins p.777-78, 9 ed. p. 763-64, f-17-12)

H. pylori organisms can be found in:

- **Superficial mucus** overlying the **epithelial cells** Q
- Luminal surfaces of **foveolar** and **mucous neck cells** Q
- **Gastric pits** Q

Note Q: ***H. pylori*** shows **tropism** for **gastric epithelia** and is **not found** in association with **gastric intestinal metaplasia** Q or in **duodenal epithelium** Q

Ans. 31) A. Antral (Ref: 8 ed. Robbins p.777-78, 9 ed. p. 764)

- Within **stomach**, *H. pylori* are found in the **antrum** Q
- Thus, **antral biopsy** Q is preferred for evaluation of *H. pylori* gastritis

Ans. 32) C. A+B (Ref: 8 ed. Robbins p.777-78, 9 ed. p. 764, f-17-12)

Microscopy of ***H. pylori* gastritis**:

- **Intraepithelial neutrophils** Q and **sub-epithelial plasma cells** Q are characteristic features
- **Neutrophils** accumulate in gastric pits to form **pit abscesses** Q
- **Lymphoid aggregates with germinal centers** Q **(mucosa-associated lymphoid tissue**, or **MALT)** can be seen, which can transform into **lymphoma**

Ans. 33) D. All of the above (Ref: 8 ed. Robbins p.778, 9 ed. p. 764)

- **Non-invasive serologic** Q tests includes – **antibodies to *H. pylori***, fecal bacterial detection and **urea breath test**
- **Gastric biopsy specimens** can also be analyzed by the **rapid urease test, bacterial culture**, or **bacterial DNA detection** by **PCR**

Ans. 34) D. All of the above (Ref: 8 ed. Robbins p.778-779, 9 ed. p. 764-65)

Pathogenesis of Autoimmune gastritis Q:

a) Loss of **parietal cells** (which secretes gastric acid and intrinsic factor)
b) Absence of acid production stimulates **gastrin release**, resulting in **hypergastrinemia**
c) Lack of intrinsic factor leads to **Vitamin B 12 deficiency** and **megaloblastic anemia**
d) Associated with **achlorhydria, *H. pylori* gastritis** can cause **hypochlorhydria**

Ans. 35) C. Its sequelae (Ref: 8 ed. Robbins p.778-779, 9 ed. p. 764-66, t-17-3)

- All the options mentioned in the question differentiate between *H. pylori* gastritis and autoimmune gastritis except **its sequelae** Q

- The risk of **adenocarcinoma is more** in **autoimmune gastritis** than ***H. pylori* gastritis** [Q], however it can be seen in both

	***H. pylori*–Associated**	**Autoimmune**
Location	Antrum	Body
Inflammatory infiltrate	Neutrophils, sub epithelial plasma cells	Lymphocytes, macrophages
Acid production	Increased to slightly decreased	Decreased
Gastrin levels	Normal to decreased	Increased
Other lesions	Hyperplastic/inflammatory polyps	Neuroendocrine hyperplasia
Serology	Antibodies to *H. pylori*	Antibodies to parietal cells (H^+, K^+-ATPase, intrinsic factor)
Sequelae	Peptic ulcer, adenocarcinoma	Atrophy, pernicious anemia, adenocarcinoma, carcinoid tumor
Associations	Low socioeconomic status, poverty, residence in rural areas	Autoimmune disease; thyroiditis, diabetes mellitus, Graves disease

Ans. 36) D. All of the above (Ref: 8 ed. Robbins p.779, 9 ed. p. 765)

Autoimmune gastritis is associated with:

- **Hashimoto thyroiditis, insulin-dependent (type I) diabetes mellitus, Addison disease,** Primary ovarian failure, hypoparathyroidism, **Graves disease**, vitiligo, myasthenia gravis and Lambert-Eaton syndrome [Q]

Ans. 37) A. Crohn disease (Ref: 8 ed. Robbins p.780, 9 ed. p. 766)

Granulomatous Gastritis:

- **Crohn disease** [Q] is the most common cause in western countries
- Other causes – **Sarcoidosis** [Q] and **infections** including **mycobacteria, fungi, CMV** and ***H. pylori***

Ans. 38) A. Duodenum (Ref: 8 ed. Robbins p.780-81, 9 ed. p. 766, f-17-14)

- Peptic ulcers are **four times** [Q] more common in **proximal duodenum** [Q] (anterior duodenal wall) than in the stomach

Ans. 39) B. Lesser curvature (Ref: 8 ed. Robbins p.780-81, 9 ed. p. 766-67, f-17-14)

- **Gastric peptic ulcers** [Q] are located along the **lesser curvature** [Q] near the interface of the body and antrum

Ans. 40) B. Heaped up margin (Ref: 8 ed. Robbins p.780-81, 9 ed. p. 767, f-17-14)

Heaped-up margins [Q] are more characteristic of **carcinomas** [Q]

Peptic ulcer [Q]:

- Is a round to oval, sharply **punched-out defect** [Q]
- Mucosal margin may **overhang the base** slightly
- **Base of peptic ulcers** is **smooth and clean** [Q]
- **Malignant transformation** of peptic ulcers is very **rare** [Q]

Ans. 41) D. Antrum is most commonly affected (Ref: 8 ed. Robbins p.782, 9 ed. p. 768-69, f-17-15, t-17-5)

Menetrier Disease [Q]

- Due to increased secretion of **transforming growth factor α (TGF-α)**
- In children, it follows **respiratory infection** and is **self-limited**
- Patients have **increased risk** of **gastric adenocarcinoma** [Q]

Morphology [Q]:

- **Irregular enlargement** of **gastric rugae**
- Most commonly affects **body and fundus, antrum is spared** [Q]
- **Microscopy**: **Most characteristic feature** is hyperplasia of **foveolar mucous cells**

Ans. 42) C. Most commonly occurs in stomach (Ref: 8 ed. Robbins p.782-83, 9 ed. p. 769)

Gastrinomas Q

- May lead to **Zollinger-Ellison syndrome** Q
- Most commonly found in **small intestine or pancreas** Q
- In stomach, there occurs a **marked increase** in number of **parietal cells** Q
- **Gastrin overproduction** leads to proliferation of endocrine cells
- 60% to 90% of gastrinomas are **malignant** Q
- Forms a component of **multiple endocrine neoplasia type I (MEN-1)** Q

Ans. 43) B. Parietal cells (Ref: 8 ed. Robbins p.782, 9 ed. p. 769, t-17-5, f-17-15)

- In **Zollinger-Ellison syndrome**, there is increase in the **number** of **parietal cells** Q
- In **Menetrier disease, mucous cells** are predominantly **seen**

Note: In **Zollinger-Ellison syndrome**, association with **adenocarcinoma** is **not** seen

Ans. 44) D. Associated with adenocarcinoma (Ref: 8 ed. Robbins p.783-84, 9 ed. p. 770, t-17-5)

Fundic gland polyps:

- Has an association with **familial adenomatous polyposis (FAP)** Q
- Risk factors include – **proton pump inhibitor** Q therapy
- Five times **more common in women** Q
- **Doesn't** increase the risk of **adenocarcinoma** Q

Ans. 45) D. Gastric adenomas (Ref: 8 ed. Robbins p.784, 9 ed. p. 770-71, t-17-5, f-17-16)

Gastric Adenomas Q:

- **Males** are affected **three times** more often than females
- **More common** in patients with **FAP** Q
- **Increased risk of adenocarcinoma** Q in **gastric adenoma** patients (in lesions greater than **2 cm** in **diameter**)
- **Most common** in **antrum** Q
- Characteristic feature includes **epithelial dysplasia** Q

Ans. 46) D. Cancer of gastric antrum is on rise (Ref: 8 ed. Robbins p.784-85, 9 ed. p. 771)

Epidemiology:

Gastric cancer incidence is reduced due to:

- Decreased consumption of **dietary carcinogens**, such as **N-nitroso compounds** and **benzopyrene**
- **Reduced use** of salt and smoking for food preservation due to widespread availability of **refrigeration**
- Intake of **green, leafy vegetables** and **citrus fruits** (containing **vitamin C, vitamin E and beta-carotene** Q)

Points to Remember:

- **Partial gastrectomies** done for **Peptic Ulcer Disease** patients have high risk of developing cancer in the **residual gastric stump** Q
- **Early gastric cancer** are tumors limited to the **mucosa and submucosa** Q
- Due to **increased incidence** of **Barrett esophagus**, cancer of the **gastric cardia** Q is on the rise and **not of antrum**

Ans. 47) A. CDH1 (Ref: 8 ed. Robbins p.785, 9 ed. p. 771)

Lauren classified gastric cancer into **Diffuse** Q and **Intestinal type** Q

Pathogenesis Q:

- **Diffuse gastric cancers** Q are more common in individuals with **germline mutations** in **CDH1** Q, which encodes **E-cadherin** Q and also with **BRCA-2 mutations**

- **Intestinal type gastric cancers** are **more common** in individuals with **Familial Adenomatosis Polyposis**Q and in which mutations in **β-catenin** as well as **microsatellite instability** are also seen

Ans. 48) C. Most commonly, it involves greater curvature (Ref: 8 ed. Robbins p.785-86, 9 ed. p. 772, f-17-17,18)

Morphology of Gastric Cancers Q

- Most common site involved is **gastric antrum** Q
- **Lesser curvature** Q is most commonly involved

Intestinal type Q

- Produces an **exophytic mass** or an **ulcerated tumor** composed of **glandular structures**

Diffuse type Q

- Produces an **infiltrative growth pattern**, composed of **signet-ring cells**
- **Linitis plastica** Q: **Desmoplastic reaction** imparts a **leather bottle appearance** to gastric mucosa

Ans. 49) B. Diffuse type cancer has reduced incidence (Ref: 8 ed. Robbins p.786, 9 ed. p. 772-73)

Salient Features of Gastric Cancer Q

- Incidence of **intestinal type** Q **gastric cancers** is reduced due to ***H. pylori* eradication** (due to reduced incidence of **atrophic gastritis** Q and **intestinal metaplasia**)
- **Precursor lesion** of **intestinal type gastric cancer** includes **flat dysplasia** and **adenomas** Q
- **Prognostic indicators** Q: **Depth of invasion** and **extent of nodal and distant metastasis**
- Can metastasize to the **supraclavicular sentinel lymph node (Virchow's node)** Q or to periumbilical region (**Sister Mary Joseph** Q nodule)

Ans. 50) D. All of the above (Ref: 9 ed. Robbins p.771)

Gastric Cancer Q **can metastasize to**:

- Supraclavicular sentinel lymph node (**Virchow node**)
- Periumbilical lymph nodes (**Sister Mary Joseph nodule**)
- Left axillary lymph node (**Irish node**)
- Ovary (**Krukenberg tumor**)
- Pouch of Douglas (**Blumer shelf**)

Ans. 51) C. GIT (Ref: 8 ed. Robbins p.786, 9 ed. p. 773)

Extra-nodal lymphomas:

- Most commonly seen is **GI tract**, particularly **stomach** Q
- **Risk factors** Q – Allogeneic bone marrow transplantation and organ transplant recipients
- In the gut, these are referred to as **lymphomas of mucosa-associated lymphoid tissue (MALT)**, or **MALTomas** Q
- **Second most common** primary lymphoma of gut is **Diffuse large B-cell lymphoma** Q

Ans. 52) D. Any of the above (Ref: 8 ed. Robbins p.786-87, 9 ed. p. 773, f-17-19)

Pathogenesis Q **of Extra-nodal marginal zone B-cell lymphomas** Q:

- Arises at the sites of **chronic inflammation**
- **Most common** cause of inflammation in stomach is **chronic *H. pylori*** Q **infection**
- Translocations associated with **gastric MALTomas** include **t(11;18), t(1;14)** and **t(14;18)** Q
- **FISH (fluorescent in situ hybridization)** Q: Used to identify tumors with translocations

Ans. 53) A. CD5 (Ref: 8 ed. Robbins p.787, 9 ed. p. 773)

MALTomas:

- Express **B-cell markers CD19 and CD20** Q, shows **CD43** Q positivity
- **Do not** express **CD5** and **CD10**, which are **T-cell markers**

Ans. 54) B. Most common site is tracheobronchial tree and lungs (Ref: 8 ed. Robbins p.787-88, 9 ed. p. 773-75, t-17-6)

Carcinoid Tumors Q

- **Well-differentiated neuroendocrine carcinomas** Q
- Most common site is **GI tract** Q and **> 40%** occur in the **small intestine** Q
- **Tracheobronchial tree** Q and **lungs** Q are the **second most common site**
- **Gastric carcinoids** may be associated with **endocrine cell hyperplasia, chronic atrophic gastritis** and **Zollinger-Ellison syndrome**
- **Carcinoids** within the GI tract arise from the **endocrine cells**

Ans. 55) B. Jejunum and ileum (Ref: 8 ed. Robbins p.787-88, 9 ed. p. 774, t-17-6)

In GIT:

- **Most common** site of **carcinoid** in **small intestine** is **jejunum and ileum** Q **(40%)**
- **Next common site** is **appendix and colorectum** Q
- **Stomach carcinoid tumors** are associated with **atrophic gastritis, MEN-1** Q
- **Proximal duodenal carcinoids** are associated with **Zollinger-Ellison syndrome**

Ans. 56) D. Any of the above (Ref: 8 ed. Robbins p.788, 9 ed. p. 774, t-17-6)

- In **jejunum and ileum**, carcinoid can occur **throughout the mucosa** Q
- In **appendix**, most common site is **tip** Q
- **Rectum** is more commonly involved than **cecum** Q in colon

Ans. 57) D. Occurs when tumors are confined to intestine (Ref: 8 ed. Robbins p.788-89, 9 ed. p. 773-75)

Carcinoid Syndrome Q

- **Ileal tumors** Q i.e. **mid-gut carcinoid** Q tumors may cause **carcinoid syndrome**
- Occurs due to **vasoactive substances** secreted by the tumor into the systemic circulation
- **Clinical features** Q – Cutaneous flushing, sweating, bronchospasm, colicky abdominal pain, diarrhea and right-sided cardiac valvular fibrosis
- In tumors confined to the intestine, **vasoactive substances** released are metabolized to inactive substances by **liver** Q
- Thus, this syndrome is **strongly associated with metastatic disease**

Ans. 58) B. Mid-gut carcinoid (Ref: 8 ed. Robbins p.789, 9 ed. p. 775)

- **Most important prognostic factor** for **GI carcinoid tumors** is its **location** Q
- **Mid-gut carcinoid tumors (jejunum and ileum)** are often **multiple** and tend to be **aggressive** Q

Ans. 59) A. Gastrointestinal Stromal Tumor (Ref: 8 ed. Robbins p.789-90, 9 ed. p. 775)

- **GI stromal tumor (GIST)** Q is the most common **mesenchymal tumor** of the abdomen
- Most common site is **stomach** Q followed by **small intestine, colorectum** and **esophagus**

Differential diagnosis of **mesenchymal tumors** Q includes:

- Leiomyoma, leiomyosarcoma, Schwannoma, glomus tumors, solitary fibrous tumor, fibromatosis, spindle cell carcinoma and mesothelioma

Ans. 60) C. Interstitial cells of Cajal (Ref: 8 ed. Robbins p.789-90, 9 ed. p. 775-76, f-17-21)

Pathogenesis of GIST:

- Arises from the **interstitial cells of Cajal** Q, located in the **muscularis propria** which serve as **pacemaker cells** for gut peristalsis
- **Gain-of-function mutation** of **the gene** encoding the tyrosine kinase ***c-KIT* (CD117)** Q are most commonly seen
- Mutations in **platelet-derived growth factor receptor α (PDGFRA)** can also be seen

Ans. 61) D. All of the above (Ref: 8 ed. Robbins p.789-90, 9 ed. p. 776-77, f-17-21)

Morphology of **GISTs** Q

- **Solitary, well-circumscribed, fleshy mass** Q
- Can be **submucosal** (60%), **sub-serosal** (30%) or **intramural** (10%)

Microscopy Q

- GISTs can be of **spindle cell type** (thin elongated cells) or **epithelioid type**
- **Most useful diagnostic marker** is **c-KIT** Q, detectable in 95% of **gastric GIST**
- **Multiple serosal nodules** Q are seen throughout the **peritoneal cavity** due to metastases

Ans. 62) B. Small intestinal GIST are less aggressive than gastric GIST (Ref: 8 ed. Robbins p.789-90, 9 ed. p. 775-77)

Prognosis in **GIST's** Q

- Correlates with **tumor size**, **mitotic index** and **location**
- **Tumor size** – GISTs under **5 cm** rarely metastasize, but **>10 cms** Q can metastasize
- **Mitotic index** – Mitosis **>5/50 hpf** and **size >10cms** can **metastasize**
- **Location** Q – **Gastric GISTs** behaves **less aggressively** than those arising in the **small intestine**

Ans. 63) D. Neurofibromatosis (Ref: 8 ed. Robbins p.789)

Carney triad Q:

- Seen primarily in **young females** Q and includes **gastric GIST**, **Paraganglioma** and **Pulmonary chondroma**

Points to remember:

- **Type 1 Neurofibromatosis** Q patients has increased incidence of gastric GIST's
- **Carney-Stratakis syndrome** Q – Germline **loss of SDH function** (SDH mutation), which confers an **increased risk** for **GIST** and **Paraganglioma**

Ans. 64) D. Sigmoid colon is most common site (Ref: 8 ed. Robbins p.790, 9 ed. p. 777)

- Most common site is **small intestine** Q because of its **narrow lumen**

Ans. 65) A. Sigmoid colon (Ref: 8 ed. Robbins p.791, 9 ed. p. 778, f-17-22)

- **Volvulus** is defined as **complete twisting of bowel loop** about its mesenteric base of attachment
- **Sites** – Most frequently involves **sigmoid colon** Q, followed by cecum, small bowel, stomach, or, rarely transverse colon

Ans. 66) C. Both A & B (Ref: 8 ed. Robbins p.792, 9 ed. p. 779)

- **Intestinal segments** at the end of their respective arterial supplies are susceptible to ischemia. They are called as **Watershed zones** Q and include:
  a) **Splenic flexure** – Superior and inferior mesenteric arterial circulations terminate
  b) **Recto-sigmoid** –Inferior mesenteric, pudendal and iliac arterial circulations terminate

Ans. 67) C. Ischemic bowel disease (Ref: 8 ed. Robbins p.792, 9 ed. p. 779)

Ischemic Bowel Disease:

- Intestinal capillaries supplies alongside the glands, from crypt to surface which allows **crypts** to be **well oxygenated** but leaves surface epithelium prone to ischemia
- **Grossly** Q – presents as **transmural infarction**
- **Morphology** Q – **surface epithelial atrophy** or **necrosis and sloughing**, with **normal** or **hyper proliferative crypts**

Ans. 68) Cecum (Ref: 8 ed. Robbins p.793, 9 ed. p. 780-81)

- Most common site of **Angiodysplasia** includes **right colon and cecum**
- Cause – Cecum has the largest diameter and develops the greatest wall tension, which might lead to **angiodysplasia**

Ans. 69) D. Maize (Ref: 8 ed. Robbins p.795, 9 ed. p. 782)

Celiac disease (celiac sprue or gluten-sensitive enteropathy):

- **Immune-mediated enteropathy** due to ingestion of gluten-containing cereals, **wheat**, **rye**, or **barley** Q

Ans. 70) A. HLA-DQ8 (Ref: 8 ed. Robbins p.795, 9 ed. p. 782-83, f-17-25,26)

- **HLA-DQ2** Q or **HLA-DQ8** Q **allele** are seen in patients with **celiac disease**

Morphology Q

- **Biopsy sites –duodenum** (second portion) or **proximal jejunum** (as they are exposed to the highest concentrations of dietary **gluten**) Q
- **Histopathology** – Increased number of **intraepithelial lymphocytes, crypt hyperplasia and villous atrophy** Q

Ans. 71) B. In infants the symptoms develop soon after birth (Ref: 8 ed. Robbins p.795, 9 ed. p.783)

Celiac Disease:

- **In children,** it begins between **6 and 24 months** of age, after introduction of **gluten** to the diet
- **Extra-intestinal complaints** include arthritis, seizure disorders, aphthous stomatitis, iron deficiency anemia, pubertal delay and short stature
- **Dermatitis herpetiformis** Q is seen in **10%** of patients

Noninvasive serologic tests Q:

- **Sensitive test – IgG/IgA antibodies** to **tissue transglutaminase** or **deamidated gliadin** Q
- **Specific test** include – **Anti-endomysial antibodies** Q

Note:

- Cancers associated – **Enteropathy – associated T-cell lymphoma** Q followed by **small intestinal adenocarcinoma**

Ans. 72) C. Due to mutation in MTP (Ref: 8 ed. Robbins p.796-97, 9 ed. p. 784)

Abetalipoproteinemia Q:

- **Autosomal recessive** disease, caused by mutation in **microsomal triglyceride transfer protein (MTP)** Q
- Characterized by an inability to secrete triglyceride rich lipoproteins

Autoimmune enteropathy Q:

- **X-linked disorder** characterized by severe persistent diarrhea, which occurs most often in **young children**
- ***IPEX*** (immune dysregulation, polyendocrinopathy, enteropathy and X-linkage) – severe familial form, occurs due to germline mutation in the **FOXP3 gene** Q

Ans. 73) D. All of the above (Ref: 8 ed. Robbins p.799-800, 9 ed. p. 786-87, f-17-28)

Campylobacter jejuni Q:

- Cause of **traveler's diarrhea**
- Infection can lead to **reactive arthritis**, in patients with **HLA-B27**
- **Extra-intestinal complications: Erythema nodosum** and **Guillain-Barre syndrome** Q

Morphology Q:

- **Comma-shaped, flagellated, Gram-negative** Q organisms
- **Cryptitis** Q (neutrophil infiltration of the crypts) and **crypt abscesses** Q (crypts with accumulations of luminal neutrophils) are commonly seen

Ans. 74) C. Shigella (Ref: 8 ed. Robbins p.800-01, 9 ed. p. 787-88)

Complications of **Shigella infection** Q includes:

a) **Reiter syndrome**: Triad of **sterile arthritis** Q, **urethritis** Q and **conjunctivitis** Q, affecting **HLA-B27-positive** men

b) **Hemolytic-uremic syndrome** Q: Associated with ***Enterohemorrhagic E. coli*** **(EHEC)** Q

Ans. 75) D. Non caseating granulomas (Ref: 8 ed. Robbins p.801-02, 9 ed. p. 788-89)

- *Salmonella typhi* is responsible agent for **typhoid fever** in endemic countries
- *Salmonella paratypi* infection is more common in **travelers** Q

Morphology Q:

- Enlarged **Peyer's patches** in the terminal ileum
- Can lead to **oval ulcers, along the axis of the ileum** Q, which may **perforate**
- In liver, **hepatocytes** are replaced by **macrophage aggregates**, called as **typhoid nodules** Q

Ans. 76) D. Yersinia (Ref: 8 ed. Robbins p.802, 9 ed. p. 789-90)

- **Yersinia infection** Q is a differential diagnosis for **Crohn disease**

Ans. 77) A. Enterotoxigenic E. Coli (Ref: 8 ed. Robbins p.802, 9 ed. p. 790)

- **Enterotoxigenic E. Coli (ETEC)** Q organisms: Major cause of **traveler's diarrhea** Q
- **Enterohemorrhagic E. Coli (EHEC) – E. coli O157:H7** and **non-O157:H7** serotypes: Produces **Shiga-like toxins**
- **Enteroaggregative E. Coli** can also be a cause of **traveler's diarrhea**

Ans. 78) D. All of the above (Ref: 8 ed. Robbins p.803, 9 ed. p. 791, f-17-29)

Pseudomembranous Colitis:

- Also known as **antibiotic-associated colitis** or antibiotic-associated diarrhea
- Caused by ***Clostridium difficile*** Q
- **Third-generation cephalosporins** Q are **most commonly** implicated
- ***C. difficile*–associated colitis** leads to formation of **pseudo-membranes** Q
- Most commonly seen in hospitalized patients
- **Metronidazole** or **vancomycin** are generally effective therapies

Ans. 79) D. Cannot differentiate histologically from tuberculosis (Ref: 8 ed. Robbins p.803-04, 9 ed. p. 791-92, f-17-30)

- **Acid fast bacilli stain (AFB stain)** Q helps to differentiate between **mycobacteria** and **T. whippelli.** The former is **AFB positive**, while later is not
- Thus we can differentiate between the two histologically using **special stains**

Morphology of **Whipple disease** Q:

- Caused by **Gram-positive actinomycete** i.e. **Tropheryma whippelii** Q
- Hallmark is dense accumulation of **distended, foamy macrophages** Q in the small intestine, which are **PAS positive**Q and **diastase resistant**
- A similar infiltrate of **foamy macrophages** is also seen in **intestinal tuberculosis** (which also shows **PAS-positivity**)
- **Acid-fast stain** Q can be used to distinguish between them, since **mycobacteria stain positively** while *T. whippelii* do not

Ans. 80) A. Cecum (Ref: 8 ed. Robbins p.806, 9 ed. p. 795, f-17-31)

- **Amebiasis** is most commonly seen in **cecum** Q and **ascending colon** Q, although sigmoid colon, rectum and appendix can also be involved

Ans. 81) D. All of the above (Ref: 8 ed. Robbins p.806, 9 ed. p. 795, f-17-31)

- **Entamoeba histolytica** Q is the causative agent for **Amebiasis**
- Has a characteristic **flask-shaped ulcer** Q with narrow neck and broad base
- Parasites may penetrate **splanchnic vessels** and embolize to liver producing **Amebic liver abscesses** Q
- **Metronidazole** is the most effective treatment

Ans. 82) D. IL-23 (Ref: 8 ed. Robbins p.808-09, 9 ed. p. 797)

Increased susceptibility of **Crohn disease** Q occurs due to **following mutations:**

- **NOD2** (nucleotide oligomerization binding domain 2) polymorphisms
- **ATG16L1** (autophagy-related 16-like)
- **IRGM** (immunity-related GTPase M)

Note:

- Polymorphisms in **ECM1 (extracellular matrix protein 1)** [Q], which inhibits **matrix metalloproteinase 9** [Q], are associated with **ulcerative colitis**
- Polymorphisms of **IL-23 receptor** [Q] are **protective** in both **Crohn disease and ulcerative colitis** [Q]

Ans. 83) A. Crohn disease (Ref: 8 ed. Robbins p.808-09, 9 ed. p. 798-800, f-17-32-35)

Differentiating features macroscopically, microscopically and clinically

Feature	Crohn Disease	Ulcerative Colitis
Bowel region	Ileum ± colon	Colon only
Distribution	Skip lesions	Diffuse
Stricture	Present	Absent
Wall appearance	Thick	Thin
Inflammation	Transmural	Limited to mucosa
Pseudo polyps	Moderate	Marked
Ulcers	Deep, knife-like	Superficial, broad-based
Lymphoid reaction	Marked	Moderate
Fibrosis	Marked	Mild to none
Serositis	Marked	Mild to none
Granuloma	Present	Absent
Fistulae/sinuses	Present	Absent
Perianal fistula	Yes (in colonic disease)	No
Fat/vitamin malabsorption	Seen	Not seen
Malignant potential	With colonic involvement	Yes
Toxic megacolon	Not seen	Seen
Recurrence after surgery	Common	No

Ans. 84) D. Rectum (Ref: 8 ed. Robbins p.810-11, 9 ed. p. 799, f-17-34)

- In **Crohn disease** [Q], the most common sites involved are the **terminal ileum**, **ileocecal valve** and **cecum** [Q]

Ans. 85) A. Aphthous ulcer (Ref: 8 ed. Robbins p.810-11, 9 ed. p. 799, f-17-34-35)

Morphology of Crohn Disease [Q]**:**

- Earliest lesion is an **aphthous ulcer** [Q]
- Present as **elongated, serpentine ulcers** oriented along the axis of the bowel
- **Cobblestone appearance** [Q] is seen as the diseased tissue is depressed below the level of normal mucosa
- **Fissures** [Q] can develop between mucosal folds, which may extend deeply to become **fistula tracts**
- **Features of chronicity** – Thickened intestinal wall, **submucosal fibrosis**, **stricture** [Q] formation, **Paneth cell metaplasia** (in left colon) and mucosal atrophy
- **Creeping fat** [Q] – Due to **extensive transmural disease**, mesenteric fat extends around the serosal surface
- **Non caseating granuloma** [Q] – Hallmark of Crohn disease
- **Metastatic Crohn disease** – Cutaneous granulomas forming nodules

Ans. 86) D. All of the above (Ref: 8 ed. Robbins p.810-11, 9 ed. p. 800)

Extra-intestinal manifestations [Q] of **Crohn disease** includes:

- Uveitis, migratory polyarthritis, sacroiliitis, ankylosing spondylitis, erythema nodosum, clubbing of the fingertips

- Pericholangitis and primary sclerosing cholangitis can occur in Crohn disease, though are more common in ulcerative colitis

Ans. 87) B. Transmural (Ref: 8 ed. Robbins p.811-12, 9 ed. p. 800, f-17-36,37)

- **Transmural involvement** Q is a feature of Crohn disease

Morphology of Ulcerative Colitis Q

Gross Q:

- Always involves the **rectum** Q and extends proximally in a **continuous fashion**
- **Pan-colitis** Q – entire colon is involved
- **Backwash ileitis** Q – mucosal inflammation of the distal ileum
- **Abrupt transition** between diseased and uninvolved colon
- **Pseudo-polyps** Q occurs due to islands of **regenerating mucosa**, which bulge into the lumen
- **Chronic disease** – mucosal atrophy, toxic megacolon

Microscopic Features: Q

- Inflammatory infiltrates, crypt abscesses, crypt distortion and pseudopyloric epithelial metaplasia
- **Inflammatory process** is limited to the **mucosa** and **superficial submucosa**

Ans. 88) B. Anti- Saccharomyces cerevisiae antibody (Ref: 8 ed. Robbins p.813, 9 ed. p. 801)

Serological studies used to differentiate between **Ulcerative Colitis** and **Crohn disease**:

- **Perinuclear anti-neutrophil cytoplasmic antibodies** Q are positive in **75% of individuals** with **ulcerative colitis** and only 11% with **Crohn disease**
- **Anti-Saccharomyces cerevisiae** Q antibodies are often present in **Crohn disease**

Ans. 89) C. Dense sub-epithelial collagen layer (Ref: 8 ed. Robbins p.814, 9 ed. p. 802, f-17-39)

Microscopic colitis Q is of two types:

Collagenous colitis Q:

- Occurs primarily in middle-aged and older women
- Characterized by the presence of a dense **sub-epithelial collagen layer**
- Increased number of **intraepithelial lymphocytes**, mixed inflammatory infiltrate within **the lamina propria**

Lymphocytic colitis Q:

- **Sub-epithelial collagen layer** is of **normal thickness**
- **Intraepithelial lymphocytes** exceed **one T-lymphocyte per five colonocytes**
- Strong association with **celiac disease** and **autoimmune diseases**, including thyroiditis, arthritis and autoimmune or lymphocytic gastritis

Hence, **dense sub-epithelial collagen layer** is characteristic feature of **collagenous colitis** and not lymphocytic colitis

Ans. 90) A. Adenoma (Ref: 8 ed. Robbins p.815, 9 ed. p. 804)

- Most common **neoplastic polyp** is **adenoma** Q, which can progress to **cancer**
- **Non-neoplastic polyps** can be further classified as **inflammatory** Q, **hamartomatous** Q, or **hyperplastic** Q

Ans. 91) A. Inflammatory polyp (Ref: 8 ed. Robbins p.815-16, 9 ed. p. 804-05, f-17-42)

Solitary rectal ulcer syndrome Q:

- Example of a **purely inflammatory lesion**
- Presents as **rectal bleeding, mucus discharge** and **inflammatory lesion** of the **anterior rectal wall**

Ans. 92) D. Dysplasia is not seen (Ref: 8 ed. Robbins p.816-17, 9 ed. p. 805-06, f-17-43, t-17-10)

Juvenile Polyps Q:

- Example of **Hamartomatous polyp**

- Can be sporadic or syndromic
- Seen in children less than 5 years of age and are located in the **rectum** Q
- **Juvenile polyposis – Autosomal dominant** syndrome and patients have **3 to 100 hamartomatous polyps**
- **Extra-intestinal manifestation** includes **Pulmonary arteriovenous malformations** Q
- **SMAD4** Q is the **most common** identified **mutation** followed by BMPR1A
- **Dysplasia** can be seen in **juvenile polyps** Q
- **Juvenile polyposis syndrome** is associated with an increased risk of **colonic adenocarcinoma** Q

Ans. 93) D. Hamartomatous lesion leads to increased risk of carcinomas (Ref: 8 ed. Robbins p.817-18, 9 ed. p. 806-07, f-17-44, 17-10)

- **Hamartomas** Q are not **preneoplastic precursor lesions**

Peutz-Jeghers Syndrome Q

- **Autosomal dominant** syndrome
- Presents with **multiple GI hamartomatous polyps** and **mucocutaneous hyperpigmentation** Q
- Associated with **increased risk of cancers** Q of the colon, pancreas, breast, lung, ovaries, uterus, testicles and sex cord tumors
- Occurs due to **loss-of-function mutations** in the gene **LKB1/STK11** Q
- **Most common site** of **polyps – small intestine** Q, followed by stomach, colon, bladder and lungs

Ans. 94) B. Gastrointestinal cancer (Ref: 8 ed. Robbins p.818, 9 ed. p. 806, t-17-10)

Cowden Syndrome Q

- Associated with loss-of-function mutation in **PTEN** Q
- Characterized by macrocephaly, intestinal hamartomatous polyps and benign skin tumors i.e. **trichilemmomas, papillomatous papules** and **acral keratoses** Q
- **Does not** increase the risk of GI malignancy
- Increased predisposition to **breast carcinoma, follicular carcinoma of the thyroid** and **endometrial carcinoma** Q

Ans. 95) A. Sessile serrated adenoma (Ref: 8 ed. Robbins p.818-19, 9 ed. 808, f-17-45-46)

Hyperplastic Polyps Q:

- Occurs due to decreased **epithelial cell turnover** and **delayed shedding** of surface epithelial cells
- Results in **"piling up"** of **goblet cells** and absorptive cells
- **Lack malignant potential**
- Must be **distinguished** from **sessile serrated adenomas**, which have **malignant potential** Q

Ans. 96) B. Hamartomatous polyp (Ref: 8 ed. Robbins p.816, 9 ed. p. 806, t-17-10)

Tuberous Sclerosis:

- Associated with **Hamartomatous polyps** Q
- **TSC1 and TSC2 genes** Q are most commonly mutated
- **Extra-intestinal manifestations** include – facial angiofibroma, cortical tubers and **renal angiomyolipoma**

Ans. 97) D. All of the above (Ref: 8 ed. Robbins p.819, 9 ed. p. 807-08)

Neoplastic Polyps:

- Most common **neoplastic polyps** are **colonic adenomas** Q, precursors of colorectal adenocarcinomas
- Adenomas can be small, **pedunculated polyps** to large **sessile lesions**
- 3 types – tubular, tubulovillous or villous
- Colorectal adenomas are characterized by the presence of **epithelial dysplasia** Q

Ans. 98) C. Serrated surface confined to the surface (Ref: 8 ed. Robbins p.819-20, 9 ed. p. 808-09, f-17-45,46)

Sessile Serrated Adenomas Q

- Most commonly found in the **right colon**
- **Lack** Q typical cytologic features of **dysplasia**, found in other adenomas

Microscopy Q

- **Serrated architecture** throughout the full length of the glands, including the **crypt base**, associated with lateral growth and crypt dilation
- In **hyperplastic polyps**, serrated architecture is confined to the **mucosal surface**

Ans. 99) B. Invasion of lamina propria or muscularis propria is seen (Ref: 8 ed. Robbins p.820, 9 ed. p. 808-09, f-17-47)

Intramucosal Carcinoma Q

- Dysplastic epithelial cells breach the basement membrane to invade the **lamina propria** or **muscularis mucosa**
- Has little or no metastatic potential
- Treatment requires complete polypectomy

Note:

- **Invasive adenocarcinoma** shows invasion beyond the **muscularis mucosa** Q

Ans. 100) C. 100% patients have mutations in APC gene (Ref: 8 ed. Robbins p.820-21, 9 ed. p. 809-10, t-17-10, f-17-48)

Familial adenomatous polyposis (FAP) Q

- **Autosomal dominant** Q disorder in which patients develop numerous **colorectal adenomas**
- Caused by the mutations of **adenomatous polyposis coli or APC gene**
- At least **100 polyps** are necessary for diagnosis
- **Colorectal adenocarcinoma** Q develops in **100%** of untreated patients, before age of 30 years
- **Prophylactic colectomy** Q is treatment of choice for individuals carrying **APC mutations**
- **Extra-intestinal manifestations** Q include – **Congenital hypertrophy of the retinal pigment epithelium**
- **<10% of patients** show mutations of the **base-excision repair** gene ***MUTYH***

Ans. 101) D. CNS tumors (Ref: 8 ed. Robbins p.821, 9 ed. p. 809, t-17-11)

Patients with **FAP gene mutation** are at increased risk of developing –

a) **Gardner syndrome** Q – Intestinal polyps, **osteomas** of mandible, skull and long bones, **epidermal cysts, desmoid tumors**, thyroid tumors and dental abnormalities

b) **Turcot syndrome** Q is characterized by **intestinal adenomas** and **CNS tumors (Medulloblastoma and Glioblastoma)**

Ans. 102) C. Cancer arises in left colon (Ref: 8 ed. Robbins p.821-22, 9 ed. p. 810, t-17-11)

Hereditary non-polyposis colorectal cancer (HNPCC) / Lynch syndrome Q:

- **Autosomal Dominant** Q disorder, example of **microsatellite instability**
- Increased risk of cancers in **colorectum** Q, endometrium, stomach, ovary, ureters, brain, small bowel, hepatobiliary tract and skin
- **Colon cancers** occur at **younger age** and are located in the **right colon** Q
- Occurs due to **inherited mutations** in **mismatch repair genes – MSH2 and MLH1** Q

Ans. 103) D. Any of the above (Ref: 8 ed. Robbins p.822-23, 9 ed. p. 810-11)

Epidemiology of Carcinoma Colon:

- **Dietary factors** Q associated with increased risk of colorectal cancer – **low intake of vegetable fiber** and **high intake** of refined **carbohydrates and fat**
- **Deficiencies** of **vitamins A, C and E** Q

- **NSAIDs** [Q] have **protective effect** due to inhibition of **cyclooxygenase-2 (COX-2)**, which is expressed in **colorectal carcinomas** and **adenomas**

Ans. 104) E. All of the above (Ref: 8 ed. Robbins p.823-24, 9 ed. p. 811-12, f-17-49, 50, t-17-11)

Classic **adenoma-carcinoma sequence** [Q] includes the following mutation:

- **APC** gene mutation
- **KRAS** mutations
- **SMAD2** and **SMAD4** mutations
- **p53** is mutated in 70% to 80% of **colon cancers**
- Increased **telomerase** expression in advanced lesions

Ans. 105) C. K-RAS and p 53 mutation is commonly involved (Ref: 8 ed. Robbins p.824, 9 ed. p. 812, f-17-50)

- **DNA mismatch repair deficiency** [Q] occurs due to loss of mismatch repair genes **i.e. MLH-1, MSH2**
- **Microsatellite instability** [Q] – Mutations accumulate in microsatellite repeats
- These mutations are generally **silent** [Q] as **microsatellites** are seen in **noncoding regions**
- **TGF-β receptor mutation** and **loss of BAX**, leads to uncontrolled growth of cells
- But, **KRAS** and **p53** are **not mutated** in mismatch repair pathway of colon cancer

Ans. 106) A. Right colon (Ref: 8 ed. Robbins p.824, 9 ed. p. 812)

Microsatellite Instability [Q]:

- Can lead to development of cancers in **right colon** [Q]
- Shows prominent **mucinous differentiation** and **peri-tumoral lymphocytic infiltrates**

Ans. 107) A. Tumors of the right side causes napkin like constriction (Ref: 8 ed. Robbins p.824-25, 9 ed. p. 812-15, f-17-51,52)

Morphology:

- Tumors in the **proximal colon (cecum and ascending colon)** or right colon, grow as polypoid, exophytic masses and **rarely cause obstruction** [Q]
- Carcinomas in the **distal colon** or left side are annular lesions and produce **"napkin-ring" constrictions** and luminal narrowing can lead to **obstruction** [Q]

Ans. 108) C. Both of the above (Ref: 8 ed. Robbins p.825, 9 ed. p. 813-14)

Clinical Features of Colon Cancer

Right-sided colon cancers –

- Presents with fatigue and weakness due to **iron deficiency anemia** [Q]
- Iron deficiency anemia in an older man or postmenopausal woman occurs due to GIT cancer until proven otherwise

Left-sided colorectal adenocarcinomas [Q]:

- Presents with **occult bleeding, changes in bowel habits**, or cramping left lower quadrant discomfort

Note:

- Two most important **prognostic factors** are **depth of invasion** [Q] and the **presence or absence of lymph node metastases** [Q]

Ans. 109) A. Idiopathic (Ref: 8 ed. Robbins p.829, 9 ed. p. 817)

Ormond Disease [Q] (Sclerosing retro peritonitis or idiopathic retroperitoneal fibrosis):

- Characterized by **dense fibrosis** [Q] that can involve the mesentery
- **Unknown cause**, but is thought to be an inflammatory process

Ans. 110) D. All of the above (Ref: 8 ed. Robbins p.829, 9 ed. p. 817)

Tumors involving peritoneum:

- **Mesotheliomas** [Q] (Primary tumors arising from peritoneal lining)
- **Desmoplastic small round cell tumor (soft-tissue tumor** [Q] can develop rarely)
- **Metastasis** (common in peritoneal cavity)

Ans. 111) B. Adenomatous (Ref: Robbins 9 ed. 770-71) Refer Q 45 for details

Ans. 112) A. Sigmoid colon (Ref: Schwartz 9 ed. p. 1991)

- Sigmoid colon is the most common site for diverticulosis

Ans. 113) C. Chromosome 13 (Ref: Robbins 9 ed. p. 850)

Wilson Disease

- Autosomal Recessive disorder
- Due to mutation of the ATP7B gene
- ATP 7 B gene is located on chromosome 13

Ans. 114) D. Increased risk of adenocarcinoma of esophagus (9th ed. Robbins p. 329, 763)

H. Pylori infection leads to:

1) Duodenal ulcer
2) Gastric ulcer
3) Chronic superficial gastritis
4) Chronic atrophic gastritis
5) Gastric adenocarcinoma
6) Lymphoproliferative disease (MALT)
7) Gastro esophageal reflux disease

Ans. 115) B. MSH 2 (Ref: 9th ed. Robbins p. 810) Refer Q 105 for details

Ans. 116) B. High propensity of malignant change (Ref: 9 ed. Robbins p.775-77) Also, Refer Q 59-63

- Recurrence or metastasis is common for tumors which are mitotically active and are more than 10 cm

Ans. 117) B. Involves only colon (9 ed. Robbins p. 800) Refer Q 87 for details

Ans. 118) A. Lamina propria (Ref: 9 ed. Robbins p. 773) Refer Q 51-53 for details

- Histologically, gastric MALToma takes the form of a dense lymphocytic infiltrate in the lamina propria

Ans. 119) D. Ileocecal junction (Ref: 10 ed. Ackerman)

- Ileocecal region is the most common site of involvement
- Tuberculous ulcers are multiple and circumferential

Ans. 120) A. Gastrin secreting tumor (Ref: 9 ed. Robbins p. 769) Refer Q 42 for details

Ans. 121) C. Rectosigmoid

8 ed. Robbins: Adenocarcinoma of colon are distributed equally over the entire length of colon

7ed. Robbins: Recto sigmoid is the most common site for adenocarcinoma colon

Ans. 122) D. GIST (Ref: 9 ed. Robbins p. 763) Refer Q 27-33 for details

Ans. 123) C. Ileo-jejunum (Ref: 9 ed. Robbins p. 773-775) Refer Q 55 for details

Ans. 124) A. Gastric carcinoma (Ref: 9 ed. Robbins p. 771) Refer Q 46 for details

Ans. 125) B. HLA-DQ2 (Ref: 9 ed. Robbins p. 782-83) Refer Q 70 for details

Ans. 126) B. Crohn disease (Ref: 9 ed. Robbins p. 978-800) Refer Q83 for details

Ans. 127) D. Stomach (Ref: 9 ed. Robbins p. 775) Refer Q 59 for details

Ans. 128) D. Non-caseating granuloma (Ref: 9 ed. Robbins p. 978-800) Refer Q 83, 84 and 85 for details

Ans. 129) B. Autosomal dominant (Ref: 9 ed Robbins p. 809) Refer Q 101 for details

- Gardner syndrome is inherited as Autosomal dominant disorder

Ans. 130) A. Chronic non-specific ulcerative colitis (Ref: 9 ed. Robbins p. 800) Refer Q 87 for details

Ans. 131) D. Gardener syndrome (Ref: 9 ed Robbins p. 809) Refer Q 101 for details

Ans. 132) A. Sigmoid colon

Ans. 133) A. Absence of nerves (Ref: 9 ed. Robbins p. 753-54)

- Primary achalasia – due to distal esophageal inhibitory neuronal (ganglion cell) degeneration
- Secondary achalasia – seen in Chagas disease, in which Trypanosoma cruzi infection causes destruction of the myenteric plexus

Ans. 134) A. CD 117 (Ref: 9 ed. Robbins p. 775-76) Refer Q 60 for details

Ans. 135) B. Associated with achlorhydria/hypochlorhydria (Ref: 9 ed. Robbins p. 771) Refer Q 46 for details

Ans. 136) A. Transient decrease in pressure at LES (Ref: 9 ed. Robbins p. 755)

- Most common cause of gastro-esophageal reflux is transient lower esophageal sphincter relaxation

Ans. 137) A. Intestinal metaplasia Refer to answer 11 for details

Ans. 138) B. Stomach (Ref: 9 ed. Robbins p. 771) Refer Q 46 for details

Ans. 139) D. ALK mutation is seen in most cases (Ref: 9 ed. Robbins p. 775-76) Refer Q 60-62

Ans. 140) A. Hamartomatous polyp (Ref: 9 ed. Robbins p. 805) Refer Q 92 for details

Ans. 141) D. Barrett's esophagus, mucin stain, dysplasia (Ref: 9 ed. Robbins p. 757-58) Refer Q 11, 12, 14, 16, 46 for details

16 Liver and Biliary Tract

How to go about this chapter?

- **One should be thorough with the following topics:**
  - **Liver failure, Hepatic encephalopathy, Cirrhosis**
  - **Laboratory evaluation of liver diseases**
  - **Portal hypertension**
  - **Jaundice**
  - **Cholestasis**
  - **Hepatitis A, B, C, D, E, G**
  - **Chronic hepatitis, Autoimmune hepatitis**
  - **Drug- and Toxin-Induced Hepatic Injury, Steatosis**
  - **Alcoholic Liver Disease, Non-Alcoholic Fatty Liver Disease**
  - **Hemochromatosis, Primary Biliary Cirrhosis, Primary Sclerosing Cholangitis**
  - **Acute fatty liver of pregnancy**
  - **Focal nodular hyperplasia, Hepatocellular adenomas, Hepatoblastoma**
  - **Hepatocellular carcinoma, Klatskin tumors**

GENERAL FEATURES OF LIVER DISEASE

1) All are TRUE about microscopic anatomy of liver EXCEPT:

a) Divided into concepts of hepatic lobule and hepatic acinus
b) Histopathology of liver is discussed on basis of lobular architecture
c) Space of Disse represent mononuclear phagocyte system
d) Canals of Hering connect bile canaliculi to bile ductules in periportal region

2) Acute liver failure occurs when encephalopathy develops within ..... weeks of initial liver injury.

a) 6 weeks b) 16 weeks
c) 26 weeks d) 36 weeks

3) Morphological changes seen in brain in hepatic encephalopathy include(s):

a) Gliosis
b) Astrocyte swelling
c) Both of the above
d) None of the above

4) Cirrhosis is defined by the following morphological feature(s):

a) Fibrosis
b) Parenchymal nodules
c) Disruption of liver architecture
d) All of the above

5) In cirrhosis, following collagen types is/are deposited in space of Disse:

a) Type I b) Type III
c) Both of above d) Type IV

6) Fibrosis occurs due to proliferation of:

a) Hepatic stellate cells
b) Portal fibroblasts
c) Fibrocytes
d) Endothelial cells

7) In cirrhosis, contraction of myofibroblasts is brought about by:

a) ET-1
b) PDGF
c) TGF
d) MMP-2

8) All of the following tests indicate damage to bile canaliculcus EXCEPT:

a) Serum alkaline phosphatase
b) Serum γ-glutamyl transpeptidase
c) Serum 5' -nucleotidase
d) Serum bilirubin

9) **All are the post hepatic causes of portal hypertension EXCEPT:**
a) Right heart failure
b) Obstructive thrombosis
c) Constructive pericarditis
d) Hepatic vein outflow obstruction

10) **Clinical consequences of Portal hypertension include(s):**
a) Ascites
b) Congestive splenomegaly
c) Hepatic encephalopathy
d) All of the above

11) **Ascites is defined when at least...... ml of fluid is deposited in peritoneal cavity.**
a) 100 ml b) 500 ml
c) 1 liter d) 1.5 liter

12) **Sites of porto-systemic shunts include(s):**
a) Rectum
b) Esophagogastric junction
c) Retro peritoneum
d) All of the above

13) **Mutation of the following leads to hereditary unconjugated hyperbilirubinemias:**
a) UGT1A1 b) UGT1A2
c) UGT1A3 d) Any of the above

14) **TRUE about unconjugated bilirubin in the pathophysiology of jaundice includes all EXCEPT:**
a) Unconjugated bilirubin is insoluble in water
b) Unconjugated bilirubin is found attached to serum albumin
c) Unconjugated bilirubin can be excreted in urine
d) Unconjugated bilirubin may diffuse into brain of newborn

15) **All are the causes of unconjugated bilirubinemias EXCEPT:**
a) Gilbert syndrome
b) Crigler-Najjar syndrome
c) Hemolytic anemia
d) Rotor syndrome

16) **Jaundice becomes evident when serum bilirubin levels rise above:**
a) 0.2-1.2 mg/dl b) 1-2-2 mg/dl
c) 2-2.5 mg/dl d) Any of the above

17) **All are TRUE about Dubin-Johnson syndrome EXCEPT:**
a) Autosomal Recessive disorder
b) Cause of conjugated hyperbilirubinemias
c) Due to absence of MDRP-2
d) Hepatocytes are swollen and shows inflammation

18) **In Crigler-Najjar syndrome following drug can improve bilirubin glucuronidation:**
a) Phenobarbital b) Acetaminophen
c) Propranolol d) All of the above

19) **TRUE about cholestasis is/are:**
a) Can be extra or intra hepatic
b) Accumulation of bile pigment in hepatic parenchyma
c) Hepatocytes may show feathery degeneration
d) All of the above

20) **Progressive familial intrahepatic cholestasis (PFIC) showing increased levels of GGT:**
a) PFIC-1 b) PFIC-2
c) PFIC-3 d) PFIC-4

INFECTIOUS DISORDERS

21) **Which of the following viruses has longest incubation period?**
a) Hepatitis A b) Hepatitis B
c) Hepatitis C d) Hepatitis E

22) **Which of the following virus is a double stranded DNA virus?**
a) Hepatitis A b) Hepatitis B
c) Hepatitis C d) Hepatitis D

23) **All are TRUE about Hepatitis A virus infection EXCEPT:**
a) Incubation period of 3-6 weeks
b) After one week of onset of jaundice, virus is shed in feces
c) Virus can be detected in serum and saliva
d) IgG antibody against HAV appears in the blood after onset of symptoms

24) **Healthy carrier state in Hepatitis B virus infection is defined by:**
a) Positive HBsAg >6 months
b) HBeAg negative
c) Serum HBV DNA <10^5 copies/mL
d) All of the above

25) **Which of the following is implicated in pathogenesis of liver cancer in HBV infection?**
a) HBsAg b) HBcAg
c) HBeAg d) HBx

26) **Which of the following serum marker indicates infectivity?**
a) HBsAg b) HBeAg
c) Anti-HBc d) None of the above

27) **Which of the following is the basis of current vaccination strategies for Hepatitis B infection?**
a) HBsAg b) Anti-HBs
c) Anti-HBe d) Anti-HBc

28) **Risk for acquiring the Hepatitis C virus infection by needle stick injury is:**
a) 0.1% b) 0.3%
c) 1.8% d) 2.5%

29) All are TRUE about the Hepatitis C virus infection EXCEPT:
a) Incubation period between 2-26 weeks
b) Episodic elevations of serum aminotransferases
c) HCV RNA is detectable in blood for 1 – 3 weeks
d) Elevated levels of anti-HCV IgG after acute infection confer immunity

30) Most common cause of acute hepatitis in India is:
a) Hepatitis A virus b) Hepatitis B virus
c) Hepatitis C virus d) Hepatitis E virus

31) Which of the following virus replicates in bone marrow?
a) Hepatitis C b) Hepatitis D
c) Hepatitis E d) Hepatitis G

32) Cryoglobulinemia is associated with following:
a) Hepatitis B b) Hepatitis C
c) Hepatitis D d) Hepatitis E

33) Ground glass hepatocytes is characteristic feature of:
a) Hepatitis A b) Hepatitis B
c) Hepatitis C d) Hepatitis D

34) Macrovesicular steatosis is a feature of:
a) Hepatitis A b) Hepatitis B
c) Hepatitis C d) None of the above

35) Morphological features of Acute hepatitis include(s):
a) Ballooning degeneration
b) Cholestasis
c) Bridging necrosis
d) All of the above

36) Causes of cirrhosis include(s):
a) Viral hepatitis
b) Autoimmune hepatitis
c) Cryptogenic
d) All of the above

37) TRUE about echinococcal liver abscess:
a) Cystic structure
b) Wall is laminated
c) Hooklets and intact organisms can be identified
d) All of the above

38) All are seen in Type 1 autoimmune hepatitis EXCEPT:
a) Antinuclear antibody
b) Anti-smooth muscle antibody
c) Anti-actin antibody
d) Anti-liver kidney microsome-1 antibody

39) Characteristic cell/s seen in autoimmune hepatitis:
a) Neutrophils
b) Lymphocytes
c) Lymphocytes and plasma cells
d) Eosinophils

40) Clinical features of Autoimmune hepatitis includes all EXCEPT:
a) Elevated serological markers of viral infection
b) Elevated serum IgG
c) Elevated γ-globulin levels
d) High titers of antibodies

41) Oral contraceptive pill causes the following patterns of hepatic injury EXCEPT:
a) Hepatic adenoma
b) Cholestatic injury
c) Budd-Chiari syndrome
d) Peliosis hepatitis

42) Reye's syndrome is characterized by:
a) Microvesicular steatosis
b) Macrovesicular steatosis
c) Both of the above
d) None of the above

ALCOHOLIC LIVER DISEASE

43) Alcoholic hepatitis is characterized by:
a) Hepatocyte swelling
b) Mallory-Denk bodies
c) Neutrophilic reaction
d) All of the above

44) Mallory-Denk bodies represent:
a) RNA
b) DNA
c) Glycogen
d) Intermediate filaments

45) Alcoholic hepatitis is characterized by all EXCEPT:
a) Hyperbilirubinemia
b) Elevated serum aminotransferases
c) Elevated alkaline phosphatase
d) ALT : AST > 2:1

METABOLIC LIVER DISEASE

46) All are TRUE about Non-Alcoholic fatty liver disease EXCEPT:
a) Can progress to cirrhosis
b) Associated with obesity
c) Most common cause of cryptogenic cirrhosis
d) Doesn't progress to hepatocellular carcinoma

47) All are TRUE about Non-Alcoholic Steatohepatitis EXCEPT:
a) Liver biopsy is the most reliable diagnostic tool
b) Serum AST and ALT are elevated
c) AST/ALT ratio > 2-2.5
d) Cardiovascular disease is a frequent cause of death

48) Morphology of Non-Alcoholic Fatty liver disease include(s):
a) Steatosis b) Steatohepatitis
c) Cirrhosis d) All of the above

49) All are TRUE about hemochromatosis EXCEPT:
a) Autosomal Recessive
b) Disease manifests when > 20 gm. of iron is deposited in liver
c) Hepcidin plays a role in iron absorption
d) Transcription of Hepcidin is increased by iron deficiency

50) Cause(s) for hereditary hemochromatosis include(s) mutation in:
a) Hemojuvelin
b) Transferrin receptor-2
c) HFE
d) All of the above

51) TRUE about morphology of hereditary hemochromatosis includes all EXCEPT:
a) Most common organ involved is liver
b) Can progress to cirrhosis
c) Pancreatic fibrosis is frequently seen
d) Marked inflammation is seen

52) Extra-hepatic hemosiderin deposition can be detected by:
a) Buccal biopsy
b) GI biopsy
c) Both of the above
d) None of the above

53) All are TRUE about biochemical tests for Wilson disease EXCEPT:
a) Increase in hepatic copper levels
b) Decrease in serum ceruloplasmin
c) Increased urinary excretion of copper
d) Increased serum copper levels

54) α_1AT gene is located on following chromosome:
a) Chromosome 6
b) Chromosome 10
c) Chromosome 12
d) Chromosome 14

CHOLESTATIC DISEASES

55) Causes of neonatal cholestasis include/s:
a) Biliary atresia
b) Infection
c) Drugs
d) All of the above

56) Causes of "perinatal" biliary atresia include all EXCEPT:
a) Viral infection
b) Autoimmune reactions
c) Aberrant intrauterine development of extra-hepatic biliary tree
d) Genetic causes

57) TRUE about primary biliary cirrhosis includes all EXCEPT:
a) Has female predominance
b) Presents with pruritus
c) Antimitochondrial antibodies are seen in 90% of patients
d) No risk of hepatocellular carcinoma

58) All are TRUE about primary sclerosing cholangitis EXCEPT:
a) M:F=2:1
b) Inflammation and obliterative fibrosis of bile ducts
c) P-ANCA directed against myeloperoxidase is seen
d) Elevation of serum Alkaline phosphatase

59) Bile duct hamartoma is another name of the following disorder:
a) Von Meyenburg complex
b) Polycystic liver disease
c) Caroli disease
d) Hepatic fibrosis

60) Which of the following anomalies of biliary tract are associated with polycystic kidney disease?
a) Polycystic liver disease
b) Bile duct hamartoma
c) Caroli disease
d) All of the above

61) Jagged-1 mutation is associated with:
a) Congenital hepatic fibrosis
b) Caroli disease
c) Allagile syndrome
d) Von Meyenburg complex

CIRCULATORY DISORDERS

62) Nutmeg liver represent areas of:
a) Hypoperfusion in liver
b) Congestion of liver
c) Both of the above
d) None of the above

63) Causes of hepatic vein thrombosis include(s):
a) Polycythemia Vera
b) Antithrombin deficiency
c) Antiphospholipid antibody syndrome
d) All of the above

HEPATIC DISEASE ASSOCIATED WITH PREGNANCY

64) Fatal outcome of which hepatitis can occur in pregnancy?
a) Hepatitis B
b) Hepatitis C
c) Hepatitis E
d) None of the above

65) TRUE about Acute fatty liver of pregnancy:
a) Presents in second trimester
b) Macrovesicular steatosis

c) Morphologically, distinction from viral hepatitis is difficult
d) Conservative management

66) All are TRUE about intrahepatic cholestasis of pregnancy EXCEPT:
a) Presents with pruritus in third trimester
b) Serum bilirubin >10 mg%
c) ALP is elevated
d) Biopsy shows mild cholestasis without necrosis

NODULES AND TUMORS

67) Focal nodular hyperplasia is associated with use of:
a) OCP
b) Anabolic steroids
c) Both of the above
d) None of the above

68) Nodular regenerative hyperplasia can be seen in:
a) Renal transplantation
b) Vasculitis
c) HIV infection
d) All of the above

69) Most common benign neoplasm affecting liver:
a) Cavernous hemangioma
b) Hepatic adenoma
c) Hepatoblastoma
d) None of the above

70) Which subtypes of hepatic adenoma has highest malignant potential?
a) HNF1-α Inactivated hepatocellular adenomas
b) β-Catenin Activated Hepatocellular adenomas
c) Inflammatory hepatocellular adenomas
d) All of the above

71) Angiosarcoma of liver is associated with:
a) Vinyl chloride b) Arsenic
c) Thorotrast d) All of the above

72) TRUE about Hepatoblastoma:
a) Most common liver tumor of young childhood
b) Activation of WNT pathway
c) Associated with FAP
d) All of the above

73) Disease(s) which can give rise to hepatocellular carcinoma:
a) Hereditary hemochromatosis
b) Alpha -1 Anti-trypsin deficiency
c) NAFLD
d) All of the above

74) Following mutation(s) are associated with Hepatocellular carcinoma:
a) Activation of β-catenin
b) Inactivation of p53
c) IL-6/JAK/STAT pathway
d) All of the above

75) Which of the following is/are premalignant lesions of hepatocellular carcinoma?
a) Large cell change
b) Small cell change
c) Dysplastic nodules
d) Any of the above

76) All are TRUE about Fibro lamellar carcinoma EXCEPT:
a) Occurs in young adults
b) Prognosis is good
c) Occurs in patients with chronic liver disorders
d) Presents as scirrhous tumor

77) Serum alpha-fetoprotein is elevated in:
a) Hepatocellular carcinoma
b) Yolk sac tumor
c) Cirrhosis
d) All of the above

78) Which drug(s) can prolong the life of individuals with advanced hepatocellular carcinoma?
a) Sorafenib
b) Imatinib
c) Cyclophosphamide
d) All of the above

79) Risk factors for cholangiocarcinoma include(s):
a) Opisthorchis sinensis
b) Primary sclerosing cholangitis
c) Hepatitis C
d) All of the above

80) Klatskin tumors arise from:
a) Junction of right and left hepatic ducts
b) Junction of the common bile duct and cystic duct
c) Junction of common hepatic duct and cystic duct
d) Junction of common bile duct and common hepatic duct

81) Perineural invasion is seen in:
a) Hepatocellular carcinoma
b) Cholangiocarcinoma
c) Intraductal papillary biliary neoplasm
d) Mucinous cystic neoplasm

82) Most common primary lymphoma affecting liver is:
a) Diffuse large B-cell lymphoma
b) MALT lymphoma
c) Hepatosplenic delta gamma lymphoma
d) Mantle cell lymphoma

GALLBLADDER

83) All are predisposing conditions for formation of pigmented gall stones EXCEPT:
a) Chronic hemolytic anemia
b) Ileal dysfunction
c) Bacterial contamination of biliary tree
d) Hypomotility of gall bladder

84) Venous congestion of liver affects: (NEET 2014)
a) Midzone
b) Perihepatic zone
c) Centrilobular zone
d) All of the above

85) In hemochromatosis iron is not deposited in: (NEET 2014)
a) Heart b) Pituitary
c) Testis d) Skin

86) Which cells of the mononuclear phagocyte system are present in liver? (NEET 2014)
a) Kupffer cells b) Merkel cells
c) Gittle cells d) Berger cells

87) Patient with cirrhosis is positive for HBs Ag and has increased levels of alpha fetoprotein. What is the most probable diagnosis? (NEET 2014)
a) Sub-massive hepatic necrosis
b) Hepatocellular carcinoma
c) Massive hepatic necrosis
d) None of the above

88) PAS positive diastase resistant intrahepatic granules are seen in: (NEET 2014)
a) Alpha 1 antitrypsin deficiency
b) Dystrophic calcification
c) Metastatic calcification
d) Glucocerebrosidase

89) Marker of level of liver injury in cases of hepatitis B: (NEET 2014)
a) HBsAg b) HBVDNA
c) Anti HBeAg d) Anti HBc

90) What accumulates in tissues in hemochromatosis? (NEET 2014)
a) Iron b) Copper
c) Ceruloplasmin d) Lipofuscin

91) Following is/are the risk factors for cholangiocarcinoma: (NEET 2014)
a) Primary sclerosing cholangitis
b) Clonorchis sinensis infection
c) Both a and b
d) None of the above

92) Under Blood safety programme compulsory tests done are all EXCEPT: (NEET 2014)
a) HIV b) VDRL
c) Malaria d) Hepatitis E

93) Mallory hyaline body is made of: (NEET 2014, 2013)
a) Keratin b) Myosin
c) Reticulin d) Fibrin

94) Which of the following is premalignant to cholangiocarcinoma? (NEET 2014)
a) Biliary intraepithelial neoplasia
b) Mucinous cystic neoplasms
c) Intraductal papillary biliary neoplasia
d) All of the above

95) Centrilobular necrosis is seen in following EXCEPT: (NEET 2014)
a) Cardiac failure
b) CCl4 toxicity
c) Chloroform toxicity
d) Alcoholic hepatitis

96) Copper is mainly transported by: (NEET 2013)
a) Ceruloplasmin b) Albumin
c) Haptoglobin d) Globulin

97) Gene of Wilson's disease is: (NEET 2013)
a) ATP 7A b) ATP7B
c) ADP7A d) ADP7B

98) Pathological manifestation of chronic alcoholism include all of the following EXCEPT: (NEET 2013)
a) Piecemeal necrosis
b) Ballonning degeneration
c) Microvesicular fatty changes
d) Central hyaline sclerosis

99) Thorium induced tumor: (NEET 2013)
a) Angiosarcoma of liver
b) Renal cell carcinoma
c) Lymphoma
d) Astrocytoma

100) Which is a risk factor for cholangiocarcinoma? (NEET 2013)
a) Obesity
b) Primary sclerosing cholangitis
c) Salmonella carrier state
d) HBV infection

101) All of the following are risk factors for carcinoma gallbladder, EXCEPT: (NEET 2013)
a) Typhoid carriers
b) Adenomatous gall bladder polyps
c) Choledochal cysts
d) Oral contraceptives

102) The following parasitic infections predispose to malignancies: (NEET 2013)
a) Pargibunuasus
b) Guinea worm infection
c) Clonorchiasis
d) Schistosomiasis

103) Hemochromatosis is a defect in metabolism of: (NEET 2013)
a) Iron
b) Copper
c) Magnesium
d) Calcium

104) Which does not cause Macrovesicular steatosis? (NEET 2013)
a) Alcoholic fatty liver
b) Tetracycline toxicity
c) Acute fatty liver of pregnancy
d) Reyes syndrome

105) Primary biliary cirrhosis is positive for: (NEET 2013)
a) PANCA
b) Anti-mitochondrial antibody
c) Anti-nuclear antibody
d) Anti-microsomal antibody

106) Central stellate scar is seen in: (NEET 2013)
a) Focal nodular hyperplasia
b) Chronic regenerative hyperplasia
c) Hepatoblastoma
d) Hepatocellular carcinoma

107) Histopathology of chronic hepatitis: (NEET 2013)
a) Ballooning b) Councilman bodies
c) Bridging necrosis d) All of the above

108) Centrilobular necrosis of liver may be seen with: (NEET 2013)
a) Phosphorus b) Arsenic
c) CCl4 d) Ethanol

109) Unconjugated hyperbilirubinemia is seen in: (NEET 2013)
a) Dubin Johnson syndrome
b) Gilbert's syndrome
c) Both of the above
d) None of the above

110) A 40-year-old obese lady with RUQ pain and recurrent jaundice. What is seen in liver pathology? (AIIMS May 2014)
a) NASH
b) Peliosis hepatitis
c) Autoimmune hepatitis
d) None of the above

111) Following Histopathological figure depicts: (AIIMS Nov 2015)

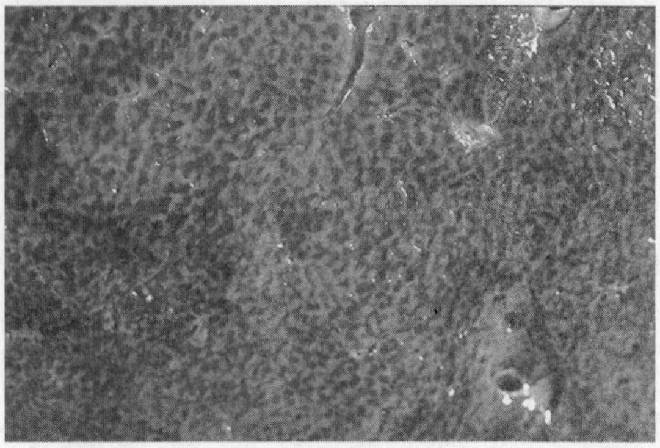

a) Nutmeg liver with dark areas of perivenular dead hepatocytes and gray areas of periportal viable hepatocytes
b) Nodular regenerative hyperplasia of liver induced due to OCP's
c) Nutmeg liver with pale areas of necrosis and dark congested areas of perivenular viable hepatocytes
d) Cirrhotic liver with fibrotic nodules

112) Klatskin tumor is: (NEET 2013)
a) Nodular type of cholangiocarcinoma
b) Fibrolamellar hepatocellular carcinoma
c) Gallbladder carcinoma
d) Hepatocellular carcinoma

CHAPTER 16 – LIVER AND BILIARY TRACT

Ans. 1) **C. Space of Disse represent mononuclear phagocyte system (Ref: 8 ed. Robbins p. 834-35, 9 ed. p. 821-22, f-18-1,5)**

Hepatic Microarchitecture is divided according to:

Lobular model [Q]:

- Liver is divided into 1 to 2 mm diameter hexagonal lobules around the terminal hepatic vein and the portal tracts are at the periphery of the lobule
- Hepatocytes in close proximity to terminal hepatic vein are called **centrilobular** [Q]
- Hepatocytes in close proximity to portal tract are called **periportal** [Q]

Acinar model [Q]:

- In **acinus**, liver parenchyma is divided into three zones:

Zone 1 – Closest to the vascular supply

Zone 2 – Intermediate

Zone 3 – Near the terminal hepatic venule and farthest from afferent blood supply

Note: Histopathology of the liver is discussed on the basis of a lobular architecture

Normal morphology:

- Hepatocytes are arranged into **anastomosing sheets** or **plates**
- **Vascular sinusoids** lie between the plates of hepatocytes, which are lined by fenestrated **endothelial cells** [Q]
- Deep to the endothelial cells lies **space of Disse** [Q]
- **Kupffer cells** are attached to the endothelial cells
- **Hepatic stellate cells (HSCs)** are **found** in the **space of Disse** [Q]
- Intervening the hepatocytes are **bile canaliculi** which drain into the **canals of Hering** (ductular structures that connect **bile canaliculi** to **bile ductules** in **periportal region**)

Thus, **Kupffer cells** forms a part of **mononuclear phagocyte system** and not space of Disse, which contains **quiescent stellate cell**

Ans. 2) **C. 26 weeks (Ref: 9 ed. Robbins p.835, 9 ed. p. 825, f-18-6)**

Acute liver failure [Q] or **Fulminant liver failure**:

- Acute liver illness associated with **encephalopathy** and **coagulopathy**
- Occurs within **26 weeks** [Q] of the initial liver injury in **absence** of pre-existing liver disease
- Occurs due to **massive hepatic necrosis**, induced by **drugs or toxins**
- Accidental or deliberate ingestion of **acetaminophen** is the **most common cause** [Q]

Ans. 3) **B. Astrocyte swelling (Ref: 8 ed. Robbins p. 836, 9 ed. p. 826)**

Hepatic Encephalopathy [Q]

- Associated with **elevated ammonia levels** in blood and central nervous system
- **Minor morphologic changes** in the brain, includes **astrocyte swelling** [Q]
- **Reversible,** if the underlying hepatic condition is corrected

Ans. 4) **D. All of the above (Ref: 8 ed. Robbins p. 837, 9 ed. p. 827, f-18-5,7,8)**

Cause of cirrhosis – Alcohol abuse, viral hepatitis, non-alcoholic steatohepatitis (NASH)

Cirrhosis is defined by **three main morphologic characteristics**:

- **Bridging fibrous septa** [Q]: Delicate bands or broad scars linking portal tracts with one another and portal tracts with **terminal hepatic veins**
- **Parenchymal nodules** [Q]: Micro-nodules (<0.3 cm) to macro-nodules (several centimeters)
- **Disruption** of the **liver architecture** [Q]

Ans. 5) **C. Both of the above (Ref: 8 ed. Robbins p.837, 9 ed. p. 827)**

- In **normal liver, interstitial collagens (types I and III)** Q are seen in **portal tracts** and around **central veins** and **type IV collagen** is present in **space of Disse**
- In cirrhosis, **types I and III collagen** Q are deposited in **space of Disse**, creating fibrotic septal tracts

Ans. 6) **A. Hepatic stellate cells (Ref: 8 ed. Robbins p.837, 9 ed. p. 827, f-18-5)**

- **Mechanism of fibrosis** in **cirrhosis** – Predominantly due to the proliferation of **hepatic stellate cells** Q and their activation into highly fibrogenic cells

Ans. 7) **A. ET-1 (Ref: 8 ed. Robbins p.837-38, 9 ed. p. 823-24, f-18-5)**

Cytokines and chemokines which play a role in **cirrhosis of liver:**

a) **Platelet – Derived growth factor receptor β (PDGFR-β)** in **stellate cells** – proliferation and **activation** of **hepatic stellate cells** into **myofibroblasts** Q

b) **Transforming growth factor β (TGF-β)**, **metalloproteinase 2 (MMP-2)** and tissue inhibitors of metalloproteinase 1 and 2 **(TIMP-1 and -2)** – Fibrogenesis by stellate cells

c) **Endothelin-1 (ET-1)** Q – Contraction of **myofibroblasts**

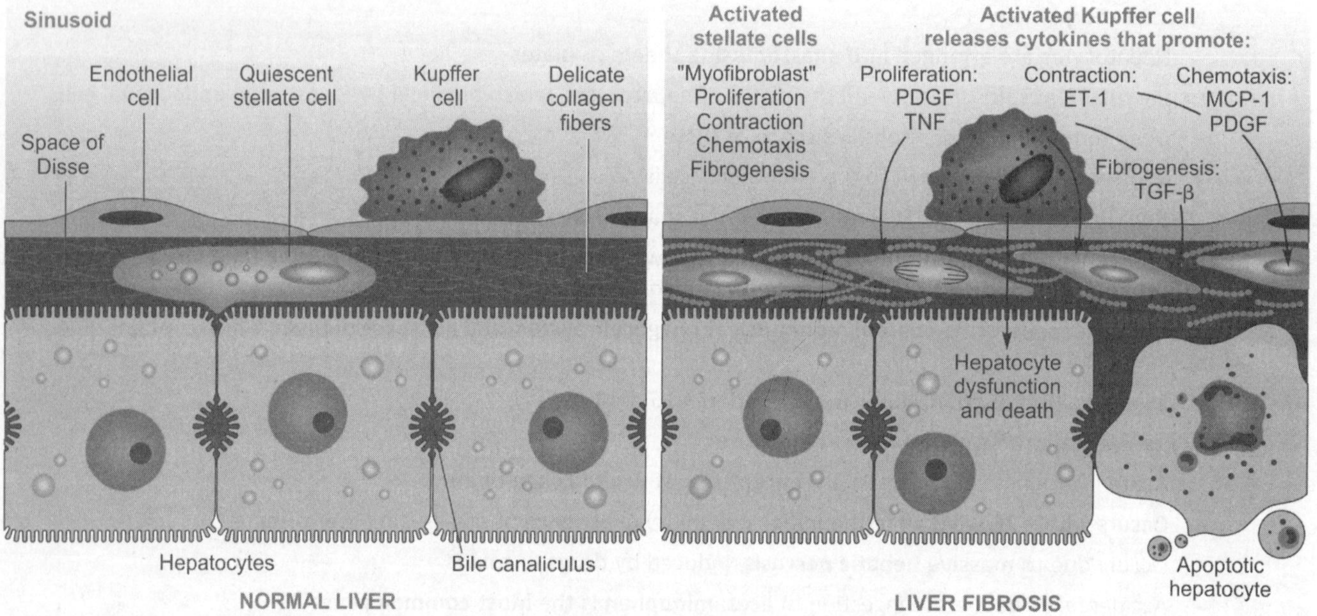

Stellate cell activation and liver fibrosis

Ans. 8) **D. Serum bilirubin (Ref: 8 ed. Robbins p.835, 9 ed. p. 822, t-18-1)**

Following **enzymes** are produced resulting from **damage to bile canaliculus** Q

- Serum **alkaline phosphatase**
- Serum **γ-glutamyl transpeptidase**
- Serum **5' -nucleotidase**

Laboratory evaluation of liver disease:

Test Category	Serum Measurement	Levels in Liver Disease
Hepatocyte integrity	**Cytosolic hepatocellular enzymes:** Serum aspartate aminotransferase (AST) Serum alanine aminotransferase (ALT) Serum lactate dehydrogenase (LDH)	 Increased Increased Increased
Biliary excretory function	Substances normally secreted in bile: **Serum bilirubin** - Total: Unconjugated plus conjugated - Direct: Conjugated only **Urine bilirubin** **Serum bile acids** **Plasma membrane enzymes (from damage to bile canaliculus)** - **Serum alkaline phosphatase, Serum γ-glutamyl transpeptidase (GGT)**	 Increased Increased Increased Increased
Hepatocyte synthetic function	**Proteins secreted into the blood** - Serum albumin - Coagulation factors: Prothrombin (PT) and partial thromboplastin (PTT) times (fibrinogen, prothrombin, factors V, VII, IX and X) **Hepatocyte metabolism** Serum ammonia Aminopyrine breath test (hepatic demethylation)	 Decreased Prolonged Increased Decreased

Ans. 9) **B. Obstructive thrombosis (Ref: 8 ed. Robbins p.838, 9 ed. p. 828-29, f-18-9)**

Portal hypertension – Increased resistance to portal blood flow

Can be divided into **3 types** on basis of etiology:

Prehepatic causes [Q]

- Obstructive thrombosis, narrowing of the portal vein before it ramifies in the liver, or massive splenomegaly with increased splenic vein blood flow

Intrahepatic causes [Q]

- Cirrhosis (most common), schistosomiasis, massive fatty change, diffuse fibrosing granulomatous disease such as sarcoidosis and nodular regenerative hyperplasia

Post hepatic causes [Q]

- Severe right-sided heart failure, constrictive pericarditis and hepatic vein outflow obstruction

Ans. 10) **D. All of the above (Ref: 8 ed. Robbins p.839, 9 ed. p. 829, f-18-9)**

Four major clinical consequences of **portal hypertension** [Q]

- **Ascites**
- **Porto-systemic venous shunts**
- **Congestive splenomegaly**
- **Hepatic encephalopathy**

Ans. 11) **B. 500 ml (Ref: 8 ed. Robbins p.839, 9 ed. p. 829)**

Ascites

- Accumulation of excess fluid in the **peritoneal cavity** [Q]
- Most common cause is **cirrhosis** [Q]
- **Ascites** can be detected when at least **500 mL** [Q] of fluid have accumulated
- Fluid is serous, with **< 3 gm/dl of protein (albumin)** and serum to ascitic fluid albumin gradient **≥ 1.1 gm/dL**

Ans. 12) D. All of the above (Ref: 8 ed. Robbins p. 839, 9 ed. p;. 830, f-18-9)

- Increased **portal pressure** leads to reversal of blood flow from **portal to systemic circulation,** which leads to **formation of collateral vessels** and **new vessels**

Principal sites involved are:

- **Rectum** Q (manifest as hemorrhoids)
- **Esophagogastric junction** Q (producing varices)
- Retro peritoneum
- Falciform ligament of the liver (involving **periumbilical** Q and **abdominal wall collaterals** Q)

Important **clinical hallmark** of **portal hypertension:**

- **Abdominal wall collaterals** Q appear as **dilated subcutaneous veins**, which extend from umbilicus towards the rib margin (**caput medusae** Q)

Ans. 13) A. UGT1A1 (Ref: 8 ed. Robbins p.839-40, 9 ed. p. 852-53, f-18-27)

UGT1A1 Q:

- Responsible for **bilirubin glucuronidation** Q
- Mutation leads to **unconjugated hyperbilirubinemias** Q: Crigler-Najjar syndrome types I and II and Gilbert syndrome

Note: Bile salts are **taurine or glycine** Q **conjugated salts** of **human bile acids** i.e. **cholic acid** and **chenodeoxycholic acid** Q

Ans. 14) C. Unconjugated bilirubin can be excreted in urine (Ref: 8 ed. Robbins p.839-40, 9 ed. p. 852-53)

Bilirubin can be of two types – **unconjugated** and **conjugated**

Unconjugated Bilirubin Q

- **Insoluble in water**
- Exists in combination with **albumin complexes**
- Not excreted in urine
- Can diffuse and accumulate in the brain of infants leading to **kernicterus**
- Seen in **hemolytic disease of newborn (erythroblastosis fetalis)** Q

Conjugated Bilirubin Q

- **Water-soluble**, nontoxic and can be excreted in urine

Ans. 15) D. Rotor syndrome (Ref: 8 ed. Robbins p.840-41, 9 ed. p. 853, t-18-8)

Causes of Jaundice Q:

A) Unconjugated hyperbilirubinemias Q

Excess production of bilirubin

- Hemolytic anemia
- Resorption of blood from internal hemorrhage (e.g. alimentary tract bleeding, hematomas)
- Ineffective erythropoiesis (e.g. pernicious anemia, thalassemia)

Impaired bilirubin conjugation

- Physiologic jaundice of the newborn (decreased UGT1A1 activity)
- Breast milk jaundice
- Genetic deficiency of UGT1A1 activity (Crigler-Najjar syndrome types I and II)
- Gilbert syndrome
- Diffuse hepatocellular disease (e.g. viral or drug-induced hepatitis, cirrhosis)

B) Conjugated hyperbilirubinemias Q

- Dubin-Johnson syndrome, Rotor syndrome

- Impaired bile flow due to duct obstruction

Ans. 16) C. 2-2.5 mg/dL (Ref: 8 ed. Robbins p.841, 9 ed. p. 853)

- **Serum bilirubin levels** in normal adult vary between **0.3 and 1.2 mg/dL** [Q]
- **Jaundice becomes evident** when the serum bilirubin levels rise above **2.0 to 2.5 mg/dL** [Q]

Ans. 17) D. Hepatocytes are swollen and shows inflammation (Ref: 8 ed. Robbins p.841-42, f-18-5, 9 ed. p. 853, t-18-9)

Dubin-Johnson Syndrome [Q]

- **Autosomal recessive** disorder
- Results in **conjugated hyperbilirubinemia** [Q]
- Due to mutation in the canalicular **multidrug resistance protein 2 (MRP2)** [Q]
- **Microscopy** – Liver shows **darkly pigmented granules** [Q] within the cytoplasm of hepatocytes
- Most of patients are asymptomatic and have a normal life expectancy

Ans. 18) A. Phenobarbital (Ref: 8 ed. Robbins p.841, 9 ed. p. 853)

- In **Crigler-Najjar syndrome, phenobarbital** can improve **bilirubin glucuronidation** by inducing hypertrophy of the hepatocellular endoplasmic reticulum [Q]

Ans. 19) D. All of the above (Ref: 8 ed. Robbins p.842-43, 9 ed. p. 853-55, f-18-28)

Cholestasis [Q]:

- Accumulation of **bile pigment** in hepatic parenchyma
- Due to **extra-hepatic** or **intrahepatic obstruction** of **bile channels**
- Patients present with **jaundice, pruritus, skin xanthomas**
- **Intestinal malabsorption** leads to deficiency of **fat-soluble vitamins A, D or K**
- **Elevated serum alkaline phosphatase** [Q] and **γ-glutamyl transpeptidase (GGT)** [Q] are characteristic finding

Morphology [Q];

- **Feathery degeneration** [Q]: Fine foamy appearance of hepatocytes due to the accumulation of **bile pigment droplets**
- Elongated **green-brown plugs** of bile are seen in dilated bile canaliculi
- **Kupffer cells** contain **bile pigments**
- Proliferation of bile ductular epithelial cells
- Portal tract edema and **periductular infiltrates** of **neutrophils**

Complications – Portal tract fibrosis and biliary cirrhosis

Ans. 20) C. PFIC-3 (Ref: 8 ed. Robbins p.843)

Progressive Familial Intrahepatic Cholestasis (PFIC) [Q] is of 3 types:

Progressive familial intrahepatic cholestasis 1 (PFIC 1)

- Cholestasis begins in infancy
- Patients present with severe pruritus
- Progresses to liver failure before adulthood
- Due to **mutation of ATP8B1 gene** [Q]

Progressive familial intrahepatic cholestasis 2 (PFIC 2)

- Presents with **pruritus, growth failure** and **progression to cirrhosis** in first decade
- Patients have **higher risk** for **cholangiocarcinoma** [Q]
- Due to **mutation** in hepatocyte canalicular **bile salt export pump (BSEP)**, encoded by the **ABCB11 gene** [Q]

Progressive familial intrahepatic cholestasis 3 (PFIC-3)

- Due to mutations in the **ABCB4 gene**
- Associated with **increased GGT levels** [Q]

Ans. 21) B. Hepatitis B (Ref: 8 ed. Robbins p.844, t-18-4, 9 ed. p. 832)

Mean incubation period [Q] of:

Hepatitis A virus – 2–4 weeks

Hepatitis B virus – 1–4 months (2-26 weeks)

Hepatitis C virus – 7–8 weeks

Hepatitis D virus – Same as HBV

Hepatitis E virus – 4–5 weeks

Ans. 22) B. Hepatitis B (Ref: 8 ed. Robbins p.844-46, t-18-4, 9 ed. p. 831-33)

Important Properties of Hepatitis Viruses [Q]

Virus	Hepatitis A	Hepatitis B	Hepatitis C	Hepatitis D	Hepatitis E
Type of virus	ssRNA	Partially ds DNA	ssRNA	Circular defective ssRNA	ssRNA
Viral family	Hepatovirus; related to picornavirus	Hepadnavirus	Flaviridae	Subviral particle in Deltaviridae family	Calicivirus
Route of transmission	Fecal-oral	Parenteral, sexual contact, perinatal	Parenteral	Parenteral	Fecal-oral
Mean incubation period	2–4 weeks	1–4 months	7–8 weeks	Same as HBV	4–5 weeks
Frequency of chronic liver disease	Never	10%	~80%	5% (coinfection); ≤70% for superinfection	Never

Ans. 23) D. IgG antibody against HAV appears in blood after onset of symptoms (Ref: 8 ed. Robbins p.844, t-18-4, 9 ed. p. 831)

- **IgM anti-HAV antibody** appears in blood at the **onset of symptoms**
- **IgM** levels, decline in few months and is followed by appearance of **IgG anti-HAV** [Q], which persists for years and confers lifelong immunity against re-infection

Ans. 24) D. All of the above (Ref: 8 ed. Robbins p. 845-46, 9 ed. p. 831-33, f-18-12)

Healthy carrier state [Q] in **Hepatitis B infection**:

- Positive HBsAg > 6 months
- **HBeAg negative**, with presence of Anti-HBe
- **Serum HBV DNA <10^5 copies/mL**
- **Normal AST** and **ALT levels**
- Absence of significant inflammation and necrosis on liver biopsy

However, **recovery** [Q] from chronic hepatitis is indicated by **negative test for HBsAg**

Ans. 25) D. HBx (Ref: 8 ed. Robbins p. 846, 9 ed. p. 832, f-18-12)

HBV genome [Q] contains:

- Nucleocapsid "core" protein – **HBcAg (hepatitis B core antigen)**
- Pre-core and core region – **HBeAg (hepatitis B "e" antigen)**
- Envelope glycoprotein – **HBsAg (hepatitis B surface antigen)**
- A **polymerase (Pol)** – Which has both **DNA polymerase activity** and **reverse transcriptase activity**
- **HBx protein** [Q] – Necessary for virus replication and plays an important role in pathogenesis of **liver cancer** in **HBV infection**

Ans. 26) B. HBeAg (Ref: 8 ed. Robbins p.846-47, 9 ed. p. 832-33, f-18-12)

Serum markers Q helpful in Hepatitis B:

- **HBsAg** Q – Appears before the onset of symptoms and returns to normal levels in **3 to 6 months**
- **Anti-HBs antibody** – Rise when the acute disease is over and is detectable after disappearance of HBsAg
- **HBeAg, HBV-DNA and DNA polymerase** Q – Signify **active viral replication**
- **Persistence of HBeAg** is an important indicator of **continued viral replication, infectivity** and progression to **chronic hepatitis**
- **IgM anti-HBc** Q is detectable before the onset of symptoms and its level rises simultaneously with **serum aminotransferase levels**
- **IgM anti-Hbc** Q is replaced by **IgG anti-HBc** over period of months

Ans. 27) B. Anti-HBs (Ref: 8 ed. Robbins p.846-47, 9 ed. p. 833)

Anti-HBs Q:

- Levels rise after disappearance of HBsAg and **persist** for life
- **Anti-HBs** confers **protection** and form basis for the **current vaccination strategies**
- **Vaccination** induces a protective **anti-HBs antibody** Q response in 95% of infants, children and adolescents

Ans. 28) C. 1.8% (Ref: 8 ed. Robbins p.847, 9 ed. p. 834)

- Risk of acquiring **Hepatitis C Virus (HCV)** by **needle stick is six times** higher than that for HIV **(1.8 vs 0.3%)** Q

Ans. 29) D. Elevated levels of anti-HCV IgG after acute infection confer immunity (Ref: 8 ed. Robbins p.847-48, 9 ed. p. 833-35, f-18-13)

Salient features of **Hepatitis C virus infection** Q:

- **Incubation period** for HCV ranges from **2 to 26 weeks** Q
- **HCV RNA** is **detectable** in blood for **1 to 3 weeks** and coincide with **elevations in serum transaminases** Q
- In **acute HCV infection, 50% to 70%** of patients show **anti-HCV antibodies (IgM)**
- Elevated titers of **anti-HCV IgG** Q occurring after an **active infection do not** consistently confer **effective immunity**
- **Hallmark** of **HCV infection** Q: Persistent infection and chronic hepatitis, which may lead to **cirrhosis**
- **HCV RNA levels** Q are performed to assess and confirm the diagnosis of **chronic HCV** infection
- **Characteristic feature** of **chronic HCV infection** is **episodic elevations in serum aminotransferases** Q

Ans. 30) D. Hepatitis E virus (Ref: 8 ed. Robbins p.849, 9 ed. p. 835)

Hepatitis E Virus Infection:

- Accounts for more than **30% to 60%** Q of cases of **acute hepatitis** in India
- Has **high mortality rate** among **pregnant women** Q

Ans. 31) D. Hepatitis G (Ref: 8 ed. Robbins p.849)

Hepatitis G virus:

- Is not hepatotropic and **does not** cause elevations in serum aminotransferases
- Appears to **replicate** in the **bone marrow** and spleen

Ans. 32) B. Hepatitis C (Ref: 8 ed. Robbins p.850, 9 ed. p. 836)

- Due to the presence of circulating **antibody-antigen complexes, HBV** and **HCV** leads to **immune complex disease** Q **(vasculitis** and **glomerulonephritis)**
- **Cryoglobulinemia** Q is seen in individuals with **chronic hepatitis C** Q
- **HCV** is the **most common** cause of **chronic viral hepatitis** Q
- Treatment of Hepatitis C virus infection – **IFN-α** and **ribavirin**

Ans. 33) **B. Hepatitis B (Ref: 8 ed. Robbins p.851-52, 9 ed. p. 837, f-18-14,15)**

- **Ground-glass hepatocytes** are seen in **HBV infected hepatocytes** Q, which shows cytoplasm packed with spheres and tubules of **HBsAg**

Ans. 34) **C. Hepatitis C (Ref: 8 ed. Robbins p. 851-52, 9 ed. p. 837-38, f-18-14,16)**

Morphology of liver in **chronic HCV** Q infection:

- **Lymphoid aggregates** and **bile duct reactive changes** in the portal tracts
- Mild to moderate **macrovesicular steatosis** Q, in **HCV genotype 3 infections** Q
- **Panlobular** microvesicular and macrovesicular steatosis are seen in **toxic hepatitis** Q

Ans. 35) **D. All of the above (Ref: 8 ed. Robbins p.851-52, 9 ed. p. 837, f-18-14)**

Morphological features of acute hepatitis Q include:

- **Ballooning degeneration** – due to diffuse swelling of hepatocytes
- **Cholestasis** – bile plugs in canaliculi and brown pigmentation of hepatocytes
- **Apoptosis** of hepatocytes
- **Bridging necrosis – necrosis of hepatocytes**, connecting portal-to-portal, central-to-central, or portal-to-central regions of adjacent lobules
- Hypertrophy and hyperplasia of **Kupffer cells**
- Inflammatory infiltration of **portal tracts**
- **Interface hepatitis** – Inflammatory infiltrate may spill over into the adjacent parenchyma, leading to **apoptosis** of **periportal hepatocytes**

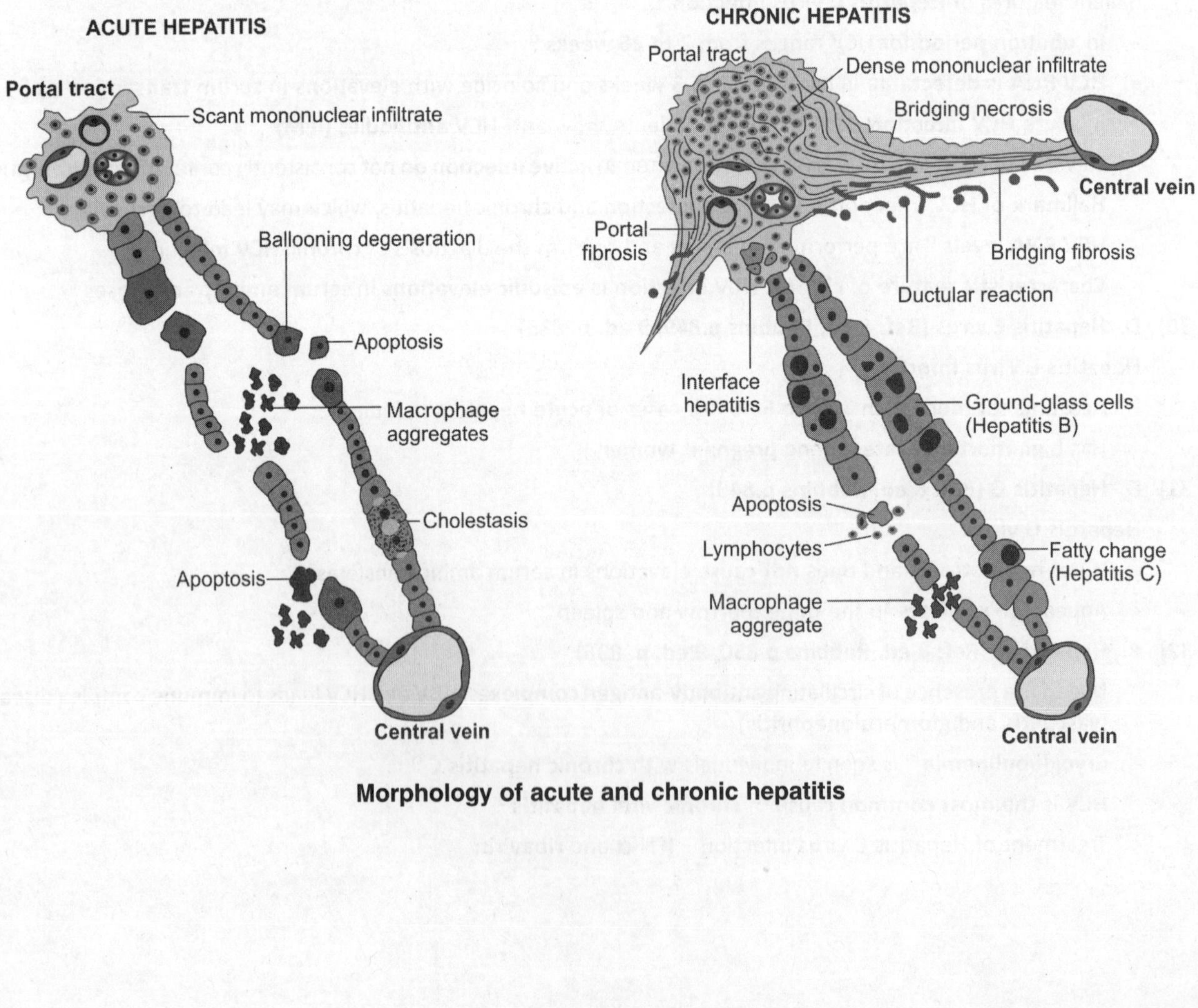

Morphology of acute and chronic hepatitis

Ans. 36) D. All of the above (Ref: 8 ed. Robbins p. 853, 9 ed. p. 827)

- **Hallmark** of **chronic liver damage** is deposition of **fibrous tissue**
- **Continued loss of hepatocytes** and **fibrosis** results in **cirrhosis** Q

Causes of Cirrhosis Q:

- Viral hepatitis
- Autoimmune hepatitis
- Hepatotoxins (carbon tetrachloride, mushroom poisoning)
- Pharmaceutical drugs (acetaminophen, α-methyldopa)
- Alcohol

Cryptogenic Cirrhosis Q – When no cause is found for cirrhosis

Ans. 37) D. All of the above (Ref: 8 ed. Robbins p.854-55, f-18-20, 9 ed. p. 839)

Liver Abscess:

- Occur as solitary or multiple lesions
- **Echinococcal infection** causing liver abscess has **cystic structure** and **laminated** wall with **hooklets** and **intact organisms**
- Viable cyst contains **colorless fluid**, which contains **daughter cysts** and **brood capsules** with **scolices** (with **hooklets** of 20-40 μm length)

Ans. 38) D. Anti-liver kidney microsome-1 antibody (Ref: 8 ed. Robbins p.855-56, 9 ed. p. 839-40, t-18-4)

Autoimmune Hepatitis:

- More common in **females** but can be seen in children and adults
- Classified into type 1 and 2 on basis of circulating antibody pattern
- **Type 1** Q **autoimmune hepatitis** show following antibodies – **antinuclear (ANA)**, **anti–smooth muscle (SMA)**, **anti–actin (AAA)** and **anti–soluble liver antigen/liver-pancreas antigen (anti-SLA/LP)**
- **Type 2** Q **autoimmune hepatitis** – Characterized by **anti–liver kidney microsome-1 (ALKM-1)** antibodies and **anti–liver cytosol-1 (ACL-1)** antibodies

Ans. 39) D. Lymphocytes and plasma cells (Ref: 8 ed. Robbins p.855-56, 9 ed. p. 839-40, f-18-17)

Morphology Q **of liver** in **autoimmune hepatitis**:

- **Cluster of plasma cells** and **lymphocytes** in interface of **portal tracts and hepatic lobules** Q
- **Interface hepatitis –** Lymphocytic/lymphoplasmacytic infiltrates in portal tracts and extending in the lobule
- **Hepatic rosette** formation
- Can progress to **cirrhosis** and may coexist with **autoimmune cholangitis**

Ans. 40) A. Elevated serological markers of viral infection (Ref: 8 ed. Robbins p.855-56, f-18-21)

Salient Features of **autoimmune hepatitis:**

- Absence of serologic markers of **viral infection** Q
- **Elevated serum IgG** and **γ-globulin levels**
- High serum titers of **autoantibodies** Q

Ans. 41) D. Peliosis hepatis (Ref: 8 ed. Robbins p.856-57,872, 9 ed. p. 841, t-18-5)

Oral Contraceptive Q can lead to following hepatic injuries:

- **Hepatic adenomas, cholestatic injury, Budd-Chiari syndrome, sinusoidal dilatation**

Peliosis hepatis Q (blood-filled cavities, not lined by endothelial cells) occurs due to:

- **Anabolic steroids** Q and **tamoxifen** Q
- Cancer, Tuberculosis, AIDS, or post-transplantation immunodeficiency

Ans. 42) A. Microvesicular steatosis (Ref: 8 ed. Robbins p.857, 9 ed. p. 841, t-18-5)

Reye Syndrome Q

- **Mitochondrial dysfunction** seen throughout the body, seen commonly in children
- Characterized by **extensive accumulation of fat droplets** within the **hepatocytes (microvesicular steatosis)** Q
- Associated with administration of **acetylsalicylic acid (aspirin)** Q for relief of **fever**

Drug- and Toxin-Induced Hepatic Injury Q

Pattern of Injury	Associated Drugs
Cholestatic	Contraceptive and anabolic steroids, antibiotics, HAART
Cholestatic hepatitis	Antibiotics, phenothiazine, statins
Hepatocellular necrosis	Methyldopa, phenytoin, Acetaminophen, halothane, Isoniazid
Microvesicular steatosis	**Valproate**, tetracycline, **aspirin (Reye syndrome)**, HAART
Steatohepatitis with Mallory-Denk bodies	Ethanol, Amiodarone
Fibrosis and cirrhosis	Alcohol, methotrexate, enalapril, vitamin A and Retinoids
Granulomas	Sulfonamides, amiodarone, isoniazid, Allopurinol
Budd-Chiari syndrome	Oral contraceptives
Peliosis hepatis	Anabolic steroids, tamoxifen
Hepatocellular adenoma	**Oral contraceptives, anabolic steroids**
Hepatocellular carcinoma	Alcohol, Thorotrast
Cholangiocarcinoma	Thorotrast
Angiosarcoma	Thorotrast, **vinyl chloride**

Ans. 43) D. All of the above (Ref: 8 ed. Robbins p.857-58, 9 ed. p. 842-43, f-18-19, 20)

Alcoholic hepatitis Q **(Alcoholic Liver Disease)** is characterized by:

- Hepatocyte swelling and necrosis
- Mallory-Denk bodies
- Neutrophilic reaction
- Fibrosis

Ans. 44) D. Intermediate filaments (Ref: 8 ed. Robbins p.857-58, 9 ed. p. 842-43, f-18-20)

Mallory Bodies:

- Tangled skeins of cytokeratin **intermediate filaments** Q
- Visible as **eosinophilic cytoplasmic clumps/inclusions** Q in hepatocytes
- **Characteristic** feature of **alcoholic liver disease** Q
- Can also be seen in **Non-Alcoholic Fatty Liver Disease, Primary Biliary Cirrhosis, Wilson disease, chronic cholestatic syndromes** and **hepatocellular tumors**

Ans. 45) D. ALT : AST > 2:1 (Ref: 8 ed. Robbins p.860, 9 ed. p. 844-45)

Laboratory Features of **Alcoholic hepatitis** Q:

- **Hyperbilirubinemia, elevated serum aminotransferases** and **alkaline phosphatase** and **neutrophilic leukocytosis**
- **Serum AST** to **serum ALT ratio** is **2:1** or **higher** in alcoholic liver disease patients

Note: Also see answer 47

Ans. 46) D. Doesn't progress to hepatocellular carcinoma (Ref: 8 ed. Robbins p. 860-61, 9 ed. p. 845-46, f-18-22)

Non-Alcoholic Fatty Liver Disease (NAFLD) Q

- Includes **hepatic steatosis, inflammation** and **non-alcoholic steatohepatitis (NASH)**
- **Main components** of **NASH** are **hepatocyte ballooning, lobular inflammation** and **steatosis**, which can progress to **cirrhosis**

- NASH is **strongly associated** with **obesity, dyslipidemia**, hyperinsulinemia and insulin resistance
- **Most common cause** of so-called **cryptogenic cirrhosis** Q (cirrhosis of "unknown" origin)
- NAFLD contributes to the progression of **HCV** infection, **HBV** infection and **Hepatocellular carcinoma** Q

Ans. 47) C. AST/ALT ratio > 2-2.5 (Ref: 8 ed. Robbins p. 860-61, 9 ed. p. 845-46)

Salient Features of **NASH**

- **Liver biopsy** Q is the **most reliable diagnostic tool**
- **Serum AST and ALT** Q are **elevated**
- **AST/ALT ratio** is usually **less than 1** Q, in contrast to **alcoholic steatohepatitis** in which the ratio is **above 2.0 to 2.5** Q
- **Cardiovascular disease** Q is **most common cause** of **death** due to its association with metabolic syndrome

Ans. 48) D. All of the above (Ref: 8 ed. Robbins p. 860-61, 9 ed. p. 846, f-18-22)

Morphology of liver in NAFLD Q**:**

Steatosis

- Macrovesicular and Microvesicular change

Steatohepatitis (NASH)

- **Steatosis** and **multifocal parenchymal inflammation**, mainly **mononuclear cells** Q
- Mallory-Denk bodies (less prominent) , hepatocyte death and fibrosis (sinusoidal and within portal tracts and around terminal hepatic venules)
- **Cirrhosis** in chronic cases

Note: Greater than 90% of "cryptogenic cirrhosis" (i.e., cirrhosis of unknown cause) is now thought to represent "burned out" NAFLD

Ans. 49) D. Transcription of Hepcidin is increased by iron deficiency (Ref: 8 ed. Robbins p.861-63, 9 ed. p. 847-49, t-18-7)

Salient Features of **Hemochromatosis** Q:

- First described by von Recklinghausen
- **Primary or hereditary** form: **Homozygous-recessive** Q inherited disorder and is caused by **excessive iron absorption**
- **Secondary hemochromatosis (Hemosiderosis)** Q: Due to accumulation of iron in tissues due to parenteral administration of iron
- Regulation of intestinal absorption of **dietary iron** is **abnormal**
- **0.5 to 1.0 gm/year of iron accumulation** occurs in **liver**
- Disease manifests typically after **20 gm** of **stored iron** have accumulated
- **Hepcidin** Q is the **main regulator** of iron absorption
- **Hepcidin levels** are increased by **inflammatory cytokines** and **iron** Q and **decreased** by **iron deficiency, hypoxia** and **ineffective erythropoiesis** Q
- **Hepcidin lowers** plasma **iron levels** Q and **deficiency** of Hepcidin causes **iron overload** Q

Ans. 50) D. All of the above (Ref: 8 ed. Robbins p.861-63, 9 ed. p. 848, f-18-24)

- Mutations in **hepcidin, hemojuvelin (HJV), transferrin receptor 2 (TfR2)** and **HFE** proteins can lead to **hemochromatosis**
- **Mutations** of ***HAMP*** **and** ***HJV*** cause **juvenile hemochromatosis** Q
- Mutations of **HFE** and **TfR2** cause **classic form** of **hereditary hemochromatosis** Q
- **Adult form of hemochromatosis**: Caused by **mutations** of ***HFE*** Q (gene located on the short arm of **chromosome 6** Q)

Ans. 51) D. Marked inflammation is seen (Ref: 8 ed. Robbins p.861-63, 9 ed. p. 848-49, f-18-25)

Morphology of Hemochromatosis Q

- Deposition of **hemosiderin** occurs in **liver (most commonly)** Q
- **Hemosiderin** deposition can also be seen in pancreas, myocardium, pituitary gland, adrenal gland, thyroid and parathyroid glands, joints and skin
- **Cirrhosis** and **pancreatic fibrosis** are frequent **complications** Q
- In **liver, hemosiderin** is seen as **golden-yellow granules** Q in the cytoplasm of **periportal hepatocytes**
- **Iron** stains **blue** Q with **Prussian blue stain**
- **Inflammation is characteristically absent** Q
- **Pseudo-gout** Q – Due to excessive deposition of **calcium pyrophosphate**
- Small and atrophic **testes** (due to derangement of **hypothalamic-pituitary axis)**

Ans. 52) A. Buccal biopsy (Ref: 8 ed. Robbins p.863, 9 ed. p. 849)

- **Extra-hepatic hemosiderin deposition** Q is detected by **buccal biopsy** Q

Ans. 53) D. Increased serum copper levels (Ref: 8 ed. Robbins p.864, 9 ed. p. 849-50)

Biochemical diagnosis of **Wilson disease** Q is based on:

- **Decrease** in **serum ceruloplasmin** Q **levels**
- **Increase** in **hepatic copper content** Q (**most sensitive** and **accurate test**)
- **Increased** urinary excretion of **copper** (**most specific screening test**)
- **Serum copper levels** are of **no diagnostic value**, since they may be low, normal or elevated

Note:

In liver biopsy, excess copper deposition is demonstrated by special stains: Rhodamine stain for copper and Orcein stain for copper-associated protein

Ans. 54) D. Chromosome 14 (Ref: 8 ed. Robbins p.864, 9 ed. p. 850)

α_1-Antitrypsin deficiency Q:

- **Autosomal recessive** disorder of **protein folding**
- **Low levels** of circulating **α_1-Antitrypsin (α_1AT)**
- Leads to development of **pulmonary emphysema**
- Gene for **α_1-Antitrypsin** is located on **chromosome 14** Q
- **PiMM** Q – **Most common** genotype, occurring in **90% of individuals**

PiZ Q:

- **Most common** clinically significant **mutation** Q
- **Homozygotes** for the **PiZZ protein** Q have **10%** of normal circulating **α_1AT levels**

Ans. 55) D. All of the above (Ref: 8 ed. Robbins p.866, 9 ed. p. 856-57, t-18-10, f-18-34)

Major Causes of Neonatal Cholestasis Q:

- Bile duct obstruction – **Extra-hepatic biliary atresia**
- **Neonatal infection** – Cytomegalovirus, Bacterial sepsis, Urinary tract infection, Syphilis
- **Toxic** – Drugs, Parenteral nutrition
- **Metabolic disease** – Tyrosinemia, Niemann-Pick disease, Galactosemia, Defective bile acid synthetic pathways, α1-Antitrypsin deficiency, Cystic fibrosis
- **Miscellaneous** – Shock/hypoperfusion, Indian childhood cirrhosis, Alagille syndrome (paucity of bile ducts)
- Idiopathic neonatal hepatitis

Ans. 56) C. Aberrant Intrauterine development of extrahepatic biliary tree (Ref: 9 ed. Robbins p.857)

Biliary atresia are of two forms:

A) Fetal form:

- Associated with situs inversus, malrotation of abdominal viscera, interrupted inferior vena cava, polysplenia and congenital heart disease
- **Cause** – Aberrant intrauterine development of extrahepatic biliary tree

B) Perinatal form:

- Associated with **viral infection** (Reovirus, rotavirus and cytomegalovirus)
- **Autoimmune reactions**
- **Biliary atresia** with organ malformations have genetic basis

Ans. 57) D. No risk of hepatocellular carcinoma (Ref: 8 ed. Robbins p. 866-69, 9 ed. p. 858-59, f-18-35-37, t-18-11)

Primary Biliary Cirrhosis (PBC) [Q]

- **Autoimmune** inflammatory **disease** with **F : M** [Q] ratio in excess of **6 : 1**
- **Clinical features** [Q] – Fatigue, **pruritus**, hepatomegaly, eyelid **xanthelasmas**, hyperpigmentation, inflammatory **arthropathy** and **cirrhosis** in chronic cases
- **Antimitochondrial antibodies** [Q] are present in **90% to 95% of patients**
- **Elevated levels** of **Alkaline phosphatase** and **γ-glutamyltransferase** [Q] (markers of cholestasis)
- **Increased risk** of developing **hepatocellular carcinoma** [Q]

Extra hepatic manifestations [Q]

- Sjögren syndrome, systemic sclerosis, thyroiditis, rheumatoid arthritis, Raynaud phenomenon, membranous glomerulonephritis and celiac disease

Ans. 58) C. P-ANCA directed against myeloperoxidase is seen (Ref: 8 ed. Robbins p.869, 9 ed. p. 859-60, f-18-39)

Primary Sclerosing Cholangitis (PSC) [Q]

- Characterized by **inflammation** and **obliterative fibrosis** of intrahepatic and extrahepatic bile ducts
- Seen in 70% of chronic **ulcerative colitis** [Q] patients
- Male : Female = 2 : 1

Antibodies [Q] seen in **PSC**:

- Anti-smooth muscle antibodies
- Anti-nuclear antibodies (ANAs)
- Rheumatoid factor
- **Atypical p-ANCA** – Directed against **nuclear envelope protein**, instead of **myeloperoxidase** (typical of p-ANCA antibodies) – Seen in 65% of patients

Morphology [Q]:

- **Concentric periductal fibrosis** around **affected ducts ("onion-skin fibrosis")**

Clinical features [Q]:

- Fatigue, pruritus, jaundice, persistent elevation of **serum alkaline phosphatase**
- **Increased incidence** of chronic pancreatitis, **hepatocellular carcinoma** and **cholangiocarcinoma** [Q]

Hence, in PSC, **atypical P-ANCA** rather than typical P-ANCA is seen

Ans. 59) A. Von Meyenburg complex (Ref: 8 ed. Robbins p.869-70, 9 ed. p. 861, f-18-40)

- **Von Meyenburg Complexes** are often referred as **"bile duct hamartoma"**

Ans. 60) D. All of the above (Ref: 8 ed. Robbins p.869-70, 9 ed. p. 861-62)

Diseases associated with **Polycystic kidney disease**:

- **Von Meyenburg complexes, Polycystic liver disease, Congenital hepatic fibrosis, Caroli disease** Q
- Most frequent **extra-renal manifestation** Q of **autosomal-dominant polycystic kidney** disease – **single or multiple liver cysts** (due to mutation in **PKD1**)
- Most frequent association with **autosomal recessive** Q **polycystic kidney disease – Congenital hepatic fibrosis** Q

Ans. 61) C. AllagilLe syndrome (Ref: 8 ed. Robbins p.870)

Alagille Syndrome Q

- Characterized by **absence** of **bile ducts** in portal tracts
- Caused by **mutations** of the gene encoding **Jagged1** (located on **chromosome 20p**) and mutations of **Notch 2 receptor** Q

Clinical Features Q

- Chronic cholestasis, peripheral stenosis of the pulmonary artery, butterfly-like vertebral arch defects, posterior embryotoxon and hypertelic facies

Ans. 62) C. Both of above (Ref: 8 ed. Robbins p.872, 9 ed. p. 864-65, f-18-48)

Morphology of liver in venous congestion:

- **Right-sided cardiac decompensation** Q leads to **passive congestion of liver** Q
- **Left-sided cardiac failure** or **shock** Q may lead to **centrilobular necrosis**
- Combination of **hypoperfusion** and **congestion** acts synergistically to cause **centrilobular hemorrhagic necrosis** Q

Cut Surface:

- Liver shows **variegated mottled appearance**, reflecting **hemorrhage and necrosis** in **centrilobular regions**, which is termed as **nutmeg liver** Q

Ans. 63) D. All of the above (Ref: 8 ed. Robbins p.873, 9 ed. p. 863-64, f-18-46)

Causes of Hepatic Vein Thrombosis Q:

- **Budd-Chiari syndrome**: Due to obstruction of two or more major **hepatic veins**
- Primary myeloproliferative disorders (Polycythemia Vera)
- Inherited disorders of coagulation (e.g. deficiencies in Antithrombin, protein S or protein C or mutations of factor V)
- Antiphospholipid syndrome
- Paroxysmal Nocturnal Hemoglobinuria
- Intra-abdominal cancers, particularly HCC
- Idiopathic

Ans. 64) C. Hepatitis E (Ref: 8 ed. Robbins p.874-75, 9 ed. p. 866)

- **HEV infection** Q, in pregnant patients has fatality rates of 10% to 20%

Ans. 65) C. Morphologically, distinction from viral hepatitis is difficult (Ref: 8 ed. Robbins p.875, 9 ed. p.866)

Acute Fatty Liver of Pregnancy (AFLP) Q

- Presents in **third trimester** Q of pregnancy
- On biopsy, there is diffuse **microvesicular steatosis** Q of hepatocytes
- Difficult to distinguish from **viral hepatitis** Q
- Can progress to hepatic failure and death within days
- Primary treatment includes **termination of pregnancy** Q

Ans. 66) B. Serum bilirubin >10mg% (Ref: 8 ed. Robbins p.875, 9 ed. p.866-67)

Intrahepatic Cholestasis of Pregnancy Q

- Presents with **pruritus** in **third trimester** Q
- **Serum bilirubin** (mostly conjugated) rarely exceeds **5 mg/dL** Q
- **Alkaline phosphatase** and **bile salts** can be elevated
- **Increased incidence** of fetal distress, stillbirths and prematurity

Ans. 67) C. Both of the above (Ref: 8 ed. Robbins p.875-76, 9 ed. p. 867, f-18-51)

Focal Nodular Hyperplasia Q

- Seen in young to middle-aged adults
- Long term use of **anabolic hormones** and **oral contraceptive pills** have been implicated in its development

Ans. 68) D. All of the above (Ref: 8 ed. Robbins p.876, 9 ed. p.867)

Nodular Regenerative Hyperplasia Q

- Looks similar to **micro nodular cirrhosis** Q, but without fibrosis
- Occurs in association with **solid-organ (renal) transplantation, hematopoietic stem cell transplantation** and **vasculitis** Q
- Seen in **HIV**-infected persons and patients of **SLE** Q

Ans. 69) A. Cavernous hemangioma (Ref: 8 ed. Robbins p. 876, 9 ed. p. 867, f-18-52)

Cavernous Hemangiomas Q

- **Most common** Q benign liver tumor
- Appear as discrete red-blue, soft nodules, **less than 2 cm** in diameter
- Can be mistaken radiographically or intra-operatively for **metastatic tumors**

Ans. 70) D. β-Catenin Activated Hepatocellular Adenomas (Ref: 8 ed. Robbins p.876-77, 9 ed. p.867-69, f-18-53-54)

Subtypes of Hepatocellular Adenoma Q:

A) HNF1-α inactivated hepatocellular adenomas:

- Most commonly found in **women, no risk** of malignant transformation Q
- **Liver fatty acid binding protein (LFABP)** Q: Constitutively expressed in all normal hepatocytes, but is **absent** in these tumors

B) β-Catenin activated Hepatocellular adenomas:

- High risk for **malignant transformation** Q and are associated with **oral contraceptive** and **anabolic steroid** use
- **Immunostain** for **β-catenin** shows nuclear translocation
- **Diffuse positivity** of **glutamine synthetase** in hepatocytes is also seen

C) Inflammatory hepatocellular adenomas:

- Associated with **non-alcoholic fatty liver disease (NAFLD)** Q
- Characterized by **activating mutations in gp130** (co-receptor for **IL-6**)
- Leads to constitutive **JAK-STAT signaling** and overexpression of **acute phase reactants (C-reactive protein and serum amyloid A)** Q

Ans. 71) D. All of the above (Ref: 8 ed. Robbins p.877)

- **Angiosarcoma** is associated with exposure to **vinyl chloride**, **arsenic** or **Thorotrast** Q

Ans. 72) D. All of the above (Ref: 8 ed. Robbins p.877-78, 9 ed. p.869-70, f-18-55)

Hepatoblastoma Q:

- **Most common** Q liver tumor of early childhood
- **Two variants** are: **Epithelial type, epithelial and mesenchymal type** Q
- Frequent activation of **WNT signaling pathway**

- Most commonly seen in patients with **Familial adenomatous polyposis** Q
- **FOXG1** Q (of the TGF-β pathway) is **highly expressed** in **some tumors**
- **Associated** with **Beckwith-Wiedemann syndrome** Q

Ans. 73) D. All of the above (Ref: 8 ed. Robbins p.878, 9 ed. p.870-71, f-18-55)

Risk factors for **hepatic cancers:**

- **Viral infections (HBV, HCV)** and toxic injuries (**aflatoxin, alcohol**) Q
- **Hereditary hemochromatosis, α1AT deficiency, Wilson disease** and **Metabolic syndrome** (obesity, diabetes mellitus and nonalcoholic fatty liver disease) Q

Ans. 74) D. All of the above (Ref: 8 ed. Robbins p.878, 9 ed. p.871, f-18-55)

Molecular changes seen in **hepatocellular carcinoma** Q:

- **β-catenin activation**
- **p53** inactivation
- **IL-6/JAK/STAT** signal pathway activation

Ans. 75) D. Any of the above (Ref: Robbins 9 ed. p.871-73, f-18-57-58, t-18-12)

Precursor Lesions of HCC:

- **Cellular Dysplasias** (**small cell change** Q and **large cell change**) – Seen in **chronic liver disease**
- **Low-grade** Q and **High-grade** Q **dysplastic nodules** – Seen in **cirrhosis**

Precursor Lesions of Hepatocellular Carcinoma

	Hepatocellular Adenoma	Small Cell Change	Large Cell Change	Low Grade Dysplastic Nodule	High Grade Dysplastic Nodule
Premalignant	Yes	Yes	In HBV infection	Uncertain	Yes
Association with cirrhosis	Rare	Common	Common	Usual	Usual
Occurrence without predisposing condition	Occasional	No	No	No	No
Requirement for cancer screening	Depends on predisposing condition	Yes	Yes	Yes	Yes

Ans. 76) C. Occurs in patients with chronic liver disorders (Ref: 8 ed. Robbins p.879, 9 ed. p.873, f-18-59)

Fibro lamellar carcinoma Q:

- **Most commonly** seen in **young adults** Q
- **No gender predilection** Q
- Patients **don't** have an underlying **chronic liver disease** Q
- Usually presents as single large, **hard "scirrhous" tumor** Q with fibrous bands coursing through it

Ans. 77) D. All of the above (Ref: 8 ed. Robbins p.879-880)

Serum α-fetoprotein levels are **elevated** Q in:

- **Hepatocellular carcinoma**
- **Yolk-sac tumors**

Non-neoplastic conditions:

- Cirrhosis, Massive liver necrosis, Chronic hepatitis (HCV infection), Normal pregnancy, Fetal distress or death and Fetal neural tube defects such as anencephaly and spina bifida

Ans. 78) A. Sorafenib (Ref: 8 ed. Robbins p.880)

- **Sorafenib** Q (kinase inhibitor) can prolong the life of individuals with advanced-stage **Hepatocellular carcinoma**

Ans. 79) D. All of the above (Ref: 8 ed. Robbins p.880, 9 ed. p.874, f-18-60)

Risk factors for **cholangiocarcinoma** Q:

- Infestation by **liver flukes (Opisthorchis and Clonorchis species)** Q
- **Chronic inflammatory disease** of the large bile ducts – Primary sclerosing cholangitis, hepatolithiasis and fibro polycystic liver disease
- **Hepatitis B and C** and **Non-alcoholic fatty liver disease** Q

Ans. 80) A. Junction of right and left hepatic ducts (Ref: 8 ed. Robbins p.880, 9 ed. p.874)

- **Klatskin tumors** Q – Extrahepatic tumors (perihilar), located at the **junction of the right and left hepatic ducts** Q
- **Cholangiocarcinoma** can be **intrahepatic** Q or **extrahepatic** Q

Note: Questions have been asked whether Klatskin tumors are benign or malignant.

Answer – Remember it is a malignant tumor Q

Ans. 81) B. Cholangiocarcinoma (Ref: 8 ed. Robbins p.881, 9 ed. p.874, f-18-60)

- **Extrahepatic cholangiocarcinoma** – Appear as firm, gray nodules within the bile duct wall
- **Intrahepatic cholangiocarcinoma** – Occur in the noncirrhotic liver

Note: Lymphovascular and **perineural invasion** Q are common, leading to extensive intrahepatic and extrahepatic metastases

Ans. 82) A. Diffuse large B-cell lymphoma (Ref: 9 ed. p.875)

- Most common **lymphomas** Q affecting liver are **– Diffuse large B-cell lymphomas** Q, followed by **MALT lymphomas**
- **Hepatosplenic delta-gamma T cell lymphoma,** are most common in young adult males Q

Ans. 83) D. Hypo motility of gallbladder (Ref: 8 ed. Robbins p.883-84, 9 ed. p.876)

Conditions that lead to formation of **cholesterol gallstones** Q:

- **Super saturation of bile** with cholesterol
- **Hypo motility** of the gallbladder
- Accelerated cholesterol crystal nucleation
- **Hyper secretion of mucus** in gallbladder

Conditions that lead to formation of **pigment stones** Q (increased **unconjugated bilirubin** in bile):

- **Chronic hemolytic anemia**
- Severe Ileal dysfunction
- Infection of the biliary tract with **Escherichia coli, Ascaris lumbricoides** or the liver fluke, **C. sinensis**

Ans. 84) C. Centrilobular zone (Ref: Robbins 9 ed. p. 864) Refer Q 62 for details

Ans. 85) C. Testis (Ref: 9 ed. Robbins p. 848-49) Refer Q 51 for details

Ans. 86) A. Kupffer cells (Ref. 9 ed. Robbins p. 821-22) Refer Q 1 for details

Ans. 87) B. Hepatocellular carcinoma (Ref: Harrison's 18th ed. p. 777)

Cirrhosis, hepatitis B positivity and alpha fetoprotein strongly suggests hepatocellular carcinoma

Ans. 88) A. Alpha 1 antitrypsin deficiency (Ref: 9th ed. Robbins p. 851, f-18-26)

Morphology of α1AT Deficiency:

- Round to oval cytoplasmic globular inclusions in hepatocytes
- These inclusions are strongly periodic acid–Schiff (PAS)-positive and diastase-resistant

Ans. 89) B. HBV DNA (Ref: 9 ed. p. 832-33) Also, Refer Q 26 for details

- HBV DNA is most sensitive and specific marker of virus replication
- HBeAg, HBV-DNA and DNA polymerase– signify active viral replication

Ans. 90) A. Iron (Ref: 9 ed. Robbins p. 847) Refer Q 49 for details

Ans. 91) C. Both a and b (Ref: 9 ed. Robbins p. 874) Refer Q 79 for details

Ans. 92) D. Hepatitis E (Ref: 9 ed. Robbins p. 835-36)

Hepatitis E Virus (HEV):

- Enterically transmitted, water-borne infection
- Occurs in young to middle-aged adults

Ans. 93) A. Keratin (Ref: 9 ed. Robbins p. 34) Refer Q 44 for details

Ans. 94) D. All of the above (Ref: 9 ed. Robbins p. 874)

Premalignant Lesions for Cholangiocarcinoma:

- Most important – Biliary intraepithelial neoplasia (low to high grade, BiliN-1,-2, or -3)
- Rare – Mucinous cystic neoplasms and Intraductal papillary biliary neoplasia

Ans. 95) D. Alcoholic hepatitis (Ref: 9 ed. Robbins p. 874)

Ans. 96) A. Ceruloplasmin (Ref: 9 ed. Robbins p. 849-50)

- **In liver, copper binds to α_2-globulin (apoceruloplasmin) to form ceruloplasmin, which is secreted into the blood**

Ans. 97) B. ATP 7B (Ref: 9 ed. Robbins p. 849-50)

- Wilson disease is caused by mutation of the ATP7B gene

Ans. 98) A. Piecemeal necrosis (Ref: 9 ed. Robbins p. 842-43) Refer Q 43 for details

- Piecemeal necrosis is seen in acute hepatitis

Ans. 99) A. Angiosarcoma of liver (Ref: 9 ed. Robbins p. 875)

- Angiosarcoma of liver has associations with vinyl chloride, arsenic, or Thorotrast

Ans. 100) B. Primary sclerosing cholangitis (Ref: 9 ed. Robbins p. 859-60) Refer Q 58 for details

Ans. 101) D. Oral contraceptives (Ref: 9 ed. Robbins p. 879-880)

Ans. 102) C. Clonorchiasis & D. Schistosomiasis (Ref: 9 ed. Robbins p. 871)

- **Clonorchis sinensis: Predisposes to liver, bile duct (cholangiocarcinoma) and pancreas (adenocarcinoma)**
- **Schistosoma haematobium: predisposes to urinary bladder (squamous cell carcinoma)**

Ans. 103) A. Iron (Ref: 9 ed. Robbins p. 847-49) Refer Q 49 and 50 details

Ans. 104) A. Alcoholic fatty liver (Ref: 9 ed. Robbins p. 841) Refer Q42, 46, 48 and 65 for details

Ans. 105) A. Anti mitochondrial antibody (Ref: 9 ed. Robbins p. 858) Refer Q 57 for details

Ans. 106) A. Focal nodular hyperplasia (Ref: 9 ed. Robbins p. 867)

Morphology:

- There is a central gray-white, depressed stellate scar from which fibrous septa radiate to the periphery

Ans. 107) C. Bridging necrosis (Ref: 9 ed. Robbins p. 837-38) Refer Q 35 for details

Ans. 108) C. CCl4

Centrizonal (centrilobular) necrosis: Seen in the cells surrounding central hepatic vein. E.g. – Cardiac failure or shock, Chloroform toxicity, Carbon tetrachloride toxicity (CCl4), viral hepatitis

Ans. 109) C. Gilbert syndrome (Ref: 9 ed. Robbins p. 853) Refer Q15 for details

Ans. 110) A. NASH (Ref: Rosai and Ackerman's Surgical Pathology 10th ed. p. 872, 881 & 905; 9 ed. Robbins p. 621, 634)

Nonalcoholic Fatty Liver Disease (NAFLD):

- Seen in persons who do not drink alcohol
- Liver shows steatosis, steatohepatitis and cirrhosis
- Associated with insulin resistance, metabolic syndrome, Type 2 diabetes, Obesity, dyslipidemia, Hypertension
- Most common cause of elevation of serum transaminases
- Liver biopsy is essential for diagnosis

Autoimmune Hepatitis:

- Histological features are indistinguishable from chronic viral hepatitis

Salient Features include:

- Female predominance (70%)
- Absence of serologic evidence of viral infection
- Elevated serum IgG (levels greater than 2.5 g/dL)
- Association with other autoimmune diseases like rheumatoid arthritis, thyroiditis, Sjögren syndrome and ulcerative colitis
- Most patients have circulating antinuclear antibodies, anti-smooth muscle antibodies, liver/kidney microsomal antibody and/or anti-soluble liver/pancreas antigen

Peliosis Hepatis:

- Consists of presence of cystic blood-filled spaces in the liver parenchyma
- Lesions range from less than one to several millimeters in diameter
- Associated with wasting diseases, malignancy, liver or renal transplantation, treatment with steroid hormones and antitumor chemotherapy
- Peliotic lesions in immunosuppressed patients (e.g. AIDS) are caused by rickettsia organisms

So, the history and clinical features suggest NASH as diagnosis, hence is the answer

Ans. 111) A. Nutmeg liver with dark areas of perivenular dead hepatocytes and gray areas of periportal viable hepatocytes (Ref: 9 ed. Robbins p. 864-65) Refer Q 62 for details

Ans. 112) A. Nodular type of cholangiocarcinoma (Ref: 9 ed. Robbins p. 874) Refer Q 80 for details

17 The Pancreas

How to go about this chapter?

- **One should be thorough with the following topics:**
  - **Ectopic pancreas**
  - **Hereditary pancreatitis**
  - **Autoimmune pancreatitis**
  - **Pancreatic pseudocysts**
  - **Serous cystic neoplasms of pancreas**
  - **Mucinous cystic neoplasms of pancreas**
  - **Intraductal papillary mucinous neoplasms, Solid-pseudo papillary neoplasm**
  - **Pancreatic cancer**

1) **All are TRUE about Pancreas Divisum EXCEPT:**
a) Most common congenital anomaly of pancreas
b) Duct of Wirsung is very short
c) Pancreas is drained mostly by duct of Santorini
d) Can lead to pancreatic cancer

2) **Most favored site for ectopic pancreas includes:**
a) Duodenum
b) Jejunum
c) Meckel diverticula
d) Ileum

3) **Most commonly seen mutation in acute pancreatitis:**
a) PRSS1 b) SPINK1
c) CFTR d) None of the above

4) **Chemokines involved in the pathogenesis of chronic pancreatitis include(s):**
a) TGF-β
b) PDGF
c) Both of the above
d) None of the above

5) **Features of autoimmune pancreatitis include(s):**
a) Inflammatory cell infiltrate
b) Venulitis
c) Increased plasma cells
d) All of the above

6) **TRUE about pseudocysts:**
a) Arise after an episode of acute pancreatitis
b) Most commonly involve lesser omental sac
c) Wall is formed by fibrin and granulation tissue
d) All of the above

7) **All are TRUE about serous cystic neoplasms of pancreas EXCEPT:**
a) Arises most commonly in tail of pancreas
b) Occurs more commonly in females
c) Malignant transformation is commonly seen
d) Inactivation of VHL gene is most common genetic abnormality detected

8) **All are TRUE about mucinous cystic neoplasm of pancreas EXCEPT:**
a) Arise in body of or tail of pancreas
b) Cyst is lined by columnar mucinous epithelium
c) Stroma is similar to ovarian stroma
d) Doesn't undergo malignant change

9) **All are TRUE about Intraductal papillary mucinous neoplasm EXCEPT:**
a) Arise frequently in men
b) Involves head of pancreas
c) Does not involve pancreatic duct
d) Lack dense ovarian stroma

10) **Which of the following mutation is seen in solid-pseudo papillary neoplasm?**
a) p53
b) β-catenin
c) K-RAS
d) SMAD4

11) **All cystic neoplasms of pancreas occurs in women EXCEPT:**
a) Serous cystadenomas
b) Mucinous cystadenomas
c) Intraductal papillary mucinous neoplasm
d) Solid pseudo papillary tumor

12) Earliest abnormality predisposing to pancreatic cancer:
a) Telomere shortening
b) p16 inactivation
c) p53 inactivation
d) SMAD4 mutation

13) Most frequently inactivated tumor suppressor gene in pancreatic cancer:
a) K-RAS
b) p16
c) SMAD4
d) P53

14) Greatest predisposition to pancreatic cancer is associated with:
a) Peutz-Jeghers syndrome
b) Hereditary pancreatitis
c) Familial breast and ovarian cancers
d) HNPCC

15) Most common site of pancreatic cancer includes:
a) Head
b) Body
c) Tail
d) Entire gland

16) Carcinoma arising from the following site presents early:
a) Head
b) Body
c) Tail
d) Entire gland

17) Following marker is most commonly used for pancreatic cancer detection:
a) Alpha fetoprotein
b) CA-19-9
c) CA-15-3
d) PSA

CHAPTER 17 – THE PANCREAS

Ans. 1) **D. Can lead to pancreatic cancer (Ref: 8 ed. Robbins p.892, 9 ed. p.883, f-19-1)**

Pancreas Divisum Q

- **Most common congenital anomaly** Q of the pancreas
- **Main pancreatic duct** (duct of **Wirsung)** Q joins the common bile duct at the papilla of Vater
- Accessory pancreatic duct (the duct of **Santorini)** Q drains into the duodenum through a separate minor papilla
- In Pancreas Divisum, **duct of Wirsung** Q drains only a small portion of the head of the gland
- Increased susceptibility of **pancreatitis** Q

Ans. 2) **A. Duodenum (Ref: 8 ed. Robbins p.893, 9 ed. p.883)**

Ectopic Pancreas Q

- Pancreatic tissue is found outside the pancreas
- Favored sites for ectopic pancreas: **Stomach and duodenum** Q, followed by the jejunum, Meckel diverticula and ileum

Ans. 3) **A. PRSS1 (Ref: 8 ed. Robbins p.893-94, 9 ed. p.886, t-19-2)**

Hereditary Pancreatitis Q:

- Due to the mutations that **increases or sustains the activity of trypsin** and leads to recurrent attacks of severe **acute pancreatitis**
- Cause – **Gain-of-function mutations** in the **trypsinogen gene** (i.e. **PRSS1)** Q
- Other genetic mutations – **SPINK1 (Serine peptidase inhibitor, Kazal type 1)** Q and **CFTR (Cystic fibrosis transmembrane conductance regulator)** Q

Ans. 4) **C. Both of the above (Ref: 8 ed. Robbins p.896-98, 9 ed. p.888-89, f-19-5,6)**

Fibrogenic cytokines in chronic pancreatitis:

- **Transforming growth factor β (TGF-β)** and **platelet-derived growth factor** Q, which leads to activation and proliferation of periacinar **myofibroblasts (pancreatic stellate cells)** Q, resulting in deposition of **collagen** and **fibrosis**

Ans. 5) **D. All of the above (Ref: 8 ed. Robbins p.897, 9 ed. p.888-89, f-19-5,6)**

Autoimmune Pancreatitis Q:

- Characterized by a **mixed inflammatory cell infiltrate** around the ducts, **venulitis**, and **increased numbers** of **IgG4-secreting plasma cells**

Ans. 6) **D. All of the above (Ref: 8 ed. Robbins p.898, 9 ed. p.889-90, f-19-7)**

Predisposing factors Q for pseudocysts:

- Acute pancreatitis or chronic alcoholic pancreatitis

Most common sites Q include:

- **Lesser omental sac**, pancreas, retro peritoneum between the stomach and transverse colon or between the stomach and liver or **sub-diaphragmatic**

Note – Cyst **lacks true epithelial lining** and is lined by **fibrin** and **granulation tissue** Q

Ans. 7) **C. Malignant transformation is commonly seen (Ref: 8 ed. Robbins p.899, 9 ed. p.890, f-19-8)**

Serous cystic neoplasms (serous cystadenomas)

- Most common in the **tail of the pancreas** Q
- Cysts are small, and are lined by **cuboidal cells**, and contain clear, thin, straw-colored fluid
- Most commonly seen in **women** Q
- Almost always **benign** Q and surgical resection is **curative**
- **Inactivation** of **VHL tumor suppressor gene** Q is common

Ans. 8) D. Doesn't undergo malignant change (Ref: 8 ed. Robbins p.899, 9 ed. p.890-91, f-19-9)

Mucinous Cystic Neoplasms:

- Most common in **women**
- **Site – Tail of the pancreas** Q
- Cystic cavities are filled with **thick, tenacious mucin** and epithelium is lined by **columnar mucin** and with a **dense stroma** similar to **ovarian stroma** Q
- There is an associated **invasive adenocarcinoma** Q

Ans. 9) C. Don't involve pancreatic duct (Ref: 8 ed. Robbins p.899, 9 ed. p.891, f-19-11)

Intraductal papillary mucinous neoplasms (IPMNs) Q

- **Mucin-producing neoplasms** that involve the larger duct of the pancreas
- Most commonly affect **men**
- Most common site: **Head of the pancreas** Q
- **Absence** of **dense "ovarian" stroma** Q
- Involve the **pancreatic duct** and can progress to **invasive cancer** Q

Ans. 10) B. β-catenin (Ref: 8 ed. Robbins p.900, 9 ed. p.891)

Solid-pseudo papillary neoplasm Q:

- Seen most commonly in **young women**
- Associated with **hyper activation** of the **Wnt signaling pathway** due to activating mutations of the **β-catenin** Q oncogene
- **Surgical resection** is the treatment of choice

Ans. 11) C. Intraductal papillary mucinous neoplasm (Ref: 8 ed. Robbins p.899-900, 9 ed. p.890-91)

- **Intraductal papillary mucinous neoplasms (IPMNs)** Q most commonly affect **men** Q
- Rest tumors most commonly affect **women**

Ans. 12) A. Telomere shortening (Ref: 8 ed. Robbins p.900, 9 ed. p.892, f-19-11,12)

- **Invasive pancreatic cancers** arise from **noninvasive precursor lesions** in small ducts – **pancreatic intraepithelial neoplasia (PanIN)**
- Earliest lesion in the **epithelial cells** of PanIN shows **telomere shortening** Q

Ans. 13) B. p16 (Ref: 8 ed. Robbins p.900-01, 9 ed. p.892-93, t-19-3)

Molecular pathogenesis of pancreatic cancer:

- **KRAS (chromosome 12p)** Q mutation occurs early
- **CDKN2A gene (chromosome 9p)** Q is most frequently **inactivated tumor suppressor gene** which encodes **p16/ INK4a** and **ARF**
- Other tumor suppressor genes altered – SMAD4, p53 and BRCA2 in **higher grade lesions**
- As the question asks particularly, **tumor suppressor gene** and thus answer here is **p16** Q

Ans. 14) A. Peutz-Jeghers syndrome (Ref: 8 ed. Robbins p.902, 9 ed. p.894, t-19-4)

- **Peutz-Jeghers syndrome** has highest inherited predisposition to pancreatic cancer and shows **LKB1 (19p13) mutation** Q

Inherited Predisposition to Pancreatic Cancer with involved gene:

- Peutz-Jeghers syndrome (STK11)
- Hereditary pancreatitis (PRSS1, SPINK1)
- Familial atypical multiple-mole melanoma syndrome (CDKN2A)
- Hereditary breast and ovarian cancer (BRCA1, BRCA2, PALP2, BRCA2)
- Hereditary non-polyposis colorectal cancer (HNPCC) (MLH1, MSH2)

Ans. 15) A. Head (Ref: 8 ed. Robbins p.902-03, 9 ed. p.893-94, f-19-13)

- **Most common site** of **pancreatic cancer** is the **head of the gland** [Q] followed by body, tail and the entire gland

Ans. 16) A. Head (Ref: 8 ed. Robbins p.902-03, 9 ed. p.893-94, f-19-13)

- Carcinoma of **head of the pancreas** [Q] obstructs the **distal common bile duct** and patients presents with early **jaundice**
- Carcinomas of **body and tail** of the pancreas **do not involve biliary tract** [Q] and hence remain **silent** and are widely disseminated at time of presentation
- Point to remember – **Perineural invasion** [Q], lymphatic and large vessel invasion is common in pancreatic cancer

Ans. 17) B. CA-19-9 (Ref: 8 ed. Robbins p.903, 9 ed. p.894-95)

- Serum levels of **Carcinoembryonic antigen** [Q] and **CA19-9 antigen** [Q] are elevated in pancreatic cancer and are useful in patient's response to treatment
- **Note – Migratory thrombophlebitis/Trousseau sign** [Q] is seen in **pancreatic cancer**

18

The Kidney

How to go about this chapter?

- **One should be thorough with the following topics:**
  - **End stage renal disease**
  - **Post streptococcal glomerulonephritis**
  - **Rapidly progressive glomerulonephritis**
  - **Lupus nephritis**
  - **Nephrotic syndrome, Minimal change disease, Membranous nephropathy**
  - **Collapsing glomerulopathy, Focal segmental Glomerulosclerosis**
  - **Membranoproliferative glomerulonephritis, Dense deposit disease**
  - **IgA Nephropathy, Hereditary nephritis**
  - **Chronic glomerulonephritis**
  - **Diabetic kidney, Acute tubular injury, Acute and Chronic Pyelonephritis**
  - **Xanthogranulomatous pyelonephritis, Benign Nephrosclerosis**
  - **Multicystic renal dysplasia, Polycystic Kidney Disease**
  - **Angiomyolipomas, Renal cell carcinoma**

GLOMERULAR DISEASES

1) In End stage renal disease, Glomerular Filtration Rate is:
a) <5% b) 20-25%
c) <50% d) >50%

2) Glomerular basement membrane (GBM) contains following collagen:
a) Type II b) Type III
c) Type IV d) None of the above

3) Which cell in glomerulus lays down collagen framework:
a) Mesangial cells
b) Visceral epithelial cells
c) Endothelial cells
d) Parietal epithelial cells

4) Following is/are responsible for formation of crescents:
a) Fibrin b) Tissue factor
c) IL-1 d) All of the above

5) Sclerosis is accumulation of Extra Cellular Matrix within:
a) Mesangial areas b) Capillary loops
c) Both of the above d) None of the above

6) Linear pattern of immunofluorescence is seen in:
a) Heyman nephritis
b) Anti-GBM disease
c) Circulating immune complex diseases
d) Any of the above

7) GBM antigen responsible for Anti-GBM disease:
a) Type II collagen b) Type III collagen
c) Type IV collagen d) None of the above

8) All are TRUE about Anti-GBM antibody induced glomerulonephritis EXCEPT:
a) Antibodies against component of GBM proper
b) Antibodies can cross react with antibodies of basement membrane of lung
c) Antibodies against type IV collagen
d) Results in granular pattern of staining on Immunofluorescence

9) Sub-epithelial immune complex deposits are formed due to:
a) Cationic antigens b) Anionic antigens
c) Both of the above d) None of the above

10) Post infectious glomerulonephritis is characterized by:
a) Granular immune complex deposits
b) Sub-epithelial deposits/humps on EM

c) Elevation of ASO titers
d) All of the above

11) Crescents in Rapidly Progressive Glomerulonephritis (RPGN) is formed by proliferation of:
a) Parietal epithelial cells
b) Visceral epithelial cells
c) Mesangial cells
d) Endothelial cells

12) Treatment of choice for Type I RPGN include:
a) Plasmapheresis
b) Anti-TTG
c) Corticosteroids
d) Methotrexate

13) Causes of Pauci-immune RPGN includes all EXCEPT:
a) Idiopathic
b) Wegener's granulomatosis
c) Lupus nephritis
d) Microscopic polyangiitis

14) Immunofluorescence (IF) microscopy reveals linear pattern in:
a) Lupus nephritis
b) Henoch-Schönlein Purpura
c) Microscopic polyangiitis
d) Goodpasture syndrome

15) Nephrotic syndrome is characterized by:
a) Massive proteinuria
b) Hypoalbuminemia
c) Generalized edema
d) All of the above

16) All are seen in Nephrotic syndrome EXCEPT:
a) Highly selective proteinuria
b) Decreased synthesis of lipoproteins in liver
c) Urine shows oval fat bodies
d) Renal vein thrombosis

17) Most important cause of Nephrotic syndrome in children:
a) Minimal change disease
b) Membranous nephropathy
c) Membranous proliferative GN
d) Focal Segmental Glomerulosclerosis

18) Most important cause of Nephrotic syndrome in adults:
a) Minimal change disease
b) Membranous Nephropathy
c) IgA Nephropathy
d) Membranous Proliferative Glomerulonephritis (MPGN)

19) Sub-epithelial deposits producing irregular spikes on silver stain is seen in:
a) Membranous Nephropathy
b) Rapid proliferative Glomerulonephritis
c) Membranous Proliferative Glomerulonephritis
d) Focal Segmental Glomerulosclerosis

20) Following is seen in glomeruli in Minimal Change Disease on Electron Microscopy (EM):
a) Granular deposits
b) Linear deposits
c) Diffuse effacement of foot processes
d) None of the above

21) Features of lipoid nephrosis are all EXCEPT:
a) Normal glomeruli by light microscopy
b) Effacement of foot processes on EM
c) Excellent response to corticosteroid therapy
d) IF shows IgG deposits

22) Minimal change disease in adults is most commonly associated with:
a) HIV
b) Hodgkin lymphoma
c) Non Hodgkin lymphoma
d) NSAID therapy

23) Collapsing glomerulopathy is associated with:
a) HIV
b) Hodgkin disease
c) Non Hodgkin lymphoma
d) Sickle cell anemia

24) All are TRUE about NPHS1 gene mutation EXCEPT:
a) NPHS1 maps on chromosome 19
b) Gives rise to steroid resistant nephrotic syndrome
c) Encodes the protein nephrin
d) Gives rise to congenital nephrotic syndrome of Finnish type

25) NPHS2 gene encodes the following protein:
a) Nephrin
b) Podocin
c) CD2AP
d) None of the above

26) Tubuloreticular inclusions within endothelial cells is a feature of:
a) HIV
b) Hodgkin disease
c) Non Hodgkin Lymphoma
d) Post streptococcal glomerulonephritis

27) Following is associated with Type I MPGN:
a) HIV b) Hepatitis A
c) Hepatitis B d) CMV

28) C3NeF is associated with:
a) Type I MPGN
b) Dense deposit disease
c) Focal segmental glomerulosclerosis
d) Minimal change disease

29) Tram track appearance/Split membrane is a feature of:
a) MPGN
b) Membranous nephropathy

c) IgA nephropathy
d) Focal segmental glomerulosclerosis

30) Sub-endothelial and basement membrane deposits are seen in:
a) Mesangiocapillary glomerulonephritis
b) Membranous glomerulonephritis
c) Focal segmental glomerulosclerosis
d) IgA nephropathy

31) Secondary MPGN is seen with:
a) SLE
b) Hepatitis B
c) Cryoglobulinemia
d) All of the above

32) Recurrent hematuria is commonly seen in:
a) IgA nephropathy
b) Alport's syndrome
c) Benign familial hematuria
d) Post streptococcal glomerulonephritis

33) Alport's syndrome is characterized by:
a) Hematuria
b) Nerve deafness
c) Posterior cataract
d) All of the above

34) Following mutation in X-linked Alport syndrome predisposes to end stage renal disease:
a) COL4A5 b) COL4A3
c) COL4A4 d) None of the above

35) Normal glomerular basement width is:
a) 100-200 nm b) 200-300 nm
c) 300-400 nm d) 400-500 nm

36) Least associated with chronic glomerulo-nephritis:
a) Rapid Progressive Glomerulonephritis
b) Focal Segmental Glomerulosclerosis
c) Post streptococcal glomerulonephritis
d) Membranous nephropathy

37) All are TRUE about morphology of kidney in chronic glomerulonephritis EXCEPT:
a) Asymmetrical contracted kidney
b) Granular cortical surface
c) Obliteration of glomeruli by collagen
d) Cortex is thinned

38) Morphological changes seen in diabetic kidney include(s):
a) Capillary basement membrane thickening
b) Diffuse mesangial sclerosis
c) Nodular glomerulosclerosis
d) Any of the above

39) Glomerulosclerosis seen in Diabetes is due to deposition of:
a) Collagen IV b) Fibronectin
c) Increased ROS d) Any of the above

TUBULAR AND INTERSTITIAL DISEASES

40) Cause(s) of acute tubular necrosis include(s):
a) Ischemia
b) Drugs
c) Urinary obstruction
d) All of the above

41) Tam-Horsfall protein is secreted by:
a) Ascending thick limb of the Henle
b) Distal convoluted tubule
c) Proximal convoluted tubule
d) Both a and b

42) Mercuric poisoning most commonly affects:
a) Proximal convoluted tubule
b) Distal convoluted tubule
c) Collecting ducts
d) Loop of Henle

43) Ethylene glycol poisoning leads to deposition of.......in tubule lumens.
a) Eosinophilic granular material
b) Calcium oxalate crystals
c) Neutral lipids
d) None of the above

44) Which of the following phase of Acute kidney injury is associated with increase in urine volume?
a) Initiation phase
b) Maintenance phase
c) Recovery phase
d) None of the above

45) Intra-renal reflex most commonly involves which portion of renal parenchyma?
a) Upper pole
b) Lower pole
c) Both a and b
d) Mid pole

46) Complications of acute pyelonephritis:
a) Papillary necrosis
b) Pyonephrosis
c) Perinephric abscess
d) Any of the above

47) Thyroidisation of renal tubules is seen in:
a) Chronic glomerulonephritis
b) Chronic pyelonephritis
c) Acute kidney disease
d) Any of the above

48) Following can be grossly confused with renal cell carcinoma:
a) Chronic pyelonephritis
b) Xanthogranulomatous pyelonephritis
c) Chronic glomerulonephritis
d) None of the above

49) Analgesic nephropathy is characterized morphologically by:
a) Renal papillary necrosis
b) Acute interstitial nephritis
c) Minimal change disease
d) All of the above

50) Analgesic nephropathy predisposes to:
a) Clear cell renal cell carcinoma
b) Urothelial carcinoma of renal pelvis
c) Chromophobe renal cell carcinoma
d) Sarcomatoid renal cell carcinoma

51) Papillary necrosis is associated with:
a) Diabetes mellitus
b) NSAID's
c) Sickle cell disease
d) All of the above

52) Renal damage in light chain nephropathy can occur due to:
a) Bence Jones proteinuria
b) Amyloidosis
c) Hypercalcemia
d) All of the above

VASCULAR DISORDERS

53) All are TRUE about benign nephrosclerosis EXCEPT:
a) Kidneys can be normal in size
b) Kidneys can be moderately reduced in size
c) The cortical surfaces have fine even granularity
d) GFR is markedly reduced

54) TRUE about Accelerated nephrosclerosis:
a) Seen in malignant hypertension
b) Kidney has a flea bitten appearance
c) Fibrinoid necrosis of arterioles
d) All of the above

55) Most common cause of renal artery stenosis:
a) Atheromatous plaque
b) Fibromuscular dysplasia
c) Hypertensive crisis
d) Diabetes mellitus

56) Thrombotic microangiopathies is characterized by:
a) Microangiopathic hemolytic anemia
b) Thrombocytopenia
c) Renal failure
d) All of the above

57) Most common agent responsible for typical Hemolytic uremic syndrome (HUS):
a) E. coli
b) Streptococcus
c) Shigella
d) Staphylococcus

58) Most common cause of Atypical HUS:
a) Factor H deficiency
b) C3 NeF deficiency
c) Complement Factor I
d) CD46 (membrane cofactor protein)

59) Thrombotic Thrombocytopenic Purpura is characterized by all EXCEPT:
a) Fever, microangiopathic hemolytic anemia
b) Thrombocytopenia
c) Genetic deficiency of ADAMTS 13
d) Absence of neurological symptoms

CYSTIC DISEASES OF THE KIDNEY

60) Most common cause of abdominal mass in newborns:
a) Nephroblastoma
b) Nephrogenic rests
c) Multicystic renal dysplasia
d) Polycystic kidney disease

61) TRUE about the genetics of polycystic kidney disease:
a) PKD1 gene encodes Polycystin-1
b) PKD2 gene encodes Polycystin-2
c) Polycystin-1 is localized to tubular epithelial cells
d) All of the above

62) Extra-renal congenital anomalies of Polycystic kidney include(s):
a) Polycystic liver disease
b) Mitral valve prolapse
c) Berry aneurysms
d) All of the above

63) Congenital hepatic fibrosis is seen in:
a) Autosomal Dominant Polycystic Kidney Disease
b) Autosomal Recessive Polycystic Kidney Disease
c) Both of the above
d) None of the above

64) Which of the following increases the risk of Renal cell carcinoma?
a) Autosomal Dominant Polycystic Kidney disease
b) Medullary sponge kidney
c) Nephronophthisis
d) Acquired cystic disease

OBSTRUCTIVE UROPATHY

65) Obstructive uropathy occurs due to:
a) Congenital anomalies
b) Urinary calculi
c) Benign prostatic hyperplasia
d) All of the above

66) Increased concentration of all of the following leads to stone formation EXCEPT:
a) Uric acid
b) Oxalic acid
c) Calcium
d) Nephrocalcin

67) Struvite stones are another name of:
a) Calcium oxalate stones
b) Magnesium ammonium phosphate stones

c) Uric acid stones
d) Cysteine stones

68) Infection predisposes to the following type of stones:
a) Calcium oxalate stones
b) Magnesium ammonium phosphate stones
c) Uric acid stones
d) Cysteine stones

NEOPLASMS OF KIDNEY

69) Angiomyolipoma patients can have following associated mutation:
a) VHL b) TSC-1
c) P53 d) All of the above

70) Cell of origin of renal oncocytoma:
a) Proximal tubule b) Distal tubule
c) Collecting duct d) None of the above

71) Risk factor(s) for developing renal cell carcinoma include(s):
a) Cigarette smoking
b) Hypertension
c) Obesity
d) All of the above

72) Renal cell carcinoma has an association with:
a) Von Hippel-Lindau (VHL) syndrome
b) Hereditary papillary carcinoma
c) Birt-Hogg-Dubé syndrome
d) All of the above

73) Most common histological type of Renal cell carcinoma:
a) Clear cell carcinoma
b) Papillary carcinoma
c) Chromophobe carcinoma
d) Collecting duct carcinoma

74) Sporadic or familial clear cell carcinoma of kidney is associated with deletion of the following chromosome:
a) 3p b) 4q
c) 17p d) 22q

75) Papillary carcinoma cytogenetically involve(s):
a) Trisomy 7 b) Trisomy 17
c) Loss of Y d) All of the above

76) Chromophobe renal cell carcinoma arises from the following:
a) Distal convoluting tubule
b) Proximal convoluted tubule
c) Collecting ducts
d) Any of the above

77) Which of the following has excellent prognosis:
a) Clear cell carcinoma
b) Papillary carcinoma
c) Chromophobe carcinoma
d) None of the above

78) Following Paraneoplastic syndrome(s) is/are associated with renal cell carcinoma:
a) Polycythemia b) Hypercalcemia
c) Hypertension d) All of the above

79) Metastasis of renal cell carcinoma into ...... reduces the 5 years survival rate drastically.
a) Liver b) Lung
c) Renal vein d) Adrenals

80) Xp11 translocation carcinoma leads to over-expression of:
a) Hepatocyte growth factor
b) Scatter factor
c) TFE3
d) Any of the above

81) Rhabdoid tumor of kidney is associated with the following mutation/s:
a) P53 b) INI-1
c) RB d) All of the above

82) Which of the following tumor is more commonly seen in sickle cell patients:
a) Papillary renal cell carcinoma
b) Medullary renal cell cancer
c) Chromophobe RCC
d) Multicystic nephroma

83) Which of the following tumor(s) can show regression without treatment?
a) Choriocarcinoma
b) Renal cell carcinoma
c) Neuroblastoma
d) All of the above

84) Chromophobe renal cell carcinoma cells show positivity of :
a) PAS stain b) Perl's stain
c) Hale colloidal iron d) Mucicarmine

85) Mutations in COL 4A5 gene manifests as: (NEET 2014)
a) Alport's syndrome
b) HNPCC
c) Goodpasture
d) Vitiligo

86) Glomerulonephritis associated sensory neural deafness is seen in: (NEET 2014)
a) Nail patella syndrome
b) Alport syndrome
c) Down syndrome
d) Fabry's disease

87) PSGN is: (NEET 2014)
a) Dense deposit disease
b) Rapidly progressive glomerulosclerosis
c) Nephrotic syndrome
d) Nephritic syndrome

88) Frequency of renal involvement in HSP: (NEET 2013)
a) 20-40% b) >80%
c) 40-60% d) 10%

89) Malignant hypertension causes: (NEET 2013)
a) Flea bitten kidney
b) Irregular granular contracted kidney
c) Large white kidney
d) No change in kidney

90) Oncocytic carcinoma arises from: (NEET 2013)
a) Perivascular
b) Glomerulus
c) Loop of Henle
d) Collecting duct

91) Renal papillary necrosis is almost always associated with one of the following conditions: (NEET 2013)
a) Diabetes-mellitus
b) Analgesic-nephropathy
c) Chronic pyelonephritis
d) Post streptococcal GN

92) Alport's syndrome is: (NEET 2013)
a) X-linked
b) Co-dominant
c) AD
d) AR

93) Most common cause of nephrotic syndrome in adults: (NEET 2013)
a) Membranous glomerulonephritis
b) Minimal change disease
c) Acute GN
d) Mesangiocapillary GN

94) Most common cause of nephritic syndrome in adults: (NEET 2013)
a) Rapidly Progressive glomerulonephritis
b) Focal Segmental Glomerulonephritis
c) Membranous glomerulonephritis
d) Minimal change disease

95) Podocytes are seen in: (NEET 2013)
a) Bowman's capsule
b) Proximal convoluted tubule
c) Distal convoluted tubule
d) Collecting tubule of the kidney

96) All of the following decrease in Nephrotic syndrome EXCEPT: (NEET 2013)
a) Fibrinogen b) Thyroxin
c) Transferrin d) Albumin

97) Chromophobe variant of renal cell carcinoma is associated with: (AIPGMEE 2010)
a) VHL gene mutations
b) Trisomy of 7 and 17 (+7, +17)
c) 3 p deletions (3p-)
d) Monosomy of 1 and Y (-1, -Y)

98) Electron microscopy is diagnostic in: (AIPGMEE 2010)
a) Goodpasture's syndrome
b) Alport's syndrome
c) Wegener's syndrome
d) Churg-Strauss syndrome

99) Hypercoagulation in nephrotic syndrome is caused by: (AIPGMEE 2010)
a) Loss of Antithrombin III
b) Decreased fibrinogen
c) Decreased metabolism of vitamin K
d) Increase in protein C

100) All are TRUE about Xanthogranulomatous inflammation EXCEPT? (AIPGMEE 2011)
a) Presence of foamy macrophages
b) Presence of tuberculous infection
c) Multinucleated giant cell
d) Presence of yellow nodules

101) A 7-year-old girl is brought with complaints of generalized swelling of the body. Urinary examination reveals grade 3 proteinuria and the presence of hyaline and fatty casts. She has no history of hematuria. Which of the following statements about her condition is TRUE? (AIIMS MAY 2011)
a) No IgG deposits or C3 deposition on renal biopsy
b) Her C3 levels will be low
c) IgA nephropathy is the likely diagnosis
d) Alport's syndrome is the likely diagnosis

102) Primary cause of edema in Nephrotic Syndrome is: (AIIMS May 2012)
a) Na+ and Water retention
b) Increased venous pressure
c) Protein loss
d) Hyperlipidemia

103) Most common nephropathy associated with malignancy: (AIIMS May 2015)
a) Membranous
b) MCD
c) IgA
d) FSGS

104) Most common gene defect in idiopathic Steroid Resistant Nephrotic syndrome (SRNS): (AIIMS Nov 2011)
a) ACE
b) NPHS
c) HOX 1
d) PAX

105) A person with radiologically confirmed reflux nephropathy develops nephritic range proteinuria, which of the following would be the most likely histologic finding in the patient: (Nov 2011)

a) Focal segmental glomerulosclerosis
b) Nodular glomerulosclerosis
c) Membranous glomerulopathy
d) Proliferative glomerulonephritis with crescents

106) Markers of acute kidney injury include all of the following EXCEPT: (AIIMS Nov 2013)
a) Micro RNA-122
b) Cystatin C
c) N-gal
d) Kim-1

107) A patient with a history of recurrent ureteric stones presented with fever. Right sided Nephrectomy was done. What is your diagnosis? (Image based question) (AIIMS Nov 2014)
a) Adult polycystic kidney disease
b) Renal cell carcinoma
c) Cystic dysplastic kidney
d) Hydronephrosis with chronic pyelonephritis

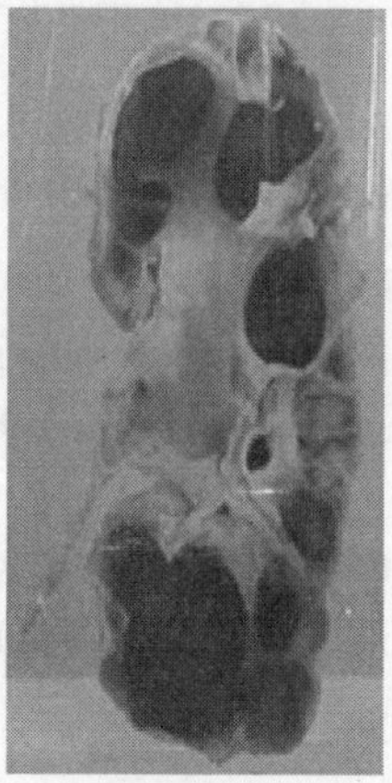

108) Which is not related to immunity? (NEET 2014)
a) MPGN
b) PSGN
c) Diabetic nephropathy
d) IgA nephropathy

CHAPTER 18 – THE KIDNEY

Ans. 1) **A. <5% (Ref: 8 ed. Robbins p.907, 9 ed. p.898-99)**

- **End-stage renal disease (ESRD)** is characterized by **GFR < 5%** ᑫ of normal

Ans. 2) **C. Type IV (Ref: 8 ed. Robbins p.909-10, 9 ed. p.900-02, f-20-1,2)**

- **Glomerular basement membrane (GBM)** consists of **Type IV collagen (most common)** ᑫ, laminin, proteoglycans (heparan sulfate), fibronectin, entactin

Ans. 3) **A. Mesangial cells (Ref: 8 ed. Robbins p.910, 9 ed. p.900, f-20-1)**

- Glomerular tuft is supported by **mesangial cells** ᑫ
- **Functions** – Mesenchymal cells are **contractile**, **phagocytic**, capable of proliferation, and lays down **matrix and collagen** ᑫ

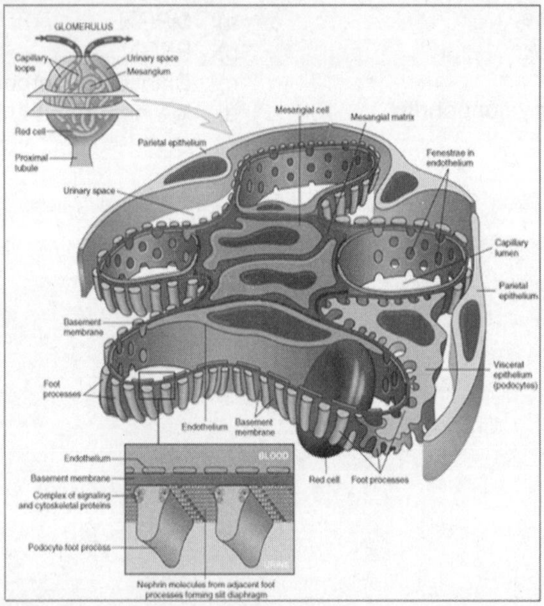

Ans. 4) **D. All of the above (Ref: 8 ed. Robbins p.911, 9 ed. p.902)**

- **Crescents** are formed due to proliferating **parietal epithelial cells** ᑫ and infiltrating leucocytes
- **Mediators** responsible for **crescent formation – fibrin** ᑫ (most important), **IL-1, tissue factor, TNF, IFN-γ**

Ans. 5) **C. Both of above (Ref: 8 ed. Robbins p.911, 9 ed. p.903)**

- **Sclerosis** is characterized by deposition of **extracellular collagenous matrix**, which can be seen in **mesangial areas** ᑫ (diabetic glomerulosclerosis) or **capillary loops** ᑫ

Ans. 6) **B. Anti-GBM disease (Ref: 8 ed. Robbins p.912-14, 9 ed. p.903-05, f-20-4,5, t-20-4)**

Antibody-Mediated Injury:

A) Linear pattern of staining ᑫ on **Immunofluorescence**:

- Seen in **anti-GBM (glomerular basement membrane) nephritis** ᑫ, in which antibodies are formed against **NC1 domain of type IV collagen antigen** ᑫ

B) Granular pattern ᑫ of staining:

- Seen in **membranous glomerulopathy** ᑫ, **Heyman nephritis**, planted antigen disease and circulating immune Complex Disease

Ans. 7) **C. Type IV collagen (Ref: 8 ed. Robbins p.912-14, 9 ed. p.903-05, f-20-4, t-20-4)**

Anti-GBM antibody-induced glomerulonephritis and **Goodpasture syndrome** ᑫ**:**

- Antibodies are formed against the **noncollagenous (NC1) domain of α3 chain of type IV collagen** ᑫ

Ans. 8) **D. Results in granular pattern of staining on Immunofluorescence (Ref: 8 ed. Robbins p.912-14, 9 ed. p.903-05, f-20-4)**

Anti-GBM antibody induced glomerulonephritis: [Q]

- Deposition of antibodies along the entire length of **GBM** results in **Diffuse linear pattern** [Q] of staining on **IF**
- Antibodies can cross react with **basement membrane** in the **lung alveoli**, resulting in simultaneous lung and kidney lesions **(Goodpasture syndrome)** [Q]

Note: As discussed earlier, **antibodies** are directed against **Type IV collagen** [Q] of the **basement membrane**

Ans. 9) **A. Cationic antigens (Ref: 8 ed. Robbins p.912-14, 9 ed. p.903-05, f-20-4,5)**

Immune complex deposits may lie in: (as depicted in figure)

- **Mesangium** [Q] i.e. between endothelial cells and GBM **(sub-endothelial deposits)** [Q]
- Between the outer surface of the GBM and podocytes **(sub-epithelial deposits)** [Q]

Factors which affect **localization of immune complexes** include:

- **Molecular charge** and **size** of antigen
- **Highly cationic antigens** tend to cross GBM, and are found in **sub-epithelial** [Q] location
- **Highly anionic antigens** are trapped **subendothelially** [Q]
- **Antigens with neutral charge** tend to accumulate in the **mesangium** [Q]

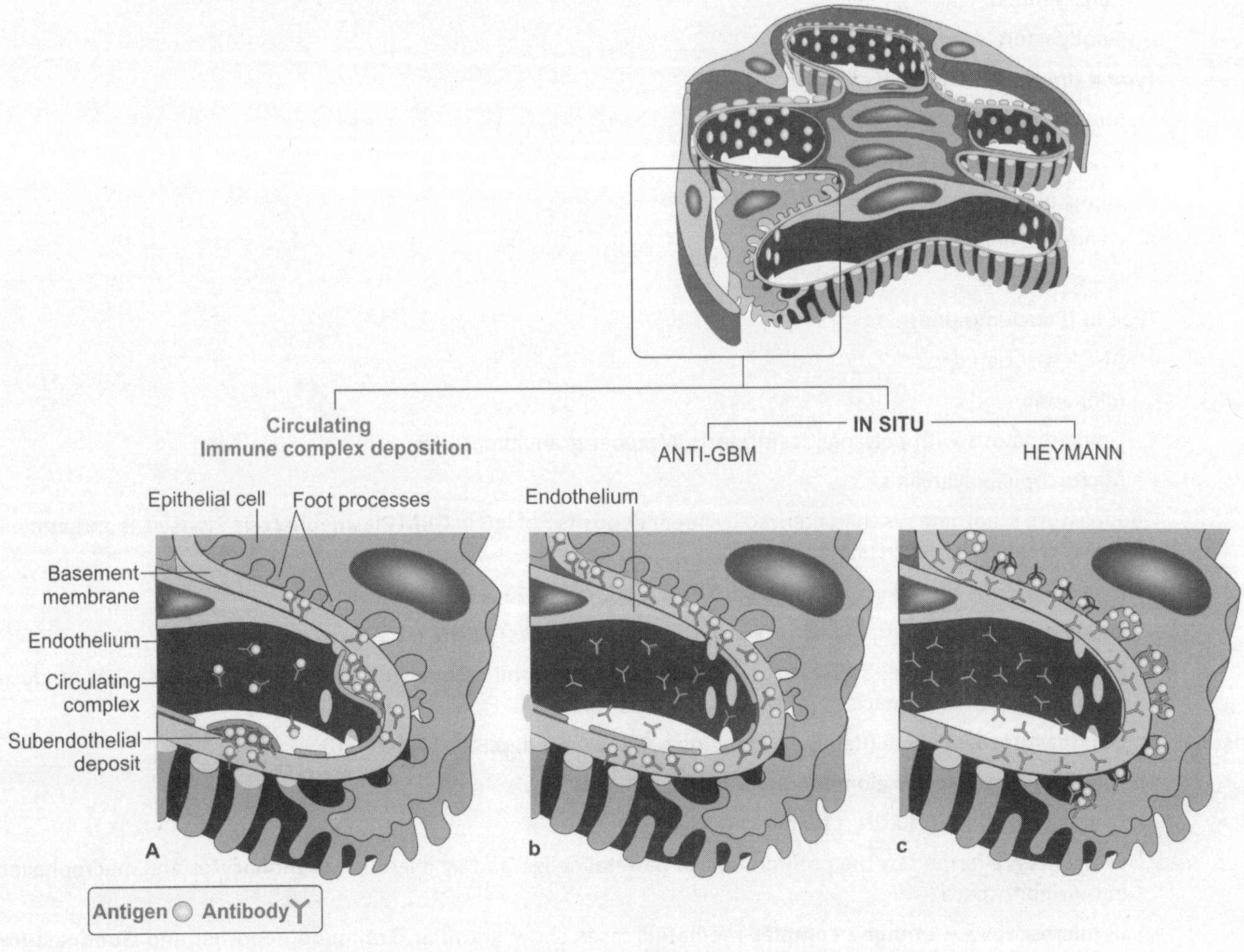

Patterns of antibody-mediated glomerular injury

Ans. 10) D. All of the above (Ref: 8 ed. Robbins p.917-20, 9 ed. p.909-12, f-20-9)

Post-Streptococcal Glomerulonephritis [Q]

- Appears **1 to 4 weeks** [Q] after **streptococcal infection** of the pharynx or skin (impetigo)
- Most common between **6 to 10 years** of age
- Caused by **group A β-hemolytic streptococci** [Q] (types 12, 4, and 1)
- **IF** – shows **granular deposits** [Q] of IgG and C3 in **mesangium** and along the **GBM**
- **EM** – discrete, amorphous, **sub-epithelial "humps"** [Q] are seen
- **Laboratory findings: Elevation** of **anti-streptococcal antibody** [Q] titers and decline in **serum concentration of C3**

Ans. 11) A. Parietal epithelial cells (Ref: 8 ed. Robbins p.920-21, 9 ed. p.912-13, t-20-6)

Rapidly Progressive Glomerulonephritis (RPGN) [Q]:

- Characterized by the presence of **crescents** in most of the glomeruli **(crescentic glomerulonephritis)** [Q]
- Occurs due to the proliferation of **parietal epithelial cells** [Q]

Ans. 12) A. Plasmapheresis (Ref: 8 ed. Robbins p.920-21, 9 ed. p.912-13, t-20-6)

Classification of RPGN [Q]

Type I (Anti-GBM Antibody)

- Renal limited
- Goodpasture syndrome

Type II (Immune Complex)

- Idiopathic
- Post infectious glomerulonephritis
- Lupus nephritis
- Henoch-Schönlein purpura
- IgA nephropathy

Type III (Pauci-Immune)

- ANCA-associated
- Idiopathic
- Granulomatosis with polyangiitis (formerly Wegener granulomatosis)
- Microscopic polyangiitis

Goodpasture syndrome [Q] is characterized by **linear deposits** [Q] of **IgG** in **GBM Plasmapheresis** [Q] is used as a treatment modality to remove the circulating antibodies

Ans. 13) C. Lupus nephritis (Ref: 8 ed. Robbins p.920-21, 9 ed. p.912-13, t-20-6)

- **Lupus nephritis** is associated with **Type II (Immune complex) RPGN** [Q]
- **Type III (Pauci-immune) RPGN** has circulating **anti-neutrophil cytoplasmic antibodies (ANCAs)** [Q] that produce cytoplasmic (c) or perinuclear (p) staining pattern

Ans. 14) D. Goodpasture syndrome (Ref: 8 ed. Robbins p.920-21, 9 ed. p.912-12, f-20-10)

Morphology of crescentic glomerulonephritis [Q]:

- Histologic picture of RPGN is dominated by **crescents**
- Crescents are formed by the **proliferation of parietal cells** [Q] and by migration of **monocyte**s and **macrophages** into **urinary space**
- **IF microscopy** [Q] – **immune complex-mediated** cases show **granular** [Q] immune deposits; and **Goodpasture syndrome** show **linear** [Q] fluorescence pattern

Ans. 15) D. All of the above (Ref: 8 ed. Robbins p.922, 9 ed. p.914)

Manifestations of **Nephrotic Syndrome** [Q]:

- **Massive proteinuria**, with daily loss of **3.5 gm.** or more of protein
- **Hypoalbuminemia**, with plasma albumin levels less than **3 gm/dL**
- Generalized edema
- Hyperlipidemia and lipiduria
- Characterized by **highly selective proteinuria** Q which consists of **low-molecular-weight proteins – albumin and transferrin**

Ans. 16) B. Decreased synthesis of lipoproteins in liver (Ref: 8 ed. Robbins p.922, 9 ed. p.914)

- In Nephrotic syndrome patients there is **increased synthesis** of **lipoproteins** Q in liver
- Hyperlipidemia
- **Lipiduria** – Lipid appears in urine either as **free fat** or **oval fat bodies**
- **Thrombotic** and **thromboembolic complications (Renal vein thrombosis)** Q occur due to loss of endogenous anticoagulants (**Antithrombin III**) in urine

Ans. 17) A. Minimal change disease (Ref: 8 ed. Robbins p.922-23, 9 ed. p.914-15, t-20-7)

- Most common cause of **Nephrotic syndrome** in **children**: **Minimal-change disease** Q

Ans. 18) B. Membranous Nephropathy (Ref: 8 ed. Robbins p.922-23, 9 ed. p.914-15, t-20-7)

- Most common cause of N**ephrotic syndrome** in adults: **Focal Segmental Glomerulosclerosis** Q followed by **Membranous Nephropathy** Q

But in the question, FSGS is not an option so the answer here is Membranous Nephropathy

Ans. 19) A. Membranous Nephropathy (Ref: 8 ed. Robbins p.922-24, 9 ed. p.915-16, f-20-12)

Morphology of **membranous nephropathy**:

- **Light microscopy** – Diffuse thickening of **glomerular capillary wall**
- **Electron microscopy** Q – Irregular **sub-epithelial** Q **electron dense deposits**, with **effacement** of **podocyte foot processes**
- **Silver stain** shows **irregular spikes** Q protruding from the GBM
- **Immunofluorescence microscopy** demonstrate **granular deposits** Q

Ans. 20) C. Diffuse effacement of foot processes (Ref: 8 ed. Robbins p.923-26, 9 ed. p.917-18, f-20-13)

Minimal-Change Disease Q

- Characterized by **diffuse effacement of foot processes** of **podocytes** on **electron microscopy** Q
- Glomeruli appear **normal** Q by **light microscopy**
- Age group – between **2 and 6 years**

Ans. 21) D. IF shows IgG deposits (Ref: 8 ed. Robbins p.923-26, 9 ed. p.917-18, f-20-13)

Features of Lipoid Nephrosis Q

- Glomeruli are **normal** Q by light microscopy
- Shows dramatic response to **corticosteroid therapy** Q
- **Visceral epithelial cells**, shows diffuse **effacement of foot processes**
- **No immune complex deposits** are seen on Electron Microscopy

Ans. 22) B. Hodgkin lymphoma (Ref: 8 ed. Robbins p.923-26, 9 ed. p.917-18, f-20-13)

- **Hodgkin lymphoma** Q patients have **increased incidence** of developing **Minimal-change disease** Q

Ans. 23) A. HIV (Ref: 8 ed. Robbins p.926-27, 9 ed. p.919, f-20-15)

Collapsing Glomerulopathy Q:

- Morphologic variant of **FSGS**
- Characterized by **retraction and/or collapse** of the **glomerular tuft**
- Proliferation and hypertrophy of **glomerular visceral epithelial cells**

- **Prominent tubular injury**, with formation of **micro cysts**
- **Seen most commonly in HIV-associated nephropathy** Q
- Has **poor prognosis**

Ans. 24) B. Gives rise to steroid resistant nephrotic syndrome (Ref: 8 ed. Robbins p.926-27, 9 ed. p.918)

Mutations associated with **Focal segmental Glomerulosclerosis:**

NPHS1 gene mutation Q**:**

- Maps on **chromosome 19q13** and encodes the protein **nephrin** Q
- Leads to **Congenital nephrotic syndrome of the Finnish type** Q

NPHS2 gene mutation Q**:**

- Maps on **chromosome 1q25-q31** and encodes the protein product **Podocin** Q
- Leads to **steroid-resistant nephrotic syndrome** Q of childhood onset

Ans. 25) B. Podocin (Ref: 8 ed. Robbins p.926-27, 9 ed. p.918)

- Refer to explanation of answer number 24

Ans. 26) A. HIV (Ref: 8 ed. Robbins p.928, 9 ed. p.919-20)

HIV-associated nephropathy Q (severe form of **collapsing variant of FSGS**):

- Characterized by presence of **large numbers of tubulo-reticular inclusions** Q within **endothelial cells**, detected by **electron microscopy**

Ans. 27) C. Hepatitis B (Ref: 8 ed. Robbins p.928, 9 ed. p.920)

- Proteins derived from **infectious agents** such as **Hepatitis C** and **B viruses** Q are the antigens involved in **Membranoproliferative Glomerulonephritis**

Ans. 28) B. Dense deposit disease (Ref: 8 ed. Robbins p.928-929, 9 ed. p.922, f-20-18)

Dense-deposit disease (type II MPGN) Q:

- Characterized by **excessive activation** of **alternative complement pathway** Q
- Patients have circulating autoantibody termed **C3 nephritic factor (C3NeF)** Q, resulting in persistent C3 activation and **hypocomplementemia**

Ans. 29) A. MPGN (Ref: 8 ed. Robbins p.928-929, 9 ed. p.920-922, f-20-16,17)

Morphology of MPGN Q**:**

- Glomeruli are large and **hyper-cellular** (**mesangial** and **endocapillary proliferation**)
- GBM is thickened, and shows a **"double-contour"** or **"tram-track" appearance** Q
- **"Duplication"** of the basement membrane (**splitting**) Q

Ans. 30) A. Mesangiocapillary glomerulonephritis (Ref: 8 ed. Robbins p.928-929, 9 ed. p.920-922, f-20-16,17)

- **Mesangiocapillary/Membranoproliferative glomerulonephritis** is associated with both **sub-endothelial** and **basement membrane** deposits Q
- **Immunofluorescence – granular** or **linear** pattern of staining

Ans. 31) D. All of the above (Ref: 8 ed. Robbins p.929, 9 ed. p. 922)

Secondary MPGN Q can be seen with:

A) Chronic immune complex disorders:

- SLE; **hepatitis B** Q; **hepatitis C** Q, **Cryoglobulinemia**; endocarditis; infected ventriculoatrial shunts; chronic visceral abscesses; HIV infection and schistosomiasis

B) α1-Antitrypsin deficiency

C) Malignant diseases – Chronic Lymphocytic Leukemia Q

Ans. 32) A. IgA nephropathy (Ref: 8 ed. Robbins p.929-31, 9 ed. p. 923-24, f- 20-19)

Salient Features of IgA Nephropathy (Buerger Disease) Q**:**

- **Most common** Q type of glomerulonephritis worldwide
- Characterized by **recurrent hematuria** Q and **prominent IgA deposits** in the mesangial regions
- IgA deposits are also present in **Henoch-Schönlein purpura** Q
- Occurs with **increased frequency** in individuals with **gluten enteropathy (celiac disease)** Q
- Immunofluorescence shows **mesangial deposition of IgA**

Ans. 33) D. All of the above (Ref: 8 ed. Robbins p.931-32, 9 ed. p. 924, f-20-20)

Hereditary nephritis includes:

- **Alport's syndrome** and **Benign Familial hematuria**

Alport Syndrome Q:

- Characterized by **hematuria, nerve deafness** and **eye disorders**, including lens dislocation, posterior cataracts and corneal dystrophy

Electron Microscopy Q:

- Glomerular basement membrane shows **alternate foci of thickening with attenuation** (thinning) and **splitting** and lamination of the lamina densa, producing a distinctive **basket-weave appearance** Q

Ans. 34) A. COL4A5 (Ref: 8 ed. Robbins p.931-32, 9 ed. p. 924, f-20-20)

- Patients with **deletions** in **Collagen IV α5 chain (COL4A5)** Q are at risk for developing **end stage renal disease** at an earlier age

Ans. 35) C. 300-400 nm (Ref: 8 ed. Robbins p.932, 9 ed. p. 925)

- Normal basement membrane width is **300 to 400 nm** in healthy adults

Thin Basement Membrane Lesion (Benign Familial Hematuria):

- Characterized by **familial asymptomatic hematuria** Q
- Characterized by **diffuse thinning of the GBM** to width between **150 and 225 nm** Q

Ans. 36) C. Post streptococcal glomerulonephritis (Ref: 8 ed. Robbins p.932-33, 9 ed. p. 925, f-20-21)

Conditions which **predispose** to **chronic glomerulonephritis** Q:

- Crescentic glomerulonephritis (RPGN)
- Focal Segmental Glomerulosclerosis
- Membranoproliferative glomerulonephritis
- Membranous nephropathy
- IgA nephropathy

Post-streptococcal glomerulonephritis is **least** Q associated with development of **chronic glomerulonephritis**

Ans. 37) A. Asymmetrical contracted kidney (Ref: 8 ed. Robbins p.933, 9 ed. p. 925, f-20-21)

Morphology of kidney in **chronic glomerulonephritis**:

- **Symmetrically contracted** Q
- **Diffusely granular cortical surfaces** Q of the kidney
- **Cortex is thinned** Q with **obliteration of glomeruli** by acellular eosinophilic masses

Ans. 38) D. All of the above (Ref: 8 ed. Robbins p.934-35, 9 ed. p. 1118-19, f-24-37,38,39)

Glomerular lesions in **diabetic patients** include:

- **Capillary basement membrane thickening, diffuse mesangial sclerosis**, and **nodular glomerulosclerosis** Q

Ans. 39) D. Any of the above (Ref: 8 ed. Robbins p.934-35)

Diabetic Glomerulosclerosis Q

- Occurs due to **increased** amounts of **type IV collagen** Q, **fibronectin** and **reactive oxygen species** and **decreased** heparin sulfate

Ans. 40) D. All of the above (Ref: 8 ed. Robbins p.935-36, 9 ed. p. 927)

ATI (Acute tubular injury) predisposing factors include [Q]:

- **Ischemia**, due to decreased or interrupted blood flow
- Direct **toxic injury** to the tubules by **drugs** or dyes
- **Urinary obstruction** by tumors, prostatic hypertrophy

Ans. 41) D. Both a & b (Ref: 8 ed. Robbins p.937, 9 ed. p. 929)

Tamm-Horsfall Protein [Q]

- Urinary glycoprotein secreted by the cells of **ascending thick limb** [Q] and **distal tubules** [Q]

Ans. 42) A. Proximal convoluted tubule (Ref: 8 ed. Robbins p.937-38, 9 ed. p. 929)

- **Toxic Acute Tubular Injury** [Q] most commonly affects **Proximal Convoluted Tubules** [Q]. E.g. **mercuric chloride poisoning** [Q]

Ans. 43) B. Calcium oxalate crystals (Ref: 8 ed. Robbins p.938, 9 ed. p. 929)

- **Carbon tetrachloride poisoning** [Q] – Characterized by accumulation of **neutral lipids** [Q] in injured cells
- **Ethylene glycol** [Q] poisoning produces vacuolar degeneration of **proximal convoluted tubules** [Q] and **calcium oxalate crystals** [Q] are found in tubular lumens

Ans. 44) C. Recovery phase (Ref: 8 ed. Robbins p.938, 9 ed. p. 929)

Clinical course of ATI can be divided into **three stages**:

a) **Initiation phase** – Characterized by **oliguria** [Q]

b) **Maintenance phase** – Oliguria, salt and water overload, rising BUN concentrations, hyperkalemia, metabolic acidosis

c) **Recovery phase** – Increase in **urine volume** up to **3 L/day** [Q] and **hypokalemia** [Q]

Ans. 45) C. Both a & b (Ref: 8 ed. Robbins p.939-41, 9 ed. p. 930-34, f-20-31)

- **Most common cause** of **Pyelonephritis** include **Ascending Infection** [Q] i.e. the spread of infection from urethra to bladder and kidneys

Mechanisms by which the infection moves from **bladder to kidney**:

Urinary tract obstruction and stasis of urine [Q]

Vesicoureteral reflux [Q]

Intra-renal reflux [Q]:

- Infected bladder urine can propel into the renal pelvis
- **Most common** [Q] in the **upper and lower poles** [Q] of the kidney, where **papillae** tend to have **flattened** or **concave tips** [Q]
- Can be demonstrated **radiographically** by **voiding cystourethrogram** [Q]

Ans. 46) D. Any of the above (Ref: 8 ed. Robbins p.941-42, 9 ed. p. 931-32, f-20-27-29)

Complications of **acute pyelonephritis:**

- **Papillary necrosis** [Q] – Seen in diabetics, sickle cell disease, urinary tract obstruction
- **Pyonephrosis** [Q]
- **Perinephric abscess** [Q]

Ans. 47) B. Chronic pyelonephritis (Ref: 8 ed. Robbins p.942-44, 9 ed. p. 933-35, f-20-31,32)

Morphology of Chronic Pyelonephritis [Q]:

- **Asymmetric** and **irregular scarring of kidneys** [Q]
- In contrast, however in **chronic glomerulonephritis** [Q], both kidneys are **diffusely and symmetrically** scarred [Q]
- **Coarse, discrete, corticomedullary scars** [Q] present over the **dilated, blunted, or deformed calyces**, with flattening of the papillae
- **Scars** are most commonly located in **upper** [Q] and **lower poles** [Q]

Microscopy ᵠ:

- Tubules show **atrophy** ᵠ in some areas and **hypertrophy or dilation** ᵠ in others
- **Dilated tubules** are filled with casts resembling **thyroid colloid (Thyroidisation)** ᵠ

Ans. 48) B. Xanthogranulomatous pyelonephritis (Ref: 8 ed. Robbins p.943, 9 ed. p. 934)

Xanthogranulomatous pyelonephritis ᵠ:

- Rare form of **chronic pyelonephritis**
- Characterized by accumulation of **foamy macrophages** ᵠ and plasma cells, lymphocytes, polymorphs and occasional giant cells
- Associated with **Proteus infection** ᵠ and obstruction
- Lesions produce **large, yellowish** ᵠ orange nodules and on **gross examination** can be confused with **renal cell carcinoma** ᵠ

Ans. 49) D. All of the above (Ref: 8 ed. Robbins p.944-46, 9 ed. p. 935-36)

NSAID-associated renal syndromes ᵠ include:

- **Acute kidney injury**
- Acute hypersensitivity **interstitial nephritis**
- Acute interstitial nephritis and **minimal-change disease**
- **Membranous nephropathy**

Ans. 50) B. Urothelial papillary carcinoma of renal pelvis (Ref: 8 ed. Robbins p.946, 9 ed. p. 936)

- **Analgesic nephropathy** predisposes to **Urothelial carcinoma of the renal pelvis – 9 ed.**
- Patients with **analgesic nephropathy** develop **Transitional papillary carcinoma** of the **renal pelvis – 8 ed.**

Ans. 51) D. All of the above (Ref: 8 ed. Robbins p.946, 9 ed. p. 936, t-20-9)

Papillary necrosis ᵠ **is associated with**:

- **Analgesic nephropathy, Diabetes mellitus, Urinary tract obstruction**, **Sickle cell disease** or trait and **renal tuberculosis** (focally)

Ans. 52) D. All of the above (Ref: 8 ed. Robbins p.948, 9 ed. p. 937-38, f-20-35)

Renal damage in **Light-Chain Cast Nephropathy ("Myeloma Kidney")** ᵠ occurs due to:

- Deposition of **Bence-Jones protein** ᵠ in renal tubular epithelial cells
- **Amyloidosis (AL type)** ᵠ – Formed from free light chains (usually of λ type)
- **Light-chain deposition disease – light chains** (of κ type) deposit in GBMs and mesangium
- Hypercalcemia and hyperuricemia

Ans. 53) D. GFR is markedly reduced (Ref: 8 ed. Robbins p.949, 9 ed. p. 938-39, f-20-36)

Benign Nephrosclerosis ᵠ:

- Associated with **hypertension** ᵠ
- Associated with **sclerosis of renal arterioles and small arteries**

Morphology:

- Kidneys are either **normal** or **moderately reduced** ᵠ in size
- Cortical surface have a fine granularity that resembles **grain leather** ᵠ
- **Histologic examination** ᵠ – Narrowing of the lumens of arterioles, due to thickening and hyalinization of the walls (**hyaline arteriolosclerosis**) ᵠ

Ans. 54) D. All of the above (Ref: 8 ed. Robbins p.949-51, 9 ed. p. 939-40, f-20-37,38)

Malignant or Accelerated Hypertension:

- **Malignant nephrosclerosis** is associated renal vascular disorder
- **Hyperplastic arteriolosclerosis** ᵠ is a characteristic feature
- Patients have markedly **elevated levels** of plasma **renin**

Morphology ^{Q}:

- **Small, pinpoint petechial hemorrhages** appear on the **cortical surface** resulting in **"flea-bitten" appearance** ^{Q} of kidney
- **Fibrinoid necrosis** ^{Q} of the arterioles – Producing smudgy eosinophilic appearance due to fibrin deposition of the vessel wall
- **Hyperplastic arteriolitis/onion-skinning** ^{Q} of the vessel wall

Ans. 55) A. Atheromatous plaque (Ref: 8 ed. Robbins p.951-52, 9 ed. p. 940-41, f-20-39)

Renal Artery Stenosis ^{Q}:

- **Most common cause** – Narrowing of the renal artery by **Atheromatous plaque** ^{Q}, occurs more frequently in **men**
- **Second most frequent** cause is **Fibromuscular dysplasia** ^{Q} of the **renal artery**, more common in **women** and occurs in younger age group

Ans. 56) D. All of above (Ref: 8 ed. Robbins p.952-54, 9 ed. p. 941-43, f-20-40)

Thrombotic Microangiopathies ^{Q}:

- Characterized by – **Microangiopathic hemolytic anemia, thrombocytopenia, renal failure** and thrombotic lesions in capillaries and arterioles

Ans. 57) A. E. coli (Ref: 8 ed. Robbins p.952-54, 9 ed. p. 941-43)

Typical hemolytic uremic syndrome ^{Q} – Occurs following intestinal infection with strains of **E. coli** (the most common being **O157:H7**) ^{Q} that produce **Shiga-like toxins**

Ans. 58) A. Factor H deficiency (Ref: 8 ed. Robbins p.952-54, 9 ed. p. 941-43)

Atypical HUS:

- Occurs due to **inherited deficiency** of complement regulatory proteins; most commonly **Factor H** ^{Q}, which inhibits C3 convertase
- Other protein deficiency which can be seen – **Complement Factor I** and **CD46 (membrane cofactor protein)**

Ans. 59) D. Absence of neurological symptoms (Ref: 8 ed. Robbins p.952-54, 9 ed. p. 941-43)

TTP ^{Q}:

- Manifested by the **pentad** of **fever, neurologic symptoms, microangiopathic hemolytic anemia, thrombocytopenia and renal failure** ^{Q}
- Most common cause is **deficient ADAMTS13 activity** ^{Q}
- **ADAMTS 13** is a **negative regulator of vWF** ^{Q}
- Deficiency of ADAMTS 13 permits the formation of abnormally **large multimers of vWF**

Ans. 60) C. Multicystic renal dysplasia (Ref: 8 ed. Robbins p.955-56, 9 ed. p. 949, f-20-46)

Multicystic Renal Dysplasia ^{Q}:

- **Most common form** of **cystic renal disease** in children
- **Most common cause** of **abdominal mass in newborns** ^{Q}
- Can be **unilateral** or **bilateral**

Important Points to Remember:

- **Neuroblastoma** is the **most common extra-cranial solid tumor** ^{Q} of childhood, seen in **infancy** ^{Q}
- **Wilms Tumor** – Most common **primary renal tumor of childhood** ^{Q}
- **Mesoblastic nephroma** is a **congenital renal neoplasm** ^{Q} that is discovered before 6 months of age

Ans. 61) D. All of the above (Ref: 8 ed. Robbins p.956-59, 9 ed. p. 945-47)

Genetics of Autosomal Dominant (Adult) Polycystic Kidney Disease ^{Q}:

- **PKD1 gene** is located on **chromosome 16p** and encodes **polycystin-1**
- **Polycystin-1** is expressed in **tubular epithelial cells**
- **PKD2 gene** is located on **chromosome 4q**, and encodes **polycystin-2**

Ans. 62) D. All of the above (Ref: 8 ed. Robbins p.958, 9 ed. p. 947)

Extra-renal congenital anomalies Q seen in patients with **polycystic kidney disease**:

- **Polycystic liver disease**
- Cysts occur much less frequently in **spleen, pancreas and lungs**
- **Intracranial berry aneurysms** Q
- **Mitral valve prolapse** Q

Ans. 63) B. Autosomal Recessive Polycystic Kidney Disease (Ref: 8 ed. Robbins p.959, 9 ed. p. 947-48)

Autosomal recessive (childhood) polycystic kidney disease Q:

- Caused by **mutations** of the **PKHD1 gene**, located on **chromosome 6p** Q
- **PKHD1 gene** encodes **fibrocystin** Q
- Associated with **congenital hepatic fibrosis** Q

Ans. 64) D. Acquired cystic disease (Ref: 8 ed. Robbins p.960, 9 ed. p. 949)

Acquired (Dialysis-Associated) Cystic Disease Q:

- In patients undergoing dialysis, there is **increased risk of renal cell carcinoma** Q

Ans. 65) D. All of the above (Ref: 8 ed. Robbins p.960-62, 9 ed. p. 950-51, f-20-47,48)

Common causes of obstructive uropathy Q include:

- **Congenital anomalies**: Posterior urethral valves, urethral strictures, meatal stenosis
- Urinary calculi, Benign prostatic hypertrophy
- **Tumors**: Carcinoma of the prostate, bladder tumors, retroperitoneal lymphoma, carcinoma of the cervix or uterus
- **Inflammation**: Prostatitis, ureteritis, urethritis, retroperitoneal fibrosis
- Sloughed papillae or blood clots, Pregnancy, Uterine prolapse and cystocele
- Functional disorders: Neurogenic (spinal cord damage or diabetic nephropathy)

Ans. 66) D. Nephrocalcin (Ref: 8 ed. Robbins p.962-63, 9 ed. p. 951-52)

- Predisposing factors for stone formation in urine: **Hypercalciuria** Q, **Hyperoxaluria** Q and **Hyperuricosuria** Q
- **Inhibitors of crystal formation** Q in urine includes – **Pyrophosphate, diphosphonate**, citrate, **glycosaminoglycan, osteopontin**, and a glycoprotein called **nephrocalcin** Q

Ans. 67) B. Magnesium ammonium phosphate stones (Ref: 8 ed. Robbins p.962-63, 9 ed. p. 951-52, t-20-12)

Magnesium ammonium phosphate stones Q or **Struvite stones**:

- Occurs due to **infection** by **urea-splitting bacteria (e.g. Proteus)** Q that convert **urea to ammonia**
- **Alkaline urine** Q causes the precipitation of **magnesium ammonium phosphate salts**
- Large stones are called as **staghorn calculi** Q

Ans. 68) B. Magnesium ammonium phosphate stones (Ref: 8 ed. Robbins p.962-63, 9 ed. p. 951-52, t-20-12)

- Refer to above question for explanation

Ans. 69) B. TSC-1 (Ref: 8 ed. Robbins p.963, 9 ed. p. 952-53)

Angiomyolipomas Q:

- Associated with **tuberous sclerosis** Q (due to **loss-of-function mutations** in the **TSC1 or TSC2 suppressor genes** Q)

Tuberous sclerosis patients may predispose to:

- **Facial angiofibroma, pulmonary lymphangiomyomas, sub ependymal giant astrocytoma** and **cardiac rhabdomyomas** Q

Ans. 70) C. Collecting duct (Ref: 8 ed. Robbins p.964, 9 ed. p. 953)

- **Oncocytoma** Q is thought to arise from the **intercalated cells of collecting ducts** Q

Ans. 71) D. All of the above (Ref: 8 ed. Robbins p.964, 9 ed. p. 953)

Risk factors Q for developing **renal cell carcinoma** Q:

- **Cigarette smoking (most common)** Q, **obesity**, hypertension, estrogen therapy

- Exposure to asbestos, petroleum products and heavy metals
- **Increased risk** in patients with **end stage renal disease**, chronic kidney disease, acquired cystic disease and tuberous sclerosis

Ans. 72) D. All of the above (Ref: 8 ed. Robbins p.964, 9 ed. p. 953)

Following increases the **risk** for **renal cell carcinoma**:

- **Von Hippel-Lindau (VHL) syndrome** Q – In development of familial and sporadic clear cell carcinomas
- **Hereditary leiomyomatosis** and **renal cell cancer syndrome** (HLRCC) Q – Due to **mutation** of the **FH gene**, which expresses **fumarate hydratase**
- **Hereditary papillary carcinoma** Q – ***MET* proto-oncogene** mutation
- **Birt-Hogg-Dubé syndrome** Q – Due to mutations involving the **BHD gene**, which expresses **folliculin**

Ans. 73) A. Clear cell carcinoma (Ref: 8 ed. Robbins p.964, 9 ed. p. 954, f-20-50)

Clear Celi Carcinoma Q:

- **Most common type** Q of renal cell carcinoma
- Associated with **deletion of chromosome 3p**, which harbors VHL gene
- **VHL gene** acts as **tumor suppressor gene** Q in both **sporadic** and **familial** cancers

Ans. 74) A. 3p (Ref: 8 ed. Robbins p.964, 9 ed. p. 954, f-20-50)

- Refer to answer 73 for details

Ans. 75) D. All of the above (Ref: 8 ed. Robbins p.964, 9 ed. p. 953, f-20-50)

Cytogenetics of Papillary Carcinoma Q:

- **Most common** Q cytogenetic abnormalities are **Trisomy 7 and 17, loss of Y** in male patients in **sporadic form** and **trisomy 7** in **familial form**
- Chromosome 7 encodes proto-oncogene **MET** Q
- MET encodes the receptor for **hepatocyte growth factor (scatter factor)** Q

Ans. 76) C. Collecting ducts (Ref: 8 ed. Robbins p.964-65, 9 ed. p. 954)

- **Chromophobe carcinoma** arises from **intercalated cells of collecting ducts** Q
- **Clear cell carcinomas** arise from **proximal tubular epithelium** Q
- **Papillary carcinomas** are thought to arise from **distal convoluted tubules** Q and are multifocal and bilateral

Ans. 77) C. Chromophobe carcinoma (Ref: 8 ed. Robbins p.965, 9 ed. p. 954)

- **Chromophobe carcinoma** has **excellent prognosis** Q

Ans. 78) D. All of the above (Ref: 8 ed. Robbins p.966, 9 ed. p. 955)

Paraneoplastic syndromes associated with **Renal cell carcinomas** Q:

- **Polycythemia**, **hypercalcemia**, hypertension, hepatic dysfunction, feminization or masculinization, **Cushing syndrome**, eosinophilia, Leukemoid reactions and **amyloidosis**

Ans. 79) C. Renal vein (Ref: 8 ed. Robbins p.966, 9 ed. p. 955)

- **RCC metastasizes to the lungs and bones** Q followed by the regional lymph nodes, liver, adrenal and brain
- RCC can **invade** the **renal vein** Q, which leads to decreased survival rates

Ans. 80) C. TFE3 (Ref: 9 ed. Robbins p.955)

Xp11 translocation carcinoma Q:

- Occurs in **young patients**
- Defined by translocations of ***TFE3* gene** located at Xp11.2, which result in **overexpression of the TFE3** Q transcription factor

Ans. 81) B. INI-1 (Ref: 10 ed. Ackerman, p.1182-83)

- **Rhabdoid tumors of kidney** results from **biallelic alteration** (deletion or mutation) of **hSNF5/INI1 locus** Q at chromosome **22q11.2**

Ans. 82) B. Medullary renal cell cancer (Ref: 10 ed. Ackerman, p.1189)

- **Renal medullary carcinoma** is a rare **malignant renal neoplasm**, which occurs in young black patients with **sickle cell disease** Q

Ans. 83) D. All of the above (Ref: 10 ed. Ackerman, p.1184)

Following tumors can show **occasional regression** without treatment:

- **Renal cell carcinoma (RCC)** [Q], gestational choriocarcinoma, malignant melanoma, and neuroblastoma

Ans. 84) C. Hale colloidal iron (Ref: 10 ed. Ackerman, p.1189)

- **Chromophobe RCC** cells shows cytoplasmic **vesicles**, which stain for **Hale colloidal iron** [Q]

Ans. 85) A. Alport's syndrome (Ref: 9 ed. Robbins p. 924) Refer Q 34 for details

Ans. 86) B. Alport's syndrome (Ref: 9 ed. Robbins p. 924) Refer Q 33 for details

Ans. 87) D. Nephritic syndrome (Ref: 9 ed. Robbins p. 909-913) Refer Q 10 for details

Ans. 88) C. 40-60% (Ref: Heptinstall Pathology of the kidney volume-1, p. 463)

- Pediatric renal involvement in HSP is between 20-56% and in adults – 50-78%

Ans. 89) A. Flea-bitten kidney (Ref: 9 ed. Robbins p. ed. p. 939-40) Refer Q 54 for details

Ans. 90) D. Collecting ducts (Ref: 9 ed. Robbins p. 954) Refer Q 76 & 77 for details

Ans. 91) A. Diabetes Mellitus> B. Analgesic nephropathy

Ans. 92) A. X-linked (Ref: 9 ed. Robbins p. 924)

Ans. 93) A. Membranous glomerulonephritis (Ref: 9 ed. Robbins p. 914-15) Refer Q 18 for details

Ans. 94) A. Rapidly Progressive Glomerulonephritis

- Most common cause of Nephritic Syndrome: Rapidly progressive glomerulonephritis (Post streptococcal and nonstreptococcal glomerulonephritis

Ans. 95) A. Bowman's capsule (Ref: 9 ed. Robbins p. 900)

- In Bowman's capsule, visceral epithelial cells (podocytes) become an intrinsic part of the capillary wall, separated from endothelial cells by a basement membrane

Ans. 96) A. Fibrinogen (Ref: 9 ed. Robbins p. 914) Refer Q 15 & 16 for details

Ans. 97) D. Monosomy of 1 and Y (-1, -Y) (Ref: 9 ed. Robbins p. 953, Refer Q 72, 73 & 75 for details of Cytogenetics of RCC. After going through several books and Internet, option D becomes an answer of exclusion

Ans. 98) B. Alport's syndrome (Ref: 9 ed. Robbins p. 924) Refer Q 33 for details, Q 40 (Ch. 15) for Good pasture syndrome

Ans. 99) A. Loss of Antithrombin III (Ref: 9 ed. Robbins p. 914) Refer Q 16 for details

Ans. 100) B. Presence of tuberculous infection (Ref: 9 ed. Robbins p. 934) Refer Q 48 for details

Ans. 101) A. No IgG deposits or C3 deposition on renal biopsy (Ref: 9 ed. Robbins p. 914) Refer Q 15 for details

Ans. 102) C. Protein loss (Ref: 9 ed. Robbins p.914) Refer Ans 15 for details

Ans. 103) A. Membranous (Ref: 9 ed. Robbins p.914-15)

Membranous nephropathy is the most common cause of adult-onset nephrotic syndrome and is associated with:

- Drugs (penicillamine, captopril, gold, nonsteroidal anti-inflammatory drugs (NSAIDs)
- Carcinomas of lung and colon and melanoma
- SLE
- Infections (chronic hepatitis B, hepatitis C, syphilis, schistosomiasis, malaria)
- Autoimmune disorders (thyroiditis)

Ans. 104) B. NPHS (Ref: 9 ed. Robbins p.918) Refer Q 24 for details

Ans. 105) A. Focal segmental glomerulosclerosis (Ref: 9 ed. Robbins p.914-15) Refer Q 18 for details

Ans. 106) A. Micro RNA -122 (Ref: Ackerman 10 ed p. 1308, internet)

Acute kidney injury:

Biomarker Types	Biomarkers
Functional markers	SCr and plasma/serum Cystatin C
Up-Regulated markers	NGAL,KIM-1, L-FABP, IL-18
Low molecular weight proteins	Urine Cystatin C

Biomarkers of acute kidney injury (AKI):

Neutophil Gelatinase Associated Lipocalin (NGAL)	- Excellent biomarker in urine and plasma - For early prediction of AKI - For prognosis of AKI - For monitoring of clinical trials in AKI
Kidney Injury Molecule-1 (KIM-1)	- Detectable in urine soon after AKI
Cystatin C	- Serum Cys-C is sensitive serum marker of GFR - Urinary Cys-C levels have been found to be elevated in individuals with known tubular dysfunction

Ans. 107) D. Hydronephrosis with chronic pyelonephritis (Ref: 9 ed. Robbins p. 933-35) Refer Q 47 for details

Ans. 108) C. Diabetic nephropathy (Ref: 9 ed. Robbins p. 1117)

- Manifestation of chronic diabetes on kidneys is due to increased levels of blood glucose levels and are not immune mediated

19 The Lower Urinary Tract and Male Genital System

How to go about this chapter?

- **One should be thorough with the following topics:**
  - **Malakoplakia**
  - **Urothelial cancer of bladder**
  - **Bowen disease**
  - **Cryptorchidism**
  - **Intra-tubular germ cell neoplasia**
  - **Seminoma, Embryonal carcinoma, Yolk sac tumor, Leydig Cell Tumor**
  - **Benign prostatic hyperplasia, Prostatic cancer**

URETER

1) Hemorrhagic cystitis can be seen due to following infection:
a) Adenovirus b) Chlamydia
c) Mycoplasma d) Tuberculosis

URINARY BLADDER

2) All are TRUE about Malakoplakia of bladder EXCEPT:
a) Soft yellow mucosal plaques
b) Microscopy shows infiltrating large foamy macrophages
c) Michaelis-Gutmann bodies is a characteristic feature
d) Mycobacterium tuberculosis is the causative agent

3) In Urothelial cancer, prognosis is worse when there is invasion of:
a) Lamina propria
b) Muscularis mucosa
c) Muscularis propria
d) Any of the above

4) Loss of polarity and cohesiveness in urothelium/ transitional epithelium is seen in all EXCEPT:
a) Urothelial papilloma
b) High grade Papillary Urothelial cancer
c) Carcinoma in situ
d) Invasive Urothelial cancer

5) Pagetoid spread of tumor cells are seen in:
a) Carcinoma In Situ
b) Papillomas
c) Papillary urothelial cancers
d) Squamous cell carcinomas

6) Schistosomiasis of the bladder predisposes to:
a) Squamous cell carcinoma
b) Transitional cell carcinoma
c) Adenocarcinoma
d) Small cell carcinoma

7) Following is/are the risk factors for developing bladder cancer:
a) Cigarette smoking
b) Exposure to cyclophosphamide
c) Analgesics
d) All of above

8) Superficial papillary tumors of bladder is/are associated with:
a) 9p deletion
b) 17p deletion
c) p53 mutation
d) Any of the above

9) Most common sarcoma of the bladder in adults:
a) Leiomyosarcoma
b) Embryonal rhabdomyosarcoma
c) Synovial sarcoma
d) Pleomorphic sarcoma

URETHRA

10) Most common agent responsible for Non-Gonococcal urethritis:
a) E. coli
b) Chlamydia
c) Mycoplasma
d) Proteus

11) **Tumors in proximal urethra show(s):**
a) Urothelial differentiation
b) Squamous cell differentiation
c) Glandular differentiation
d) None of the above

PENIS

12) **Condyloma Acuminatum is most commonly associated with following infection:**
a) HPV-6 b) HPV-16
c) HPV-18 d) HPV-11

13) **Bowen disease is most commonly associated with following infection:**
a) HPV-6
b) HPV-16
c) HPV-18
d) HPV-11

14) **Bowenoid papulosis all are TRUE EXCEPT:**
a) Occurs in sexually active adults
b) Occurs at a younger age
c) Associated with HPV-16 infection
d) Can develop into invasive cancer

TESTIS AND EPIDIDYMIS

15) **FALSE about Cryptorchidism:**
a) Testicular descent is hormonally dependent
b) Histological changes in affected testes begin to appear at 2 years of age
c) Orchiopexy is treatment of choice
d) Contralateral testis never shows malignant change

16) **Most common causative agent for epididymitis in younger individuals:**
a) C. trachomatis
b) E. Coli
c) Pseudomonas
d) Any of the above

17) **Most common benign para testicular tumor:**
a) Adenomatoid tumor
b) Mesothelioma
c) Liposarcoma
d) Rhabdomyosarcoma

18) **Most common risk factor for the development of Mediastinal germ cell tumors:**
a) Exposures to pesticide
b) Exposure to non-steroidal estrogen
c) Cryptorchidism
d) Klinefelter syndrome

19) **TRUE about intra-tubular germ cell neoplasia:**
a) Precursor lesion of testicular germ cell tumors
b) Cells express OCT3/4 and NANOG
c) Shows reduplication of the chromosome 12p
d) All of the above

20) **All are TRUE about seminoma of testes EXCEPT:**
a) Most common germ cell tumor
b) Cut surface of tumor shows extensive necrotic areas
c) Sheets of tumor cells divided into lobules by delicate fibrous septa
d) May contain synctiotrophoblastic cells

21) **All are TRUE about spermatocytic seminoma EXCEPT:**
a) Occurs in older age group
b) Associated with poor prognosis
c) Lack lymphocytes and granulomas
d) Spireme chromatin pattern

22) **Marker(s) to differentiate seminoma from embryonal cancer include(s):**
a) CD30
b) OCT3/4
c) PLAP
d) Any of the above

23) **Most common testicular tumor in young children:**
a) Mature teratoma
b) Immature teratoma
c) Choriocarcinoma
d) Endodermal sinus tumor

24) **TRUE about teratoma testes:**
a) Second most common testicular neoplasm in children
b) In children it follows a benign course
c) In post-pubertal males it has malignant behavior
d) All of the above

25) **TRUE about biomarkers of testicular tumors:**
a) LDH levels are used to assess tumor burden
b) AFP levels are elevated in yolk sac tumors
c) HCG levels are elevated in choriocarcinoma
d) All of the above

26) **Gynecomastia is the most common symptom of following testicular tumor:**
a) Leydig cell tumor
b) Sertoli cell tumor
c) Seminoma
d) Teratoma

27) **Crystalloids of Rinke are seen in following testicular tumor:**
a) Sertoli cell tumor
b) Leydig cell tumor
c) Gonadoblastoma
d) Testicular lymphoma

28) **Most common testicular neoplasm in individuals above 60 years of age:**
a) Non-Hodgkin lymphoma
b) Spermatocytic seminoma
c) Sertoli-Leydig cell tumor
d) Yolk sac tumor

PROSTATE

29) Prostatic carcinoma arises most commonly from:
a) Peripheral zone
b) Transitional zone
c) Central zone
d) Peri-urethral zone

30) Enzyme(s) responsible for benign prostatic hyperplasia:
a) Type 1 5 α-reductase
b) Type 2 5 α-reductase
c) Both of the above
d) None of the above

31) All of the following prevents prostatic cancer EXCEPT:
a) Lycopenes
b) Red meat
c) Vitamin D
d) Soy products

32) Most common epigenetic alteration seen in prostatic cancer:
a) GSTP-1 gene hyper methylation
b) RB gene
c) CDKN2A gene
d) APC gene

33) Metastasis arising in prostatic cancer are:
a) Osteoblastic
b) Osteoclastic
c) Both of the above
d) None of the above

34) Most common bone involved by prostatic cancer:
a) Lumbar spine
b) Proximal femur
c) Ribs
d) Thoracic spine

35) Benign glands of prostate are differentiated from malignant glands by presence of:
a) Basal cells
b) Perineural invasion
c) Vascular invasion
d) Lymphatic invasion

36) All are TRUE about Gleason grading system EXCEPT:
a) Divided into primary and secondary grades
b) Most well differentiated tumors have grade 2
c) Least differentiated tumors have grade 10
d) Higher the grade, better the prognosis

37) Advanced metastatic prostatic cancer is treated by:
a) Orchiectomy
b) LHRH agonists
c) Both of the above
d) Brachytherapy

38) Urine biomarker useful for patients with elevated PSA levels, but negative biopsy for cancer:
a) PCA3
b) TMPRSS-2 – ERG fusion gene
c) Both of above
d) None of the above

39) Secondary involvement of prostate is seen in:
a) Urothelial cancer of bladder
b) Adenomatoid tumor of epididymis
c) Penile cancer
d) Colorectal cancer

40) Most common bladder cancer: (NEET 2014)
a) Secondaries
b) Transitional cell carcinoma
c) Sarcoma
d) Lymphoma

41) Rokitanski protuberances are seen in: (NEET 2014)
a) Mucinous carcinoma
b) Teratoma
c) Epidermal Cystadenoma
d) Papillary carcinoma

42) Transitional cell carcinoma bladder caused by: (NEET 2013)
a) Schistosomiasis
b) Ascariasis
c) Malaria
d) None of the above

43) Which of the following tumors show increased c-kit? (NEET 2013)
a) Yolk sac tumor
b) Embryonal carcinoma
c) Choriocarcinoma
d) Seminoma

44) Which of the following germ cell tumor is malignant? (NEET 2013)
a) Leydig cell tumor
b) Sertoli cell tumor
c) Seminoma
d) Dermoid cyst

CHAPTER 19: THE LOWER URINARY TRACT AND MALE GENITAL SYSTEM

Ans. 1) **A. Adenovirus (Ref: 8 ed. Robbins p.974-75, 9 ed. p.962)**

- **Common causes** of cystitis: **Escherichia coli** Q, Proteus, Klebsiella and Enterobacter

Hemorrhagic cystitis:

- Occurs due to **Adenovirus** Q **infection** and patients receiving **cyclophosphamide**

Ans. 2) **D. Mycobacterium tuberculosis is the causative agent (Ref: 8 ed. Robbins p.975, 9 ed. p.963, f-21-4,5)**

Malakoplakia Q

Etiology Q:

- **Chronic inflammatory reaction** which occurs due to **acquired defects** in **phagocyte function** Q
- Most commonly by infection e.g. – **E. coli** Q or **Proteus** species
- Occurs in **immunosuppressed** transplant recipients
- Grossly – Occurs as **soft, yellow**, slightly raised **mucosal plaques** Q
- **Microscopy** – Plaques contain **large, foamy macrophages** Q mixed with **multinucleate giant cells** Q and lymphocytes
- **Michaelis-Gutmann bodies** Q – Laminated mineralized concretions due to deposition of calcium in enlarged lysosomes, which are present in **macrophages**

Ans. 3) **C. Muscularis propria (Ref: 8 ed. Robbins p.976, 9 ed. p.964, t-21-2,3,4)**

- In **urothelial cancer, invasion of muscularis propria (detrusor muscle)** Q implies worse prognosis
- **Muscularis mucosa** is **superficial layer** and **muscularis propria** is **detrusor muscle**, the later when invaded is associated with decrease in survival
- **Muscle invasion** Q is the most important prognostic marker

Ans. 4) **A. Urothelial papilloma (Ref: 8 ed. Robbins p.977-78, 9 ed. p.965-66, f-21-6-11)**

Urothelial tumors: Arise from **lateral** or **posterior walls** at **bladder base**

- **Papillomas**: Show central core of **loose fibrovascular tissue**, which is covered by epithelium that is histologically identical to **normal urothelium** Q
- **Low-grade papillary urothelial carcinomas** Q: Show orderly **architecture** and **cytologic appearance**. The cells maintain polarity and are **cohesive**
- **High grade papillary urothelial carcinomas, Carcinoma In situ, Invasive urothelial cancers** Q are associated with loss of polarity and cohesiveness of tumor cells

Ans. 5) **A. Carcinoma in situ (Ref: 8 ed. Robbins p.978, 9 ed. p.966, f-21-11)**

Carcinoma in situ (CIS, or flat urothelial carcinoma) Q:

- Defined by the **presence of cytological malignant cells** Q within a flat urothelium
- Cells show **full-thickness cytologic atypia** and **scattered malignant cells** in the urothelium (termed as **Pagetoid spread** Q)
- **Lack of cohesiveness** Q leads to **shedding of malignant cells** into the **urine**
- **50% to 75%** of **CIS** can progress to invasive cancer if left untreated

Ans. 6) **A. Squamous cell carcinoma (Ref: 8 ed. Robbins p.979, 9 ed. p.967)**

- **Urinary schistosomiasis** Q predisposes to **squamous cell carcinomas** Q

Ans. 7) **D. All of the above (Ref: 8 ed. Robbins p.979-80, 9 ed. p.964-65)**

Factors predisposing to bladder cancer Q:

- Cigarette smoking
- Industrial exposure to **aryl amines**
- Schistosoma haematobium infection

- Long-term use of **analgesics** and exposure to **cyclophosphamide** Q
- Irradiation

Ans. 8) **A. 9p deletion (Ref: 8 ed. Robbins p.980, 9 ed. p.965)**

- **9p deletions** Q are present in **superficial noninvasive papillary tumors**
- **Low-grade, noninvasive tumors** show mutations in **HRAS oncogene** Q
- **Invasive urothelial cancers** show **chromosome 17p** Q deletion and **p53** mutation

Ans. 9) **A. Leiomyosarcoma (Ref: 8 ed. Robbins p.981, 9 ed. p.968)**

- **Most common** sarcoma affecting bladder in **infancy** Q or childhood: **embryonal rhabdomyosarcoma** Q
- **Most common sarcoma** of bladder in adults is **leiomyosarcoma** Q

Ans. 10) **B. Chlamydia (Ref: 9 ed. Robbins p.969)**

- **Chlamydia trachomatis** Q is responsible for **25% to 60%** of **non-gonococcal urethritis** Q in men

Ans. 11) **A. Urothelial differentiation (Ref: 8 ed. Robbins p.982, 9 ed. p.969)**

- Tumors arising within the **proximal urethra** Q shows **urothelial differentiation** Q
- Lesions found within **distal urethra** Q are more often **squamous cell carcinomas** Q

Ans. 12) **A. HPV-6 (Ref: 8 ed. Robbins p.983, 9 ed. p.970, f-21-15,16,17)**

Condyloma Acuminatum:

- Benign sexually transmitted wart caused by **Human Papillomavirus (HPV)** Q
- **HPV type 6** Q followed by **HPV type 11** are the most frequent agents

Ans. 13) **B. HPV-16 (Ref: 8 ed. Robbins p.983-84, 9 ed. p.971, f-21-18)**

- **Bowen disease** Q and **Bowenoid papulosis** Q histologically resemble features of **Carcinoma in situ (CIS)**
- Associated with **HPV type 16** Q infection

Bowen Disease Q**:**

- Occurs in the genital region of both **men** and **women**, **older** than **35 years**
- Involves the skin of the **shaft of the penis** and the **scrotum**
- Can transform into **infiltrating squamous cell carcinoma** Q

Ans. 14) **D. Can develop into invasive cancer (Ref: 8 ed. Robbins p.983-84, 9 ed. p.971)**

Bowenoid Papulosis Q**:**

- Occurs in sexually active adults
- Affects age group **younger than 35 years** Q
- Presents as **multiple reddish brown** Q papular lesions
- Associated with **HPV type 16 infection**
- Never predisposes to **invasive carcinoma**
- Can **regress spontaneously** Q

Ans. 15) **D. Contralateral testis never shows malignant change (Ref: 8 ed. Robbins p.984-85, 9 ed. p.972-73, f-21-20)**

Cryptorchidism Q**:**

- **Complete** or **partial failure** of **intra-abdominal testes** to descend into the **scrotal sac**
- Testicular descent is **hormone dependent**
- Occurs in two phases: **transabdominal** and **inguinoscrotal** phase
- **Most common** site of testicular arrest is **inguinal canal** Q
- Histological changes in the **undescended testis** begin as early as **2 years** Q of age
- **Orchiopexy (placement in the scrotal sac)** Q – Surgical procedure of choice, which is performed at 6 months to 1 year of age

- **Undescended testis** is at a greater risk for developing **testicular cancer** ᵠ
- Cancer can also develop in the **contralateral/normally descended testis** ᵠ

Ans. 16) A. C. trachomatis (Ref: 8 ed. Robbins p.986, 9 ed. p.973-74)

- In sexually active men **younger than 35 years** ᵠ, most frequent pathogens includes ***C. trachomatis*** and ***Neisseria gonorrhoeae***
- In men **older than 35 years, *E. coli*** and ***Pseudomonas***, are responsible for most of the infections

Ans. 17) A. Adenomatoid tumor (Ref: 8 ed. Robbins p.987, 9 ed. p.975)

- Most common **benign** paratesticular tumor is **Adenomatoid tumor** ᵠ
- Most common **malignant** paratesticular tumor: **Rhabdomyosarcoma** in **children** and **Liposarcoma** in **adults**

Ans. 18) D. Klinefelter syndrome (Ref: 8 ed. Robbins p.988, 9 ed. p.975)

Major risk factors for **Testicular germ cell tumors**:

- **Cryptorchidism** ᵠ
- Exposures to **pesticides** and **nonsteroidal estrogens** In utero
- **Klinefelter syndrome** ᵠ (patients are also at increased risk for developing **Mediastinal germ cell tumors** ᵠ)

Ans. 19) D. All of the above (Ref: 8 ed. Robbins p.988, 9 ed. p.975-76)

Intra-tubular germ cell neoplasia (ITGCN) ᵠ:

- **Precursor lesion** of **testicular germ cell tumors** ᵠ
- Cells expresses the transcription factors **OCT3/4** ᵠ and **NANOG** ᵠ
- Shows **reduplication** of chromosome 12p, in form of an **isochromosome i(12p)** ᵠ
- Activating mutation of ***C-KIT*** can be seen

Ans. 20) B. Cut surface of tumor shows extensive necrotic areas (Ref: 8 ed. Robbins p.988-89, 9 ed. p.976, f-21-23,24)

Seminomas ᵠ:

- **Most common type** ᵠ of germ cell tumor, which occurs in **third decade**
- Similar to ovarian **Dysgerminoma** ᵠ
- Contain **isochromosome 12p** ᵠ and express **OCT3/4** and **NANOG**
- Can show ***C-KIT*** ᵠ activating mutation

Morphology ᵠ:

- **Grossly** ᵠ – **Homogeneous, gray white, lobulated cut surface, devoid** of **hemorrhage or necrosis** ᵠ
- **Microscopically** ᵠ – Composed of **sheets of uniform cells**, which is divided into lobules by **delicate fibrous septa** (which has lymphocytic infiltrate)
- 15% of seminomas contain **syncytiotrophoblasts** ᵠ
- May show an ill-defined **granulomatous reaction**

Ans. 21) B. Associated with poor prognosis (Ref: 8 ed. Robbins p.989, 9 ed. p.976-77)

Spermatocytic Seminoma:

- Affects individuals older than **65 years** ᵠ and has **excellent prognosis** ᵠ
- **Cut surface** – Soft, pale gray and reveal mucoid cysts
- Shows **three cell populations** – medium-sized cells, smaller cells resembling secondary spermatocytes and scattered giant cells
- Chromatin pattern in tumor cells is similar to non-neoplastic spermatocytes **(spireme chromatin)** ᵠ
- **Lack lymphocytes** ᵠ, granulomas, syncytiotrophoblasts and admixture with other tumors
- Shows an **association with ITGCN** ᵠ

Ans. 22) A. CD30 (Ref: 8 ed. Robbins p.989, 9 ed. p.977, f-21-25,26)

- **Embryonal carcinomas** ^Q^ and **seminomas** ^Q^ both are positive for **OCT 3/4** and **PLAP**
- **Embryonal carcinomas** show **positivity** for **cytokeratin** ^Q^ and **CD30** ^Q^, but are negative for **KIT**

Salient Features of **Embryonal Carcinomas:**

- Occurs in age group of **20-30 years** ^Q^ and are **more aggressive** than **seminomas**
- **Cut surface** ^Q^ – tumor is **variegated** and **punctuated** by foci of **hemorrhage** or **necrosis**

Microscopy ^Q^:

- Cells grow in **alveolar** or **tubular patterns**
- Tumor cells are large and anaplastic with hyperchromatic nuclei with prominent nucleoli
- **Mitotic figures** and **tumor giant cells** are frequently seen

Ans. 23) D. Endodermal sinus tumor (Ref: 8 ed. Robbins p.989-90, 9 ed. p.977)

Endodermal sinus tumor/yolk sac tumor ^Q^

- **Most common testicular tumor** in **infants** and **children** up to **3 years** ^Q^

Microscopy:

- **Endodermal sinuses (Schiller-Duval bodies)** ^Q^ are seen, which resemble **primitive glomeruli**
- Intra and extra-cytoplasmic **hyaline-like globules** ^Q^, which show **α-fetoprotein (AFP)** and **α_1-antitrypsin** positivity
- Good prognosis

Ans. 24) D. All of the above (Ref: 8 ed. Robbins p.989-90, 9 ed. p.977)

- **Pure forms** of **teratoma** are **second most common** ^Q^ testicular tumor in infants and children after **yolk sac tumors**
- **Malignant non–germ cell tumors** ^Q^ may arise in **teratoma** and is called as "teratoma with malignant transformation", most commonly **squamous cell carcinoma** ^Q^
- In children, **differentiated mature teratoma** usually follow a **benign course** ^Q^
- However, in **post-pubertal male**, teratoma should be considered as **malignant** ^Q^

Ans. 25) D. All of the above (Ref: 8 ed. Robbins p.992, 9 ed. p.979)

Germ cell tumors of the testis secrete following hormones and enzymes:

- **Lactate dehydrogenase** ^Q^ – Correlates with the **tumor mass** ^Q^ and provides a tool to assess **tumor burden** ^Q^
- Elevated **serum AFP** levels are seen in **yolk sac tumor** ^Q^
- Elevated **serum HCG** levels are seen in **choriocarcinoma** ^Q^

Uses of Serum Markers ^Q^:

- In **staging** of testicular germ cell tumors
- For assessing the **tumor burden**
- In monitoring the **response to therapy**

Ans. 26) A. Leydig cell tumor (Ref: 8 ed. Robbins p.992, 9 ed. p.980)

Leydig Cell Tumors ^Q^:

- **Age group** ^Q^ – 20 and 60 years
- Elaborate **androgens**, **estrogens**, corticosteroids
- Most common symptom is **testicular swelling**
- **Gynecomastia** ^Q^ is the first symptom
- In children, **sexual precocity** is commonly seen

Ans. 27) B. Leydig cell tumor (Ref: 8 ed. Robbins p.992, 9 ed. p.980)

Morphology of Leydig Cell Tumors ^Q^:

- Circumscribed nodule, **< 5 cm** in diameter

- **Cut surface** – Distinctive **golden brown**, homogeneous appearance
- **Microscopy** – Cytoplasm of **neoplastic Leydig cells** contains rod-shaped **crystalloids of Reinke** Q

Ans. 28) A. Non-Hodgkin lymphoma (Ref: 8 ed. Robbins p.992, 9 ed. p.980)

- **Non-Hodgkin lymphomas** Q: **Most common** Q testicular neoplasm in men older than age **60 years**

Most common NHL (in decreasing order of frequency) affecting testes:

- **Diffuse large B-cell lymphoma** Q, Burkitt lymphoma and EBV-positive extra nodal NK/T cell lymphoma

Ans. 29) A. Peripheral zone (Ref: 8 ed. Robbins p.993, 9 ed. p.981, f-21-30)

- **Prostatic hyperplasia** Q arise in the **transitional zone** Q i.e. the **inner periurethral** zone of the prostate
- **Prostatic carcinomas** Q originate in the **peripheral zone** Q

Ans. 30) B. Type 2 5α-reductase (Ref: 8 ed. Robbins p.994-95, 9 ed. p.983-83, f-21-32)

- **Type 1 5α-reductase** is **not detected** in prostate
- **Dihydrotestosterone (DHT)** Q is the **main androgen** in the prostate
- **DHT** is derived from testosterone by the action of **type 2 5α-reductase** Q

Ans. 31) A. Red meat (Ref: 8 ed. Robbins p.997, 9 ed. p.984)

Prostatic Cancer:

- **Increased risk** – consumption of fats or carcinogens present in **red meats** Q
- Dietary products which **prevent** or **delay** prostate cancer – **Lycopenes** Q (found in tomatoes), **soy products** and **vitamin D**

Ans. 32) A. GSTP-1 gene hyper methylation (Ref: 8 ed. Robbins p.997, 9 ed. p.985)

- **Most common epigenetic alteration** in prostate cancer is **hyper-methylation of glutathione S-transferase (GSTP1) gene** Q, located on chromosome **11q13**
- Genes which are silenced include – *RB, CDKN2A, MLH1, MSH2* and *APC*
- Increased risk is seen with germline mutations of **BRCA2** and **HOXB13 (homeobox gene)**
- **Most common** chromosomal rearrangement in prostatic cancer leads to **ERG - TMPRSS2** Q fusion

Ans. 33) Osteoblastic (Ref: 8 ed. Robbins p.998, 9 ed. p.986, f-21-35)

- Metastasis from the prostate reaching the bones are **osteoblastic** Q

Ans. 34) A. Lumbar spine (Ref: 8 ed. Robbins p.998, 9 ed. p.986)

- Prostatic cancer can metastasize to the following bones (descending order): **lumbar spine** Q, proximal femur, pelvis, thoracic spine and ribs
- Tumor spread occurs via **Batson's vertebral** Q venous system

Ans. 35) A. Basal cells (Ref: 8 ed. Robbins p.999, 9 ed. p.986, f-21-36)

- **Benign prostatic glands** contain **basal cells** Q
- Basal cells are **absent** Q in **prostatic cancer**
- **α-methylacyl-coenzyme A-racemase (AMACR)** Q, also known as **P504S**, is the **most sensitive immunohistochemical marker** Q of prostate cancer

Ans. 36) D. Higher the grade, better the prognosis (Ref: 8 ed. Robbins p.999-1000, 9 ed. p.987-88, f-21-37,38)

- **Grade and stage** are the **best prognostic predictors** Q of prostate cancer
- For grading prostate cancer **Gleason system** Q is used
- **Grade 1** – Most well differentiated tumors
- **Grade 5** – Tumors show no glandular differentiation
- **Primary pattern** and **secondary pattern**, each of them are graded from 1 to 5, thus **1+1(2)** Q, represents **well differentiated cancer** Q and **5+5(10)** Q represents **poorly differentiated cancer** Q
- Thus, **higher** the grade, **poorer** the prognosis

Ans. 37) C. Both of the above (Ref: 8 ed. Robbins p.1002, 9 ed. p.989)

- Advanced prostatic cancer is treated by **androgen deprivation** ^{Q} therapy
- **Androgen deprivation** ^{Q} is achieved by **orchiectomy** ^{Q}, or by **luteinizing hormone-releasing hormone (LHRH) analogues** ^{Q}, which leads to **pharmacologic orchiectomy**

Ans. 38) A. PCA3 (Ref: 9 ed. Robbins p.989)

- **PCA3** ^{Q} is overexpressed in 95% of **prostate cancers**
- **Urine PCA3** ^{Q} is useful in patients suspected to have **prostate cancer** because of elevated PSA, but those with **negative prostate biopsy** ^{Q}
- Combination of **urinary PCA3** screening of urine for **TMPRSS2-ERG fusion DNA** ^{Q} have increased sensitivity and specificity for diagnosing **prostatic cancer**

Ans. 39) A. Urothelial cancer of bladder (Ref: 8 ed. Robbins p.1002, 9 ed. p.990)

- **Most common** tumor to secondarily involve the prostate is **urothelial cancer** ^{Q}

Note: Most aggressive variant of prostate cancer is **small-cell cancer** ^{Q} (neuroendocrine carcinoma)

Ans. 40) B. Transitional cell carcinoma (Ref: 9 ed. Robbins p. 964)

Ans. 41) B. Teratoma (Ref: 9 ed. Robbins p.977)

- Rokitanski protuberances are seen in mature benign teratoma

Ans. 42) A. Schistosomiasis (Ref: 9 ed. Robbins p.967) Refer Q 6 & Q7 for details

Ans. 43) D. Seminoma (Ref: 9 ed. Robbins p. 976) Refer Q 19, 20 for details

Ans. 44) C. Seminoma (Ref: 9 ed. Robbins p.976-77)

20 The Female Genital Tract

How to go about this chapter?

- **One should be thorough with the following topics:**
  - **Infections of female genital tract: Herpes Simplex Virus, Condyloma Acuminatum**
  - **Embryonal Rhabdomyosarcoma of vagina**
  - **HPV infection in cervical cancer**
  - **Cervical Intraepithelial Neoplasia and Squamous cell carcinoma of cervix**
  - **Endometriosis, Endometrial hyperplasia, Endometrial carcinoma, Leiomyosarcoma**
  - **Ovarian neoplasms (serous and mucinous), Germ cell tumors**
  - **Benign teratomas, Dysgerminoma, Yolk Sac Tumor of ovary, Ovarian fibromas**
  - **Leydig cell tumors, Krukenberg tumor, Ectopic pregnancy, Complete mole**
  - **Choriocarcinoma, Placental Site Trophoblastic Tumor (PSTT)**

1) **All of the following arises from the mullerian ducts EXCEPT:**
a) Fallopian tubes b) Uterus
c) Cervix d) Gartner duct

INFECTIONS

2) **All are TRUE about Herpes simplex virus infection EXCEPT:**
a) HSVs are RNA viruses
b) HSV-1 typically results in oropharyngeal infection
c) HSV-2 involves genital mucosa and skin
d) HSV-2 infection enhances acquisition of HIV-1

3) **Strawberry cervix occurs as a result of following infection:**
a) Trichomonas vaginalis
b) Gardnerella vaginalis
c) Candidiasis
d) Molluscum contagiosum

4) **Most common cause of Pelvic Inflammatory Disease:**
a) N. gonorrhoeae b) Chlamydia
c) Streptococcus d) C. perfringens

VULVA

5) **Causes of leukoplakia of vulva:**
a) Lichen sclerosis
b) Keratosis
c) Paget's disease
d) All of the above

6) **All are TRUE about Condyloma Acuminatum EXCEPT:**
a) Also known as genital warts
b) Caused by HPV-6
c) Presents as exophytic mass
d) Can progress into carcinoma

7) **All are TRUE about Extramammary Paget disease involving vulva EXCEPT:**
a) Intraepithelial proliferation of malignant cells
b) Cells stain with Mucicarmine and Alcian blue
c) Cells express cytokeratin-7
d) Has associated underlying vulvar carcinoma

VAGINA

8) **All are TRUE about embryonal rhabdomyosarcoma of vagina:**
a) Arises in anterior vaginal wall
b) Occurs in girls older than 5 years of age
c) Can cause obstruction of the urinary tract
d) Tumor cells underneath cambium layer is a characteristic feature

CERVIX

9) **TRUE about cervical lining epithelium:**
a) Ecto-cervix is lined by stratified squamous epithelium
b) Endo-cervix is lined by columnar, mucus-secreting epithelium
c) Transformation zone is similar to squamo-columnar junction
d) All of the above

10) HPV infection most commonly affects:
a) Ectocervix
b) Endocervix
c) Transformation zone
d) Any of the above

11) HPV most commonly implicated in cancer cervix:
a) HPV-16 b) HPV-18
c) HPV-6 d) HPV-11

12) All are TRUE about cervical intraepithelial neoplasia EXCEPT:
a) Moderate and severe dysplasia are classified as High grade Squamous Intraepithelial Lesion (HSIL)
b) Low grade Squamous Intraepithelial Lesion (LSIL) occurs due to HPV infection
c) LSIL can progress to invasive carcinoma
d) LSIL are more common than HSIL

13) Cervical epithelium showing full thickness diffuse atypia is termed as:
a) CIN I b) CIN II
c) CIN III d) LSIL

14) TRUE about HPV infection:
a) Highest viral loads are seen in maturing keratinocytes
b) Ki-67 expression is increased in the upper portion of the epithelium
c) Overexpression of p16 is seen
d) All of the above

15) In Microinvasive carcinoma, depth of stromal invasion is:
a) ≤ 5 mm b) ≤ 10 mm
c) ≤ 15 mm d) ≤ 20 mm

16) Most common histological subtype of carcinoma cervix:
a) Squamous cell carcinoma
b) Adenocarcinoma
c) Adenosquamous
d) Neuroendocrine cancer

17) All of the following are common causes of death in carcinoma cervix EXCEPT:
a) Distant metastasis
b) Uremia
c) Ureteral obstruction
d) Pyelonephritis

ENDOMETRIUM

18) Prominent spiral arterioles in endometrium occurs during following days:
a) 21-22 b) 22-23
c) 23-24 d) 24-25

19) Causes of chronic endometritis include(s):
a) PID b) IUCD
c) Tuberculosis d) All of the above

20) All are TRUE regarding endometriosis EXCEPT:
a) Most commonly involves ovaries
b) Occurs most commonly in post-menopausal women
c) Consists of both endometrial glands and stroma
d) It may lead to infertility

21) Most probable explanation of endometriosis includes:
a) Regurgitation theory
b) Benign metastatic theory
c) Metaplastic theory
d) Stem cell theory

22) Increased production of .... leads to development of endometriosis:
a) Progesterone b) Aromatase
c) PGE2 d) MMP's

23) Adenomyosis is the presence of endometrial tissue in:
a) Ovary b) Myometrium
c) Cervix d) Uterine ligaments

24) Administration of following drug(s) can result in endometrial polyp:
a) Tamoxifen
b) Rituximab
c) Cyclophosphamide
d) Any of the above

25) Endometrial hyperplasia is associated with:
a) Obesity
b) Menopause
c) PCOS
d) Any of the above

26) Most common gene mutated in endometrial hyperplasia and carcinoma:
a) p53 b) APC
c) PTEN d) Rb

27) Which of the following has maximum chance of going into endometrial cancer?
a) Simple hyperplasia
b) Simple hyperplasia with atypia
c) Complex hyperplasia
d) Complex hyperplasia with atypia

28) Treatment of choice for complex hyperplasia with atypia/atypical hyperplasia in menopausal female:
a) Hysterectomy
b) Progestin therapy
c) Close follow up
d) None of the above

29) Complex hyperplasia with atypia/ atypical hyperplasia progresses to endometrial cancer in ..... % of cases.
a) 1% b) 3%
c) 8% d) 23-48%

30) Most common type of endometrial carcinoma:
a) Endometrioid cancer
b) Clear cell carcinoma
c) Serous cell carcinoma
d) Malignant mixed mullerian tumor

31) Following are the risk factors for endometrioid cancers EXCEPT:
a) Obesity b) Multi-parity
c) Diabetes d) Hypertension

32) Poorly differentiated endometrioid cancers/ Type II endometrial cancer show following genetic mutation:
a) p53 b) KRAS
c) PTEN d) MSI

33) Most common type II endometrial cancer:
a) Serous cancer
b) Clear cell cancer
c) Malignant mixed mullerian tumor
d) Endometrioid type

34) TRUE about type II endometrial cancers:
a) Develops in patients with endometrial atrophy
b) Patients with predisposing conditions for estrogen exposure
c) Are well differentiated cancers
d) No precursor lesions are seen

35) For diagnosing leiomyosarcoma, order of significance of morphological features:
a) Coagulative necrosis, mitotic activity, pleomorphism, cellularity
b) Cellularity, high mitotic activity, pleomorphism, coagulative necrosis
c) High mitotic activity, coagulative necrosis, pleomorphism and cellularity
d) Pleomorphism, coagulative necrosis, high mitotic activity and cellularity

OVARY

36) Most common ovarian tumor which present bilaterally:
a) Serous tumors
b) Mucinous tumors
c) Endometrioid tumors
d) Clear cell tumors

37) Most common ovarian tumors are:
a) Surface epithelial – Stromal tumors
b) Sex cord – Stromal tumors
c) Germ cell tumors
d) Metastasis

38) Most common malignant ovarian tumors:
a) Serous carcinomas
b) Mucinous carcinomas
c) Endometrioid carcinoma
d) Transitional cell carcinoma

39) Risk factors for developing ovarian serous carcinoma includes all EXCEPT:
a) Nulliparity
b) Family history
c) Gonadal dysgenesis
d) Oral contraceptive pills

40) Psammoma bodies characterize which ovarian tumors?
a) Serous tumors
b) Mucinous tumors
c) Endometrioid tumors
d) Teratoma

41) PAX-8 positivity is characteristically seen in:
a) Serous tumors
b) Mucinous tumors
c) Endometrioid tumors
d) All of the above

42) Pseudomyxoma peritonei can be an associated finding with following ovarian tumor(s):
a) Serous tumors
b) Mucinous tumors
c) Endometrioid tumors
d) Clear cell tumors

43) TRUE about endometrioid cancers of ovary:
a) Associated with endometrial cancer
b) Associated with endometriosis
c) Good prognosis
d) All of the above

44) Most common ovarian tumor(s) in children:
a) Germ cell tumors
b) Sex-cord stromal tumors
c) Surface epithelial tumors
d) Any of the above

45) TRUE about ovarian teratomas:
a) Also called as dermoid cysts
b) Seen in young females of reproductive age group
c) May be associated with Paraneoplastic syndrome
d) All of the above

46) All are TRUE about morphology of teratoma EXCEPT:
a) Bilateral in 10-15% cases
b) Three germ layers components are seen
c) 1% or dermoid can transform into malignancy
d) Most common malignancy seen is thyroid carcinoma

47) TRUE about Dysgerminoma:
a) Ovarian counterpart of seminoma
b) Occurs most commonly in second and third decades
c) Most commonly occurs unilaterally
d) All of the above

48) **Schiller-Duval body is a feature of:**
a) Embryonal carcinoma
b) Yolk sac tumor
c) Choriocarcinoma
d) Teratoma

49) **All are TRUE about granulosa cell tumors of ovary:**
a) Occurs in post-menopausal females
b) Call-Exner bodies are distinct morphological feature
c) Considered to be benign
d) Increased serum levels of inhibin are seen

50) **Meig's syndrome is associated with:**
a) Ovarian fibroma
b) Ovarian thecoma
c) Ovarian teratoma
d) Any of the above

51) **Reinke crystalloids are characteristically seen in:**
a) Leydig cell tumors
b) Sertoli cell tumors
c) Gonadoblastoma
d) Cystic teratoma

52) **Primary site of Krukenberg tumor of ovary:**
a) Gastric cancer
b) Colon cancer
c) Breast cancer
d) None of the above

53) **Most common site of ectopic pregnancy:**
a) Extra-uterine Fallopian tube
b) Ovary
c) Abdominal cavity
d) Cornual end of fallopian tube

GESTATIONAL AND PLACENTAL DISORDERS

54) **TRUE about complete mole:**
a) Genetic material is completely paternally derived
b) 46XX is the most common karyotype
c) Increased risk of choriocarcinoma
d) All of the above

55) **Choriocarcinoma may arise in:**
a) Complete mole
b) Abortions
c) Normal pregnancy
d) All of the above

56) **All are TRUE about morphology of choriocarcinoma EXCEPT:**
a) Soft fleshy tumor
b) Areas of necrosis and hemorrhage
c) Chorionic villi
d) Cytotrophoblasts and syncytiotrophoblasts are seen

57) **Proliferation of the following is seen in Placenta site trophoblastic tumor (PSTT):**
a) Cytotrophoblasts
b) Syncytiotrophoblasts
c) Intermediate trophoblast
d) Any of the above

58) **Most common ovarian tumor in young lady is: (NEET 2014)**
a) Dysgerminoma
b) Ovarian Mucinous Cystadenocarcinomas
c) Ovarian Serous Cystadenocarcinomas
d) Fibroid

59) **Inhibin is tumor marker for: (NEET 2014)**
a) Granulosa cell tumor
b) Malignant melanoma
c) Prolactinoma
d) Breast carcinoma

60) **Vaginal adenosis is evident in women who had exposure to in utero: (NEET 2014)**
a) DES
b) Asbestos
c) Cadmium
d) Nickel

61) **Leiomyosarcoma most common age group: (NEET 2014)**
a) 20-40 years
b) 30-50 years
c) 40-60 years
d) 50-70 years

62) **Signet ring appearance is seen in: (NEET 2014)**
a) Granulosa cell tumor
b) Krukenberg tumor
c) Teratoma
d) Dysgerminoma

63) **Early age of sex is risk factor for: (NEET 2014)**
a) Carcinoma Cervix
b) Carcinoma vulva
c) Carcinoma vagina
d) Carcinoma ovary

64) **Which is not a risk factor of endometrial carcinoma? (NEET 2013)**
a) Obesity
b) Smoking
c) Infertility
d) Tamoxifen

65) **Which of the following is the ovarian counterpart of testicular seminoma? (NEET 2013)**
a) Brenner's tumor
b) Endodermal sinus tumor
c) Dermoid
d) Dysgerminoma

66) **Most common tumor of ovary: (NEET 2013)**
a) Dermoid
b) Serous epithelial tumor
c) Mucinous
d) Dysgerminoma

67) Endometrial cancer, which of the following tumor suppressor gene occur? (NEET 2013)

a) P53 b) Rb
c) PTEN d) APC

68) Call exner bodies are seen in: (NEET 2013)

a) Dysgerminoma
b) Granulosa cell tumor
c) Thecoma
d) Arrhenoblastoma

69) Most common malignancy of fallopian tube: (NEET 2013)

a) SCC
b) Serous CA
c) Teratoma
d) Choriocarcinoma

70) Psammoma bodies are seen in following EXCEPT: (NEET 2013)

a) Serous Cystadenoma of ovary
b) Mucinous Cystadenoma of ovary
c) Meningioma
d) Papillary carcinoma of thyroid

71) Clue cell are seen in: (AIPGMEE 2012)

a) Bacterial vaginosis
b) Bacterial candidiasis
c) Chlamydial vaginosis
d) Trichomoniasis

72) Which of the following is a marker for granulosa cell tumor? (Nov 2011)

a) Alkaline phosphatase
b) Inhibin
c) CA 19-9
d) CA 5

CHAPTER 20: THE FEMALE GENITAL TRACT

Ans. 1) D. Gartner duct (Ref: 8 ed. Robbins p.1006-07, 9 ed. p.992, f-22-1)

Mullerian Ducts [Q]:

- **Unfused upper portion** of mullerian ducts mature into the **fallopian tubes** [Q]
- **Fused lower portion** develops into the **uterus**, **cervix** and **upper vagina** [Q]

Mesonephric Ducts [Q]:

- **Regresses** in adult females, but may persist as small **epithelial inclusions** [Q] adjacent to the **ovaries**, **tubes** and **uterus**
- In the cervix and vagina, these rests are termed as **Gartner duct cysts** [Q]

Ans. 2) A. HSVs are RNA viruses (Ref: 8 ed. Robbins p.1008-09, 9 ed. p.993, f-22-2)

Herpes Simplex Virus:

- **DNA viruses** [Q] and include, **HSV-1** and **HSV-2**
- **HSV-1** [Q] results in **oropharyngeal infection**
- **HSV-2** [Q] usually involves **genital mucosa** and skin
- Virus can migrate to the **regional nerve** ganglia and establishes a **latent infection** [Q]
- **HSV cytopathic changes** [Q]: **Multinucleated squamous cells** containing eosinophilic to basophilic viral inclusions with a **"ground-glass" appearance** [Q]
- **Cesarean section** is indicated in **mothers** with HSV infection of the genital tract
- **HSV-2 infection** enhances **HIV-1** acquisition and transmission

Ans. 3) A. Trichomonas vaginalis (Ref: 8 ed. Robbins p.1008-09, 9 ed. p.993-94, f-22-3)

Salient features of the infections of the **lower vaginal tract**:

- **Molluscum contagiosum** [Q] – Caused by **poxvirus** [Q], presents as **pearly**, **dome-shaped papules** and contains cells with **cytoplasmic viral inclusions** [Q]
- **Candidiasis – Filamentous fungal hyphae** in **wet KOH mounts** of the discharge or on Papanicolaou (Pap) smear
- **Trichomonas vaginalis** [Q] – Vaginal and cervical mucosa has **fiery-red appearance**, termed as **"strawberry cervix"** [Q]
- **Gardnerella vaginalis** [Q] – Leads to **bacterial vaginosis** [Q], present with thin, green-gray, **malodorous (fishy)** vaginal discharge
- Ureaplasma urealyticum and Mycoplasma hominis – Leads to **chorioamnionitis** [Q]

Ans. 4) A. *N. gonorrhoeae* (Ref: 8 ed. Robbins p.1009-10, 9 ed. p.994-95, f-22-4)

- ***Neisseria gonorrhoeae*** [Q] is the most common cause of **Pelvic Inflammatory Disease(PID)**
- Staphylococci, streptococci, coliforms and Clostridium perfringens most commonly results in **puerperal infections**

Ans. 5) D. All of the above (Ref: 8 ed. Robbins p.1011-12, 9 ed. p.996-97, f-22-5)

Causes of **Leukoplakia** [Q] involving vulva:

- Inflammatory dermatoses (e.g., psoriasis, chronic dermatitis)
- **Lichen sclerosis** and **squamous cell hyperplasia**
- **Neoplasms** – Vulvar intraepithelial neoplasia (VIN), Paget disease and Invasive carcinoma

Ans. 6) D. Can progress into carcinoma (Ref: 8 ed. Robbins p.1012, 9 ed. p.997, f-22-6)

Condyloma Acuminatum [Q]:

- **Benign genital warts** caused by **HPV type 6 and 11** [Q]
- **Not precancerous lesions** [Q]

Microscopy [Q]:

- Surface epithelium shows **viral cytopathic change** i.e. **koilocytic atypia** [Q] (features of which includes **nuclear enlargement**, **hyperchromasia** and cytoplasmic perinuclear halo)

Ans. 7) **D. Has associated underlying vulvar carcinoma (Ref: 8 ed. Robbins p.1014, 9 ed. p.999, f-22-9)**

Extra-mammary Paget Disease (vulva) [Q]:

- Presents as a pruritic, red, crusted, area, usually on labia majora

Morphology of Paget Disease:

- **Intraepithelial proliferation** of **malignant cells** [Q]

Paget Cells:

- Larger than surrounding **keratinocytes** and are seen **singly** or in **small clusters** within the **epidermis**
- Have **pale cytoplasm** which stains with **periodic acid–Schiff (PAS)**, **Alcian blue**, or **Mucicarmine stains** and also express **cytokeratin 7** [Q]

Note:

- **Vulvar Paget disease** is **not associated** with **underlying cancer**

Note: Paget disease of breast is associated with underlying **breast cancer** [Q]

Ans. 8) **B. Occurs in girls older than 5 years of age (Ref: 8 ed. Robbins p.1017, 9 ed. p.1001, f-22-11)**

Embryonal Rhabdomyosarcoma/Sarcoma Botryoides [Q]:

- Most frequently found in infants and in children **younger than 5 years** [Q] of age
- Tumors tend to grow as **grape like clusters (botryoides)** [Q]
- Death occurs due to spread into the peritoneal cavity or by obstruction of the urinary tract

Characteristic Feature [Q]:

- Tumor cells surround the **blood vessels** or are beneath the vaginal epithelium, later is termed as the **cambium layer** [Q] of Nicholson

Ans. 9) **D. All of the above (Ref: 8 ed. Robbins p.1017-19, 9 ed. p.1001, f-22-12)**

- **Ectocervix** is lined by mature **squamous epithelium** [Q]
- **Endocervix** is lined by **columnar** [Q], mucus-secreting epithelium
- **Squamocolumnar junction/transformation zone** [Q] – Junction where the squamous and columnar epithelium meet

Ans. 10) **C. Transformation zone (Ref: 8 ed. Robbins p.1017-19, 9 ed. p.1001, f-22-12)**

- **HPV** [Q] **infection** affects the immature squamous metaplastic epithelial cells in the **transformation zone** [Q]
- **Transformation zone** is the region where **in-situ (precursor) cervical lesions** [Q] and **cancers** [Q] develop

Ans. 11) **A. HPV-16 (Ref: 8 ed. Robbins p.1019, 9 ed. p.1002)**

- **HPV-16** [Q]: Most commonly implicated in cervical cancer followed by **HPV-18**
- HPVs infect **immature basal cells** [Q] of **squamous epithelium** or **immature metaplastic squamous cells** present at the **squamocolumnar junction**
- Although **HPV** infects immature **squamous cells, viral replication** occurs in **maturing squamous cells**

How does HPV bring about tumorogenesis?

- **HPV E6 and E7** [Q], interfere with the activity of **tumor suppressor proteins** [Q]
- **HPV E7 protein** promotes **degradation of RB** [Q] protein and **inhibits p21 and p27** [Q] (cyclin-dependent kinase inhibitors)
- **HPV E6** promotes **degradation of RB** and **up-regulates** the expression of **telomerase**
- Thus resulting in **increased proliferation of cells**, which further can acquire additional mutations

Ans. 12) **C. LSIL can progress to invasive carcinoma (Ref: 8 ed. Robbins p.1019-21, 9 ed. p.1003-04, f-22-14,15, t-22-1)**

Cervical Intraepithelial Neoplasia Q:

- **CIN I** corresponds to low grade squamous intraepithelial lesion **(LSIL)** Q
- **CIN II** and **CIN III** are combined into one category i.e. high grade squamous intraepithelial lesion **(HSIL)** Q
- **LSIL** Q is associated with **HPV infection** Q, may **regress spontaneously** or progress to HSIL, but **does not** Q **progress** to **invasive carcinoma**
- **HSILs** are at **high risk** Q for progression to **carcinoma**

Ans. 13) C. CIN III (Ref: 8 ed. Robbins p.1019-21, 9 ed. p.1003-04, f-22-14,15, t-22-1)

Grading of SIL:

- **LSIL (CIN I)** Q – If immature squamous cells are confined to **lower one third** Q of the epithelium
- **HSIL (CIN II & III)** Q – If immature squamous cells involve **upper two thirds** Q of the epithelial thickness
- **CIN III** is characterized by **diffuse atypia** Q, loss of maturation and **expansion of the immature basal cells** to the **epithelial surface** Q

Ans. 14) D. All of the above (Ref: 8 ed. Robbins p.1020, 9 ed. p.1003, f-22-15)

HPV related changes in cervical epithelium:

- **HPV in situ hybridization** shows that the **highest viral loads** are found in **maturing keratinocytes** Q
- **Ki-67** (marker of actively dividing cells) is seen in the **upper portion of epithelium** (which is normally confined to the **basal layer** of the epithelium)
- **Overexpression of p16 (cyclin-dependent kinase inhibitor)**
- Ki-67 activity and p16 overexpression are useful for **confirmation of the diagnosis** of **Squamous Intraepithelial Lesion (SIL)**

Ans. 15) A. ≤ 5 mm (Ref: 10 ed. Ackerman p.1446-47, f-19-81,82)

- **Microinvasive carcinoma** Q – Invasive squamous cell carcinomas in which the depth of stromal invasion is minimal i.e. **less than or equal to 5 mm** Q

Ans. 16) A. Squamous cell carcinoma (Ref: 8 ed. Robbins p.1021, 9 ed. p.1004, f-22-16,17)

- **Squamous cell carcinoma** Q is the **most common** histologic subtype of cervical cancer followed by **adenocarcinoma**

Ans. 17) A. Distant metastasis (Ref: 8 ed. Robbins p.1023, 9 ed. p.1006)

- Death in advanced cervical cancer occurs due to consequences of **local tumor invasion** (e.g. **ureteral obstruction, pyelonephritis and uremia** Q) and not by distant metastases

Ans. 18) A. 21-22 (Ref: 8 ed. Robbins p.1025, 9 ed. p.1008, f-22-19)

- **Progesterone** Q brings endometrial stromal changes in the **late secretory phase** of menstrual cycle
- **Prominent spiral arterioles** Q appear by **days 21 to 22** Q of menstrual cycle

Ans. 19) D. All of the above (Ref: 8 ed. Robbins p.1027-28, 9 ed. p.1010)

Causes of chronic endometritis Q:

- Chronic **pelvic inflammatory disease (PID)**
- Retained gestational tissue
- Intrauterine contraceptive devices
- Tuberculosis

Diagnosis of **chronic endometritis** Q is made on identification of **plasma cells** Q in the stroma

Ans. 20) B. Occurs most commonly in post-menopausal women (Ref: 8 ed. Robbins p.1028, 9 ed. p.1010)

Endometriosis:

- Definition: Presence of **"ectopic" endometrial tissue** Q outside the uterus
- Ectopic tissue includes both **endometrial glands** Q and **stroma** Q

- **Most common sites** Q (in **decreasing order** of **frequency**) – **Ovaries**, uterine ligaments, rectovaginal septum, cul de sac, pelvic peritoneum, large and small bowel and appendix, mucosa of the cervix, vagina, fallopian tubes and laparotomy scars
- **Common** in women in **active reproductive life** Q
- May result in infertility, dysmenorrhea (painful menstruation), pelvic pain

Ans. 21) A. Regurgitation theory (Ref: 8 ed. Robbins p.1028, 9 ed. p.1010-11)

Following theories have been proposed for **etiology** of endometriosis:

A) Regurgitation theory Q
- Endometrial tissue implants occurs at ectopic sites due to retrograde flow of menstrual endometrium
- **Widely accepted** Q theory

B) Benign metastases theory
- From uterus, endometrial tissue can spread to **distant sites (e.g., bone, lung and brain)** through **blood vessels** and **lymphatic channels**

C) Metaplastic theory
- Endometrium arises directly from **coelomic epithelium** (mesothelium of pelvis or abdomen)

D) Extra-uterine stem/progenitor cell theory
- **Stem/progenitor cells** from the **bone marrow** differentiate into endometrial tissue

Ans. 22) B. Aromatase (Ref: 8 ed. Robbins p.1028-29, 9 ed. p.1011, f-22-22)
- **In endometriosis, increased estrogen production** by **endometriotic stromal cells** occurs due to high level of **aromatase** Q (absent in normal endometrial stroma)
- Thus, **inhibitors of aromatase** are **beneficial** in the treatment of **endometriosis**

Ans. 23) B. Myometrium (Ref: 8 ed. Robbins p.1029, 9 ed. p.1012)
- **Adenomyosis** Q – **Defined** as the **presence of endometrial tissue** within the **uterine wall** Q (myometrium)
- **Ovarian endometriosis** leads to formation of **chocolate cysts** Q or endometriomas
- **Ovarian endometriosis** Q (Atypical endometriosis) has an association with **ovarian cancer** Q (endometrioid and clear cell types)

Ans. 24) A. Tamoxifen (Ref: 8 ed. Robbins p.1029-30, 9 ed. p.1012)
- **Tamoxifen** Q administration (used in the treatment of **breast cancer**) – Increases the risk of **Endometrial polyps** Q

Ans. 25) D. Any of the above (Ref: 8 ed. Robbins p.1030, 9 ed. p.1013)

Endometrial hyperplasia Q is associated with **prolonged estrogenic stimulation**

Causes of estrogen excess Q includes:
- Obesity (peripheral conversion of androgens to estrogens)
- Menopause
- Polycystic ovarian syndrome
- Functioning granulosa cell tumors of the ovary
- Estrogen replacement therapy

Ans. 26) C. PTEN (Ref: 8 ed. Robbins p.1030, 9 ed. p.1013)
- **Inactivation** of **PTEN tumor suppressor gene** Q – Common genetic alteration in **endometrial hyperplasia** and **endometrial carcinomas**
- Patients with **Cowden syndrome** Q (germline mutations in **PTEN**), have a high incidence of **endometrial carcinoma**Q and **breast cancer**

Ans. 27) D. Complex hyperplasia with atypia (Ref: 8 ed. Robbins p.1030-31, 9 ed. p.1013-14, f-22-23)

According to **8 ed. Robbins** hyperplasia has been classified into:
- **Simple hyperplasia** with or without atypia Q and **Complex hyperplasia** with or without hyperplasia Q

However, **9 ed. Robbins** classify it into:

- **Typical hyperplasia** Q (Simple hyperplasia and complex hyperplasia) and **atypical hyperplasia** Q (Simple hyperplasia with atypia and complex hyperplasia with atypia)

  The features of **atypical hyperplasia** overlap with those of **well-differentiated endometrioid adenocarcinoma** Q – **9 ed. Robbins**

  Hence, according to 8 ed. Robbins, answer here will be Complex hyperplasia with atypia, which is a component of atypical hyperplasia (according to 9 ed. Robbins)

Ans. 28) A. Hysterectomy (Ref: 8 ed. Robbins p.1030, 9 ed. p.1013)

- **Atypical hyperplasia** is managed by **hysterectomy** Q or, in **young women** who desire fertility, a trial of **progestin therapy** Q and **close follow-up** can be done

Ans. 29) C. 23-48% (Ref: 8 ed. Robbins p.1030, 9 ed. p.1013)

- Approximately, **1% to 3%** Q of women with **typical hyperplasia of endometrium** Q progresses to **carcinoma**
- Approximately **23% to 48%** Q of women with **atypical hyperplasia of endometrium** Q are found to have **carcinoma** when **hysterectomy** is performed

Ans. 30) A. Endometrioid cancer (Ref: 8 ed. Robbins p.1031-34, 9 ed. p.1014-18)

- **Endometrial carcinoma** has been classified into **type I** Q and **type II** Q
- **Type I (Endometrial) Carcinoma** Q – **Most common type** and are referred to as **Endometrioid carcinoma** Q

Ans. 31) B. Multi-parity (Ref: 8 ed. Robbins p.1032, 9 ed. p.1014)

Endometrial carcinomas Q like endometrial hyperplasia are associated with:

- **Obesity, diabetes, hypertension, unopposed estrogen stimulation and infertility** Q
- **Nulliparous** Q women with **anovulatory cycles** Q are also at **increased risk**

Ans. 32) A. p53 (Ref: 8 ed. Robbins p.1032-34, 9 ed. p.1015-17, f-22-24,t-22-4)

- **Loss-of-function mutations** in **TP53** Q are present in **50%** of **poorly differentiated carcinomas** Q
- **TP53** Q mutations are present in **90%** of **serous endometrial carcinoma** Q

Mutations commonly seen in **endometrioid cancers/type I endometrial cancers** Q –

- PIK3CA, KRAS, ARID1A, DNA mismatch repair genes, p53

Ans. 33) A. Serous cancer (Ref: 8 ed. Robbins p.1033-34, 9 ed. p.1017-18, f-22-26)

Type II endometrial cancers (poorly differentiated tumors Q**):**

- Most common subtype is **serous carcinoma** Q
- Other tumors include – **Clear cell carcinoma** and **malignant mixed mullerian tumor**

Ans. 34) A. Develops in patients with endometrial atrophy (Ref: 8 ed. Robbins p.1033-34, 9 ed. p.1017-18, f-22-26, t-22-4)

Salient Features of Type II endometrial carcinoma Q:

- Arises in patients with **endometrial atrophy** Q
- **Poorly differentiated tumors**
- **Most common** subtype is **serous carcinoma** Q
- **Mutations** in the tumor suppressor gene **p53** Q are commonly seen
- Precursor lesion identified is **serous endometrial intraepithelial carcinoma** Q
- **Spread beyond the uterus** Q at the time of diagnosis is commonly seen

Ans. 35) A. Coagulative necrosis, mitotic activity, pleomorphism, cellularity (Ref: 10 ed. Ackerman p.1516-17)

- **Morphologic features** in their order of significance for diagnosing **leiomyosarcoma** Q – **coagulative necrosis, high mitotic activity, pleomorphism and cellularity**

Following table shows differentiating features between Q:

- Leiomyosarcoma, STUMP (Smooth muscle tumor of unknown malignant potential), Mitotically active leiomyoma and Leiomyoma

Coagulative Necrosis	Mitotic count per 10 HPF	Atypia	Diagnosis
Present	Greater than 10	Moderate to severe (focal or diffuse) or None to mild	- Leiomyosarcoma
Present	Equal to or less than 10	- Moderate to severe (focal or diffuse) - None to mild	- Leiomyosarcoma - STUMP
Absent	Greater than 10	Moderate to severe - Diffuse - Focal	- Leiomyosarcoma - STUMP
Absent	Greater than 10	None to mild	- Mitotically active leiomyoma (up to 15 mitoses/10 HPF)
Absent	Equal to or less than 10	Moderate to severe - Diffuse - Focal	- STUMP - Leiomyoma
Absent	Equal to/or less than 10	None to mild	- Leiomyoma

Ans. 36) A. Serous tumors (Ref: 8 ed. Robbins p.1041, 9 ed. p.1023, t-22-5, 6)

- **Serous tumors (benign, borderline, malignant)** [Q] are most commonly seen **bilaterally** [Q]
- Only 5% of primary **mucinous cystadenomas/ carcinomas** are **bilateral**

Ans. 37) A. Surface epithelial – Stromal tumors (Ref: 8 ed. Robbins p.1041, 9 ed. p.1023, t-22-5,6)

- Most **primary ovarian neoplasms** arise from **mullerian epithelium** [Q]

Ans. 38) A. Serous carcinomas (Ref: 8 ed. Robbins p.1041-42, 9 ed. p.1023-24, t-22-6)

Serous Neoplasms [Q]:

- **Most common malignant ovarian tumors** [Q]
- Comprise approximately 40% of all the ovarian cancers

Ans. 39) D. Oral contraceptive pills (Ref: 8 ed. Robbins p.1042, 9 ed. p.1024)

Risk factors for **malignant serous tumors (serous carcinomas)** [Q] includes

- Nulliparity
- Family history and heritable mutations
- Gonadal dysgenesis

However, **oral contraceptives** [Q] and **tubal ligation** [Q] reduces the risk of developing ovarian cancer

Ans. 40) A. Serous tumors (Ref: 8 ed. Robbins p.1042-44, 9 ed. p.1024-26, f-22-33)

- **Concentric calcifications (psammoma bodies)** [Q] characterize **serous tumors** [Q], although they are not specific for neoplasia

Ans. 41) A. Serous tumors (Ref: 10 ed. Ackerman p.1563-67)

- **PAX8** [Q] is commonly **positive** in **serous tumors of the ovary**
- **CK20 and carcinoembryonic antigen (CEA)** [Q] are negative in serous tumors

Ans. 42) B. Mucinous tumors (Ref: 8 ed. Robbins p.1044-45, 9 ed. p.1027, f-22-35)

- In past it was thought, that **mucinous tumors of ovary** are accompanied by extensive deposits of **intra-abdominal mucin (pseudomyxoma peritonei)** [Q]
- But, now pseudomyxoma peritonei is considered **metastatic to the ovary** [Q] from **appendix** [Q]

Ans. 43) D. All of the above (Ref: 8 ed. Robbins p.1045-46, 9 ed. p.1027)

Salient features of endometrioid cancer of ovary:

- **15% to 20%** of cases of **endometrioid carcinoma** coexist with **endometriosis** [Q]
- **15% to 30%** of **ovarian endometrioid carcinomas** are accompanied by **carcinoma of the endometrium** [Q]
- Have **good prognosis** [Q]

Ans. 44) A. Germ cell tumors (Ref: 10 ED. Ackerman p.1563-67, 9th ed. Robbins p. 1029)

Germ Cell Tumors Q:

- **Most common tumors** in **children** (60–70% of all ovarian tumors in this age group)
- **Most common** are **benign cystic teratomas** Q

Note:

- **Sex cord–stromal tumors** constitute **10–25%** of cases
- **Surface epithelial tumors** represent **15–20%** of ovarian tumors in children

Ans. 45) D. All of the above (Ref: 8 ed. Robbins p.1047-48, 9 ed. p.1029)

Benign Teratomas:

- **Cystic** and are referred to as **dermoid cysts** Q
- Found in young women during **active reproductive years**
- Associated with **paraneoplastic syndrome**: **Inflammatory limbic encephalitis** Q
- **Mature cystic teratomas** can coexist with **Mucinous cystadenoma, Brenner tumor** and **Fibrothecoma**

Ans. 46) D. Most common malignancy seen is thyroid carcinoma (Ref: 8 ed. Robbins p.1047-48, 9 ed. p.1029-30, f-22-38,39)

Benign Teratomas:

- **Bilateral** in **10% to 15%** of cases
- **Unilocular cysts** containing **hair** and **sebaceous material** Q
- **Cyst wall** is lined by **epidermis** with protruding hair shafts, **tooth structures** and areas of calcification
- Tissues from other germ layers can be identified, such as **cartilage, bone, thyroid and neural tissue** Q
- **1%** of **dermoid** undergo **malignant transformation** Q, **most commonly** to **squamous cell carcinoma** Q followed by **carcinoid tumor** and **adenocarcinoma**

Ans. 47) D. All of the above (Ref: 8 ed. Robbins p.1048-49, 9 ed. p.1030-31, f-22-41)

Dysgerminoma Q:

- Ovarian counterpart of testicular seminoma, seen in **2nd - 3rd decade**
- Expresses **OCT-3, OCT4 and NANOG** Q
- One-third have activating **mutations in the KIT gene** Q

Morphology Q:

- **Unilateral tumors** Q
- **Cut surface** Q – Solid yellow-white to gray-pink appearance, soft and fleshy

Microscopically Q:

- Tumor cells grow in **sheets or cords** separated by **scant fibrous stroma** which is infiltrated by **mature lymphocytes** Q
- Tumor cells are composed of **large vesicular cells**, having **clear cytoplasm, well-defined cell boundaries** and **centrally placed regular nuclei**

Ans. 48) B. Yolk sac tumor (Ref: 8 ed. Robbins p.1049, 9 ed. p.1031, f-22-42)

Yolk Sac Tumor (endodermal sinus tumor) Q:

- Commonly seen in **children** or **young women**
- Characteristic **histologic feature**: **Glomerulus-like structure** composed of a **central blood vessel** enveloped by **tumor cells (Schiller-Duval body)** Q
- Tumor cells elaborate **α-fetoprotein** Q (similar to the normal yolk sac)
- Intracellular and Extracellular **hyaline droplets** are present in all tumors

Note:

- **Embryonal carcinoma** expresses both **α-fetoprotein** Q and **HCG** Q

Ans. 49) C. Considered to be benign (Ref: 8 ed. Robbins p.1050, 9 ed. p.1032-33, f-22-43)

Granulosa Cell Tumors [Q]:

- Two forms – **Adult** and **juvenile granulosa cell tumors**
- Two thirds occur in **postmenopausal women** [Q]
- Elaborate large amounts of **estrogen**
- Are **potentially malignant** [Q]
- **Elevated tissue** and **serum levels of Inhibin** [Q] are seen
- **Inhibin** is also useful for **monitoring patients** after treatment
- **Mutation** in **FOXL2 gene** [Q] are **most common**

Morphology [Q]:

- **Unilateral** [Q], with foci of large, solid and cystic encapsulated masses
- Tumor cells grow in **anastomosing cords, sheets, or strands**
- Tumor cells are **small, cuboidal to polygonal cells**
- Nuclei show **grooves or folds** [Q], resulting in a **coffee bean appearance** [Q]
- **Call-Exner bodies** [Q]: **Gland like structures** filled with acidophilic material

Ans. 50) A. Ovarian fibroma (Ref: 8 ed. Robbins p.1051, 9 ed. p.1033, f-22-44)

Ovarian fibromas [Q]:

- Unilateral, encapsulated, hard, gray-white masses
- **Meig's syndrome** [Q]: **Ovarian fibroma**, **hydrothorax** [Q] **(right side)** and **ascites** [Q]
- Associated with **Basal cell nevus syndrome/Gorlin syndrome** [Q]

Ans. 51) A. Leydig cell tumors (Ref: 8 ed. Robbins p.1052, 9 ed. p.1033)

Hilus cell tumors (pure Leydig cell tumors) [Q]

- Composed of **large lipid-laden leydig cells** with characteristic cytoplasmic structures called as **Reinke crystalloids** [Q]

Ans. 52) A. Gastric cancer (Ref: 8 ed. Robbins p.1052, 9 ed. p.1034)

Features of Krukenberg Tumor [Q]:

- Bilateral **ovarian metastases** [Q]
- Composed of mucin-producing, **signet-ring cancer cells** [Q]
- Most common primary sites are **stomach (most common)** [Q], large bowel, appendix and breast

Ans. 53) A. Extra-uterine Fallopian tube (Ref: 8 ed. Robbins p.1053, 9 ed. p.1036)

Ectopic Pregnancy:

- Refers to **implantation of fetus** at a site other than the normal intrauterine location
- Most common site is the **extra uterine fallopian tube** [Q]
- **Other sites** – Ovary, abdominal cavity and Cornual end of fallopian tube
- Most important predisposing condition is **pelvic inflammatory disease** [Q]

Ans. 54) D. All of the above (Ref: 8 ed. Robbins p.1058-59, 9 ed. p.1039-40, f-22-52-54)

Complete Mole [Q]:

- Results when the sperm fertilizes an empty egg (i.e. which has lost its female chromosomes)
- Genetic material is **paternally derived** [Q]
- **46, XX** [Q] is the **most common karyotype**
- Increased risk of subsequent **choriocarcinoma** and **persistent or invasive mole**

Morphology [Q]:

- Moles are delicate, translucent, cystic, **grapelike structures** [Q] (edematous villi)
- **Chorionic villi** are **enlarged, scalloped** in shape with **central cavitation (cisterns)**
- Extensive and **circumferential trophoblastic proliferation**

Partial Moles [Q]:

- Result from fertilization of an egg with two sperms
- Karyotype is **triploid (e.g., 69, XXY)** or **tetraploid (92, XXXY)**
- Fetal tissues are **present** [Q]
- Increased risk of **persistent molar disease,** but **not choriocarcinoma** [Q]

Morphology:

- **Fraction of the villi** are **enlarged** and **edematous**
- **Trophoblastic hyperplasia** is **focal** and **less marked** than in complete moles

Ans. 55) D. All of the above (Ref: 8 ed. Robbins p.1060, 9 ed. p.1041)

- **Choriocarcinoma** [Q] can occur following **complete hydatidiform mole, previous abortion** and even after **normal pregnancy**

Ans. 56) C. Chorionic villi (Ref: 8 ed. Robbins p.1060, 9 ed. p.1041, f-22-55)

Choriocarcinoma:

- Soft, fleshy, yellow-white tumor with extensive **areas of necrosis and hemorrhage** [Q]
- Metastasize to the **lungs** and **vagina** followed by brain, liver, bone and kidney

Microscopy [Q]:

- **Does not produce chorionic villi** [Q]
- Consists of **proliferating syncytiotrophoblasts and cytotrophoblasts** and abnormal mitoses

Ans. 57) C. Intermediate trophoblast (Ref: 8 ed. Robbins p.1061, 9 ed. p.1041-42)

Placental Site Trophoblastic Tumor (PSTT):

- Arises due to **neoplastic proliferations** of **extra villous trophoblasts (intermediate trophoblasts** [Q]**)**
- **Intermediate trophoblasts** are **polygonal mononuclear cells** with abundant cytoplasm and produce **human placental lactogen** [Q]

Ans. 58) A. Dysgerminoma (Ref: 9 ed. Robbins p. 1030) Refer Q 47 for details

- 75% occur in the second and third decades of life

Ans. 59) A. Granulosa cell tumor (Ref: 9 ed. Robbins p. 1032) Refer Q 49 for details

Ans. 60) A. DES (Ref: 9 ed. Robbins p. 1000) Vaginal adenosis:

- Occurs in 35% to 90% of women exposed to DES in utero
- Microscopy - columnar mucinous epithelium resembling endocervical epithelium

Ans. 61) C. 40-60 years (Ref: 9 ed. Robbins p. 1021)

- Peak incidence of leiomyosarcoma is 40 to 60 years of age

Ans. 62) B. Krukenberg tumor (Ref: 9 ed. Robbins p. 1034)

Ans. 63) A. Carcinoma cervix

Ans. 64) B. Smoking (Ref: 9 ed. Robbins p.1014-18) Refer Q 31 for details

Ans. 65) D. Dysgerminoma (Ref: 9 ed. Robbins p.1030-31) Refer Q 47 for details

Ans. 66) B. Serous epithelial tumour (Ref: 9 ed. Robbins p. 1023-24) Refer Q 38 for details

Ans. 67) C. PTEN (Ref: 9 ed. Robbins p.1015-17) Refer Q 26 for details

Ans. 68) B. Granulosa cell tumor (Ref: 9 ed. Robbins p.1032-33) Refer Q 49 for details

Ans. 69) B. Serous carcinoma (Ref: 10 ed. Ackerman)

- Serous cancers of the fallopian are the most common primary fallopian tumors followed by endometrioid cancers

Ans. 70) B. Mucinous Cystadenoma of ovary

Ans. 71) A. Bacterial vaginosis (Ref: 9 ed. Robbins p.993-94) Refer Q 3 for details

Clue cells on Pap smear suggest Bacterial vaginosis

Ans. 72) B. Inhibin (Ref: 9 ed. Robbins p.1032-33) Refer Q 49 for details

21 The Breast

How to go about this chapter?

- **One should be thorough with the following topics:**
  - **Basic lesions and their identification on mammography**
  - **Fibrocystic disease of breast**
  - **Sclerosing Adenosis of breast**
  - **Invasive breast cancers**
  - **Breast cancers (in relation to estrogen and progesterone positivity)**
  - **BRCA1 and BRCA2 mutations in breast cancers**
  - **Ductal Carcinoma in situ**
  - **Lobular Carcinoma in situ**
  - **Paget disease of the nipple**
  - **Phyllodes tumor**
  - **Angiosarcoma of breast**

CLINICAL PRESENTATIONS OF BREAST DISEASE

1) **All of the following are TRUE about mammography EXCEPT:**
a) Sensitivity and specificity increases with age
b) Radiolucent lesions are signs of breast pathology on mammography
c) Small, irregular calcifications imply malignancy
d) 10% of invasive carcinomas are not detected by mammography

BENIGN EPITHELIAL LESIONS

2) **Blue dome cysts are seen in:**
a) Fibroadenoma
b) Fibrocystic breast disease
c) Fat necrosis
d) Lactational adenoma

3) **Following is/are mimics of invasive carcinoma of breast:**
a) Sclerosing adenosis
b) Radial scar
c) Duct papilloma
d) All of the above

4) **Gynecomastia is associated with:**
a) Anabolic steroids
b) Alcohol
c) Anti-retroviral drugs
d) All of the above

CARCINOMA OF BREAST

5) **Which of the following has the highest risk for invasive carcinoma?**
a) Non proliferative breast changes
b) Proliferative disease without atypia
c) Proliferative disease with atypia
d) Carcinoma in situ

6) **All are associated with increased risk of breast cancer EXCEPT:**
a) Young age at menarche
b) Germline mutations
c) Nulliparity
d) Oophorectomy

7) **All are TRUE about familial breast cancers EXCEPT:**
a) BRCA-1 & 2 is the most common gene mutated
b) BRCA-1 mutation increases risk of ovarian cancer
c) BRCA-2 mutation is associated with male breast cancer
d) BRCA-1 is located on chromosome 13q

8) **Under molecular mechanisms of carcinogenesis, most common type of breast cancer is:**
a) ER-positive, HER-2-negative

b) HER-2-positive
c) ER-negative, HER2-negative
d) None of the above

9) Infiltrating breast cancers are most common:
a) Squamous cell carcinoma
b) Adenocarcinoma
c) Small cell carcinoma
d) Poorly differentiated carcinoma

10) All are TRUE about Ductal carcinoma in situ of breast EXCEPT:
a) Proliferation of epithelial cells limited by basement membrane
b) Lacks myoepithelial layer
c) Presents as mammographic density
d) Comedo and non-comedo types are seen

11) All are TRUE about Paget's disease of nipple EXCEPT:
a) Patients have underlying invasive carcinoma
b) Most of cancers are well differentiated cancers
c) Presents with pruritus and eczema
d) Nipple discharge is commonly seen

12) All are TRUE about lobular carcinoma in situ EXCEPT:
a) Loss of E-cadherin is seen
b) Bilateral in 20-40% cases
c) Can develop into invasive ducal carcinoma
d) HER2 overexpression is seen

13) Nottingham histological score include(s):
a) Tubule formation
b) Nuclear pleomorphism
c) Mitotic rate
d) All of the above

14) Which of the following immunohistochemical sub-type of breast cancer has worse prognosis:
a) ER-positive, HER2-negative carcinoma
b) HER2-positive carcinoma
c) ER-negative, HER2-negative carcinomas
d) None of the above

15) TRUE about breast cancer:
a) CDH1 mutation is noted in lobular carcinoma of breast
b) BRCA-1 overexpression is noted in medullary carcinoma
c) Lymphocytic infiltrate within the tumor is associated with higher survival rate
d) All of the above

16) Familial breast cancer is associated with following mutation:
a) BRCA-1
b) BRCA-2
c) E-Cadherin
d) None of the above

17) Most important prognostic factor for invasive breast cancer:
a) Distant metastasis
b) Axillary lymph node status
c) Tumor size
d) Lymphovascular invasion

18) Peau d' orange is associated with following breast cancer:
a) Inflammatory cancer
b) Invasive ductal cancer
c) Lobular cancer
d) Metaplastic cancer

STROMAL TUMORS

19) Following arise(s) from intra-lobular stroma proliferation:
a) Fibroadenoma
b) Phyllodes tumor
c) Both of the above
d) Myofibroblastoma

20) All are TRUE about Cystosarcoma Phyllodes tumor EXCEPT:
a) Arises in sixth decade
b) Most are high grade tumors
c) Lymphatic spread is rare
d) Hematogenous metastasis can be seen

21) Post radiation therapy most common malignancy arising in breast:
a) Myofibroblastoma
b) Chondrosarcoma
c) Angiosarcoma
d) Leiomyosarcoma

22) BRCA2 not associated with: (NEET 2014)
a) Breast cancer
b) Prostate cancer
c) Ovarian cancer
d) Vulval cancer

23) ER positive status in carcinoma breast indicates: (NEET 2014)
a) Prognosis
b) Etiology
c) Site
d) None of the above

24) BRCA 1 is located on which chromosome? (NEET 2014)
a) 17p
b) 17q
c) 13p
d) 13q

25) Phyllodes tumor most commonly presents in: (NEET 2014)
a) 2nd decade
b) 3rd decade
c) 4th decade
d) 6th decade

26) Bloom Richardson grading: (NEET 2014)
- a) Carcinoma breast
- b) Carcinoma lung
- c) Carcinoma prostate
- d) Carcinoma ovary

27) Molecular classification of breast cancer is based on: (AIIMS Nov 2014)
- a) Gene expression profiling
- b) Expression of hormone receptors (ER/PR)
- c) Serum hormone levels
- d) In-vitro response to chemotherapeutic agents

28) All are risk factors for breast carcinoma EXCEPT: (NEET 2013)
- a) OCP
- b) Early menstruation
- c) Family history
- d) Late menopause

29) Proliferating breast mass is: (NEET 2013)
- a) Duct ectasia
- b) Fibroadenoma
- c) Adenosis
- d) Papilloma

30) A 17-year-old female underwent fine needle aspiration cytology (FNAC) for a lump in the breast which was well defined, non-tender and mobile. The diagnosis of a benign lesion can be considered by which of the following pathological features? (AIIMS May 2013)
- a) Dyscohesive ductal epithelial cells without cellular fragments
- b) Tightly-arranged ductal epithelial cells with dyscohesive bare nuclei
- c) Stromal predominance with hyperplasia of spindle cells
- d) Polymorphism with single or arranged ductal epithelial cells

CHAPTER 21 – THE BREAST

Ans. 1) **B. Radiolucent lesions are signs of breast pathology on mammography (Ref: 8 ed. Robbins p.1068-69, 9 ed. p.1045-46)**

- Sensitivity and specificity of mammography **increases with age** Q
- In **young age**, breast appears **fibrous** and **radio-dense**, however in **older women** it appears **radiolucent** Q
- Mammographic signs of **breast carcinoma** are **densities** and **calcifications**
- **Densities** Q – Replacement of adipose tissue with **radio-dense tissue**
- **Calcifications** Q – Small, irregular, numerous and **clustered**
- **10%** of **invasive carcinomas** are **not** detected by mammography

Ans. 2) **B. Fibrocystic breast disease (Ref: 8 ed. Robbins p.1071, 9 ed. p.1048, f-23-6)**

Three principal morphological changes Q **in fibrocystic breast disease**:

- Cysts
- Fibrosis
- Adenosis

Cysts contain turbid, **semi-translucent fluid** of **brown** or **blue color (bluedome cysts)** Q

Ans. 3) **D. All of the above (Ref: 8 ed. Robbins p.1072-73, 9 ed. p.1049-50, f-23-8-10)**

Sclerosing Adenosis Q:

- **Increased number of acini**, which are compressed and distorted in the central portion of the lesion
- Mimics **invasive carcinoma**

Complex Sclerosing Lesion/Radial scar Q:

- Composed of sclerosing adenosis, papillomas and epithelial hyperplasia
- **Central nidus** of **entrapped glands** in a **hyalinized stroma** is surrounded by **long radiating projections** into the stroma
- **Not associated** with prior trauma or surgery

Papilloma Q:

- Grow within a **dilated duct** and are composed of **multiple branching fibrovascular cores**, presents as a **nipple discharge**
- Presents as **densities** or **calcifications** on **mammogram**

Ans. 4) **D. All of the above (Ref: 8 ed. Robbins p.1093, 9 ed. p.1049-50, f-23-11)**

Gynecomastia Q is associated with:

- **Drugs**: Alcohol, marijuana, heroin, antiretroviral therapy and **anabolic steroids**
- **Klinefelter syndrome** (XXY karyotype)
- **Testicular neoplasms**, i.e. **Leydig cell** or **Sertoli cell tumors**

Ans. 5) **D. Carcinoma in situ (Ref: 8 ed. Robbins p.107-74, 9 ed. p.1050-51, t-23-1)**

Relative risk for developing invasive cancer Q of breast in decreasing order:

- Carcinoma in situ > Proliferative disease with atypia > Proliferative disease without atypia > Non proliferative breast changes

Ans. 6) **D. Oophorectomy (Ref: 8 ed. Robbins p.1076-77, 9 ed. p.1053)**

Important points to remember about breast cancer risk:

- **Oophorectomy** Q reduces endogenous estrogens and reduces Q **the risk** of breast cancer
- **Lactation suppresses ovulation** Q and trigger terminal differentiation of luminal cells, thus **reducing** breast cancer risk

- **Early age at menarche, Nulliparity, Hormone replacement therapy increases** the risk of breast cancer Q
- **Oral contraceptives** Q **do not** increase the **risk of breast cancer**

Ans. 7) D. BRCA-1 is located on chromosome 13q (Ref: 8 ed. Robbins p.1077-78, 9 ed. p.1054-55, t-23-2)

- **BRCA1 and BRCA2 mutations** Q are the most common genetic mutations seen in **familial breast cancers**
- **BRCA1** is located on chromosome **17q21** Q and **BRCA2** is located on chromosome **13q12.3** Q
- **BRCA1 mutation** markedly increases the risk of developing **ovarian carcinoma** Q
- Also, **BRCA1** and **BRCA2 mutations** are at higher risk for developing **prostatic** and **pancreatic carcinoma** Q
- Other mutations noted are ***p53*** and ***CHEK2***

Ans. 8) A. ER-positive, HER-2-negative (Ref: 8 ed. Robbins p.1079-80, 9 ed. p.1055-56, f-23-16)

ER-positive, HER2-negative cancers

- Constitute about **50% to 65% of cases** Q
- Associated with germline **BRCA2** Q mutations

HER2-positive cancers

- Constitute approximately **20%** of breast cancers

ER-negative, HER2-negative cancers

- Comprise about **15%** of breast cancers
- Associated with germline **BRCA1** Q mutations

Ans. 9) B. Adenocarcinoma (Ref: 8 ed. Robbins p.1079, 9 ed. p.1057)

- **>95%** of **breast malignancies** are **adenocarcinomas** Q
- **Carcinoma in situ** refers to **neoplastic proliferation** of epithelial cells, which **has not** breached the **basement membrane** Q
- **Invasive carcinoma (infiltrating carcinoma)** has **penetrated** Q through the **basement membrane** and grows within **stroma**

Ans. 10) B. Lacks myoepithelial layer (Ref: 8 ed. Robbins p.1080-82, 9 ed. p.1057-58, f-23-17)

Ductal Carcinoma in Situ (DCIS) Q**:**

- **Malignant clonal proliferation** of **epithelial cells** Q
- Cells **do-not breach** Q the **basement membrane**
- **Myoepithelial cells** lining the ducts/lobules are **preserved**
- Presents as **vaguely palpable mass** or forms a **mammographic density**
- 2 types – **comedo** and **non-comedo**
- **Non-comedo DCIS** Q includes **cribriform**, **solid**, **micropapillary** and **papillary** pattern

Ans. 11) B. Most of cancers are well differentiated cancers (Ref: 8 ed. Robbins p.1080-82, 9 ed. p.1057-58, f-23-18)

Paget disease of the nipple Q**:**

- Presents as a **unilateral erythematous eruption** and **pruritus**
- **Paget cells** into the nipple arises from DCIS cells within the ductal system
- **Nipple discharge** Q is seen as **tumor cells** disrupt the normal epithelial barrier
- Most patients have underlying **poorly differentiated carcinomas** Q (ER-negative and HER2-positive)

Ans. 12) D. HER2 overexpression is seen (Ref: 8 ed. Robbins p.1082-83, 9 ed. p.1059-60, f-23-19)

Lobular Carcinoma In Situ Q**:**

- Characterized by **clonal proliferation of cells** within ducts and lobules
- **Bilateral** in 20% to 40% of cases
- Cells grow in a **discohesive fashion** Q, due to loss of the **E-cadherin** Q **(tumor suppressor protein)**

- **E-cadherin**, is responsible for **cohesion** of **normal epithelial cells** in the **breast** and glandular tissues
- **Expresses ER and PR** Q, but HER2 overexpression is **not** seen
- **LCIS** is a risk factor for **invasive carcinoma**, most commonly **lobular carcinoma**

Ans. 13) D. All of the above (Ref: 9 ed. Robbins p.1064)

Nottingham Histologic Score Q**: Invasive breast carcinomas** are **graded** microscopically by assessing:

- **Tubule formation**
- **Nuclear pleomorphism**
- **Mitotic rate**

Carcinomas are divided into grade I (well differentiated), grade II (moderately differentiated) and grade III (poorly Differentiated) types

Ans. 14) C. ER-negative, HER2-negative carcinomas (Ref: 9 ed. Robbins p.1060-64, t-23-3)

- **Immunohistochemistry** Q has now become the **basis for treatment** of the breast cancers

Following points should be remembered from exam point of view:

A) ER-positive, HER2-negative carcinomas Q**:**

- Majority are **well differentiated carcinoma**
- Includes **mucinous, papillary**, **cribriform** and **lobular cancers**

B) HER2-positive carcinoma Q**:**

- Majority in this group are **poorly differentiated**, with few as **moderately differentiated cancers**
- Includes **apocrine carcinomas** and **micropapillary carcinomas**

C) ER-negative, HER2-negative carcinomas Q

- Includes **poorly differentiated cancers**
- Includes **Medullary, Spindle cell, Adenosquamous and Adenoid cystic carcinoma**

Ans. 15) D. All of the above (Ref: 9 ed. Robbins p.1060-65, t-23-3)

- **Lobular carcinoma** shows **loss of expression of *CDH1*** Q (gene that encodes **E-cadherin**)
- **Medullary carcinoma** is associated with **BRCA1 mutation** Q
- Presence of **lymphocytic infiltrates** Q in tumors is associated with **higher survival rates** and a greater response to **chemotherapy**

Ans. 16) B. BRCA-2 (Ref: 8 ed. Robbins p.1094, 9 ed. p.1066)

- **BRCA2 mutation** Q is **most commonly** associated with **familial male breast cancers**

Ans. 17) A. Distant metastasis (Ref: 8 ed. Robbins p.1089, 9 ed. p.1066-67)

- In **absence** of **distant metastases** Q, **axillary lymph node status** is the most important **prognostic factor** for **invasive carcinoma**

Ans. 18) A. Inflammatory cancer (Ref: 8 ed. Robbins p.1089, 9 ed. p.1067)

Inflammatory Carcinoma Q**:**

- Presents with **breast erythema** and **skin thickening**
- **Peau d' orange** Q – **Edematous skin** mimics the surface of an **orange peel**
- **Metastatic carcinoma cells** fill **dermal lymphatics** and blocks **lymphatic drainage** resulting in **peau d' orange** Q
- Most patients have **distant metastases** and have **poor prognosis** Q

Ans. 19) C. Both of the above (Ref: 8 ed. Robbins p.1091, 9 ed. p.1069)

- **Intra-lobular stroma** proliferation – stromal proliferation within each lobule. **Each lobule** is composed of **numerous acini**
- **Interlobular stroma proliferation –** Stromal proliferation in between two lobules
- **Fibroadenoma** and **Phyllodes**: **Biphasic tumors** arising from **intra-lobular stroma** Q

- **Interlobular stroma** [Q] in breast gives rise to **Pseudoangiomatous stromal hyperplasia**, **Myofibroblastoma** and **fibrous tumors**

Ans. 20) B. Most are high grade tumors (Ref: 8 ed. Robbins p.1091-92, 9 ed. p.1069-70, f-23-28)

Phyllodes tumor/Cystosarcoma Phyllodes [Q]**:**

- Arises from **intralobular stroma** [Q], most commonly in **sixth decade**
- Associated with gain in **chromosome 1q** [Q]
- **Low-grade tumors** [Q] and can recur occasionally
- **Lymphatic spread** is **rare** and **axillary lymph node** dissection is **contraindicated**
- Rarely, **hematogenous metastases** can be seen in **high-grade lesions**

Morphology [Q]**:**

- **Phyllodes tumor** has **higher cellularity, mitotic rate, nuclear pleomorphism**, stromal overgrowth and infiltrative borders

Ans. 21) C. Angiosarcoma (Ref: 8 ed. Robbins p.1093, 9 ed. p.1070, f-23-28)

Angiosarcomas of the breast [Q]:

- Can be **sporadic** or arise as a complication of **radiation therapy**
- **Sporadic angiosarcomas** occur in **young women**
- **High grade** and have **poor prognosis**

Ans. 22) D. Vulval cancer (Ref: 9 ed. Robbins p.1054-55) Refer Q 7 for details

Ans. 23) A. Prognosis (Ref: 9 ed. Robbins p.1060-64) Refer Q 14 for details

Ans. 24) B. 17q (Ref: 9ed. Robbins p. 315, 1054) Refer Q 7 for details

Ans. 25) D. 6th decade (Ref: 9 ed. Robbins p.1069-70) Refer Q 20 for details

Ans. 26) A. Carcinoma breast

Microscopically, grading of carcinoma breast is done by using Bloom Richardson Grading

Ans. 27) A. Gene expression profiling (Ref: 9 ed. p.1060-64, 1055-56) Refer Q 8 and 14 for details

Ans. 28) A. OCP (Ref: 9 ed. Robbins p.1051-53) Refer Q 6 for details

Ans. 29) D. Papilloma

Ans. 30) B. Tightly arranged ductal epithelial cells with dyscohesive bare nuclei

Differentiation of benign and malignant breast lesions on cytological features

a) Dispersal of cells – Lack of cell-to-cell cohesion is a characteristic feature of malignancy

b) Biphasic pattern with bipolar cells – Indicates benign process

c) Nuclear membrane irregularity – Indicates malignancy

22 The Endocrine System

How to go about this chapter?

- **One should be thorough with the following topics:**
  - **Anterior and Posterior pituitary hormones**
  - **Craniopharyngiomas**
  - **Pendred syndrome**
  - **Hashimoto thyroiditis, De Quervain thyroiditis**
  - **Follicular adenomas**
  - **RET/PTC mutation**
  - **Papillary carcinoma, Follicular carcinoma of thyroid, Medullary carcinoma**
  - **Hypercalcemia, Secondary hyperparathyroidism**
  - **Diabetes mellitus, Diabetes Insipidus, Diabetic neuropathy**
  - **Diabetes Insipidus**
  - **Insulinomas, Glucagonoma**
  - **21-hydroxylase deficiency**
  - **Waterhouse-Friderichsen Syndrome Pheochromocytoma**
  - **MEN-1 and MEN-2 syndrome**

THE PITUITARY GLAND

1) Anterior pituitary secretes following hormones EXCEPT:

a) ACTH b) TSH
c) GH d) ADH

2) All are TRUE about Pituitary cell type and their hormones released EXCEPT:

a) Lactotroph – Prolactin
b) Somatotroph – ACTH
c) Thyrotroph – TSH
d) Gonadotroph – FSH

3) Most common mutation seen in pituitary adenoma:

a) Cyclin D
b) G-protein
c) P53
d) Rb

4) All of the following are pituitary macroadenomas EXCEPT:

a) FSH adenoma
b) TSH adenoma
c) Prolactinomas in male
d) ACTH secreting adenomas

5) All are TRUE about Craniopharyngiomas EXCEPT:

a) Arises from remnants of Rathke pouch
b) Bimodal age distribution
c) Have excellent prognosis
d) Adamantinomatous variant commonly seen in adults

THYROID GLAND

6) Causes of thyrotoxicosis include(s):

a) Grave's disease
b) TSH secreting pituitary adenoma
c) Toxic multinodular goiter
d) All of the above

7) All are TRUE regarding thyroid storm EXCEPT:

a) Due to abrupt onset of hyperthyroidism
b) Acute elevation of catecholamine level
c) Common in patients with Hashimoto's thyroiditis
d) It is a medical emergency

8) Pendred syndrome occurs due to the following mutation:

a) SLC26A4
b) PAX-8
c) FOXE-1
d) TSHR

9) Most sensitive screening test for hypothyroidism:
a) Free T4 levels b) TSH levels
c) T3 levels d) T4 levels

10) Genes involved in Hashimoto's thyroiditis:
a) CTLA4 b) PTPN22
c) Both of the above d) HLA-DR3

11) In Hashimoto's thyroiditis, thyroid cell death is brought about by:
a) CD-4+ T-cells
b) CD-8+ T-cells
c) Plasma cells
d) All of the above

12) Hashimoto's thyroiditis is associated with increased risk of developing:
a) Type 1 Diabetes
b) B-cell lymphoma of thyroid
c) Papillary cancer of thyroid
d) All of the above

13) All are TRUE about morphology of Hashimoto's thyroiditis EXCEPT:
a) Mononuclear inflammatory infiltrate
b) Well-developed germinal centers
c) Hurthle cells
d) Fibrosis extend beyond the capsule of gland

14) All are TRUE about Granulomatous thyroiditis EXCEPT:
a) Most common cause of thyroid pain
b) Affects men more commonly than women
c) Preceded by viral infection
d) Also known as DeQuervain thyroiditis

15) Following is a manifestation of systemic autoimmune IgG4-related disease:
a) Grave's disease
b) Hashimoto's thyroiditis
c) Riedel thyroiditis
d) Granulomatous thyroiditis

16) Most common antibody subtype in Graves' disease:
a) Thyroid stimulating immunoglobulin
b) Thyroglobulin
c) Thyroid peroxidase
d) None of the above

17) Infiltrative ophthalmopathy occurs due to:
a) Infiltration by mononuclear cells
b) Accumulation of hyaluronic acid and chondroitin sulfate
c) Increased numbers of adipocytes
d) All of the above

18) Cut surface of thyroid in Graves' disease has:
a) Beefy appearance
b) Salt and pepper appearance
c) Sausage appearance
d) None of the above

19) Features of Graves' disease include(s):
a) Hyperthyroidism
b) Infiltrative ophthalmopathy
c) Pretibial myxedema
d) All of the above

20) Goitrogen include:
a) Cabbage b) Wheat
c) Rice d) Barley

21) Incidence of malignancy in long standing multinodular goiter is:
a) 0 % b) <5 %
c) <10 % d) <20 %

22) All are TRUE regarding thyroid nodules EXCEPT:
a) Solitary nodule is more likely neoplastic than multiple nodules
b) Nodules in younger patients are likely to be neoplastic than in older patients
c) Nodules in females are likely to be neoplastic
d) Hot nodules are more likely to be benign

23) TRUE about Follicular adenomas:
a) Intact well-formed capsule encircling the tumor
b) Present as cold nodules on radionuclide scanning
c) Solitary, spherical encapsulated lesion
d) All of the above

24) All of the following thyroid cancers arises from thyroid follicular epithelium EXCEPT:
a) Papillary cancer
b) Follicular cancer
c) Medullary cancer
d) Anaplastic cancer

25) Following mutation(s) is/are seen in Papillary carcinoma of thyroid:
a) RET/PTC
b) BRAF
c) Both of the above
d) None of the above

26) Following mutation(s) is/are noted in follicular carcinoma of thyroid:
a) RAS b) PI-3K/AKT
c) PTEN d) All of the above

27) TRUE about papillary thyroid cancer morphology:
a) Branching papillae
b) Optically clear nuclei
c) Psammoma bodies
d) All of the above

28) Papillary carcinoma of thyroid most commonly metastasize through:
a) Lymphatic route
b) Hematogenous route
c) Both of the above
d) None of the above

29) Most common variant of papillary cancer thyroid:
a) Follicular b) Tall cell
c) Columnar d) Diffuse sclerosing

30) Papillary micro-carcinoma is:
a) <1 mm in size b) <1 cm in size
c) <5 mm in size d) <5 cm in size

31) Following is helpful to demonstrate the recurrence of follicular carcinoma:
a) Serum TSH
b) Serum thyroglobulin
c) Serum T3
d) Serum T4

32) TRUE about medullary carcinoma of thyroid:
a) Arises from C-cells of thyroid
b) Raised Calcitonin levels
c) Associated with MEN syndrome
d) All of the above

PARATHYROID GLAND

33) Most common cause of primary hyperparathyroidism:
a) Parathyroid adenoma
b) Primary hyperplasia
c) Parathyroid carcinoma
d) None of the above

34) In parathyroid adenomas all are seen EXCEPT:
a) Chief cells
b) Oxyphil cells
c) Non-neoplastic parathyroid tissue
d) Adipose tissue

35) In primary parathyroid hyperplasia, weight of parathyroid glands rarely exceeds:
a) 0.5 gm b) 1 gm
c) 5 gm d) 10 gm

36) Skeletal abnormalities seen in untreated primary hyperparathyroidism:
a) Osteoporosis
b) Brown tumor
c) Osteitis fibrosa cystica
d) All of the above

37) Causes of hypercalcemia with raised PTH includes all EXCEPT:
a) Parathyroid adenoma
b) Parathyroid hyperplasia
c) Familial hypocalciuric hypercalcemia
d) Hypercalcemia of malignancy

38) Most common cause of secondary hyperparathyroidism:
a) Renal failure
b) Inadequate dietary intake of calcium
c) Steatorrhea
d) Vitamin D deficiency

THE ENDOCRINE PANCREAS

39) TRUE about pancreatic cells and the hormone released:
a) β cells – insulin
b) α cells – glucagon
c) δ cells – somatostatin
d) All of the above

40) Diagnosis of diabetes include/s:
a) Fasting plasma glucose $\geq$ 126 mg/dL
b) Random plasma glucose $\geq$ 200 mg/dL
c) Glycated hemoglobin (HbA1C) level $\geq$ 6.5%
d) All of the above

41) Following HLA haplotype(s) is/are associated with Type 1 DM:
a) HLA-DR3 b) HLA-DR4
c) HLA-DQ8 d) All of the above

42) Persistent hyperglycemia leads to tissue damage by:
a) Advanced glycation end products
b) Activation of protein kinase C
c) Disturbances in polyol pathway
d) All of the above

43) Following tissue/s don't require insulin for glucose transport:
a) Nerves b) Lenses
c) Kidneys d) All of the above

44) Following changes are seen in Pancreas in Diabetes:
a) Reduction in size of pancreas
b) Leucocytic infiltrates in islets
c) Amyloid deposition
d) All of the above

45) Most common cause of death in Diabetic patients:
a) Myocardial infarction
b) Renal failure
c) Cerebrovascular insufficiency
d) Gangrene of lower extremities

46) Characteristic lesion of kidney in diabetes:
a) Glomerular lesions
b) Vascular lesions
c) Pyelonephritis
d) All of the above

47) Micro albuminuria is defined as:
a) <10 mg% of albumin in urine
b) >10 mg% of albumin in urine
c) <30 mg% of albumin in urine
d) >30 mg% of albumin in urine

48) Neovascularization in diabetic nephropathy occurs due to:
a) FGF b) TGF
c) VEGF d) All of the above

49) **Most frequent pattern of diabetic nephropathy:**
a) Distal symmetric polyneuropathy
b) Proximal symmetric polyneuropathy
c) Both of the above
d) None of the above

50) **Most common pancreatic endocrine tumor:**
a) Insulinoma b) Gastrinomas
c) Somatostatinoma d) Glucagonomas

51) **Nesidioblastosis is associated with:**
a) Maternal diabetes
b) Beckwith-Wiedemann syndrome
c) Mutation in beta cell K^+-channel protein
d) All of the above

52) **TRUE about Zollinger-Ellison syndrome:**
a) Also called as gastrinomas
b) Seen in duodenum and pancreas
c) Jejunal ulcers are commonly seen
d) All of the above

53) **Necrolytic migratory erythema is seen in:**
a) Glucagonomas
b) Gastrinomas
c) Somatostatinoma
d) Insulinoma

54) ***VIPoma* is/are associated with:**
a) Pheochromocytomas
b) Ganglioneuromas
c) Neuroblastomas
d) All of the above

ADRENAL GLANDS

55) **Most common cause of endogenous hypercortisolism:**
a) Pituitary microadenoma
b) Pituitary macroadenoma
c) Cortical cell hyperplasia
d) None of the above

56) **Ectopic ACTH production leading to Cushing syndrome is seen most commonly in:**
a) Small cell carcinoma of lung
b) Carcinoid
c) Medullary carcinoma of thyroid
d) Islet cell tumors

57) **Most common enzyme deficiency leading to congenital adrenal hyperplasia:**
a) 21 hydroxylase
b) 11 hydroxylase
c) 17 hydroxylase
d) None of the above

58) **All are TRUE regarding clinical features of "salt-wasting" syndrome EXCEPT:**
a) Deficiency of 21 hydroxylase
b) Inability to convert progesterone to deoxycorticosterone
c) Easily recognized in males at birth
d) Presents with hyponatremia, hyperkalemia

59) **Most common infection leading to Waterhouse-Friderichsen syndrome:**
a) N. meningitides
b) Pseudomonas
c) Pneumococci
d) H. influenza

60) **Addison's disease occurs due to:**
a) Autoimmune adrenalitis
b) Infections
c) Metastatic neoplasms
d) Any of the above

61) **TRUE regarding pheochromocytomas:**
a) 10% are extra adrenal
b) 10% are malignant
c) 10% are bilateral
d) All of the above

62) **Germline mutation/s seen in familial pheochromocytomas:**
a) RET
b) NF-1
c) VHL
d) All of the above

63) **Definite diagnosis of malignancy in pheochromocytoma is based on:**
a) Capsular invasion
b) Vascular invasion
c) Both a and b
d) Metastasis

64) **TRUE about MEN-1 syndrome:**
a) Primary hyperparathyroidism is most common manifestation
b) Duodenum is most common site of gastrinomas
c) Most frequent anterior pituitary tumor is prolactinoma
d) All of the above

65) **MEN 2A syndrome is characterized by all EXCEPT:**
a) Medullary carcinoma of thyroid
b) Pheochromocytoma
c) Parathyroid hyperplasia
d) Gastrinomas

66) **Most common cause of Cushing's syndrome is: (NEET 2014)**
a) Pituitary adenoma
b) Adrenal adenoma
c) Adrenal carcinoma
d) McCune Albright syndrome

67) **Most commonly seen in MEN 1: (NEET 2014)**
a) Insulinoma
b) Gastrinomas

c) Glucagonomas
d) Somatostatinoma

68) FNAC cannot diagnose: (AIIMS Nov 2014)
a) Simple cyst
b) Colloid goiter
c) Papillary carcinoma
d) Follicular carcinoma

69) Insulin resistance state causing hyperglycemia is present in: (NEET 2014)
a) Acromegaly
b) Osteomalacia
c) Liver cell carcinoma
d) Somatostatinoma

70) Medullary thyroid carcinoma is associated with: (NEET 2014)
a) MEN I
b) MEN II
c) MEN III
d) MEN IV

71) Following is TRUE about pheochromocytoma EXCEPT: (NEET 2014)
a) Extra-adrenal tumors show Zellballen pattern
b) Follows rule of 10's
c) 90% of non-familial cases are bilateral
d) 10% of pheochromocytomas are extra-adrenal

72) Which of the following is not a hereditary disease? (NEET 2014)
a) Neurofibromatosis
b) Cretinism
c) Huntington's disease
d) Hereditary spherocytosis

73) Carcinoma which arises in the thyroglosal cyst is: (NEET 2014)
a) Papillary carcinoma
b) Follicular
c) Anaplastic
d) Medullary

74) Tense and painful thyroiditis is: (NEET 2014)
a) Dequervian's thyroiditis
b) Riedel thyroiditis
c) Hashimoto thyroiditis
d) Subacute lymphocytic thyroiditis

75) Which of the following is TRUE about Reidel's thyroiditis? (NEET 2014)
a) Fibrosis involves the thyroid and surrounding neck structures
b) Patient presents with hard fixed thyroid mass
c) It may be associated with retroperitoneal fibrosis
d) All of the above

76) Which of the following is most reliable feature of malignant transformation of pheochromocytoma? (NEET 2013)
a) Presence of mitotic figures
b) Capsular invasion
c) Vascular invasion
d) Metastasis

77) Tumor that follows rule of 10 is: (NEET 2013)
a) Pheochromocytoma
b) Oncocytoma
c) Lymphoma
d) Renal cell carcinoma

78) RET gene mutation is associated with which malignancy? (NEET 2013)
a) Pheochromocytoma
b) Medullary carcinoma thyroid
c) Lymphoma
d) Renal cell carcinoma

79) Werner syndrome is: (NEET 2013)
a) MEN I
b) MEN IIA
c) MEN II B
d) AIP

80) Orphan Annie eye nuclei appearance is characteristic of: (NEET 2013)
a) Papillary carcinoma thyroid
b) Carcinoma pituitary
c) Paraganglioma
d) Meningioma

81) Which is not seen in MEN I? (NEET 2013)
a) Parathyroid adenoma
b) Pancreatic cancer
c) Prolactinoma
d) Medullary carcinoma thyroid

82) Which thyroid carcinoma has amyloid? (NEET 2013)
a) Papillary
b) Follicular
c) Medullary
d) Anaplastic

83) Which of the following gene defect is associated with development of medullary carcinoma of thyroid? (NEET 2013)
a) RET Proto oncogene
b) FAP gene
c) Rb gene
d) BRCA-1 gene

84) Psammoma bodies are seen in all EXCEPT: (AIPGMEE 2011)
a) Follicular carcinoma thyroid
b) Papillary carcinoma thyroid
c) Cystadenocarcinomas
d) Meningioma

85) Difference between follicular adenoma and follicular carcinoma: (AIPGMEE 2012)
a) Vascular invasion
b) Histological appearance
c) FNAC
d) Clinical features

86) A 27-year-old female with right sided thyroid nodule was operated. A 2 × 2 cm thyroid nodule was resected and the following histology was found. What is your diagnosis? (Image based question) (AIIMS Nov 2014)

a) Papillary carcinoma of thyroid
b) Adenomatous goiter
c) Follicular adenoma
d) Graves' disease

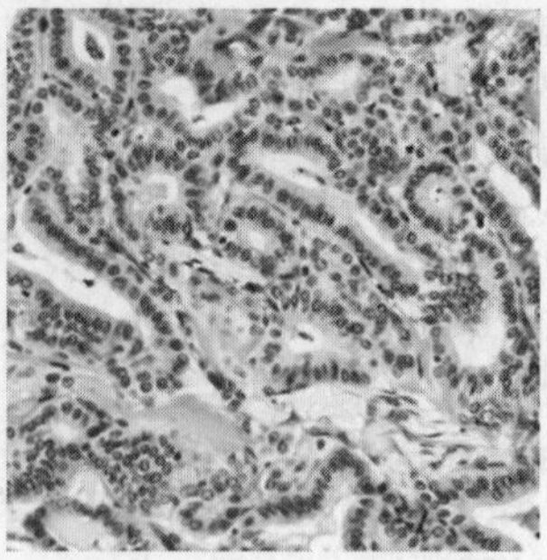

CHAPTER 22: THE ENDOCRINE SYSTEM

Ans. 1) **D. ADH (Ref: 8 ed. Robbins p.1098-99, 9 ed. p.1074, f-24-1)**

Hormones produced from **anterior pituitary** Q:

- Growth hormone (GH)
- Prolactin (PRL)
- Adrenocorticotropic hormone (ACTH)
- Pro opiomelanocortin (POMC)
- Melanocyte stimulating hormone (MSH)
- Thyroid-stimulating hormone (TSH), Follicle-stimulating hormone (FSH) and Luteinizing hormone (LH)

Hormones produced from **posterior pituitary** Q:

- Oxytocin and Antidiuretic hormone (ADH, also called **vasopressin**)

Ans. 2) **B. Somatotroph – ACTH (Ref: 8 ed. Robbins p.1100, 9 ed. p.1076, t-24-1)**

Pituitary cells and their respective hormones Q:

Pituitary Cell	Hormone
Lactotroph	Prolactin
Somatotroph	GH
Mammosomatotroph	Prolactin, GH
Corticotroph	ACTH and other POMC-derived peptides
Thyrotroph	TSH
Gonadotroph	FSH, LH

Ans. 3) **B. G-protein (Ref: 8 ed. Robbins p.1101-02, 9 ed. p.1076-77, f-24-3, t-24-2)**

- **G-protein mutations** Q are most common alterations in sporadic **pituitary adenomas**
- **Somatotroph cell adenomas** show **GNAS mutations**
- In aggressive tumors: Overexpression of **cyclin D1**, mutations of **TP53** and epigenetic silencing of retinoblastoma gene **(RB)** are seen

Ans. 4) **D. ACTH secreting adenomas (Ref: 10 ed. Ackerman p.2448)**

- **Microadenomas** are **less than 1 cm** Q in diameter, whereas **macroadenomas** are **more than 1 cms** Q
- **Prolactinomas (females), ACTH secreting adenomas** are **Microadenomas** Q
- **FSH/LH adenomas, TSH adenomas, GH adenomas, Prolactinomas in males** are Macroadenomas Q

Ans. 5) **D. Adamantinomatous variant commonly seen in adults (Ref: 8 ed. Robbins p.1106-07, 9 ed. p.1082, f-24-7)**

Craniopharyngiomas Q:

- Arises from **vestigial remnants** of **Rathke pouch** Q
- Most commonly located in **suprasellar** Q region
- **Bimodal age** distribution, first peak in children (5 to 15 years) and second peak in adults (65 years)
- Occurs due to **mutation** of the gene encoding **β-catenin** Q

Morphology:

Gross:

- 3 to 4 cm in diameter, encapsulated, **cystic** Q to solid

Two microscopic variants: Adamantinomatous craniopharyngiomas (in children) and **papillary craniopharyngiomas** (in adults)

- Tumors **less than 5 cm** in diameter, have excellent survival rates
- Malignant transformation into **squamous carcinomas** is **rare**

Adamantinomatous type [Q]

- Shows nests or cords of **stratified squamous epithelium** which shows **peripheral palisading**
- Compact, lamellar keratin formation **("wet keratin")** is a **diagnostic feature**
- **Dystrophic calcification** [Q] is commonly seen
- **Cysts** contain a cholesterol-rich, thick brownish yellow fluid **"machine oil"**

Papillary craniopharyngiomas [Q]

- Shows **solid sheets** and **papillae** lined by squamous epithelium, but lack peripheral palisading
- They **lack** keratin, calcification and cysts

Ans. 6) **D. All of the above (Ref: 8 ed. Robbins p.1108-09, 9 ed. p.1083-84, t-24-3)**

Causes of Hyperthyroidism:

Primary [Q]

- Diffuse hyperplasia (Graves' disease)
- Hyper functioning ("toxic") multinodular goiter
- Hyper functioning ("toxic") adenoma
- Iodine-induced hyperthyroidism
- Neonatal thyrotoxicosis associated with maternal Graves' disease

Secondary [Q]

- TSH-secreting pituitary adenoma (rare)

All **primary causes** are associated with **decreased TSH** [Q] levels; however, TSH-secreting pituitary adenoma is associated with increased TSH levels

Ans. 7) **C. Common in patients with Hashimoto's thyroiditis (Ref: 8 ed. Robbins p.1109, 9 ed. p.1084, t-24-3)**

Thyroid storm [Q]:

- Abrupt onset of **severe hyperthyroidism** [Q]
- Most common in patients with underlying **Graves' disease** [Q]
- Results from the **increased catecholamine levels** [Q] as seen in infection, surgery, cessation of anti-thyroid medication or stress [Q]
- Patients presents with **fever** and **tachycardia** (out of proportion of fever)
- Is a **medical emergency** [Q] and **cardiac arrhythmia** is most common cause of death

Ans. 8) **A. SLC26A4 (Ref: 8 ed. Robbins p.1110, 9 ed. p.1085, t-24-4)**

Pendred syndrome: Characterized by hypothyroidism and sensorineural deafness due to mutation in ***SCL26A4 gene*** [Q]

Common Causes of Hypothyroidism [Q]:

- Genetic defects in thyroid development **(PAX8, FOXE1, TSH receptor mutations)**
- Thyroid hormone resistance syndrome **(THRB mutations)**
- **Post ablative** – Surgery, radioiodine therapy, or external irradiation
- Autoimmune – **Hashimoto thyroiditis**
- **Iodine deficiency**
- Drugs (lithium, iodides, p-aminosalicylic acid)
- Congenital biosynthetic defect **(dyshormonogenetic goiter)**

Ans. 9) **B. TSH levels (Ref: 8 ed. Robbins p.1111, 9 ed. p.1086)**

- Measurement of the **serum TSH level** [Q] is the **most sensitive screening test** [Q] for **hypothyroidism**

- **TSH levels** are **increased** Q in **primary hypothyroidism**

Ans. 10) C. Both of the above (Ref: 8 ed. Robbins p.1111, 9 ed. p.1086)

- **Hashimoto thyroiditis** Q is associated with polymorphisms in ***cytotoxic T lymphocyte-associated antigen-4 (CTLA4)***Q and ***protein tyrosine phosphatase-22 (PTPN22)*** Q genes
- **Type 1 diabetes** is also associated with **polymorphisms** in both **CTLA4** and **PTPN22** Q
- **Polymorphisms** in the genes like **CTLA4, PTPN22 and HLA-DR3 allele** are seen in **Graves' disease** Q

Ans. 11) D. All of the above (Ref: 8 ed. Robbins p.1111-12, 9 ed. p.1086-87, f-24-10)

In **Hashimoto's thyroiditis** Q, following immunologic mechanisms leads to thyroid cell death:

- **CD8+ cytotoxic** Q T cell-mediated cell death
- **Cytokine-mediated** cell death: Activation of **CD4+ T cells** Q leads to the production of **interferon-γ** and activation of **macrophages**, leading to cell death
- **Anti-thyroid antibodies** Q (anti-thyroglobulin, anti-thyroid peroxidase antibodies) leading to the destruction of follicular cells by **antibody-dependent cell mediated cytotoxicity** Q

Ans. 12) D. All of the above (Ref: 8 ed. Robbins p.1112-13, 9 ed. p.1087-88, f-24-11)

Hashimoto's thyroiditis Q is associated with:

- Type 1 diabetes, autoimmune adrenalitis, systemic lupus erythematosus, myasthenia gravis and Sjögren syndrome
- **Extra-nodal marginal zone B-cell lymphomas** Q of **thyroid gland**
- Increased risk of **papillary carcinomas** Q

Ans. 13) D. Fibrosis extend beyond the capsule of gland (Ref: 8 ed. Robbins p.1112-13, 9 ed. p.1087-88, f-24-11)

Morphology of Hashimoto's thyroiditis Q:

- Infiltration of the parenchyma by **mononuclear inflammatory infiltrate** containing **small lymphocytes, plasma cells** and well-developed **germinal centers**
- Thyroid follicle lining cells have abundant eosinophilic, granular cytoplasm – **Hurthle cells** Q
- **Fibrosis does not extend** beyond the capsule of the gland (feature of **Riedel thyroiditis**)

Ans. 14) B. Affects men more commonly than women (Ref: 8 ed. Robbins p.1113, 9 ed. p.1088, f-24-12)

Granulomatous Thyroiditis (De Quervain thyroiditis) Q

- Affects **women** more often than men (4 : 1)
- Self-limited disease, believed to be triggered by **viral infection** Q
- **Most common** cause of **thyroid pain** Q
- **Microscopy – Multinucleated giant cells** and **lymphocytic infiltrate**

Note – Remember that, all **autoimmune diseases** and thyroid disorders are most commonly seen in females

Ans. 15) C. Riedel Thyroiditis (Ref: 8 ed. Robbins p.1114, 9 ed. p.1088-89)

Riedel thyroiditis Q**:**

- Characterized by **extensive fibrosis** involving **thyroid** and neck structures
- Stony hard thyroid mass simulates **thyroid carcinoma** Q
- Associated with **retro peritoneal fibrosis** Q
- An **example** of **systemic autoimmune IgG4-related disease** Q (fibrosis and infiltration of thyroid by plasma cells producing IgG4)

Ans. 16) A. Thyroid stimulating immunoglobulin (Ref: 8 ed. Robbins p.1114, 9 ed. p.1089)

Graves' Disease Q:

- **Autoimmune disorder** characterized by the production of autoantibodies against the **TSH receptor**
- **TSH receptor antibodies** Q: can either stimulate or block TSH receptor
- **Thyroid stimulating immunoglobulin (TSI)** Q is the **most common** antibody detected in 90% of patients

- Other antibodies seen are **anti-thyroglobulin** and **anti-thyroid peroxidase**

Ans. 17) D. All of the above (Ref: 8 ed. Robbins p.1114, 9 ed. p.1089)

Causes of **infiltrative ophthalmopathy** [Q]

- Infiltration of retro-orbital space by **mononuclear cells** [Q]
- Inflammation with edema and swelling of **extra-ocular muscles** [Q]
- Accumulation of extracellular matrix components, such as **hyaluronic acid** [Q] and **chondroitin sulfate** [Q]
- Increased numbers of **adipocytes** [Q]

Ans. 18) A. Beefy appearance (Ref: 8 ed. Robbins p.1114-15, 9 ed. p.1089-90, f-24-13)

- Cut surface of **thyroid parenchyma** in Graves' disease has soft, **meaty appearance** [Q] resembling **muscle**

Ans. 19) D. All of the above (Ref: 8 ed. Robbins p.1114-15, 9 ed. p.1089-90)

Clinical Features of Graves' Disease [Q]:

- Diffuse hyperplasia of thyroid gland, ophthalmopathy and dermopathy (pretibial myxedema)
- **Laboratory findings** [Q] – Elevated free **T4** and **T3 levels** and **depressed TSH levels**

Ans. 20) A. Cabbage (Ref: 8 ed. Robbins p.1116, 9 ed. p.1091)

Goitrogens [Q]:

- Substances that interfere with thyroid hormone synthesis
- **Examples** – Vegetables belonging to the **Brassicaceae (Cruciferae) family** (e.g., cabbage, cauliflower, Brussels sprouts, turnips and cassava)
- Cassava contains thiocyanate that **inhibits iodide transport** within the thyroid

Ans. 21) B. <5% (Ref: 8 ed. Robbins p.1117-18, 9 ed. p.1092)

- **Incidence of malignancy** in long-standing **multinodular goiters** is **low (<5%)** [Q] but not zero
- **Plummer syndrome** [Q] – When in a patient of long-standing goiter, an **autonomous nodule** develops and produce **hyperthyroidism (toxic multinodular goiter)**

Ans. 22) C. Nodules in females are likely to be neoplastic (Ref: 8 ed. Robbins p.1118, 9 ed. p.1093)

Clinical criteria which gives a clue to the nature of **thyroid nodules** [Q]:

- Thyroid disorders are more common in females, bur **thyroid nodules** in **males** [Q] are more likely to be **malignant**
- **Solitary nodules**, are more likely to be **neoplastic** [Q] than are multiple nodules
- **Nodules in younger patients** are more likely to be **neoplastic** [Q]
- **Radiation treatment** to the head and neck is a risk factor for **thyroid malignancy**
- **Hot nodules** (**Functional nodules** that take up **radioactive iodine**) are likely to be **benign** [Q] than malignant

Ans. 23) D. All of the above (Ref: 8 ed. Robbins p.1118-19, 9 ed. p.1093-94,f-24-16)

Salient features of Follicular adenomas [Q]:

- Are **solitary, spherical, encapsulated lesions**, that are demarcated from the surrounding thyroid parenchyma by a **well-defined, intact capsule** [Q]
- **Capsular integrity** is critical in **distinguishing follicular adenomas** from **follicular carcinomas**, the latter demonstrates **capsular and/or vascular invasion** [Q]
- On **radionuclide scanning**, non-functioning adenomas appear as **cold nodules** [Q]
- Only, **10%** of cold nodules are **malignant** [Q]
- **Toxic adenomas** show mutations of the **TSH receptor signaling** pathway
- **Non-functioning adenomas** have **RAS or PIK3CA** mutation, or bear a **PAX8-PPARG fusion** [Q] gene

Ans. 24) C. Medullary cancer (Ref: 8 ed. Robbins p.1119, 9 ed. p.1094)

- Most **thyroid carcinomas** are derived from the thyroid follicular epithelium **except medullary carcinomas** [Q]

Ans. 25) C. Both of the above (Ref: 8 ed. Robbins p.1119-20, 9 ed. p.1094-95, f-24-18)

- Fusion genes, **RET/PTC (RET/papillary thyroid carcinoma)** Q are seen in 20-40% cases of **papillary thyroid cancers**
- **Gain-of-function mutation** in **BRAF gene** Q is seen in one third of patients

Note:

BRAF mutations in **papillary carcinomas** are associated with adverse prognosis (like **metastatic disease** and **extra-thyroidal extension**)

Ans. 26) D. All of the above (Ref: 8 ed. Robbins p.1119-21, 9 ed. p.1094-95, f-24-18)

Following mutations are seen in **Follicular carcinoma of thyroid**:

- **Gain-of function** point mutations of ***RAS*** or ***PIK3CA***
- **Loss-of function** mutations of ***PTEN***
- **PAX8 – PPARG fusion gene** Q product which leads to cell growth, differentiation and proliferation

Ans. 27) D. All of the above (Ref: 8 ed. Robbins p.1121-22, 9 ed. p.1095-97, f-24-19)

Papillary carcinomas are the **most common** Q form of thyroid cancer

Microscopy Q:

- Contain **branching papillae** with a **fibrovascular stalk** Q
- Papillae are lined by **cuboidal epithelial cells** (well differentiated to anaplastic)
- Nuclei imparts an **optically clear** or empty appearance, also known as **ground glass** or **Orphan Annie eye** Q nuclei
- **Pseudo-inclusions/intra-nuclear inclusions** Q – Due to invagination of the cytoplasm
- **Intra-nuclear grooves** Q
- **Psammoma bodies** Q – Concentrically calcified structures present within the cores of papillae

Ans. 28) A. Lymphatic route (Ref: 8 ed. Robbins p.1121-22, 9 ed. p.1095-97)

- Metastases to adjacent **cervical lymph nodes** Q can be the **first manifestation** of disease
- **Cervical lymph node metastasis** does not have a significant influence on prognosis

Ans. 29) A. Follicular (Ref: 8 ed. Robbins p.1121-22, 9 ed. p.1095-97)

Follicular Variant Q

- **Most common variant** of papillary thyroid cancer
- Has **follicular architecture** with **nuclear features** that of **papillary carcinoma**

Ans. 30) B. <1 cm in size (Ref: 8 ed. Robbins p.1121-22, 9 ed. p.1095-97)

- Papillary micro-carcinoma is defined as **papillary carcinoma less than 1 cm** Q in size

Ans. 31) B. Serum thyroglobulin (Ref: 8 ed. Robbins p.1124, 9 ed. p.1098)

- **Serum thyroglobulin levels** Q are used for **monitoring tumor recurrence**, because it is not detectable in a patient who is free of disease

Ans. 32) D. All of the above (Ref: 8 ed. Robbins p.1124-26, 9 ed. p.1090-1100, f-24-22)

Medullary Carcinoma Q:

- Derived from the **Para follicular cells**, or **C cells** of the thyroid
- Tumor cells secrete **calcitonin** Q, which plays an important role in the diagnosis and postoperative follow-up
- Other polypeptide hormones secreted are serotonin, ACTH and vasoactive intestinal peptide (VIP)
- Has an association with **MEN syndrome 2A or 2B** Q
- **RET proto-oncogene** Q mutations are seen in both familial and sporadic cases

Microscopy Q:

- Tumor cells are **polygonal to spindle-shaped** and are arranged in nests, trabeculae and follicles

- **Acellular amyloid deposits** [Q] are present in the **stroma**
- **IHC** – shows positivity for **calcitonin, chromogranin** and **CEA**

Ans. 33) **A. Parathyroid adenoma (Ref: 8 ed. Robbins p.1127, 9 ed. p.1101)**

- Most common cause of **primary hyperparathyroidism** [Q] is **solitary parathyroid adenoma** [Q]

Ans. 34) **D. Adipose tissue (Ref: 8 ed. Robbins p.1127-28, 9 ed. p.1101-03, f-24-25)**

Morphology of **Parathyroid Adenoma**:

- **Well-circumscribed** [Q], soft, encapsulated **tan to reddish-brown** nodule
- **Microscopically** – Composed of uniform, polygonal **chief cells** and few nests of larger **oxyphil cells** [Q]
- **Compressed, non-neoplastic parathyroid tissue** is seen at the periphery of the adenoma separated by a **fibrous capsule** [Q]
- In adenoma, **adipose tissue** is **inconspicuous** [Q] unlike normal parathyroid gland

Ans. 35) **B. 1 gm (Ref: 8 ed. Robbins p.1127-28, 9 ed. p.1101-03)**

- **Primary hyperplasia** [Q] – involves **all four glands** [Q] and combined weight of all glands rarely exceeds **1 gm.**
- **Typical parathyroid adenoma** averages **0.5 to 5 gm.**
- **Parathyroid carcinomas** enlarge **one parathyroid gland** and doesn't exceed **10 gm** in weight

Ans. 36) **D. All of the above (Ref: 8 ed. Robbins p.1127-28, 9 ed. p.1101-03, f-24-26)**

Untreated primary hyperparathyroidism manifests with:

- **Osteoporosis**
- **Brown tumors**
- **Osteitis fibrosa cystica**
- **Osteoporosis** results in **decreased bone mass** and involves **phalanges, vertebrae** and **proximal femur** [Q]
- **Dissecting Osteitis** [Q] – **Railroad track appearance** along the length of the trabeculae by osteoclasts
- **Brown tumor** [Q] – **Micro-fractures** and **secondary hemorrhages** with influx of macrophages and fibrous tissue
- **Osteitis fibrosa cystica (von Recklinghausen disease of bone)** [Q] – Combination of increased osteoclast activity, peritrabecular fibrosis and cystic brown tumors
- **Primary hyperparathyroidism** is associated with **"painful bones, renal stones, abdominal groans** and **psychic moans"**

Ans. 37) **D. Hypercalcemia of malignancy (Ref: 8 ed. Robbins p.1129, 9 ed. p.1103)**

Causes of Hypercalcemia [Q]:

a) **With Raised PTH**
   - Hyperparathyroidism – Primary (adenoma > hyperplasia), Secondary, Tertiary
   - Familial hypocalciuric hypercalcemia

b) **With Decreased PTH**
   - Hypercalcemia of malignancy, Vitamin D toxicity, Immobilization, Thiazide diuretics
   - Granulomatous disease (sarcoidosis)

Note: PTH-related peptide (PTHrP) [Q] secretion is responsible for **hypercalcemia** due to osteolytic tumors

Ans. 38) **A. Renal failure (Ref: 8 ed. Robbins p.1129, 9 ed. p.1103-04)**

- **Renal failure** [Q] is the **most common cause** of **secondary hyperparathyroidism**
- **Other causes** include – Inadequate dietary intake of calcium, steatorrhea and vitamin D deficiency

Ans. 39) **D. All of the above (Ref: 8 ed. Robbins p.1130-31, 9 ed. p.1105)**

- Islets of Langerhans contain **four major and two minor cell types**

Four main cell types [Q] are:

- **β cells** – secrete insulin

- **α cells** – secrete glucagon
- **δ cells** – secrete somatostatin
- **PP (pancreatic polypeptide) cells** – stimulation of secretion of gastric and intestinal enzymes and inhibition of intestinal motility
- **Two minor cell types** [Q]**: D1 cells** (secrete VIP) and **enterochromaffin cells** (secrete serotonin)

Ans. 40) D. All of the above (Ref: 8 ed. Robbins p.1131-32, 9 ed. p.1106-07)

WHO diagnostic criteria for diabetes [Q] include:

- Fasting plasma glucose ≥ **126 mg/dL**
- Random plasma glucose ≥ **200 mg/dL**
- 2-hour plasma glucose ≥ **200 mg/dL** during an oral glucose tolerance test (OGTT) with a loading dose of 75 gm
- Glycated hemoglobin **(HbA1C) level ≥ 6.5%**

Ans. 41) D. All of the above (Ref: 8 ed. Robbins p.1134, 9 ed. p.1110)

HLA haplotypes [Q] most commonly seen in **Type 1 DM**:

- HLA-DR3
- HLA-DR4
- HLA-DQ8

Non-HLA gene **"insulin"** increases the susceptibility of **Type 1 diabetes**

Ans. 42) D. All of the above (Ref: 8 ed. Robbins p.1138-39, 9 ed. p.1115-16)

Mechanisms which leads to **deleterious effects** of **persistent hyperglycemia** [Q]:

- Formation of Advanced Glycation End Products **(AGE)**
- Activation of **Protein Kinase C**
- Oxidative Stress and Disturbances in **Polyol Pathways**
- Hexosamine Pathways and Generation of **Fructose-6-Phosphate**

Role of AGE's in DM [Q]:

- Release of cytokines and growth factors, including **TGFβ** and **VEGF**, implicated in **diabetic retinopathy**
- Generation of **reactive oxygen species (ROS)** in **endothelial cells**
- Increased **procoagulant activity** on endothelial cells and macrophages
- Proliferation of **vascular smooth muscle cells** and extracellular matrix

Ans. 43) D. All of the above (Ref: 8 ed. Robbins p.1139, 9 ed. p.1116)

- Tissues that **do not require insulin** for glucose transport – **nerves, lenses, kidneys, blood vessels** [Q]
- **Sorbitol** accumulation in the lens contributes to **cataract formation** [Q]

Ans. 44) D. All of the above (Ref: 8 ed. Robbins p.1139, 9 ed. p.1117, f-24-35)

Morphology of Pancreas in Diabetes [Q]:

In Type 1 Diabetes

- Reduction in the number and size of islets
- Insulitis – Leukocytic infiltrates in the islets

In Type 2 Diabetes

- Reduction in islet cell mass
- Amyloid deposition within islets

Ans. 45) A. Myocardial infarction (Ref: 8 ed. Robbins p.1139-43, 9 ed. p.1117-19, f-24-32)

- **Macro-vascular complications** [Q] includes myocardial infarction, renal vascular insufficiency and cerebrovascular accidents
- **Myocardial infarction** [Q]: Caused by **atherosclerosis of coronary arteries**, is the **most common** cause of death in diabetics
- **Renal failure** [Q] is the **second most common** cause of death

Ans. 46) D. All of the above (Ref: 8 ed. Robbins p.1139-43, 9 ed. p.1118-19, f-24-36-40)

Lesions most commonly seen in **diabetic kidney** ᵠ – **Glomerular lesions, renal vascular lesions** and **pyelonephritis**

Morphology of Kidney in **Diabetes** ᵠ:

- Widespread **thickening** of the **glomerular capillary basement membrane (GBM)**
- Diffuse Mesangial Sclerosis
- Nodular Glomerulosclerosis or **Kimmelstiel-Wilson disease**
- **Renal atherosclerosis** and arteriolosclerosis
- **Pyelonephritis** – Necrotizing papillitis is more prevalent in diabetes

Ans. 47) D. >30 mg% of albumin in urine (Ref: 8 ed. Robbins p.1145, 9 ed. p.1120)

- Earliest manifestation of diabetic nephropathy is **microalbuminuria** ᵠ
- **Microalbuminuria** is defined as presence of **>30 mg/day** but **<300 mg/day** ᵠ of albumin in urine

Ans. 48) C. VEGF (Ref: 8 ed. Robbins p.1145, 9 ed. p.1120)

- **Fundamental lesion** of **retinopathy** is **neovascularization** ᵠ which occurs due to hypoxia-induced overexpression of **VEGF** ᵠ in the retina

Ans. 49) A. Distal symmetric polyneuropathy (Ref: 8 ed. Robbins p.1145, 9 ed. p.1120)

Diabetic Neuropathy:

- **Most frequent pattern** of involvement is **distal symmetric polyneuropathy** ᵠ of the **lower extremities**
- In later stages, **upper extremities** may be involved, creating **"glove and stocking" pattern** ᵠ of polyneuropathy

Ans. 50) A. Insulinoma (Ref: 8 ed. Robbins p.1146-47, 9 ed. p.1121-22)

β-cell tumors (insulinomas) ᵠ:

- Most common **pancreatic endocrine neoplasms**

Morphology ᵠ:

- Most often found within the **pancreas** and can be **located anywhere** in the pancreas
- Deposition of the **amyloid** is a **characteristic feature**

Clinical Features ᵠ **(Whipple's triad):**

Hypoglycemic episodes:

- Occurs when blood glucose level falls below **50 mg/dL** ᵠ of serum
- **CNS manifestations** i. e. confusion, stupor and loss of consciousness
- Precipitated by fasting and are relieved by administration of glucose

Ans. 51) D. All of the above (Ref: 8 ed. Robbins p.1146, 9 ed. p.1121)

Islet cell hyperplasia (Nesidioblastosis) ᵠ is seen in:

- Maternal diabetes (fetal islets increases in size in response to hyperglycemia)
- Beckwith-Wiedemann syndrome
- Mutations in the β-cell **K+-channel protein** or **sulfonylurea receptor**

Ans. 52) D. All of the above (Ref: 8 ed. Robbins p.1147, 9 ed. p.1122)

Zollinger-Ellison Syndrome (Gastrinomas) ᵠ:

- Can arise in **duodenum** and **pancreas**
- **Hyper secretion of gastric acid** leading to **duodenal** and **gastric** ulcers
- Form a part of **MEN-1 syndrome**
- Ulcers are also seen in **unusual locations** such as the **jejunum** ᵠ

Ans. 53) A. Glucagonomas (Ref: 8 ed. Robbins p.1147, 9 ed. p.1122)

α-cell tumors (Glucagonomas) ᵠ:

- Associated with increased serum levels of glucagon
- Most common in **pancreatic tail** ᵠ
- Features include **diabetes mellitus**, a characteristic **skin rash (Necrolytic migratory erythema)** ᵠ and **anemia**

Ans. 54) D. All of the above (Ref: 8 ed. Robbins p.1147, 9 ed. p.1122)

- Most common site of ***VIPoma*** is **pancreatic tail** [Q]
- ***VIPoma/WDHA syndrome*** [Q] – Characterized by watery diarrhea, hypokalemia and achlorhydria, which occurs due to release of **vasoactive intestinal peptide (VIP)**
- **VIPoma syndrome** [Q] – Associated with **neuroblastomas, ganglioneuroblastoma, ganglioneuromas** and **pheochromocytomas**

Ans. 55) A. Pituitary microadenoma (Ref: 8 ed. Robbins p.1148-49, 9 ed. p.1123, t-24-8)

Endogenous Hypercortisolism [Q]:

- **Cause** – ACTH producing **Pituitary adenoma (Cushing disease)** [Q]
- **Pituitary microadenoma** [Q] – Most common
- Others – Macroadenoma (less commonly) and rarely corticotroph cell hyperplasia

Note:

- **Most common cause** of hypercortisolism is **exogenous administration of steroids**

Ans. 56) A. Small cell carcinoma of lung (Ref: 8 ed. Robbins p.1148-49, 9 ed. p.1123, t-24-8)

- **Ectopic ACTH** secretion leading to **Cushing syndrome** is most commonly seen in **small-cell carcinoma of the lung** [Q]
- Other neoplasms leading to Cushing syndrome include **carcinoids, medullary carcinoma of thyroid** and **islet cell tumors**

Ans. 57) A. 21 hydroxylase (Ref: 8 ed. Robbins p.1152-54, 9 ed. p.1127-28, f-24-46)

21-hydroxylase Deficiency [Q]:

- Most common cause of **Congenital Adrenal hyperplasia**

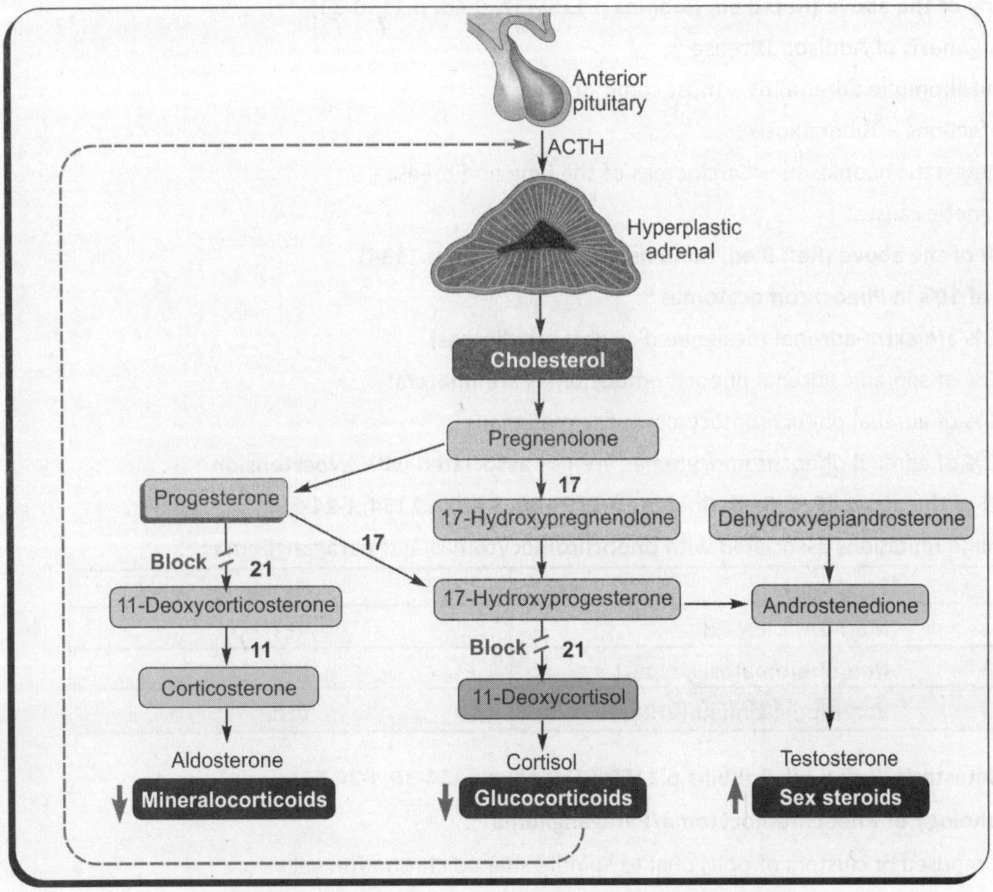

Consequences of C-21 hydroxylase deficiency

Note: 11, 17 and 21 represents 11-, 17-, and 21-hydroxylase enzymes respectively

- Impairs the synthesis of both **cortisol** and **aldosterone**
- **Increased** production of **androgens**, leads to **virilization**
- Three distinctive syndromes: (1) salt-wasting ("classic") (2) simple virilizing and (3) "non-classic" or late onset adrenal virilism

Ans. 58) C. Easily recognized in males at birth (Ref: 8 ed. Robbins p.1152-54, 9 ed. p.1127-28, f-24-46)

Salt-wasting Syndrome [Q]:

- Occurs due to the total lack of the **hydroxylase**
- Inability to convert progesterone into deoxycorticosterone
- **No synthesis of mineralocorticoids** [Q] and **deficient** synthesis of **cortisol** occur
- There is salt wasting, hyponatremia and hyperkalemia
- Excess production of **androgens**, lead to **virilization** [Q]
- **Virilization** in the female is easily recognized at **birth** [Q]
- Males are generally unrecognized at birth and present with salt wasting after 5 to 15 days

Ans. 59) A. N. meningitides (Ref: 8 ed. Robbins p.1155, 9 ed. p.1129-30, f-24-47,48)

Waterhouse-Friderichsen Syndrome [Q]:

- Most common cause – ***Neisseria meningitides*** septicemia
- Other causative agents – Pseudomonas, pneumococci, Haemophilus influenzae, staphylococci
- More common in **children**
- **Microscopy** – Hemorrhage starts within the adrenal medulla, which then spreads peripherally into the cortex

Ans. 60) D. Any of the above (Ref: 8 ed. Robbins p.1155-57, 9 ed. p.1130-31)

Pathogenesis of Addison Disease [Q]:

- **Autoimmune adrenalitis** – most common cause
- Infections – Tuberculosis
- Metastatic neoplasms – Carcinomas of the lung and breast
- Genetic causes

Ans. 61) D. All of the above (Ref: 8 ed. Robbins p.1159-60, 9 ed. p.1134)

Rule of 10's in **Pheochromocytomas** [Q]:

- 10% are **extra-adrenal** (designated as **paragangliomas**)
- 10% of sporadic adrenal pheochromocytomas are **bilateral**
- 10% of adrenal pheochromocytomas are **malignant**
- 10% of adrenal pheochromocytomas are **not associated** with **hypertension**

Ans. 62) D. All of the above (Ref: 8 ed. Robbins p.1159-60, 9 ed. p.1134, t-24-11)

Germline mutations associated with **pheochromocytomas** and **paragangliomas** [Q]:

Syndrome	Gene
MEN-2A, MEN-2B	RET
Neurofibromatosis, type 1	NF1
Von Hippel-Lindau (VHL)	VHL

Ans. 63) D. Metastasis (Ref: 8 ed. Robbins p.1159-61, 9 ed. p.1134-36, f-24-55)

Morphology of Pheochromocytoma/Paraganglioma [Q]:

- Composed of clusters of polygonal to spindle shaped chromaffin cells
- Cells are surrounded by **sustentacular cells** in **Zellballen pattern** [Q] (small nests or alveoli)

- Cells are supplied by a **rich vascular network**
- Nuclei are usually round to oval with **stippled "salt and pepper" chromatin** Q
- Tumors with **"benign"** histologic features may **metastasize** and those which are bizarrely pleomorphic may not
- **Definitive diagnosis** of malignancy is based on the presence of **metastases** Q

Ans. 64) D. All of the above (Ref: 8 ed. Robbins p.1162, 9 ed. p.1136)

MEN-1 or **Wermer syndrome** Q

- Caused by mutations in **MEN1 tumor suppressor gene**, which encodes a protein called **menin**
- Characterized by abnormalities of the **parathyroid, pancreas and pituitary glands**
- **Parathyroid**: **Primary hyperparathyroidism** is the **most common** manifestation of **MEN-1**
- **Pancreas**: **Zollinger-Ellison syndrome** (associated with **gastrinomas**) and hypoglycemia (associated with **Insulinoma**) are most common endocrine tumors
- **Pituitary**: Most frequent anterior pituitary tumor is **prolactinoma**

Note: Duodenum Q is the **most common site** of **gastrinomas** in MEN-1

Ans. 65) D. Gastrinomas (Ref: 8 ed. Robbins p.1162-63, 9 ed. p.1137)

MEN-2A or Sipple Syndrome Q:

- Characterized by **pheochromocytoma, medullary carcinoma of the thyroid and parathyroid hyperplasia**

MEN-2B syndrome:

- Characterized by **medullary thyroid carcinomas, pheochromocytomas, ganglioneuromas** (involving the skin, oral mucosa, eyes, respiratory tract and gastrointestinal tract) and **marfanoid habitus**
- **MEN-2A** and **MEN-2B** are caused by germline **gain-of-function mutations** in **RET proto-oncogene** Q
- **Loss-of-function mutations** in **RET**, result in **intestinal aganglionosis** and **Hirschsprung disease**

Ans. 66) A. Pituitary adenoma (Ref: Robbins 9 ed. p. 1123) Refer Q 55 for details

Ans. 67) B. Gastrinomas (Ref: Robbins 9 ed. p.1122) Refer Q 52 for details

Ans. 68) D. Follicular carcinoma (Ref: 9 ed. Robbins p.1093-94) Refer Q 23 for details

FNAC cannot distinguish between follicular carcinoma and a benign follicular adenoma

Ans. 69) A. Acromegaly (Ref: 9th ed. Robbins p. 1111-1112)

- Insulin resistance – Failure of target tissues to respond normally to insulin

Endocrinopathies associated with hyperglycemia and insulin resistance:

- Acromegaly, Cushing syndrome, Hyperthyroidism, Pheochromocytoma, Glucagonomas

Ans. 70) B. MEN II (Ref: 9th ed. Robbins p. 1099) Refer Q 32 for details

Ans. 71) C. 90% of Non-familial cases are bilateral (Ref: 9th ed. Robbins p. 1134-1136) Refer Q 61 for details

Ans. 72) B. Cretinism (Ref: 9 ed. Robbins p. 1086)

Cretinism refers to hypothyroidism that develops in infancy or early childhood. It is a non-heritable condition

Ans. 73) A. Papillary carcinoma (Ref: Anderson p. 1956-1958)

- Thyroid carcinomas arising after radiation or in thyroglossal cyst are papillary type

Ans. 74) A. DeQuervian's thyroiditis (Ref: 9 ed. Robbins p. 1088)

Ans. 75) D. All of the above (Ref: 9 ed. Robbins p. 1088-89)

Ans. 76) D. Metastasis (Ref: 9 ed. Robbins p. 1135) Refer Q 63 for details

- Definitive diagnosis of malignancy in pheochromocytomas is based exclusively on the presence of metastases

Ans. 77) A. Pheochromocytoma (Ref: 9 ed. Robbins p. 1134-35) Refer Q 61 for details

Ans. 78) B. Medullary carcinoma thyroid (Ref: 9 ed. Robbins p. 1095) Refer Q 32 for details

- Familial medullary thyroid carcinomas occur in multiple endocrine neoplasia type 2 (MEN-2) and are associated with germline RET mutations

Ans. 79) A. MEN I (Ref: 9 ed. Robbins p. 1136) Refer Q 65 for details

Ans. 80) A. Papillary carcinoma thyroid (Ref: 9 ed. Robbins p. 1095-97) Refer Q 27 for details

Ans. 81) D. Medullary Carcinoma of thyroid (Ref: 9 ed. Robbins p.1136) Refer Q 64 for details

Ans. 82) C. Medullary (Ref: 9 ed. Robbins p.1090-1100) Refer Q 32 for details

Ans. 83) A. RET proto oncogene (Ref: 9 ed. Robbins p. 1090-1100) Refer Q 32 for details

Ans. 84) A. Follicular carcinoma thyroid (Ref: 9 ed. Robbins p. 1024, 1095, 1315)

Ans. 85) A. Vascular invasion (Ref: 9 ed. Robbins p.1093-94) Refer Q 23 for details

Ans. 86) A. Papillary carcinoma of thyroid (Ref: 9 ed. Robbins p.1095-97) Refer Q 27 for details

23 The Skin

How to go about this chapter?

- **One should be thorough with the following topics:**
  - **Melanocytic Nevus, Dysplastic nevi**
  - **Malignant melanoma**
  - **Appendage/adnexal tumors**
  - **Squamous cell carcinoma**
  - **Familial Cancer Syndromes**
  - **Basal cell carcinoma**
  - **Dermatofibrosarcoma Protuberans**
  - **Cutaneous T-cell Lymphoma/Mycosis Fungoides**
  - **Psoriasis**
  - **Lichen Planus**
  - **Blistering disorders**
  - **Dermatitis Herpetiformis**
  - **Epidermolysis Bullosa**

1) TRUE about melanocytic nevi:
a) Activating mutations in components of the Ras signaling pathway
b) Earliest lesions are junctional nevi
c) Superficial nevus cells are large and produce melanin
d) All of the above

2) TRUE about dysplastic nevi:
a) Mutations in RAS or BRAF
b) Presents as targetoid lesions
c) Cytologic atypia and lamellar fibrosis is characteristic
d) All of the above

3) Melanomas can be seen in:
a) Skin b) Esophagus
c) Oral mucosa d) Any of the above

4) Warning signs of melanoma include(s):
a) Asymmetry
b) Irregular borders
c) Variegated color
d) All of the above

5) Following mutation(s) is/are noted in malignant melanoma:
a) CDKN2A b) BRAF
c) TERT d) All of the above

6) TRUE about the morphology of melanoma:
a) Horizontal spread of melanoma cells in radial growth phase
b) Superficial spreading is the most common type of melanoma
c) Deeper dermis invasion is seen in vertical growth phase
d) All of the above

7) Prognostic factors indicating metastatic spread of melanoma cells include(s):
a) Tumor depth
b) Number of mitosis
c) Tumor regression
d) All of the above

8) Associated with Acanthosis nigricans:
a) Obesity
b) Diabetes
c) Gastrointestinal cancers
d) Any of the above

9) All of the following are skin adnexal tumors EXCEPT:
a) Cylindroma
b) Eccrine poroma
c) Sebaceous adenoma
d) Squamous cell carcinoma

10) TRUE regarding the pathogenesis of squamous cell carcinomas:
a) DNA damage due to UV radiation
b) HPV 16 and 18 infection
c) P53 mutation is an early event
d) Old burn scars can be predisposing factor

11) Familial melanoma syndrome is associated with:
a) P16/INK4a
b) PTCH
c) PTEN
d) TSC1

12) TRUE about the pathogenesis of Basal cell carcinoma:
a) Mutations of Hedgehog signaling pathway
b) Association with Nevoid basal cell carcinoma
c) PTCH plays an important role
d) All of the above

13) TRUE about morphology of Basal cell carcinoma:
a) Present as pearly papules
b) Rodent ulcers are peculiar feature
c) Multifocal and nodular patterns are most commonly seen
d) All of the above

14) TRUE about Dermatofibrosarcoma Protuberans:
a) Associated with t(17;22) gene fusion
b) Imatinib is the treatment of choice
c) Invasion of the subcutaneous fat is common
d) All of the above

15) All are TRUE about Mycosis Fungoides EXCEPT:
a) Lymphoma of skin homing CD8+ lymphocytes
b) Evolves from patch, plaque and nodule stage
c) Sezary syndrome is a complication
d) Pautrier microabscesses is characteristic feature

16) TRUE about psoriasis:
a) Association with HLA-C
b) Presents with salmon colored plaque with silvery scale
c) Munro microabscesses can be seen
d) All of the above

17) TRUE about lichen planus:
a) Wickham's stria is a characteristic feature
b) Predisposition to squamous cell carcinoma
c) Civatte bodies are seen
d) All of the above

18) TRUE about inflammatory blistering disorders:
a) In pemphigus foliaceus, subcorneal blisters are seen
b) In Pemphigus vulgaris, suprabasal blisters are seen
c) In bullous pemphigoid, sub-epidermal blister is seen
d) All of the above

19) TRUE about pathogenesis of bullous disorders of skin:
a) In Pemphigus vulgaris, autoantibodies against Dsg1 and Dsg3 are seen
b) In Pemphigus foliaceus, autoantibodies are against Dsg1 are seen
c) In Bullous pemphigoid autoantibodies against BPAG2 are seen
d) All of the above

20) TRUE about morphology of Pemphigus diseases:
a) Acantholysis is characteristic
b) Row of tombstone appearance of intact basal cells in P. vulgaris
c) IgG deposits gives fish-net like appearance on immunofluorescence in P. vulgaris
d) All of the above

21) All are TRUE about Bullous Pemphigoid EXCEPT:
a) Linear pattern of antibody deposition along dermoepidermal junction
b) Antibodies against BPAG-1 cause blistering
c) Subepidermal non-acantholytic blisters
d) Eosinophils form content of blister cavity

22) TRUE about Dermatitis herpetiformis:
a) Associated with IgA antibodies against reticulin
b) Subepidermal blister
c) Neutrophilic microabscesses at tips of dermal papillae
d) All of the above

23) Dystrophic Epidermolysis Bullosa occurs due to mutation in:
a) Type I collagen
b) Type II collagen
c) Type IV collagen
d) Type VII collagen

24) In congenital dystrophic variety of epidermolysis bullosa, mutation is seen in the gene coding for: (AIIMS MAY 2011)
a) Laminin 4
b) Collagen type 7
c) Alpha 6 integrin
d) Keratin 14

25) Staining done for sebaceous cell carcinoma: (AIIMS NOV 2009)
a) Oil Red 0
b) PAS
c) Methanamine silver
d) KOH

26) HMB 45 is a tumor marker for: (NEET 2014)
a) Malignant melanoma
b) Mesothelioma
c) Bronchogenic carcinoma
d) Pancreatic carcinoma

27) **Sentinel lymph node biopsy is used for: (NEET 2014)**
a) Melanoma
b) Basal cell carcinoma
c) Squamous cell carcionoma
d) Thyroid carcinoma

28) **Squamous cell carcinoma marker is: (NEET 2013)**
a) Vimentin
b) Desmin
c) Cytokeratin
d) Glial fibrillary acid protein

29) **Acantholysis means: (NEET 2013)**
a) Diffuse epidermal hyperplasia
b) Loss of intercellular connections
c) Intercellular edema of the epidermis
d) Abnormal keratinization

30) **Desmoid tumor, all are TRUE EXCEPT: (NEET 2013)**
a) Cannot metastasize
b) Associated with gardener syndrome
c) Locally invasive
d) Can metastasize

31) **Most common site of a rodent ulcer is: (NEET 2013)**
a) Limbs
b) Face
c) Abdomen
d) Trunk

32) **Mutation in malignant melanoma: (NEET 2013)**
a) N-myc
b) CDK2A
c) RET
d) None

33) **A young male presented with history of fever and nodule in leg. Histopathology of the nodule reveals foamy histiocytes and neutrophilic infiltrate in dermis. Most probable diagnosis is: (AIPGMEE 2012)**
a) Sweet syndrome
b) Rosai Dorfmann disease
c) Erythema Nodosum Leprosum
d) Erythema Nodosum

CHAPTER 23: THE SKIN

Ans. 1) **D. All of the above (Ref: 8 ed. Robbins p.1169-70, 9 ed. p.1144-45, f-25-2-4)**

Melanocytic Nevus (Pigmented Nevus, Mole) Q:

- Caused by acquired mutations in **Ras signaling pathway**
- **Junctional nevus** Q – Earliest lesion and consists of **aggregates or nests** of **round cells** that grow along the **dermoepidermal junction**
- **Compound nevi** Q – Junctional nevi grow into the **dermis** as nests or cords of cells
- **Intradermal nevi** – Epidermal nests are **lost** and only **dermal nevus cells** are seen
- **Superficial nevus cells** are **larger**, produce **melanin** and grow in **nests** Q
- **Deeper nevus cells** are **smaller**, grow in cords and single cells and doesn't produce **pigment** Q
- **Neurotization/Maturation** Q – Nevus cells of **deeper dermis**, grow in fascicles resembling **neural tissue**

Ans. 2) **D. All of the above (Ref: 8 ed. Robbins p.1170-71, 9 ed. p.1145-47, f-25-5,6)**

Dysplastic Nevi Q:

- Direct precursors of **melanoma** Q
- Associated with **RAS** or **BRAF** activation and increased **CDK4 activity** Q
- Are **greater than 5 mm**, **flat macules**, slightly raised plaques or **target-like lesions** Q

Microscopy Q:

- Can involve both the epidermis and dermis
- Shows architectural and **cytologic atypia** Q (nuclear enlargement, irregular, angulated nuclear contours and hyperchromasia)
- **Lentiginous hyperplasia** Q **– Nevus cell nests** within the epidermis replace the normal basal cell layer along the **dermoepidermal junction**
- **Melanin incontinence** Q – Release of melanin from dead nevus cells into the dermis
- Dermis underlying the atypical cells shows **linear** or **lamellar fibrosis** Q

Ans. 3) **D. Any of the above (Ref: 8 ed. Robbins p.1172, 9 ed. p.1147)**

- Most commonly melanoma arises in the **skin** Q
- Other sites Q **– Oral** and **anogenital mucosal surfaces** (oropharynx, gastrointestinal and genitourinary tracts), esophagus, meninges and the uvea of the eye

Ans. 4) **D. All of the above (Ref: 8 ed. Robbins p.1172-73, 9 ed. p.1150)**

Most important warning signs **(ABCDEs) of melanoma** Q:

- **A**symmetry
- Irregular **B**orders
- Variegated **C**olor
- Increasing **D**iameter and
- **E**volution or change over time

Majority of lesions are **greater than 10 mm** Q in diameter at diagnosis

Ans. 5) **D. All of the above (Ref: 8 ed. Robbins p.1174-75, 9 ed. p.1147-49, f-25-7)**

Mutations commonly seen in **malignant melanoma** Q:

a) **CDKN2A gene mutation**:

- Encodes p15/INK4b, p16/INK4a and p14/ARF
- **p16/INK4a** inhibits CDK4 and CDK6, due to which **RB tumor suppressor gene** block cells in the **G1 phase** of the cell cycle

- **p14/ARF** enhances the activity of the **p53 tumor suppressor** by inhibiting **MDM2** Q

b) Increase in **RAS and PI3K/AKT** signaling and activating mutations in **BRAF** Q

c) ***TERT*** Q: **Most commonly mutated** and recently identified **gene**, leads to reactivation of **telomerase** activity

Ans. 6) **D. All of the above (Ref: 8 ed. Robbins p.1172-73, 9 ed. p.1149-50, f-25-8)**

Morphology of Malignant Melanoma Q:

Radial growth phase

- **Horizontal spread** of **melanoma cells** within the epidermis and superficial dermis
- Includes **lentigo maligna**, **superficial spreading** and **acral/mucosal lentiginous** melanoma
- **Superficial spreading** Q is the **most common** type of melanoma

Vertical growth phase

- Tumor cells invade downward into the **deeper dermis**
- Presents as a **nodule** and has **metastatic potential**
- **Breslow thickness** Q – Distance from superficial epidermal **granular cell layer** to the deepest **intradermal tumor cells**

Ans. 7) **D. All of the above (Ref: 8 ed. Robbins p.1173-74, 9 ed. p.1150, f-25-8)**

Prognostic factors Q used to determine **metastatic disease** in **malignant melanoma**:

- Tumor depth (**Breslow thickness**)
- Number of mitoses
- Evidence of **tumor regression** (due to the host immune response)
- Ulceration of overlying skin
- Presence and number of **tumor infiltrating lymphocytes**
- Gender
- Location (central body or extremity)

Favorable prognostic factors Q

- Thinner tumor depth, no mitoses, absence of regression and lack of ulceration, brisk tumor infiltrating lymphocyte response, female gender and location on extremity

Microscopic involvement of a **sentinel node** confers a **worse prognosis** Q

Ans. 8) **D. Any of the above (Ref: 8 ed. Robbins p.1175-76, 9 ed. p.1151-52)**

Acanthosis nigricans Q is associated with:

- **Obesity** or **endocrine abnormalities** (particularly with pituitary or pineal tumors and **diabetes**) Q
- **Gastrointestinal adenocarcinomas** Q

Note:

- Activating mutations in **"fibroblast growth factor receptor-3 (FGFR3)"** Q is seen

Ans. 9) **D. Squamous cell carcinoma (Ref: 8 ed. Robbins p.1176-78, 9 ed. p.1152-54, f-25-10,11)**

- **Appendage/adnexal tumors** Q are neoplasms which arise from **hair follicles**, **sebaceous**, **eccrine** and **apocrine glands**

Most common examples Q:

- Eccrine poroma
- Sebaceous adenoma
- Cylindroma
- Syringoma
- Pilomatricomas

Ans. 10) **B. HPV 16 and 18 infection (Ref: 8 ed. Robbins p.1180, 9 ed. p.1155, f-25-13)**

Pathogenesis of **squamous cell carcinoma (SCC)** [Q]:

- Most important cause is **DNA damage** induced by **exposure to UV light** [Q]
- Immunosuppression may lead to **HPV infection**, subtypes 5 and 8
- **Risk factors:** Industrial carcinogens (tars and oils), chronic ulcers and draining osteomyelitis, old burn scars, ingestion of arsenicals, ionizing radiation
- Tobacco and betel nut chewing (in the oral cavity)
- **p53 dysfunction** is seen early

Ans. 11) A. P16/INK4a (Ref: 8 ed. Robbins p.1182, 9 ed. p.1156, t-25-3)

Familial Cancer Syndromes with Cutaneous Manifestations [Q]

Disease	Gene/Protein
Ataxia-telangiectasia	*ATM*/ATM
Nevoid basal cell carcinoma syndrome	*PTCH*/PTCH
Cowden syndrome	*PTEN*/PTEN
Familial melanoma syndrome	*CDKN2*/p16/INK4 *CDKN2*/p14/ARF
Muir-Torre syndrome	*MSH2*/MSH2 *MLH1*/MLH1
Neurofibromatosis I	*NF1*/neurofibromin
Neurofibromatosis II	*NF2*/merlin
Tuberous sclerosis	*TSC1*/hamartin *TSC2*/tuberin
Xeroderma pigmentosum	*XPA*/XPA

Ans. 12) D. All of the above (Ref: 8 ed. Robbins p.1181-82, 9 ed. p.1155-56)

Pathogenesis of **Basal Cell Carcinoma** [Q]:

- Most common mutation is **Hedgehog signaling pathway**
- Associated with **Nevoid basal cell carcinoma syndrome** (NBCCS; also known as basal cell nevus or **Gorlin syndrome**)
- **PTCH mutation** [Q] is seen in patients with NBCCS
- NBCCS are associated with multiple basal cell carcinomas, along with **Medulloblastoma** [Q] and **ovarian fibromas**

Ans. 13) D. All of the above (Ref: 8 ed. Robbins p.1180-81, 9 ed. p.1157-58, f-25-15)

Morphology of **Basal Cell Carcinomas** [Q]:

- Presents as **pearly papules**, which contain prominent dilated sub-epidermal blood vessels **(telangiectasia)**
- **Rodent ulcers** [Q] – Advanced lesions may **ulcerate** and extensive local invasion of bone or facial sinuses may occur

Microscopy [Q]:

- **Tumor cells** resemble those in the **normal basal cell layer** of the epidermis
- Two patterns – **Multifocal growth** [Q] and **nodular lesions** [Q]
- **Peripheral palisading** [Q]: Tumor cells at the periphery of the tumor cell islands are arranged radially with their long axes in parallel alignment
- **Retraction clefts/separation artifacts** [Q] – In which the stroma retracts away from the tumor cell nests
- Metastasis is very rare

Ans. 14) D. All of the above (Ref: 8 ed. Robbins p.1182-83, 9 ed. p.1158-59, f-25-16, 17)

Dermatofibrosarcoma Protuberans Q:

- Well-differentiated, **primary fibrosarcoma** Q of the skin
- **t(17;22)** Q translocation leads to fusion of **collagen 1A1 (COL1A1)** and **platelet derived growth factor-β (PDGFB)**, leading to increased **PDGFB expression**
- **Treatment** – PDGFβ receptor tyrosine kinase inhibitor i.e. Imatinib mesylate

Microscopy Q:

- **Storiform pattern** of **radiating fibroblasts**
- **Honeycombing pattern**: Tumor cells infiltrate from dermis into **subcutaneous fat**

Ans. 15) A. Lymphoma of skin homing CD8+ lymphocytes (Ref: 8 ed. Robbins p.1184-85, 9 ed. p.1159-60, f-25-18)

Cutaneous T-cell Lymphoma/Mycosis Fungoides Q:

- **Lymphoproliferative disorder** affecting the skin, in which there is abnormal **CD4+T cells** Q proliferation
- Lesions evolve from **patch** to **plaque** to **nodular** stage
- **Sezary syndrome** Q: Characterized by diffuse **skin erythema** and scaling due to **infiltration** of the blood by **malignant T cells**

Morphology Q:

- **Histologic hallmark – Sézary-Lutzner cells** Q forming **band-like aggregates** within the superficial **dermis**
- **Pautrier microabscesses** Q – **Malignant T cells** invade the **epidermis** as **single cells** and **small clusters**
- **Tumor cells** have markedly **infolded nuclear membranes**, imparting a **hyperconvoluted** or **cerebriform** Q contour
- **Epidermotropism** Q – Marked epidermal infiltration by **Sézary-Lutzner cells**

Ans. 16) D. All of the above (Ref: 8 ed. Robbins p.1190-91, 9 ed. p.1165-66, f-25-25)

Salient Features of Psoriasis Q:

- Chronic inflammatory dermatoses, has a strong association with **HLA-C** Q
- **Koebner phenomenon** Q – Psoriatic lesions can be induced in susceptible individuals by local trauma

Morphology Q –

- Site: Elbows, knees, scalp, lumbosacral areas, intergluteal cleft and glans penis
- Presents as a **salmon-colored plaque** with loosely adherent **silver-white scale**
- **Nail changes** Q – Yellow-brown discoloration, with pitting, dimpling, **onycholysis**

Microscopy Q:

- **Acanthosis (epidermal thickening)** Q
- Downward elongation of the rete ridges described as a **test tubes in a rack** Q
- **Stratum granulosum** is **thinned** or **absent** with **parakeratosis** Q of the corneal layer
- **Auspitz sign** Q – Multiple, minute, bleeding points when the scale is lifted from the plaque
- **Munro microabscesses** – Neutrophilic aggregates in stratum corneum

Ans. 17) D. All of the above (Ref: 8 ed. Robbins p.1191-92, 9 ed. p.1166-67, f-25-26)

Lichen Planus Q:

- Characterized by pruritic, purple, polygonal, planar, papules and plaques
- Predisposes to **squamous cell carcinoma**

Morphology Q:

- Itchy, violaceous, **flat-topped papules** that may coalesce to form **plaques**
- **Wickham striae** Q – Papule with white **lacelike pattern** of lines

Microscopy Q:

- Epidermal hyperplasia with thickening of **granular cell layer (hypergranulosis)** and **stratum corneum (hyperkeratosis)**

- **Interface dermatitis** [Q] – Dense, continuous infiltrate of lymphocytes along the dermoepidermal junction
- **Sawtoothing** of **rete ridges** – Angulated zigzag contour of dermoepidermal interface
- **Colloid or Civatte bodies** [Q] – Formed due to destruction of basal keratinocytes

Ans. 18) D. All of the above (Ref: 8 ed. Robbins p.1192-94, 9 ed. p.1167-69, f-25-27)

- In **Pemphigus Vulgaris** – **Suprabasal blister** [Q] is seen, formed above the basal layer of epidermis
- In **Pemphigus foliaceus** – **Subcorneal blister** [Q] is seen and roof of bulla is formed by stratum corneum
- In **Bullous pemphigoid** – **Subepidermal blister** [Q] is seen and the entire epidermis separates from the dermis

Ans. 19) D. All of the above (Ref: 8 ed. Robbins p.1192-94, 9 ed. p.1167-69, f-25-27,28)

Pathogenesis of blistering disorders [Q]:

- **Pemphigus vulgaris** – Autoantibodies are formed against **Desmoglein-1 (Dsg1)** and **Desmoglein-3 (Dsg3)** [Q]
- **Pemphigus foliaceus** – Autoantibodies are formed against **Desmoglein-1 (Dsg1)**
- **Bullous pemphigoid** – Autoantibodies bind **BPAG2**, leading to blister formation at the **lamina lucida** of **basement membrane** [Q]

Dermatitis Herpetiformis [Q]:

- Occurs when **IgA autoantibodies** bind to the **fibrils**, that anchor hemidesmosomes to the dermis

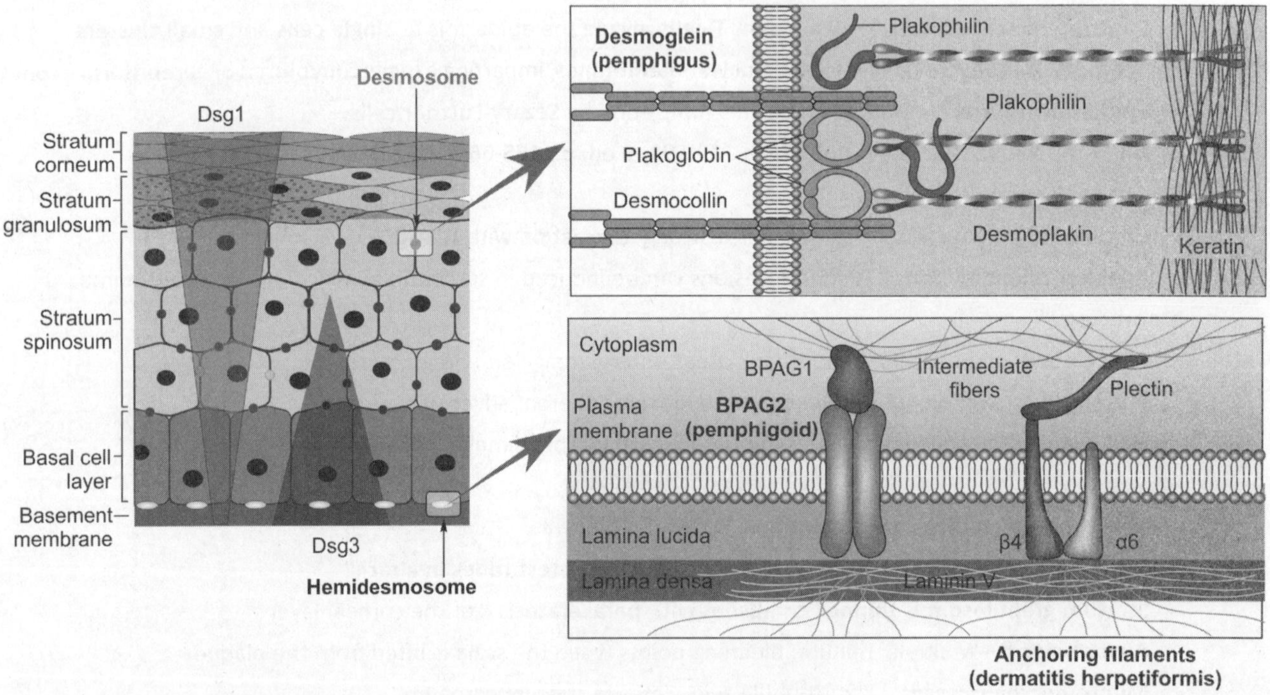

Pathogenesis of blistering disorders

Ans. 20) D. All of the above (Ref: 8 ed. Robbins p.1193-95, 9 ed. p.1169-70, f-25-29-31)

Morphology of Pemphigus [Q]:

- **Acantholysis** – Lysis of intercellular bridges between squamous epithelial cells and thus the squamous cells become round
- In **pemphigus vulgaris** and **pemphigus vegetans**, there is a **suprabasal cleft**
- **"Row of tombstones"**: Single layer of intact basal cells forming blister base
- **Reticular or fishnet-like pattern** is seen in Direct immunofluorescence in **Pemphigus vulgaris**

Ans. 21) B. Antibodies against BPAG-1 cause blistering (Ref: 8 ed. Robbins p.1195-96, 9 ed. p.1170, f-25-32,33)

Bullous Pemphigoid [Q]**:**

- Occurs due to the **autoantibodies** against the **bullous pemphigoid antigen 2 (BPAG-2)** [Q], a component of hemidesmosomes
- Antibody deposition occurs in a **linear pattern** at the **dermoepidermal junction**

Morphology [Q]**:**

- **Tense bullae** filled with **clear fluid**, which do not rupture easily
- **Microscopy**, it shows **subepidermal** blisters and **eosinophilic microabscesses** [Q] (beneath the epidermal basal cell layer)

Ans. 22) D. All of the above (Ref: 8 ed. Robbins p.1196, 9 ed. p.1170-72, f-25-34)

Dermatitis Herpetiformis [Q]**:**

- Has an association with **celiac disease** and responds to **gluten-free** diet
- **IgA antibodies** [Q] to **dietary gluten**, cross-react with **reticulin,** producing a **subepidermal blister**

Morphology [Q]**:**

- Lesions are **bilateral**, **symmetric**, involving the extensor surfaces, elbows, knees, upper back and **buttocks**
- **Neutrophilic microabscesses** [Q] at the **tips of dermal papillae**
- **Direct immunofluorescence** [Q] – shows **granular deposits** of **IgA** at the tips of **dermal papillae**

Ans. 23) D. Type VII collagen (Ref: 8 ed. Robbins p.1196-98, 9 ed. p.1171-73, f-25-35)

Epidermolysis Bullosa

- 4 types – *Simplex* type, *junctional* type, *dystrophic* type and *mixed* types
- **Dystrophic epidermolysis bullosa** [Q] results from mutations in the **COL7A1 gene** [Q], which encodes **type VII collagen**

Ans. 24) B. Collagen type 7 (Ref: 9 ed. Robbins p.1171-73) Refer Q 23 for details

Ans. 25) A. Oil red 0 (Refer: 9 ed. Lever's Histopathology of skin, p. 891-92)

- **Sebaceous carcinoma stains positively for fat with Oil Red-0**

Ans. 26) A. Malignant melanoma (Ref: 9th ed. Robbin's p. 1147-1150)

- **S-100 and HMB-45 are markers for melanoma**

Ans. 27) A. Melanoma

Sentinal biopsy is used for breast cancer and melanoma

Ans. 28) C. Cytokeratin

Important markers to remember for exam point of view:

a) **Cytokeratin** – Carcinoma, mesothelioma, Nonseminoma, GCT
b) **Vimentin** – Sarcoma (Tumor of mesenchymal origin), melanoma, seminomas, lymphoma
c) **Neurofilament** – Neural tumors
d) **Glial fibrillary acid proteins (GFAP)** – Non-neural brain tissue (Astroglial origin – Astrocytoma, ependymomas, Medulloblastoma, oligodendroglioma)
e) **Desmin** – Leiomyoma (smooth muscle) and Rhabdomyoma (skeletal muscle)

Ans. 29) B. Loss of intercellular connections (Ref: 9ed. Robbins p. 1169)

Acantholysis – Loss of intercellular connections resulting in loss of cohesion between keratinocytes

Ans. 30) D. Can Metastasize (Ref: 9 ed. Robbins p.1221-22) Refer Q 46 for details

Ans. 31) B. Face (Ref: 9 ed. Robbins p. 1157) Refer Q 25 for details

Ans. 32) B. CDK2A (Ref: 9 ed. Robbins p.1147-49) Refer Q 5 for details

Ans. 33) A. Sweet Syndrome (Ref: 9 ed. Lever's Histopathology of Skin. P. 232)

- **Neutrophils in papillary dermis in early stages**
- **In later stages, lymphocyte and histiocytes predominate**

24 Bones, Joints and Soft Tissue Tumors

How to go about this chapter?

- **One should be thorough with the following topics:**
  - **Collagen disorders**
  - **Osteopetrosis**
  - **Paget's disease**
  - **Bone disease in hyperparathyroidism**
  - **Osteomyelitis**
  - **Osteosarcoma**
  - **Osteoid osteomas**
  - **Osteoblastoma**
  - **Osteochondroma/Exostosis**
  - **Chondrosarcoma, Fibrosarcoma, Rhabdomyosarcoma, Synovial sarcoma**
  - **Ewing Sarcoma Family tumors**
  - **Giant Cell Tumor/Osteoclastoma, Chondroblastoma**
  - **Fibrous dysplasia**
  - **Osteoarthritis**
  - **Rheumatoid arthritis**
  - **Gout**
  - **Diffuse tenosynovial giant cell tumor (pigmented villonodular synovitis)**
  - **Nodular Fasciitis**

BASIC STRUCTURE AND FUNCTION OF BONE

1) **Development of bone is controlled by:**
a) Growth hormone
b) Thyroid hormone
c) Parathyroid hormone
d) All of the above

DEVELOPMENTAL DISORDERS OF BONE AND CARTILAGE

2) **Gene mutation most commonly seen in Achondroplasia:**
a) FGFR-3 b) COL2A1
c) RUNX2 d) PAX3

3) **TRUE about Osteogenesis Imperfecta (OI):**
a) Due to deficiency of type 1 collagen
b) Subtype-1 is compatible with survival
c) Associated with blue sclera
d) All of the above

4) **All are TRUE about Osteopetrosis EXCEPT:**
a) Impaired function of osteoclasts
b) Erlenmeyer flask deformity
c) Osteoclasts number are always reduced
d) Hematopoietic stem cell transplantation is treatment of choice

ACQUIRED DISORDERS OF BONE AND CARTILAGE

5) **Tumor and tumor like conditions associated with Paget's disease:**
a) Giant cell tumor
b) Giant cell reparative granuloma
c) Osteosarcoma
d) All of the above

6) **Following is/are noted in primary hyperparathyroidism:**
a) Osteoporosis
b) Brown tumors

c) Osteitis fibrosa cystica
d) All of the above

OSTEOMYELITIS

7) Most common agent responsible for developing osteomyelitis in adults:
a) Staphylococcus aureus
b) Haemophilus influenza
c) Salmonella
d) Pseudomonas

8) Complication(s) of chronic osteomyelitis:
a) Secondary amyloidosis
b) Squamous cell carcinoma in the draining sinus
c) Sarcoma of infected bone
d) All of the above

9) Most common site of involvement of tuberculous osteomyelitis:
a) Spine b) Knee
c) Hip d) Pelvis

BONE TUMORS AND TUMOR LIKE LESIONS

10) Most common primary bone cancer:
a) Osteosarcoma
b) Chondrosarcoma
c) Fibrosarcoma
d) Ewing sarcoma

11) All are TRUE regarding osteoblastoma EXCEPT:
a) Larger than 2 cms
b) Pain is unresponsive to aspirin
c) Differ morphologically from osteoid osteomas
d) Absence of reactive bone formation surrounding the lesion

12) TRUE about Osteosarcoma:
a) Most common primary malignant tumor of bone
b) Bimodal age distribution
c) Affects the metaphysis of long bones
d) All of the above

13) Following mutation(s) is/are seen in osteosarcomas:
a) Rb b) P53
c) INK4a d) All of the above

14) Codman triangle radiographically is the shadow between:
a) Cortex and medulla
b) Cortex and periosteum
c) Cortex and epiphysis
d) Epiphysis and diaphysis

15) Osteosarcomas most commonly affects:
a) Knee b) Pelvis
c) Jaws d) Shoulder

16) Metastasis from osteosarcoma is most commonly seen in:
a) Lungs b) Other bones
c) Pleura d) Heart

17) Diagnostic feature of osteosarcoma microscopically:
a) Tumor giant cells
b) Necrosis
c) Osteoid formation
d) Abnormal mitotic figures

18) TRUE about osteochondroma of bone:
a) Most common benign tumor of the bone
b) Arises from metaphysis of long bones
c) Stops growing at time of growth plate closure
d) All of the above

19) TRUE about chondroma:
a) Affects bones of hand and feet
b) Associated with Maffucci syndrome
c) Contains chondrocytes microscopically
d) All of the above

20) Which of the following chondrosarcoma can be confused with osteosarcoma:
a) Dedifferentiated chondrosarcoma
b) Clear cell chondrosarcoma
c) Mesenchymal chondrosarcoma
d) Conventional chondrosarcoma

21) TRUE regarding Ewing Sarcoma family tumor:
a) Involves the diaphysis of long bones
b) Most commonly arises in individuals younger than 20 years
c) Associated with t(11;22) translocation
d) All of the above

22) Differential diagnosis of Ewing sarcoma family tumors include(s):
a) Lymphoblastic lymphoma
b) Desmoplastic small round cell tumor
c) Embryonal rhabdomyosarcoma
d) All of the above

23) All are TRUE about Giant cell tumor of bone EXCEPT:
a) Also known as osteoclastoma
b) Arises in epiphysis of knee joint
c) Metastasis to lungs can occur
d) Osteoclastic giant cells form neoplastic component

24) Differential diagnosis of Giant cell tumor include(s):
a) Non ossifying fibroma
b) Chondroblastoma
c) Aneurysmal bone cyst
d) All of the above

25) TRUE about fibrous dysplasia:
a) Monostotic fibrous dysplasia presents in adolescence

b) Polyostotic dysplasia may lead to sarcoma
c) Polyostotic disease is commonly associated with McCune-Albright syndrome
d) All of the above

26) **Following cancers predominantly produce lytic metastasis to bone EXCEPT:**
a) Prostate
b) Lung
c) Kidney
d) Gastrointestinal tract

JOINTS

27) **Following cytokine(s) play a role in osteoarthritis:**
a) TGF-β b) TNF
c) Prostaglandins d) All of the above

28) **Most common cytokine implicated in Rheumatoid Arthritis:**
a) IFN-γ b) TNF
c) IL-17 d) IL-1

29) **In Rheumatoid Arthritis, autoantibodies is/are seen against following peptide(s):**
a) Citrullinated peptides
b) Type II collagen
c) α-enolase
d) Any of the above

30) **Histological features of Rheumatoid arthritis in joints include(s):**
a) Synovial cell hyperplasia
b) Inflammatory infiltrate
c) Pannus formation
d) All of the above

31) **Rheumatoid nodules are most commonly seen in:**
a) Elbows b) Forearm
c) Lungs d) Spleen

32) **All are the gross finding of joint in Rheumatoid Arthritis EXCEPT:**
a) Pannus
b) Eroding cartilage
c) Subchondral sclerosis
d) Bony ankylosis

33) **All are the features of Rheumatoid arthritis EXCEPT:**
a) Heberden nodes
b) Baker cyst
c) Boutonnière deformity
d) Involves metacarpophalangeal and proximal interphalangeal joints

34) **Which of the following has strongest association with HLAB-27?**
a) Reiter syndrome
b) Psoriatic arthritis
c) Rheumatoid spondylitis
d) Enteritis associated arthritis

35) **Most common agent of suppurative arthritis in children younger than 2 years of age:**
a) H. Influenza b) S. aureus
c) Salmonella d) Gonococcus

36) **Factors predisposing to gout:**
a) Duration of hyperuricemia
b) Genetic predisposition
c) Heavy alcohol consumption
d) All of the above

37) **Acute gouty arthritis most commonly affects:**
a) First metatarsophalyngeal joint
b) First metacarpophalyngeal joint
c) Ankle
d) Knee

38) **All are TRUE about Pseudo-gout crystals EXCEPT:**
a) Composed of calcium pyrophosphate crystals
b) Histologically, oval blue purple aggregates
c) Individuals crystals are rhomboid
d) Long slender, needle shaped and negatively birefringent

39) **Diffuse tenosynovial giant cell tumor most commonly involve:**
a) Knee
b) Hip
c) Ankle
d) Calcaneocuboid joints

SOFT TISSUES

40) **Most common site of soft tissue tumors:**
a) Thigh
b) Trunk
c) Upper extremities
d) Head and neck

41) **Following chromosomal abnormalities in soft tissue tumors are correctly matched EXCEPT:**
a) Ewing's sarcoma – t(11;22)
b) Extraskeletal myxoid chondrosarcoma – t(9;22)
c) Synovial sarcoma – t(x;18)
d) Clear-cell sarcoma – t(12;16)

42) **Differential diagnosis of painful cutaneous lesion(s):**
a) Angiolipoma
b) Fibrolipoma
c) Spindle cell lipomas
d) All of the above

43) **Floret cells is a feature of:**
a) Angiolipoma
b) Pleomorphic lipoma
c) Fibrolipoma
d) Spindle cell lipoma

44) **All are TRUE regarding Liposarcoma EXCEPT:**
a) Most common sarcoma of adulthood
b) t(12:16) occurs in myxoid liposarcoma

c) Amplification of 12q is characteristic of well differentiated liposarcoma
d) Pleomorphic liposarcoma has good prognosis

45) All are TRUE about Nodular fasciitis EXCEPT:
a) Involves the upper extremities
b) History of trauma is present
c) Can progress into malignancy
d) Abundant mitotic figures can be seen

46) All are TRUE about fibromatosis EXCEPT:
a) Dupuytren contracture is thickening involving palmar fascia
b) Peyronie disease involves penile shaft
c) Deep fibromatosis has an association with Gardner's syndrome
d) Desmoid tumors frequently metastasize

47) Most common soft tissue sarcoma in children and adolescents:
a) Fibrosarcoma
b) Rhabdomyosarcoma
c) Liposarcoma
d) Pleomorphic sarcoma

48) Rhabdomyosarcoma in pediatric age groups, predominantly affects:
a) Head and neck
b) Proximal extremities
c) Distal extremities
d) Trunk

49) Alveolar rhabdomyosarcoma contains the following molecular abnormalities:
a) FOXO1-PAX3
b) FOXO1-PAX7
c) Both of the above
d) None of the above

50) Sarcoma botryoides commonly involve(s):
a) Nasopharynx
b) Bile duct
c) Urinary bladder
d) Any of the above

51) Rhabdomyoblastic differentiation can be demonstrated with:
a) MYOD1 b) Desmin
c) Myogenin d) Any of the above

52) Most common site of alveolar rhabdomyosarcoma:
a) Lung
b) Extremities
c) Head and neck
d) Perirectal region

53) Which of the following has best prognosis?
a) Sarcoma botryoides
b) Alveolar rhabdomyosarcoma
c) Pleomorphic rhabdomyosarcoma
d) None of the above

54) Most common site of synovial sarcoma:
a) Lower extremity
b) Upper extremity
c) Trunk
d) Head and neck

55) All are TRUE about synovial sarcomas EXCEPT:
a) Can be monophasic or biphasic
b) Can have epithelial like differentiation
c) Shows mesenchymal differentiation
d) Presence of Rhabdoid cells indicates good prognosis

56) Herring bone pattern is a feature of:
a) Fibromatosis
b) Fibrosarcoma
c) Leiomyosarcoma
d) Rhabdomyosarcoma

57) Genetic mutation in fumarate hydratase is associated with:
a) Leiomyoma
b) Leiomyosarcoma
c) Synovial sarcoma
d) Fibrosarcoma

58) Which of the following is a type of seronegative spondyloarthropathy?
a) Rheumatoid arthritis
b) Gouty arthritis
c) CPPD
d) Reiter's disease

59) Gene affected in Ewing's sarcoma is: (NEET 2014)
a) EWS-FLI 1 b) PAX 3
c) EWS ATF 1 d) FUS-CHOP

60) Premalignant bone lesion: (NEET 2014)
a) Paget's disease
b) Osteoid osteoma
c) Osteochondroma
d) Enchondroma

61) All are features of Paget's disease EXCEPT: (NEET 2014)
a) Defect in osteoclasts
b) Common in females
c) Can cause deafness
d) Can cause osteosarcoma

62) Tadpole cells (comma shaped cells) on histopathology are seen in: (NEET 2013)
a) Trichoepithelioma
b) Spideroma
c) Rhabdomyosarcoma
d) Histiocytoma

63) Most common tumor of face in children: (NEET 2013)
a) Rhabdomyosarcoma

b) Squamous cell carcinoma
c) Basal cell carcinoma
d) Mixed parotid tumor

64) SYT-SSXI gene is associated with: (NEET 2013)
a) Liposarcoma
b) Rhabdomyosarcoma
c) Synovial sarcoma
d) Ewing's sarcoma

65) Ewing's sarcoma arises from: (NEET 2013)
a) G cells
b) Totipotent cells
c) Neuroectodermal cells
d) Neurons

66) Most common malignant bone tumor: (NEET 2013)
a) Osteogenic sarcoma
b) Secondaries
c) Osteoma
d) Enchondroma

67) HLA B27 is not seen in: (NEET 2013)
a) SLE
b) Ankylosing spondylitis
c) Reiter's syndrome
d) Psoriatic arthritis

68) Marker for rhabdomyosarcoma: (AIIMS May 2013)
a) Desmin
b) Synaptophysin
c) Keratin
d) Synaptophysin

69) Marker for bone formation is all EXCEPT: (AIIMS Nov 2011)
a) Osteocalcin
b) Alkaline phosphatase
c) Pro-collagen residue
d) Hydroxyproline

70) HLA B-27 more than 90% positivity is seen in: (AIIMS Nov 2014)
a) Ankylosing spondylitis
b) Reactive arthritis
c) Enteropathic arthritis
d) Rheumatoid disease

71) Immunohistopathological markers wrongly matched: (AIIMS Nov 2014)
a) Desmin–Carcinomas
b) Vimentin–Sarcomas
c) Leukocyte specific antigen–Lymphoma
d) S 100–Melanoma

CHAPTER 24: BONES, JOINTS AND SOFT TISSUE TUMORS

Ans. 1) **D. All of the above (Ref: 9 ed. Robbins p.1181-82)**

Development of bone is controlled by following **local and systemic factors** Q:

- Growth hormone (GH), Thyroid hormone (T3), Indian hedgehog (Ihh)
- Parathyroid hormone related protein (PTHrP)
- Wnt-β-catenin signaling pathway
- SOX9, RUNX2, Fibroblast growth factors (FGFs), Bone morphogenic proteins (BMPs)

Ans. 2) **A. FGFR-3 (Ref: 8 ed. Robbins p.1210-11, 9 ed. p.1184-85, t-26-2)**

Diseases of the Skeleton with identified **Genetic Defects** Q:

Disorder	Gene mutation
Cleidocranial dysplasia	RUNX2
Holt-Oram syndrome	TBX5
Waardenburg syndrome types 1 and 3	PAX3
Achondroplasia	FGFR3
Osteogenesis imperfecta types 1-4	COL1A1, COL1A2
Osteopetrosis, infantile form	RANKL

Achondroplasia Q:

- **Most common** skeletal dysplasia and a major cause of **dwarfism** Q
- Caused by **gain-of-function mutations** in **FGF receptor 3 (FGFR3)** Q

Thanatophoric dysplasia also occurs due to **mutation** of **FGFR3**

Ans. 3) **D. All of the above (Ref: 8 ed. Robbins p.1211-12, 9 ed. p.1185, t-26-3)**

Type 1 Collagen Diseases (Osteogenesis Imperfecta/brittle bone disease):

- Caused by the deficiencies in the synthesis of **type I collagen** Q (α1 & α2 chains)
- Primarily affects the bone, but also other tissues rich in type I collagen (joints, ears, **eyes – blue sclera** Q, skin and teeth)
- Has four major clinical subtypes
- **Type 1** patients have a **normal life span** Q
- **Type 2 variant** is uniformly **fatal in utero** Q or during the perinatal period

Ans. 4) **C. Osteoclasts number are always reduced (Ref: 8 ed. Robbins p.1212-14, 9 ed. p.1186-87, f-26-7,8)**

Osteopetrosis/Marble bone disease/Albers-Schönberg disease Q:

- Characterized by **reduced bone resorption**, leading to diffuse symmetric skeletal sclerosis due to impaired **formation** or **function of osteoclasts**

Morphology Q:

- Bone lack medullary canal, which is replaced by **primary spongiosa**, leading to the deficiency of hematopoietic marrow
- Ends of bones appear bulbous (**Erlenmeyer flask deformity**) Q
- **Number of osteoclasts** may be **normal**, **increased** or **decreased** Q

Point to be Remembered:

- Osteopetrosis was the **first genetic disease** Q treated with **hematopoietic stem cell transplantation** Q

Ans. 5) **D. All of the above (Ref: 8 ed. Robbins p.1216-18, 9 ed. p.1189-91, f-26-12-14)**

Tumor and **tumor-like conditions** that can develop in **Paget's disease** Q of bone:

- **Giant cell tumor, giant cell reparative granuloma** and extra-osseous masses of hematopoietic tissue
- **Sarcoma** – Osteosarcoma or fibrosarcoma (most dreaded complication)

Salient features of **Paget's Disease** Q:

- Occurs in **3 phases** – Osteolytic stage, mixed osteoclastic-osteoblastic stage and osteosclerotic stage
- **Histological hallmark**: **Mosaic pattern** of **lamellar bone** in the sclerotic phase

Ans. 6) D. All of the above (Ref: 8 ed. Robbins p.1218-19, 9 ed. p.1191-92, f-26-15, 16)

Primary hyperparathyroidism manifests with: **Osteoporosis, brown tumors** and **osteitis fibrosa cystica** Q

- **Osteoporosis** – Most severe in the **phalanges**, **vertebrae** and proximal femur
- **Dissecting osteitis** – Osteoclasts can dissect along the length of the trabeculae, creating the appearance of **railroad tracks**
- **Brown tumor** Q – **Microfractures** and **secondary hemorrhage** leads to influx of **macrophages** and reparative **fibrous tissue**
- **Generalized osteitis fibrosa cystica** (von Recklinghausen disease of bone) – Combination of increased bone cell activity, peritrabecular fibrosis and cystic brown tumors

Ans. 7) A. Staphylococcus aureus (Ref: 8 ed. Robbins p.1221, 9 ed. p.1195, f-26-20)

- **Staphylococcus aureus** Q is the **most common** agent responsible for **pyogenic osteomyelitis**
- **Escherichia coli**, Pseudomonas, Klebsiella are isolated from individuals with genitourinary tract infections
- In **neonates, Haemophilus influenzae** and **group B streptococci** are frequent pathogens
- **Salmonella infection** is common in individuals with **sickle cell disease** Q

Ans. 8) D. All of the above (Ref: 8 ed. Robbins p.1222, 9 ed. p.1196)

Complications of **chronic osteomyelitis** Q:

- Pathological fracture, secondary amyloidosis, endocarditis, sepsis
- **Squamous cell carcinoma** Q in the draining sinus tracts and **sarcoma** Q in the infected bone

Morphology of bone in **osteomyelitis** Q:

- **Dead bone** is called **sequestrum** Q
- Newly deposited bone forms a shell of living tissue, known as **involucrum** Q
- **Brodie abscess** Q – **Small intra-osseous abscess** that frequently involves the **cortex**
- **Sclerosing osteomyelitis of Garré** develops in the **jaw** Q

Ans. 9) A. Spine (Ref: 8 ed. Robbins p.1222-23, 9 ed. p.1196)

- **Tuberculous spondylitis (Pott disease)** Q most commonly involves **spine** Q (thoracic and lumbar) followed by knees and hips

Ans. 10) A. Osteosarcoma (Ref: 8 ed. Robbins p.1223-24, 9 ed. p.1196-97, t-26-6)

- Tumors arising from **hematopoietic cells (myeloma, lymphoma and leukemia)** Q, are **most common** primary bone tumors followed by **osteosarcoma** Q, chondrosarcoma and Ewing sarcoma
- As myeloma, lymphoma and leukemia are not in the options provided, hence the answer is **Osteosarcoma**

Note – Be thorough with the classification of bone tumors, **Robbins** 9 ed. **table 26-6**

Ans. 11) C. Differ morphologically from osteoid osteomas (Ref: 8 ed. Robbins p.1224-25, 9 ed. p.1197-98, f-26-21,22)

Osteoid Osteomas Q:

- **Less than 2 cm** in diameter, usually occur in **young men**
- Most commonly involves **femur** or **tibia**
- Presents with **severe nocturnal pain** that is **relieved by aspirin** Q

- **Radiographically** – Radiolucent central nidus, surrounded by **reactive (sclerotic) bone**
- Treatment – **Radiofrequency ablation**

Osteoblastoma Q:

- Larger than **2 cm**, involves the **posterior spine** Q (laminae and pedicles)
- Pain is **unresponsive to aspirin** Q
- **Does not** induce a marked reactive bony reaction
- Treatment – **Curettage** or **excised en bloc**

Morphology of **osteoid osteomas** and **osteoblastoma** Q:

- Composed of **interconnecting trabeculae** of **woven bone** with a rim of **osteoblasts** Q
- Stroma contains **loose connective tissue** with many dilated and congested capillaries

Hence, both these tumors look identical on microscopy

Ans. 12) D. All of the above (Ref: 8 ed. Robbins p.1225, 9 ed. p.1198, f-26-23)

Osteosarcoma Q:

- **Malignant tumor** in which the cancerous cells produce **osteoid matrix** Q
- Most common **primary malignant tumor** of bone
- **Bimodal age** distribution Q; most patients are **younger than 20 years**
- **Predisposing conditions** Q – Paget disease, bone infarcts, prior radiation
- Usually arises in the **metaphysis** of **long bones** (extremities)

Ans. 13) D. All of the above (Ref: 8 ed. Robbins p.1225, 9 ed. p.1198-99)

Following **mutations** Q are noted in osteosarcomas:

- **RB** mutation (and CDK4 overexpression)
- **TP53** gene mutation (and MDM2 overexpression)
- **INK4a** inactivation (INK4a encodes p16 and p14)

Ans. 14) D. Cortex and periosteum (Ref: 8 ed. Robbins p.1225-26, 9 ed. p.1198, f-26-23)

Radiographic features of osteosarcoma Q:

- Shows **large destructive**, **mixed lytic** and **blastic mass** with infiltrative margins
- Tumor **breaks** through the cortex and **lifts the periosteum**, resulting in **reactive periosteal bone formation**
- **Codman triangle** Q– **Triangular shadow** between the **cortex** and **raised ends of periosteum** seen radiographically

Ans. 15) A. Knee (Ref: 8 ed. Robbins p.1225-26, 9 ed. p.1198, f-26-24)

- **Osteosarcomas** arise in the **metaphysis** Q of the **long bones** of the extremities and most commonly affects the **knee** Q (i.e. distal femur or proximal tibia)

Ans. 16) A. Lungs (Ref: 8 ed. Robbins p.1226, 9 ed. p.1199-2000)

- **Metastasis** from osteosarcoma via bloodstream is seen most commonly in **lungs** Q, followed by other **bones**, **pleura** and **heart**

Ans. 17) C. Osteoid formation (Ref: 8 ed. Robbins p.1225-26, 9 ed. p.1199, f-26-25)

Microscopic Features of **Osteosarcoma** Q:

- Tumor cells frequently have large **hyperchromatic nuclei**
- **Bizarre tumor giant cells** with abnormal mitoses
- Vascular invasion and extensive necrosis can be seen
- **Formation of new bone (osteoid) by the tumor cells is diagnostic** Q
- Neoplastic bone has **fine, lace-like** architecture

Ans. 18) D. All of the above (Ref: 8 ed. Robbins p.1227, 9 ed. p.1200-01, f-26-26,27)

Osteochondroma/Exostosis [Q]:

- **Most common** benign bone tumor, commonly arises near the **knee**
- Most commonly are **solitary** [Q], but can be a part of multiple **hereditary exostosis syndrome**
- M:F : 3:1, they usually **stop growing** at the **time of growth plate closure** [Q]
- **Hereditary exostosis** is associated with **germline loss-of-function mutations** in **EXT1** or **the EXT2 gene** [Q]

Microscopy [Q]:

- **Cartilage cap** has histological appearance of **disorganized growth plate-like cartilage** and also undergoes **enchondral ossification**

Ans. 19) D. All of the above (Ref: 8 ed. Robbins p.1227-28, 9 ed. p.1201-02, f-26-28,29)

Chondroma/Enchondroma [Q]:

- Tumors arising in the **medullary cavity** are called **Enchondroma** and those on **surface** of bones are called **juxtacortical chondroma**
- Arises in the **metaphysis** of **tubular bones** of the **hands** and **feet** [Q]
- **Multiple enchondromas** are seen in **Ollier disease** [Q] and **Maffucci syndrome** [Q]
- **Heterozygous mutations** in **IDH1** and **IDH2 genes** are noted

Morphology [Q]:

- Composed of **well-circumscribed nodules** of hyaline cartilage which contain **benign chondrocytes**

Ans. 20) B. Clear cell chondrosarcoma (Ref: 8 ed. Robbins p.1230, 9 ed. p.1202, f-26-30)

Clear Cell Chondrosarcoma (Microscopy):

- Contains sheets of **large, malignant chondrocytes** with abundant clear cytoplasm, numerous **osteoclast-type giant cells**
- **Reactive bone formation** within the lesion, thus causing confusion with **osteosarcoma** [Q]

Ans. 21) D. All of the above (Ref: 8 ed. Robbins p.1232-33, 9 ed. p.1203, f-26-31)

Ewing Sarcoma Family Tumors [Q]:

- Ewing sarcoma and Primitive Neuroectodermal tumor (PNET) have been grouped together into a single category: the **Ewing sarcoma family tumors (ESFT)**
- Presents in individuals younger than **20 years** [Q]
- Arises in the **diaphysis of long bones** [Q], especially the **femur** and the **flat bones** of the pelvis
- **X-ray** [Q] shows a **destructive lytic tumor** [Q] which produces a characteristic **periosteal reaction** in an **onion-skin fashion**
- Shows **t(11;22)** [Q] translocation resulting in fusion of the EWS gene on chromosome 22 to the FLI1 gene

Microscopy [Q]:

- Composed of **sheets of uniform small, round cells** that have scant cytoplasm
- **Homer-Wright rosettes** (tumor cells surrounding **central fibrillary core**) can be seen

Ans. 22) D. All of the above (Ref: 10th ed. Ackerman p. 2048)

Differential diagnosis of **Ewing sarcoma family tumors** includes all **small round cell tumors** [Q] i.e.:

- **Lymphoblastic lymphoma, Desmoplastic small round cell tumor, Embryonal/ alveolar rhabdomyosarcoma**

Ans. 23) D. Osteoclastic giant cells form neoplastic component (Ref: 8 ed. Robbins p.1233-34, 9 ed. p.1203-04, f-26-32,33. 10th ed. Ackerman p. 2043-44)

Giant Cell Tumor (GCT)/Osteoclastoma [Q]:

- Arises in the **epiphysis** [Q]
- **Most common site**: Around the **knee** (distal femur and proximal tibia)

- Treatment includes **curettage** but, rarely tumors can **metastasize** to the **lungs**
- **Denosumab** [Q], **RANKL inhibitor** is the new drug used in the treatment, indicating the role of **RANKL receptor** in its pathogenesis

Morphology [Q]**:**

- Microscopically, tumor consists of sheets of uniform **oval mononuclear cells** and numerous **osteoclast-type giant cells** with **100** or **more nuclei** [Q]
- Nuclei of **mononuclear cells** and **osteoclasts** are **similar**, i.e. ovoid with **prominent nucleoli**
- **Mononuclear stromal cells** are considered **neoplastic** [Q] and not the **multinucleated osteoclastic giant cells**

Ans. 24) **D. All of the above (Ref: 10th ed. Ackerman p. 2045)**

Differential Diagnosis of **Giant cell tumor** of **bone** [Q]:

- Metaphyseal fibrous defect, nonossifying fibroma, chondromyxoid fibroma
- Chondroblastoma, Langerhans cell histiocytosis, solitary bone cyst, osteitis fibrosa cystica
- Giant cell reparative granuloma, aneurysmal bone cyst, osteoid osteoma and osteoblastoma

Ans. 25) **D. All of the above (Ref: 8 ed. Robbins p.1230-32, 9 ed. p.1206-07, f-26-38)**

Fibrous dysplasia [Q]**:**

- Benign tumor that has similarities to the localized developmental arrest
- Clinical patterns – Monostotic, Polyostotic, Mazabraud syndrome, McCune-Albright syndrome

Monostotic fibrous dysplasia [Q]**:**

- Presents in adolescence and grows till the **closure** of **growth plate**
- **Radiologically** – Ground-glass appearance and well-defined margins
- Most commonly involves – **Femur**, tibia, ribs, jawbones, calvarium and humerus

Polyostotic fibrous dysplasia [Q]**:**

- Involves **femur**, skull, tibia, humerus, ribs, fibula, radius, ulna, mandible and vertebrae in descending order
- **Craniofacial involvement** is commonly seen
- **Bisphosphonates** are used to reduce the severity of the bone pain
- Malignant transformation into **sarcoma** can be seen

Mazabraud syndrome: Polyostotic fibrous dysplasia and soft tissue **myxomas**

McCune-Albright Syndrome [Q]**:**

- Presents with **precocious sexual development** and polyostotic bone disease
- Skin disease – **Café-au-lait** spots
- **Endocrinopathies** – Hyperthyroidism, pituitary adenomas that secrete growth hormone and primary adrenal hyperplasia

Ans. 26) **A. Prostate (Ref: 8 ed. Robbins p.1235, 9 ed. p.1207)**

- **Metastatic tumors** [Q] are the **most frequent** malignant neoplasms of bone
- **Prostatic adenocarcinoma** produces predominantly **blastic lesions** [Q]
- Carcinomas of the **kidney, lung, gastrointestinal tract** and **malignant melanoma** produce **lytic lesions** [Q]
- **Metastases** commonly involves the **axial skeleton** [Q] (**vertebral column**, pelvis, ribs, skull and sternum)

Note: Radiographically, metastases may be purely **lytic (bone destroying)**, purely **blastic (bone forming)**, or **mixed lytic and blastic**

Ans. 27) **D. All of the above (Ref: 8 ed. Robbins p.1235-37, 9 ed. p.1208-09)**

Cytokines which have been **implicated in pathogenesis of osteoarthritis** [Q]:

- **TGF-β** [Q] (induces **matrix metalloproteinase**), **TNF**, **prostaglandins** and **nitric oxide**

- **Matrix metalloproteinase** produced by TGF, degrades **Type II Collagen** Q

Ans. 28) B. TNF (Ref: 8 ed. Robbins p.1237-39, 9 ed. p.1209-10)

Cytokines, which play a role in the **pathogenesis of Rheumatoid Arthritis (RA):**

- **IFN-γ (TH1 cells)** Q activates **macrophages** and synovial cells
- **IL-17 (TH17 cells)** Q recruits **neutrophils** and **monocytes**
- **TNF** and **IL-1 (macrophages)** Q stimulate the synovial cells to secrete proteases that **destroy hyaline cartilage**
- **RANKL** expressed on activated **T-cells** stimulates bone resorption

Out of the above, **TNF** has been **firmly implicated** Q in the **pathogenesis** of RA

Ans. 29) D. Any of the above (Ref: 8 ed. Robbins p.1237-39, 9 ed. p.1209-10)

Autoantibodies produced in **Rheumatoid Arthritis** Q:

- Are against **Citrullinated peptides (CCPs)**, Type II collagen, α-enolase and vimentin
- **Anti-CCP antibodies** Q may contribute to the chronicity of the disease
- **CCPs** are produced during **inflammation** and infection and smoking increases their levels
- **Rheumatoid factor** Q – **IgM** or **IgA autoantibodies** that bind to the Fc portions of their own **IgG**

Genetic susceptibility Q is associated with **HLA-DRB1 alleles** Q and **PTPN22 gene** Q

Ans. 30) D. All of the above (Ref: 8 ed. Robbins p.1237, 9 ed. p.1211, f-26-43)

Morphology of Joints in **Rheumatoid Arthritis** Q:

- **Synovial cell hyperplasia** and **proliferation**
- **Inflammatory infiltrate** composed of lymphocytes, plasma cells, dendritic cells and macrophages
- Increased vascularity, fibrinopurulent exudate on the synovial and joint surface
- **Pannus** Q – Composed of edematous synovium, inflammatory cells, granulation tissue and fibroblasts, which causes **erosion** of the articular cartilage
- Pannus in **early stages** is **fibrous (fibrous ankylosis)** which leads to fusion of the bones
- Pannus in later stages becomes bony (**bony ankylosis**)

Ans. 31) B. Forearm (Ref: 8 ed. Robbins p.1237, 9 ed. p.1211)

Rheumatoid Nodules:

- **Most common subcutaneous** lesions
- **Most common** sites Q – **Ulnar aspect of forearm** Q, elbows, occiput, lumbosacral area
- Less common sites – Lungs, spleen, pericardium, myocardium, heart valves, aorta and other viscera

Ans. 32) C. Subchondral sclerosis (Ref: 8 ed. Robbins p.1235-38, 9 ed. p.1210, f-26-41)

Morphological Features of **Osteoarthritis** Q:

- Bony spur, subchondral cyst, subchondral sclerosis, osteophytes, thinned and fibrillated cartilage

Morphological Features of **Rheumatoid Arthritis** Q:

- Fibrous ankylosis, bony ankylosis, inflammation, Pannus, eroding cartilage

Ans. 33) A. Heberden nodes (Ref: 8 ed. Robbins p.1235-40, 9 ed. p.1209-12, f-26-45)

Rheumatoid Arthritis:

- Involves predominantly metacarpophalangeal and **proximal interphalangeal joint** Q
- Radial deviation of wrist, ulnar deviation of fingers with flexion hyperextension of the fingers (**swan-neck deformity, boutonnière deformity**) Q
- **Baker cyst** is seen in the **posterior knee**, due to **increased intra-articular pressure**

- **Radiographic hallmarks** – Joint effusions, juxta-articular osteopenia with erosions, narrowing of the joint space and loss of articular cartilage

Heberden nodes [Q] – **Prominent osteophytes** at the **distal interphalangeal** joints, which are seen in **osteoarthritis**

Ans. 34) C. Rheumatoid spondylitis (Ref: 8 ed. Robbins p.1241, 9 ed. p.1213)

- **Ankylosing spondylitis**, also known as **rheumatoid spondylitis** and **Marie- Strümpell disease** is associated with **HLAB-27 positivity** [Q] in more than 90% of patients
- Other entities in the question also form a part of **seronegative spondyloarthropathies**
- In **psoriatic arthritis** – **Distal interphalangeal joints** of hands and feet are first affected and produce characteristic **"pencil in cup" deformity** [Q]

Ans. 35) A. H. Influenza (Ref: 8 ed. Robbins p.1242, 9 ed. p.1213)

- ***H. influenza*** [Q] arthritis predominates in children younger than **2 years** of age
- ***S. aureus*** is the causative agent of arthritis in older children and **adults**
- ***Gonococcal*** arthritis predominates in **late adolescence** and **young adulthood**, more commonly in **sexually active women** [Q]
- Individuals with **sickle cell disease** are prone to infection with **Salmonella** [Q]

Ans. 36) D. All of the above (Ref: 8 ed. Robbins p.1243, 9 ed. p.1215)

- **Hyperuricemia** (plasma **urate level > 6.8 mg/dL**) [Q] is necessary, but not sufficient, for development of **gout**

Factors which contribute to the conversion of **asymptomatic hyperuricemia** into **primary gout**:

- Age of the individual
- **Duration of hyperuricemia**: Gout appears after **20 to 30 years** of hyperuricemia
- **Genetic predisposition** [Q]**:** X-linked abnormalities of **HGPRT**, Polymorphisms in **URAT1** and **GLUT9**
- Heavy alcohol consumption, obesity
- **Drugs (e.g. thiazides)** [Q] that reduce excretion of urate
- Lead toxicity (so-called **saturnine gout** [Q])

Ans. 37) A. First metatarsophalangeal joint (Ref: 8 ed. Robbins p.1244, 9 ed. p.1216)

- **Acute arthritis** presents as **excruciating joint pain** and with **localized hyperemia, warmth**
- First attack of gout most commonly involves the **first metatarsophalangeal joint** [Q]
- **Other sites** affected in **descending order** of frequency: insteps, ankles, heels, knees, wrists, fingers and elbows

Ans. 38) D. Long slender, needle shaped and negatively birefringent (Ref: 8 ed. Robbins p.1244-46, 9 ed. p.1216-17, f-26-47,48)

Crystals in **gout** [Q]:

- **Urate crystals** are long, slender and **needle-shaped** and are **negatively birefringent**

Crystals in **Pseudo–gout** [Q]:

- **Calcium Pyrophosphate crystals** [Q] are chalky, white friable deposits, appears as **oval blue-purple aggregates** [Q] microscopically
- Individual crystals are **rhomboid** [Q], 0.5 to 5 μ in greatest dimension and are **positively birefringent**

Ans. 39) A. Knee (Ref: 8 ed. Robbins p.1247, 9 ed. p.1218-19, f-26-49)

Diffuse tenosynovial giant cell tumor (pigmented villonodular synovitis):

- Presents most commonly in **knee** [Q], followed by the hip, ankle and calcaneocuboid joints

Localized type (giant cell tumor of tendon sheath):

- **Most common** [Q] mesenchymal neoplasm of hand

- Presents as a **solitary**, slow-growing, **painless mass** that frequently involves the **tendon sheaths** along the **wrists** and **fingers** Q

Ans. 40) A. Thigh (Ref: 8 ed. Robbins p.1248, 9 ed. p.1219)

Locations of **soft tissue tumors** Q:

- 40% occur in **lower extremity,** especially **thigh** Q
- 20% occur in upper extremities
- 10% occur in head and neck
- 30% occur in trunk and retroperitoneum

Ans. 41) D. Clear-cell sarcoma – t(12;16) (Ref: 8 ed. Robbins p.1248-49, 9 ed. p.1219-20, t-26-8)

Chromosomal Abnormalities noted in **Soft Tissue Tumors** Q:

Tumor	Cytogenetic Abnormality
Ewing sarcoma family tumors	**t(11;22)**
Extraskeletal myxoid chondrosarcoma	**t(9;22)**
Desmoplastic small round-cell tumor	t(11;22)
Clear-cell sarcoma	**t(12;22)**
Liposarcoma—myxoid and round-cell type	t(12;16)
Synovial sarcoma	**t(x;18)**
Rhabdomyosarcoma—alveolar type	t(2;13)
Dermatofibrosarcoma Protuberans	t(17;22)
Alveolar soft-part sarcoma	t(X;17)
Infantile fibrosarcoma	t(12;15)
Nodular fasciitis	t(22;17)

Ans. 42) A. Angiolipoma (Ref: 8 ed. Robbins p.1249-50, 9 ed. p.1220)

Differential diagnosis of **painful cutaneous lesions** Q:

- **L** – leiomyoma
- **E** – eccrine spiroadenoma
- **N** – neuroma
- **D** – dermatofibroma
- **A** – angiolipoma
- **N** – neurilemmoma
- **E** – endrometrioma
- **G** – glomus tumor
- **G** – granular cell tumor

Ans. 43) B. Pleomorphic lipoma (Ref: 10th ed. Ackerman p. 2140-44)

Pleomorphic Lipoma:

- Contains hyperchromatic **multinucleated ('floret-like') tumor cells**
- Cells lie within the fibrous septa traversing the neoplasm

Ans. 44) D. Pleomorphic liposarcoma has good prognosis (Ref: 8 ed. Robbins p.1250, 9 ed. p.1220-21, f-26-50)

Liposarcoma Q**:**

- **Most common sarcoma** Q of adulthood
- **Most common sites** Q – Lower extremities; retroperitoneum

- **Types** – Myxoid, round cell, well-differentiated and pleomorphic
- **Myxoid liposarcoma** is characterized by the **reciprocal translocation t(12;16)** [Q]
- In well differentiated liposarcoma – ***MDM2*** gene is amplified on **chromosome 12q**
- **Pleomorphic liposarcoma** is a **highly cellular, poorly differentiated neoplasm** with **poor prognosis**

Ans. 45) C. Can progress to malignancy (Ref: 8 ed. Robbins p.1250-51, 9 ed. p.1221, f-26-51)

Nodular Fasciitis [Q]**:**

- Self-limited fibroblastic and myofibroblastic proliferation
- Occurs in **young adults** in the **upper extremity** [Q]
- In 25% of cases, there is a prior **history of trauma**
- **Regresses** spontaneously [Q] and if excised, it rarely recurs

Morphology [Q]**:**

Gross – Less than 5 cm, circumscribed, arises in deep dermis, subcutis or muscle

Microscopy [Q]**:**

- Cellular with plump, immature-appearing **fibroblasts** and **myofibroblasts**
- Cells vary in size and shape (**spindle** to **stellate**) and have conspicuous nucleoli
- Abundant **mitotic figures**, lymphocytes, collagen and **extravasated red blood cells** are commonly seen

Ans. 46) D. Desmoid tumors frequently metastasize (Ref: 8 ed. Robbins p.1251-52, 9 ed. p.1221-22, f-26-52)

Fibromatosis:

Superficial Fibromatosis:

- **Palmar (Dupuytren contracture)** [Q] – **Flexion contracture** of fourth and fifth fingers of the hand
- **Penile (Peyronie disease)** [Q] – **Palpable induration** or **mass** on the **dorsolateral aspect** of the **penis**
- Plantar contractures

Deep Fibromatosis (Desmoid tumors) [Q]**:**

- **Large, infiltrative masses** that frequently recur but **do not metastasize** [Q]
- Shows **mutation** in **APC/β-catenin genes** [Q]
- Associated with **familial adenomatous polyposis (Gardner syndrome)** [Q]
- **Microscopy – Bland fibroblasts** arranged in **broad sweeping fascicles** intermixed with **dense collagen**

Ans. 47) B. Rhabdomyosarcoma (Ref: 8 ed. Robbins p.1253-54, 9 ed. p.1222)

Rhabdomyosarcoma [Q]**:**

- **Malignant mesenchymal tumor** with **skeletal muscle** differentiation
- **3 subtypes** [Q]: Alveolar, embryonal and pleomorphic
- **Alveolar** and **embryonal** subtype – Most common **soft tissue sarcoma** [Q] of childhood and adolescence
- **Pleomorphic** [Q] subtype occurs predominantly in **adults**

Ans. 48) A. Head and neck (Ref: 8 ed. Robbins p.1253-54, 9 ed. p.1222)

- In **pediatric** age group, **rhabdomyosarcoma**, **most commonly** arises in the **sinuses**, **head and neck** [Q] and **genitourinary tract**

Ans. 49) C. Both of the above (Ref: 8 ed. Robbins p.1253-54, 9 ed. p.1222)

- **Alveolar rhabdomyosarcoma** shows fusion of **FOXO1 gene** to either the **PAX3** or the **PAX7 gene** [Q]
- **FOXO1-PAX3** gene rearrangement results from **t(2;13)** translocation and **FOXO1-PAX7** rearrangement results from **t(1;13)** translocation

Ans. 50) D. Any of the above (Ref: 8 ed. Robbins p.1253-54, 9 ed. p.1222-23, f-26-53)

Sarcoma Botryoides [Q]**:**

- Variant of embryonal rhabdomyosarcoma

- **Most common sites** Q – Hollow, mucosal-lined structures, such as the **nasopharynx, common bile duct, bladder and vagina**
- Characteristic feature – Presence of the zone of undifferentiated tumor cells immediately beneath the epithelium **i.e. Cambium layer** Q

Ans. 51) D. Any of the above (Ref: 8 ed. Robbins p.1253-54, 9 ed. p.1222-23)

- Ultrastructurally, rhabdomyoblasts contains **sarcomeres**
- **Immunohistochemically** shows staining with antibodies to the myogenic markers – **desmin, MYOD1, myogenin**Q

Ans. 52) B. Extremities (Ref: 8 ed. Robbins p.1253-54, 9 ed. p.1222-23, f-26-53)

Alveolar Rhabdomyosarcoma:

- Occurs in **early to middle adolescence**
- Most commonly involves the **extremities** Q (forearm, arm)
- **Other sites** include – Perirectal, perineal, head and neck regions
- Called as **alveolar**, because arrangement of tumor cells resembles **alveolar pattern (lung)** histologically

Ans. 53) A. Sarcoma botryoides (Ref: 8 ed. Robbins p.1253-54, 9 ed. p.1222-23)

- **Botryoid variant** of **embryonal rhabdomyosarcoma** has **best prognosis** Q
- Pleomorphic subtype has worst prognosis

Ans. 54) A. Lower extremity (Ref: 8 ed. Robbins p.1254-55, 9 ed. p.1223-24)

Synovial Sarcoma:

- Most common site includes **lower extremity** Q, especially around knee and thigh
- Other sites includes – **Chest wall, head and neck** Q
- Patient presents as a **deep-seated mass**
- Shows a characteristic chromosomal translocation **t(x;18)(p11;q11)** Q, which produces **SS18-SSX1, -SSX2, or**
- **SSX4 fusion genes** Q

Ans. 55) D. Presence of Rhabdoid cells indicates good prognosis (Ref: 8 ed. Robbins p.1254-55, 9 ed. p.1223-24, f-26-54, Ackerman 10th ed. p. 2174-77)

Morphology of **Synovial Sarcoma** Q:

- Can be **monophasic** or **biphasic** Q
- **Monophasic synovial sarcoma** Q – Uniform spindle cells with scant cytoplasm and dense chromatin growing in short, tightly packed fascicles
- **Biphasic synovial sarcoma** Q has **spindle cell component** and **gland-like structures** composed of cuboidal to columnar epithelioid cells
- **Mast cells** in monophasic synovial sarcoma gives a diagnostic clue
- **Prognosis is worse** Q when there is:

Necrosis, Mitosis >10/15 HPF, tumor size **>5 cms**, presence of rhabdoid cells, aneuploidy

Ans. 56) B. Fibrosarcoma (Ref: 8 ed. Robbins p.1252, f-26-57)

- **Most common site** – **deep soft tissues** Q of the extremities
- **Differential diagnosis** Q – Desmoid, malignant peripheral nerve sheath tumor, monophasic synovial sarcoma

Morphology:

- Characteristic feature is arrangement of **spindle shaped cells** in a **herring bone pattern** Q

Ans. 57) A. Leiomyoma (Ref: 8 ed. Robbins p.1254, 9 ed. p. 1223)

- **Hereditary leiomyomatosis and renal cell cancer syndrome (HLRCC)** are associated with: **Loss-of-function mutation** in **fumarate hydratase gene (chromosome 1q)** Q

Ans. 58) D. Reiter's disease [Ref: Robbins 9 ed. p. 1212-1213)

Ans. 59) A. EWS FLI 1 (9 ed. Robbins p. 1203) Refer Q 21 for details

Ans. 60) A. Paget's disease (Ref: 9 ed. Robbins p. 1191)

Ans. 61) B. Common in females (Ref: 9 ed. Robbins p. 1189-1191)

Clinical Features of Paget's Disease:

- More common in males
- Common sites – Pelvis and tibia
- Patients are usually asymptomatic and it is diagnosed when an X-ray is taken for some unrelated condition or there are raised serum alkaline phosphatase levels

Ans. 62) C. Rhabdomyosarcoma (Ref: 9 ed. Robbins p 1222)

- Diagnostic cell of Rhabdomyosarcoma is Rhabdomyoblast
- Rhabdomyoblast may be elongated – tadpole or strap cells

Ans. 63) A. Rhabdomyosarcoma (Ref: 9 ed. Robbins p. 1222) Refer Q 48 for details

Ans. 64) C. Synovial sarcoma (Ref: 9 ed. Robbins p. 1223-24) Refer Q 54 for details

Ans. 65) C. Neuroectodermal cells (Ref: 9 ed. Robbins p.1203) Refer Q 21 for details

Ans. 66) B. Secondaries

Most common primary malignant bone tumor – Osteogenic sarcoma

Most common benign bone tumor – Osteoma

Ans. 67) A. SLE (Ref: 9 ed. Robbins p. 1213) Refer Q 34 for details

Ans. 68) A. Desmin (Ref: 9 ed. Robbins p. 1222) Refer Q 47-53 for details

- **IHC markers of Rhabdomyosarcoma – stain with antibodies to Desmin, MYOD1 and Myogenin**

Ans. 69) D. Hydroxyproline

Markers of bone formation: Serum bone specific alkaline phosphatase, Serum propeptide/procollagen, Osteocalcin

Markers of bone resorption: Urine hydroxyproline, serum tartrate resistant acid phosphatase, urine and serum N-telopeptide and C-telopeptide, urine total free deoxypyrindinoline, serum bone sialoprotein, urine hydroxylysine glycoside

Ans. 70) A. Ankylosing spondylitis (Ref: 9 ed. Robbins p.1213)

HLA-B 27 Syndromes:

Acute Anterior Uveitis (50-60 %)

Ankylosing Spondylitis (80-90 %)

Reactive Arthritis (60-85 %)

Inflammatory Bowel Disease

Psoriatic Arthritis

Ans. 71) A. Desmin – Carcinomas (Ref: 9 ed. Robbins p.1222-23) Refer Q 51 for details

25 Peripheral Nerves and Skeletal Muscle

How to go about this chapter?

- **One should be thorough with the following topics:**
  - **Axonal Neuropathies**
  - **Demyelinating Neuropathies**
  - **Guillain-Barre Syndrome**
  - **Myasthenia Gravis**
  - **Lambert-Eaton Myasthenic Syndrome**
  - **Dermatomyositis**
  - **Toxic myopathies**
  - **Duchenne and Becker muscular dystrophy**
  - **Infantile hypotonia**
  - **Schwannoma**
  - **Neurofibroma**

DISEASES OF PERIPHERAL NERVES

1) In axonal neuropathy, axonal regeneration of Schwann cells occurs at rate of:
a) 1 mm/day b) 1 mm/hour
c) 1 cm/day d) 1 cm/hour

2) TRUE about demyelinating neuropathies:
a) Schwann cells with myelin are damaged
b) Axons are preserved
c) Schwann cells leads to new myelin formation
d) All of the above

3) Most common cause of mononeuritis multiplex:
a) Vasculitis b) Trauma
c) Infections d) Entrapment

4) Features of Acute Inflammatory Demyelinating polyneuropathy include all EXCEPT:
a) Ascending paralysis
b) Segmental demyelination of affected nerves
c) No infectious agent demonstrated in affected nerves
d) Responds well to steroids

5) Polyneuropathy common in diabetic patients:
a) Ascending distal symmetric
b) Descending distal symmetric
c) Ascending proximal symmetric
d) Descending proximal symmetric

6) Most common paraneoplastic neuropathy:
a) Sensorimotor neuronopathy
b) Chronic inflammatory demyelinating polyradiculoneuropathy
c) Autonomic neuropathy
d) None of the above

DISEASES OF THE NEUROMUSCULAR JUNCTION

7) All are TRUE about Myasthenia Gravis EXCEPT:
a) Autoantibodies against acetylcholine receptor
b) Antibodies against muscle-specific receptor tyrosine kinase
c) 10% of patients have thymoma
d) Electrophysiological studies shows an increase in muscle response with repeated stimulation

8) Lambert-Eaton Myasthenic Syndrome is associated with:
a) Neuroendocrine carcinoma of lung
b) Adenocarcinoma of lung
c) Papillary carcinoma of thyroid
d) Hepatocellular carcinoma

9) Dermatomyositis is associated with the following:
a) Anti-Mi2 antibody
b) Anti-Jo1 antibody
c) Anti-P155/140 antibodies
d) Any of the above

10) **All of the following are commonly seen in Dermatomyositis EXCEPT:**
a) Heliotrope rash
b) Gottron papules
c) Cardiac failure
d) Interstitial lung disease

11) **Which of the following is the morphological feature of Polymyositis?**
a) Endomysial mononuclear inflammatory infiltrate
b) Perimyseal mononuclear inflammatory infiltrate
c) Perifascicular pattern of muscle atrophy
d) Rimmed vacuoles

12) **Most common cause of toxic myopathy:**
a) Statins
b) Alcohol
c) Chloroquine
d) Thyrotoxic myopathy

13) **Duchenne and Becker muscular dystrophy occurs due to following mutation:**
a) Laminin 2
b) Dystrophin
c) Syntrophins
d) Caveolin

14) **Following is/are the morphological features of X-linked muscular dystrophy:**
a) Myofiber degeneration
b) Fatty replacement
c) Myofiber atrophy
d) All of the above

15) **Differential diagnosis of floppy infant syndrome includes:**
a) Congenital myasthenic syndrome
b) Congenital myotonia
c) Spinal muscular atrophy
d) Any of the above

16) **Congenital myopathies include(s):**
a) Central core disease
b) Nemaline myopathy
c) Centronuclear myopathy
d) All of the above

PERIPHERAL NERVE SHEATH TUMORS

17) **All are TRUE regarding Schwannoma EXCEPT:**
a) Component of Neurofibromatosis 2
b) Un-encapsulated masses
c) Most commonly occurs at cerebellopontine angle
d) Shows S 100 positivity

18) **Shredded carrot appearance is a characteristic feature of:**
a) Cutaneous Neurofibroma
b) Plexiform Neurofibroma
c) Schwannoma
d) None of the above

19) **Associated with NF-2:**
a) Bilateral Schwannoma and meningiomas
b) Ependymoma of spinal cord
c) NF-2 gene is located on Chromosome 22q12
d) All of the above

20) **Inheritance pattern of myotonic dystrophy is: (NEET 2014)**
a) Autosomal recessive
b) Autosomal dominant
c) X-linked dominant
d) X-linked recessive

21) **Pseudohypertrophy is seen in: (NEET 2014)**
a) Duchenne muscular dystrophy
b) Facioscpulohumeral dystrophy
c) Emery Dreifuss muscular dystrophy
d) Myotonic dystrophy

22) **Most common posterior mediastinal tumor is: (NEET 2014)**
a) Thymoma
b) Neurogenic tumor
c) Hemangioma
d) Sarcomas

23) **Neurofibroma is: (NEET 2013)**
a) Autosomal dominant
b) Autosomal recessive
c) X-linked recessive
d) X-linked dominant

24) **Myasthenia gravis is associated with: (NEET 2013)**
a) Thymoma
b) Thymic carcinoma
c) Thymic hyperplasia
d) Lymphoma

25) **Perifascicular atrophy of muscle fibres is seen in: (NEET 2013)**
a) Steroid myopathy
b) Dermatomyositis
c) Inclusion body myositis
d) Nemaline myopathy

26) **Which of the following is not X-linked condition? (NEET 2013)**
a) Duchenne muscular dystrophy
b) Emery-Dreifuss muscular dystrophy
c) Facioscapulohumeral muscular dystrophy
d) Becker muscular dystrophy

27) **Verocay body is seen in: (AIIMS May 2014)**
a) Schwannoma
b) Meningioma
c) Hemangioma
d) Medulloblastoma

28) **Schwannoma histopathological feature: (AIIMS Nov 2014)**
a) Antoni a and b

b) Storiform pattern
c) Bundles of cells
d) Target cells

29) The following microscopic appearance is that of a Schwannoma–a nerve sheath tumor, most commonly involving the cerebellopontine angle. What does the area marked with red arrow represent? (AIIMS Nov 2105)

a) Myxoid tissue
b) Antony A pattern
c) Antony B pattern-veruccay cells
d) Antony C pattern-veruccay cells

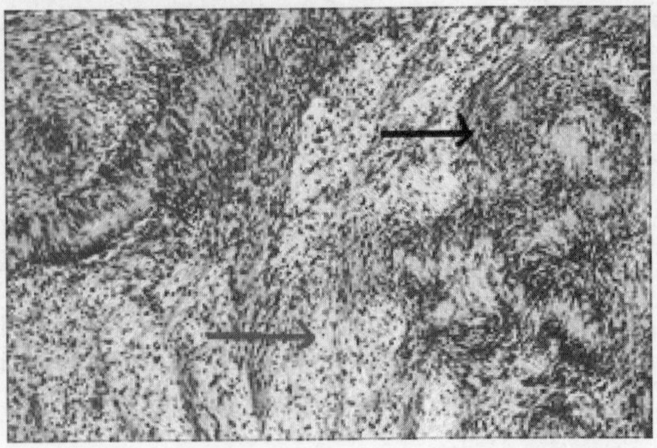

CHAPTER 25: PERIPHERAL NERVES AND SKELETAL MUSCLES

Ans. 1) **A. 1 mm/day (Ref: 8 ed. Robbins p.1258-59, 9 ed. p. 1228-29, f-27-2)**

Axonal Neuropathies Q:

- **Wallerian degeneration** Q – Morphological pattern of axonal injury produced by cutting a peripheral nerve
- In a day, **distal axon**, leads to **regeneration** of **axonal fibers** with help of **Schwann cells** and forms myelin sprouts at rate of **1 mm/day** Q
- **Traumatic neuroma** – Whorled proliferation of axons and schwann cells

Ans. 2) **B. All of the above (Ref: 8 ed. Robbins p.1258-59, 9 ed. p. 1228-30, f-27-2)**

Demyelinating Neuropathies Q:

- **Schwann cells** with their **myelin sheaths** are the **primary targets** of **damage**
- **Axons** are preserved in **demyelinating neuropathies**
- **Schwann cells** initiate repair by formation of **new myelin sheath**

Ans. 3) **A. Vasculitis (Ref: 9 ed. Robbins p. 1230)**

Causes of Mono-neuropathies Q: Trauma, entrapment and infections

Mononeuritis multiplex Q – **Vasculitis** is a common cause

Ans. 4) **D. Responds well to steroids (Ref: 8 ed. Robbins p.1261-62, 9 ed. p. 1230-31, f-27-5)**

Guillain-Barre Syndrome (Acute Inflammatory Demyelinating Polyneuropathy) Q:

- **Acute-onset**, immune-mediated **demyelinating neuropathy**
- Associated with **infections** Q by Campylobacter jejuni, Cytomegalovirus, Epstein-Barr virus and Mycoplasma pneumoniae, or by prior vaccination
- **Plasmapheresis** and **intravenous immunoglobulin** are beneficial

Morphology Q:

- **Segmental demyelination** Q affecting peripheral nerves is the **most prominent lesion**
- **Inflammation** of peripheral nerves is seen Q
- **Axonal damage** is also seen

Chronic Inflammatory Demyelinating Poly (radiculo) neuropathy Q:

- Signs and symptoms must be present for at least **2 months** Q
- Responds well to **steroids** Q

Ans. 5) **A. Ascending distal symmetric (Ref: 8 ed. Robbins p.1265-66, 9 ed. p. 1232-33, f-27-6)**

- **Most common peripheral neuropathy** in Diabetes – **ascending distal symmetric sensorimotor polyneuropathy** Q
- Predominant pathologic finding is **axonal neuropathy** Q
- Presents with numbness, loss of pain sensation, difficulty with balance and paresthesias or dysesthesias Q

Ans. 6) **A. Sensorimotor neuronopathy (Ref: 8 ed. Robbins p.1266, 9 ed. p. 1233)**

Paraneoplastic Neuropathies:

- Occurs in patients before the diagnosis of tumor
- **Sensorimotor neuronopathy** Q is the **most common** paraneoplastic form
- **Most commonly** associated with **small cell lung cancer** Q

Ans. 7) **D. Electrophysiological studies shows an increase in muscle response with repeated stimulation (Ref: 8 ed. Robbins p.1275-76, 9 ed. p. 1235-36)**

Myasthenia Gravis Q:

- Associated with autoantibodies directed against **acetylcholine receptors**

- Female-to-male ratio is **2 : 1**
- **10%** of patients with myasthenia gravis have associated **thymoma** [Q]
- **30%** of patients have **thymic hyperplasia**

Pathogenesis:

- **85%** patients have autoantibodies against postsynaptic **acetylcholine receptors** [Q]
- Antibodies against **sarcolemmal protein muscle-specific receptor tyrosine kinase** are common

Clinical Features:

- Fluctuating weakness that worsens with exertion
- **Diplopia** and **ptosis** are common, which distinguish myasthenia gravis from myopathies

Diagnosis:

- Based on clinical history, physical findings and identification of autoantibodies
- **Electrophysiological studies** [Q] shows a decrement in muscle response with repeated stimulation

Ans. 8) A. Neuroendocrine carcinoma of lung (Ref: 8 ed. Robbins p.1276, 9 ed. p. 1236)

Lambert-Eaton Myasthenic Syndrome [Q]**:**

- Caused by antibodies that block the **acetylcholine release** by inhibiting presynaptic **calcium channel** [Q]
- Rapid repetitive stimulation **increases muscle response** [Q]
- Most commonly associated with **Neuroendocrine carcinoma of the lung** [Q]

Ans. 9) D. Any of the above (Ref: 8 ed. Robbins p.1273-74, 9 ed. p. 1238)

Dermatomyositis [Q]**:**

- **Immunologic disease** in which **small blood vessel** damage leads to **muscle injury**
- Muscle and skin shows deposition of complement **membrane attack complex (C5b-9)** within capillary beds

Autoantibodies in **dermatomyositis** (with clinical features):

- **Anti-Mi2 antibodies** [Q] – Strong association with prominent **Gottron papules** and **heliotrope rash**
- **Anti-Jo1 antibodies** [Q] – Associated with **interstitial lung disease**, non-erosive arthritis and skin rash described as **"mechanic's hands"**
- **Anti-P155/P140 antibodies** [Q] – Associated with **paraneoplastic** and **juvenile** cases of dermatomyositis

Ans. 10) C. Cardiac failure (Ref: 8 ed. Robbins p.1273-74, 9th ed. p. 1238-39)

Clinical Features of Dermatomyositis [Q]**:**

- **Muscle weakness** [Q] – **Proximal muscles** (getting up from a chair and climbing steps) are affected first followed by **distal muscles** (fine movements)
- **Heliotrope rash** [Q] – Lilac colored discoloration of the upper eyelids
- **Gottron papules** [Q] – Scaling erythematous eruption or dusky red patches over the knuckles, elbows and knees
- Dysphagia due to involvement of **oropharyngeal** and **esophageal muscles**
- **Interstitial lung disease** [Q]
- Cardiac involvement is common, but **cardiac failure** [Q] is rare

Ans. 11) A. Endomysial mononuclear inflammatory infiltrate (Ref: 8 ed. Robbins p.1273-75, 9 ed. p. 1238-40, f- 27-8,9)

Morphological Features of **Dermatomyositis** [Q]:

- **Mononuclear inflammatory infiltrates – perimysial** in location
- **Perifascicular pattern** of muscle atrophy

Morphological Features of **Polymyositis** [Q]:

- **Mononuclear inflammatory infiltrates – endomysial** in location

- **Inflammatory cells** infiltrating into the myofibers
- **Degenerating** and **regenerating** myofibers

Morphological features of **Inclusion body myositis** [Q]:

In addition to the morphological features of **polymyositis**, following features are seen:

- **Rimmed vacuoles** i.e. abnormal cytoplasmic inclusions
- **Tubolofilamentous inclusions** in myofibers
- **Cytoplasmic inclusions** contain proteins (associated with neurodegenerative diseases) like beta-amyloid, TDP-43 and **ubiquitin** [Q]

Ans. 12) A. Statins (Ref: 8 ed. Robbins p.1275, 9th ed. p. 1240-41)

Toxic myopathies [Q] can be due to:

- **Statins** [Q] (Myopathy is the most common complication of statins)
- Chloroquine and hydroxychloroquine
- ICU myopathy or myosin deficient myopathy
- Thyrotoxic myopathy
- Alcohol

Ans. 13) B. Dystrophin (Ref: 8 ed. Robbins p.1268-69, 9th ed. p. 1242-43, f-27-10)

- **Duchenne** and **Becker muscular dystrophy** are caused by **loss-of-function** mutations in the **dystrophin gene** [Q]
- **Duchenne muscular dystrophy** is associated with deletions or frame shift mutations that result in total absence of dystrophin
- In **Becker muscular dystrophy**, mutation leads to abnormal synthesis of **dystrophin**, thus retaining some of its function

Ans. 14) D. All of the above (Ref: 8 ed. Robbins p.1268-69, 9th ed. p. 1242-43, f-27-11)

Morphology of **Duchenne and Becker muscular dystrophy** [Q]:

- Chronic muscle damage
- Segmental myofiber degeneration and regeneration
- Myofiber atrophy
- No inflammation
- Presence of myophagocytosis
- **Fatty replacement** or **fatty infiltration** of the muscle fibers

Immunohistochemical studies for **dystrophin:**

- Shows absence of normal staining pattern in **Duchenne muscular dystrophy** and **reduced staining** pattern in **Becker muscular dystrophy**

Ans. 15) D. Any of the above (Ref: 8 ed. Robbins p.1271-72, 9th ed. p. 1245-46, t-27-2)

Differential diagnosis of **infantile hypotonia** [Q]:

- Primary diseases of skeletal muscle (e.g., congenital myasthenic syndrome, congenital myotonia, congenital myopathies and congenital muscular dystrophies)
- Abnormalities of the brain (e.g. **encephalopathy**)
- Neuronopathies (**spinal muscular atrophy** is a prototypic example)

Ans. 16) D. All of the above (Ref: 8 ed. Robbins p.1272, 9th ed. p. 1241, t-27-2)

Congenital myopathies include:

- Central-core disease (autosomal dominant)
- Nemaline myopathy (NEM)

- Centronuclear myopathy
- Congenital fiber type disproportion

All of the conditions mentioned above are causes of **"floppy infants"**

Ans. 17) B. Un-encapsulated masses (Ref: 8 ed. Robbins p.1341-42, 9th ed. 1247, f-27-14)

Schwannoma Q:

- **Benign tumors** that exhibit Schwann cell differentiation
- Most common site – **cerebellopontine angle** Q
- Associated with inactivating mutations in **NF2 gene** on **chromosome 22**

Morphology:

- **Well-circumscribed**, firm gray, **encapsulated masses** Q
- Microscopically, Schwanomma has **Antoni A** and **Antoni B areas** Q
- **Antoni A areas** – Dense eosinophilic area in which spindle cells are arranged into cellular intersecting fascicles
- **Antoni B areas** – Loose hypocellular areas
- **Verocay bodies** Q – **"Nuclear-free zones"** that lie between the regions of nuclear palisading
- **Schwann cells** have spindled elongated nucleus with **wavy** or **buckled shape**
- **S-100 positivity** Q is a characteristic feature of **Schwann cell**

Ans. 18) B. Plexiform Neurofibroma (Ref: 8 ed. Robbins p.1341, 9th ed. 1247-48, f-27-14)

Neurofibroma:

- Benign nerve sheath tumor composed of neoplastic **Schwann cells** admixed with perineural like cells, fibroblasts, **mast cells** and **CD34+ spindle cells**

Morphology Q:

Localized cutaneous Neurofibroma Q:

- **Un-encapsulated nodular lesions**, arise in dermis and subcutaneous fat
- Composed of bland **Schwann cells** admixed with **mast cells**, **perineural cells**, **CD34+ spindle cells** and **fibroblasts**

Diffuse Neurofibroma Q:

- **Tumor cells** diffusely infiltrate the **dermis** and **subcutaneous connective tissue**, entrapping the fat and appendage structures

Plexiform Neurofibroma Q:

- **Cellular composition** similar to that of Neurofibroma
- Extracellular matrix is more **collagenous** and **fibrous**
- Collagen is seen in bundles like a **"shredded carrot"**

Ans. 19) D. All of the above (Ref: 8 ed. Robbins p.1342, 9th ed. 1249)

Neurofibromatosis Type 2 (NF-2) Q:

- Associated with **bilateral eighth-nerve Schwannoma**, multiple **meningiomas**, **gliomas**, **ependymomas** of the spinal cord
- **NF-2 gene** is located on **chromosome 22q12** Q and its **gene product** is **merlin** Q

Ans. 20) B. Autosomal dominant (Ref: 9 ed. Robbin's p. 1243-44)

Ans. 21) A. Duchenne muscular dystrophy (Ref: 9 ed. Robbins p. 1243)

Pseudohypertrophy – Enlargement of muscles of the lower leg associated with its weakness

Ans. 22) B. Neurogenic tumors

Most common tumors of posterior mediastinum are neurogenic tumors: Schwannoma, Neurofibroma and ganglioneuromas

Ans. 23) A. Autosomal dominant (Ref: 9 ed. Robbins p. 298, 1249) Refer Q 18 and 19 for details

Ans. 24) A. Thymoma (Ref: 9 ed. Robbins p. 1235-36) Refer Q 7 for details

Ans. 25) B. Dermatomyositis (Ref: 9 ed. Robbins p. 1238-40) Refer Q 9, 10 and 11 for details

Ans. 26) C. Facioscapulohumeral muscular dystrophy (Ref: 9 ed. Robbins p. 1244)

- Facioscapulohumeral muscular dystrophy is an autosomal dominant disorder

Ans. 27) A. Schwannoma (Ref: 10 ed. Rosai and Ackerman's Surgical Pathology p. 2130, 9 ed. Robbins and Cotran, p. 257, 854, 1247-48)

Schwannoma (Neurilemoma):

- Solitary, encapsulated tumor
- Associated with Von Recklinghausen disease type 2
- **Common sites** – Flexor surfaces of the extremities, neck, mediastinum, retro peritoneum, posterior spinal roots and cerebellopontine angle

Microscopically – Shows Antoni A and B patterns

- Type A areas, are quite cellular, composed of spindle cells often arranged in a palisading fashion or in an organoid arrangement (Verocay bodies)
- Type B areas– Tumor cells are separated by abundant edematous fluid that may form cystic spaces

Ancient Schwannoma – In which isolated cells with bizarre hyperchromatic nuclei are seen

Meningioma:

- Are seen in middle or later adult life
- Females are more commonly affected than males
- Presents as a well-defined Dural-based masses (WHO grade I/IV)
- Atypical meningiomas (WHO grade II/IV) have prominent nucleoli, increased cellularity and often have a higher mitotic rate
- Anaplastic (malignant) meningiomas (WHO grade III/IV) are highly aggressive tumors

Hemangioma:

- Most common tumors of infancy
- Types – capillary and cavernous

Medulloblastoma:

- Seen predominantly in children and in the cerebellum
- Extremely cellular, with sheets of anaplastic ("small blue") cells
- Tumor cells are small, with little cytoplasm and hyperchromatic nuclei; mitoses are abundant
- Homer Wright rosette can be seen, characterized by primitive tumor cells surrounding central neuropil

Ans. 28) A. Antoni a and b (Ref: 9 ed. Robbins p. 1247) Refer Q 17 for details

Ans. 29) C. Antony B pattern-veruccay cells (Ref: 9 ed. Robbins, p. 1247-48) Refer Questions above

Figure represents Antoni A areas with the tumor cell nuclei aligned in palisading rows leaving anuclear zones, resulting in formation of Verocay bodies.

26 The Central Nervous System

How to go about this chapter?

- **One should be thorough with the following topics:**
  - **CNS infections**
  - **Prion diseases**
  - **Central Pontine Myelinolysis**
  - **Neurodegenerative Diseases affecting CNS**
  - **Pilocytic Astrocytoma, Pleomorphic Xanthoastrocytoma, Glioblastoma**
  - **Oligodendroglioma, Ependymomas, Myxopapillary ependymomas**
  - **Choroid plexus papilloma**
  - **Gangliogliomas, Medulloblastoma, Atypical Teratoid/Rhabdoid Tumor**
  - **Diffuse large-cell B-cell lymphomas**
  - **Meningiomas**
  - **Paraneoplastic Syndromes**
  - **Familial Tumor Syndromes**

CELLULAR PATHOLOGY OF THE CENTRAL NERVOUS SYSTEM

INFECTIONS

1) **TRUE about neuronal inclusions:**
a) Intra-nuclear inclusions are seen in herpes
b) Intra-cytoplasmic inclusions in Rabies
c) Nucleus and cytoplasmic inclusions in Cytomegalovirus
d) All of the above

2) **Negri bodies seen in the Rabies are:**
a) Intra-nuclear inclusions
b) Intra-cytoplasmic inclusions
c) None of the above
d) Both of the above

3) **HIV infects the following cell of central nervous system:**
a) Astrocytes
b) Oligodendrocytes
c) Neurons
d) Glial cells

PRION DISEASES

4) **Prion diseases affecting humans include all EXCEPT:**
a) Creutzfeldt-Jakob disease
b) Gerstmann-Sträussler-Scheinker syndrome
c) Fatal familial insomnia
d) Scrapie

DEMYELINATING DISEASES

5) **All are TRUE regarding central pontine myelinolysis EXCEPT:**
a) Complication of sudden correction of hyponatremia
b) Oligodendrocytes are damaged
c) Inflammation is a characteristic feature
d) Periventricular regions are spared

NEURODEGENERATIVE DISEASES

6) **Neurodegenerative disorder(s) associated with deposition of tau protein include(s):**
a) Alzheimer disease
b) Parkinson disease
c) Progressive supranuclear palsy
d) All of the above

7) **Microscopic abnormalities of Alzheimer disease include(s):**
a) Neuritic plaques
b) Neurofibrillary tangles
c) Cerebral amyloid angiopathy
d) All of the above

8) **First gene identified as cause of Autosomal dominant Parkinson disease (PD):**
a) α-synuclein b) PINK1
c) LRRK2 d) None of the above

GENETIC METABOLIC DISEASES

9) **Metachromatic leukodystrophy results from deficiency of:**
a) Arylsulfatase A
b) β-galactosidase
c) Both of the above
d) None of the above

TUMORS

10) **Mutation(s) seen in Glioblastoma:**
a) PTEN b) EGFR amplification
c) TP53 d) All of the above

11) **TRUE about the morphology of Glioblastoma:**
a) Necrosis
b) Endothelial cell proliferation
c) Glomeruloid body
d) All of the above

12) **TRUE about Pilocytic astrocytoma:**
a) Located in the cerebellum
b) Tp53 mutation is rare
c) Rosenthal fibers and eosinophilic granular bodies are seen
d) All of the above

13) **All are TRUE about pleomorphic xantho-astrocytoma EXCEPT:**
a) Seen in the temporal lobe of children
b) Presents with history of seizures
c) Low grade tumor
d) Presence of necrosis and mitosis

14) **Radiotherapy and chemotherapy will be beneficial in oligodendroglioma showing following mutation:**
a) 1p b) 9p
c) 10q d) Any of the above

15) **Most common site of Ependymoma in first two years of life:**
a) First ventricle
b) Second ventricle
c) Third ventricle
d) Fourth ventricle

16) **Myxopapillary ependymomas arises from:**
a) Filum terminale
b) Cauda equina
c) Cerebellum
d) Any of the above

17) **TRUE about choroid plexus papilloma:**
a) Found in lateral ventricle in children
b) In adults, they are found in the fourth ventricle
c) Choroid plexus carcinoma resemble adeno-carcinoma
d) All of the above

18) **TRUE about Ganglioglioma:**
a) Most common neuronal tumors of the CNS
b) They present with seizures
c) Arises from the temporal lobe
d) All of the above

19) **TRUE about Medulloblastoma:**
a) Occurs in cerebellum
b) Divided into four groups on the basis of molecular alterations
c) Dissemination of CSF is a common complication
d) All of the above

20) **TRUE regarding Atypical teratoid/Rhabdoid tumors (ATRT):**
a) Malignant tumor of young children
b) Occurs in supratentorial regions
c) Shows genetic alterations in chromosome 22
d) All of the above

21) **IHC stains used for ATRT includes all EXCEPT:**
a) Epithelial membrane antigen
b) Vimentin
c) Smooth muscle actin
d) Desmin

22) **Primary CNS lymphomas are of following type:**
a) B cell type
b) T cell type
c) NK cell type
d) Any of the above

23) **Most common primary CNS lymphoma:**
a) Diffuse large B-cell lymphoma
b) Anaplastic large cell lymphoma
c) Burkitt's lymphoma
d) Intravascular lymphoma

24) **Dural based tumor include(s):**
a) Meningiomas
b) Solitary fibrous tumor
c) Metastasis
d) All of the above

25) **All of the following are included in WHO Grade I meningiomas EXCEPT:**
a) Fibroblastic
b) Syncitial
c) Clear cell
d) Transitional

26) **All are TRUE about Atypical meningiomas/Grade II/IV EXCEPT:**
a) Have high rate of recurrence
b) Presence of 4/>4 mitosis/10 hpf
c) Require radiation therapy in addition to surgery
d) Psammomatous meningioma is considered Grade II meningioma

27) **Examples of Anaplastic meningioma (Grade III/IV) includes all EXCEPT:**
a) Papillary b) Rhabdoid
c) Chordoid d) None of the above

28) **Most common cytogenetic abnormality in Meningiomas:**
a) 22 q deletion b) 17q deletion
c) 1p deletion d) 13q deletion

29) **All of the following cancers show brain metastasis EXCEPT:**
a) Lung cancer
b) Breast cancer
c) Skin (melanoma)
d) Prostatic cancer

30) **Paraneoplastic syndromes associated with CNS tumor include(s):**
a) Subacute cerebellar degeneration
b) Limbic encephalitis
c) Opsoclonus
d) All of the above

31) **Familial tumor syndromes associated with CNS tumors:**
a) Cowden syndrome
b) Li-Fraumani syndrome
c) Turcot syndrome
d) All of the above

32) **Which of the following is not a pathological finding seen in Alzheimer's disease? (NEET 2014)**
a) Cortical atrophy
b) Neurofibrillary tangles
c) Neuritic plaques
d) Lewy body

33) **Which of the following is not seen in Tuberous sclerosis? (NEET 2014)**
a) Shagreen patch
b) Adenoma sebaceum
c) Mc-Callum Plaques
d) De-pigmented nevi

34) **Neurofibromatosis true is all EXCEPT: (NEET 2014)**
a) Autosomal recessive
b) Associated with cataract
c) Scoliosis
d) Multiple fibromas

35) **Smoking is not a risk factor for: (NEET 2014)**
a) Lung carcinoma
b) Osteoporosis
c) Nonunion of bones
d) Alzhiemer's disease

36) **Adrenoleukodystrophy is: (NEET 2014)**
a) AD
b) AR
c) X-linked dominant
d) X-linked recessive

37) **Tau protein seen in: (NEET 2014)**
a) Alzheimer's disease
b) Lewy body dementia
c) Pick's disease
d) Amyloidosis

38) **Receptor on neuronal membrane that induces development of glioma: (AIIMS Nov 2015)**
a) CD-117 b) CD-133
c) CD-33 d) CD-45

39) **Most common CNS neoplasm in HIV patient: (NEET 2013)**
a) Medulloblastoma
b) Astrocytoma
c) Primary CNS lymphoma
d) Ependymoma

40) **Prion disease is caused by: (NEET 2013)**
a) Misfolding of protein
b) Denaturation of proteins
c) Missense mutation
d) Non-sense mutation

41) **Spongiform degeneration of cerebral cortex occurs in: (NEET 2013)**
a) Creutzfeldt-Jakob disease
b) Sub-acute sclerosing panencephalitis
c) Fatal familial insomnia
d) Cerebral toxoplasmosis

42) **Most common site of Glioblastoma multiforme is: (NEET 2013)**
a) CP angle b) Frontal lobe
c) Brainstem d) Occipital lobe

43) **Most common cerebellar tumor in children: (NEET 2013)**
a) Astrocytoma
b) Medulloblastoma
c) Ependymoma
d) DNET

44) **Rosenthal fibers are seen in: (NEET 2013)**
a) Pilocytic astrocytoma
b) Glioblastoma
c) Medulloblastoma
d) Ependymoma

45) **What is the histological appearance of brain in Creutzfeldt-Jakob disease? (NEET 2013)**
a) Neuronophagia
b) Spongiform change in brain
c) Microabscesses
d) Demyelination

46) **Medulloblastoma most commonly metastasizes is to: (NEET 2013)**
a) Lung b) CNS
c) Liver d) Spleen

47) Which of the following tumors is not derived from meninges? (NEET 2013)

a) Hemangioblastoma
b) Meningioma
c) Fibrous tumor
d) Hemangiopericytoma

48) Perivascular lymphocytes and microglial nodules are seen in: (NEET 2013)

a) Multiple sclerosis
b) HIV encephalitis
c) CMV meningitis
d) Bacterial meningitis

49) All of the following are neuronal tumours EXCEPT: (AIPGMEE 2011)

a) Gangliocytoma
b) Ganglioglioma
c) Neuroblastoma
d) Ependymoma

50) Rosettes are not seen in: (AIIMS May 2014)

a) Retinoblastoma
b) Medulloblastoma
c) PNET
d) Neurocysticercosis

CHAPTER 26: THE CENTRAL NERVOUS SYSTEM

Ans. 1) D. All of the above (Ref: 8 ed. Robbins p.1281, 9 ed. 1252-53)

Inclusions [Q]:

- **Viral infection** can lead to abnormal **intra-nuclear inclusions** in **herpetic infection (Cowdry body)** [Q]
- Cytoplasmic inclusions are seen in **rabies (Negri body)** [Q]
- Both nucleus and cytoplasm inclusions as seen in **Cytomegalovirus infection** [Q]
- **Neuronal intra-cytoplasmic inclusions** are seen in **Neurofibrillary tangles** [Q] of **Alzheimer disease** and **Lewy bodies** of **Parkinson disease** [Q]

Ans. 2) B. Intra-cytoplasmic inclusions (Ref: 8 ed. Robbins p.1304-05, 9 ed. 1277-78, f-28-25)

- **Negri bodies** [Q] are cytoplasmic inclusions found in **neurons** of the **hippocampus** and **Purkinje cells** of the **cerebellum**

Ans. 3) D. Glial cells (Ref: 8 ed. Robbins p.1305, 9 ed. 1278)

- Microglia expresses **CD4 co-receptor** [Q] and the **chemokine receptors (CCR5 or CXCR4)** [Q], required for infection by **HIV**
- **JC polyomavirus** infects **oligodendrocytes** [Q] and leads to **Progressive multifocal leukoencephalopathy (PML)**

Ans. 4) D. Scrapie (Ref: 8 ed. Robbins p.1308, 9 ed. 1281)

Prion diseases affecting humans:

- **Examples: Creutzfeldt-Jakob disease**, **Gerstmann-Sträussler-Scheinker syndrome, Fatal familial insomnia and Kuru** [Q]
- Are associated with abnormal forms of prion proteins (PrP)
- Results after PrP undergoes a conformational change from its **normal PrPc** to an **abnormal β-pleated sheet** isoform, termed **PrP^{sc} (for scrapie)** [Q]
- PrP^{sc} accumulation in the neural tissue leads to pathologic changes in these diseases
- **Familial forms** of **prion diseases** are associated with the mutations in the gene encoding **PrPc (PRNP)** [Q]

Ans. 5) C. Inflammation is a characteristic feature (Ref: 8 ed. Robbins p.1313, 9 ed. 1286)

Central Pontine Myelinolysis:

- Acute disorder characterized by **loss of myelin**
- Most commonly arises **2 to 6 days** after **rapid correction of hyponatremia** [Q]
- Rapid increase in osmolality results in damage of **oligodendrocytes**
- Inflammation is **absent** and neurons and axons are well preserved
- **Periventricular** and **subpial regions** of brain are spared

Ans. 6) D. All of the above (Ref: 9 ed. Robbins p. 1287-88, t-28-3,4)

Relationship between **Proteins** and **Neurodegenerative Diseases:**

Protein [Q]	Diseases with Inclusions [Q]
Aβ	Alzheimer disease (AD) [Q]
Tau	Alzheimer disease, Frontotemporal lobar degeneration, Parkinson disease (with LRRK2 mutations), Progressive supranuclear palsy, Corticobasal degeneration
α-synuclein	Parkinson disease, Multiple system atrophy

Ans. 7) D. All of the above (Ref: 8 ed. Robbins p.1314-16, 9 ed. 1290-92, f-28-38)

- **Major microscopic abnormalities** of AD are **neuritic (senile) plaques** [Q] and **neurofibrillary tangles** [Q]
- In **neuritic plaques, Aβ** [Q] is the **dominant component** of **amyloid plaque core**

- **Neurofibrillary tangles** are **tau-containing bundles** of filaments in the cytoplasm of the **neurons**
- **Cerebral amyloid angiopathy** [Q] can also be seen in AD

Ans. 8) A. α-synuclein (Ref: 8 ed. Robbins p.1320-21, 9 ed. 1294-95, f-28-40)

Genetic abnormalities seen in Parkinson disease:

α-synuclein [Q]:

- **First gene** to be identified as a cause of **autosomal dominant PD**
- Major component of **Lewy body**
- Form aggregates which are toxic to neurons

Mitochondrial dysfunction:

- Mutations in the genes that encode the proteins DJ-1, PINK1 and parkin

Mutations in the gene encoding LRRK2 (leucine-rich repeat kinase 2):

- Common cause of Autosomal dominant PD

Ans. 9) A. Arylsulfatase A (Ref: 8 ed. Robbins p.1326-27, 9 ed. 1302-03)

Metachromatic Leukodystrophy [Q]:

- Results from deficiency of lysosomal enzyme – **arylsulfatase A** [Q]
- Leads to accumulation of **cerebroside sulfate**
- Macrophages with vacuolated cytoplasm are scattered throughout white matter
- These vacuoles, in combination with **toluidine blue** dye leads to **metachromasia**

Krabbe Disease:

- **Autosomal recessive** leukodystrophy resulting from deficiency of **β-galactosidase** [Q]
- **β-galactosidase** leads to catabolism of **galactocerebroside** to ceramide and galactose

Ans. 10) D. All of the above (Ref: 8 ed. Robbins p.1331-32, 9 ed. 1306-07)

Classification of Glioblastoma (into **four molecular subtypes** [Q]): **classic**, **proneural**, **neural** and **mesenchymal**

- **Classic subtype** [Q] – Mutations of the **PTEN tumor suppressor gene,** deletions of chromosome 10 and amplification of the **EGFR oncogene**
- **Proneural type** – most common type, associated with **secondary Glioblastoma**, characterized by **TP53 mutations** [Q]
- **Neural type**
- **Mesenchymal type** – deletions of the **NF1 gene** on **chromosome 17** [Q]

Ans. 11) D. All of the above (Ref: 8 ed. Robbins p.1330-31, 9 ed. 1307-08, f-28-48)

Morphology of Glioblastoma [Q]:

- Highly cellular tumor with marked **nuclear pleomorphism**
- Numerous **mitotic figures**
- **Necrosis** – **Tumor cells** surround the edges of **necrotic areas** and produce a histologic pattern referred to as **pseudo-palisading** [Q]
- **Vascular/endothelial cell proliferation** – results in formation of **ball like structure**, called as **glomeruloid body**[Q], due to **VEGF** [Q] production by **malignant astrocytes**

Ans. 12) D. All of the above (Ref: 8 ed. Robbins p.1332-33, 9 ed. 1309, f-28-49)

Pilocytic Astrocytoma [Q]:

- Seen in **children** and **young adults**
- Located in the **cerebellum** [Q]
- **TP53** mutations are **rare** [Q]
- Occur in patients with **Neurofibromatosis type 1** [Q]

Morphology Q:

- Often **cystic** Q and are composed of **bipolar cells** with long, thin "hair like" processes
- Tumor cells are **GFAP-positive** Q
- Characteristic findings – **Rosenthal fibers** Q and **eosinophilic granular bodies** Q
- Vascular cell proliferation does not indicate unfavorable prognosis

Ans. 13) D. Presence of necrosis and mitosis (Ref: 8 ed. Robbins p.1333, 9 ed. 1309)

Pleomorphic Xanthoastrocytoma Q:

- Most often site is **temporal lobe** Q
- Seen in **children** and **young adults** and presents with **seizures** Q
- **Low-grade tumor (WHO grade II/IV)**

Microscopy:

- Tumor consists of **neoplastic astrocytes**, which are filled with **lipids**
- Absence of **necrosis** and **mitotic activity** Q

Ans. 14) A. 1p (Ref: 8 ed. Robbins p.1333-34, 9 ed. 1310)

Molecular Genetics of Oligodendroglioma Q:

- **Most common mutation affects isocitrate dehydrogenase** genes (**IDH1 and IDH2**) Q
- Deletion of portions of chromosomes **1p** and **19q**
- Loss of **9p**, **10q** and mutations in **CDKN2A**
- Tumors with **co-deletion of 1p/19q**, respond **better** to **chemotherapy and radiation**

Ans. 15) D. Fourth ventricle (Ref: 8 ed. Robbins p.1334, 9 ed. 1310)

Ependymomas Q

- Most often arise next to the **ependymal-lined ventricular system**
- Most common site in first two decades of life – near the **fourth ventricle** Q
- In adults, the **most common location** Q is the **spinal cord**
- Commonly seen in patients with **Neurofibromatosis type 2 (NF2)** Q

Microscopy:

- Tumor cells form **gland-like** structures and are most commonly arranged around vessels **(perivascular pseudo rosettes)**Q
- Tumor cells have **regular**, **round to oval** nuclei with abundant **granular chromatin**
- Fibrillary background shows **GFAP expression** Q

Ans. 16) A. Filum terminale (Ref: 8 ed. Robbins p.1334, 9 ed. 1311)

- **Myxopapillary ependymomas** occurs in the **filum terminale** Q of the spinal cord

Ans. 17) D. All of the above (Ref: 8 ed. Robbins p.1335, 9 ed. 1311)

Choroid Plexus Papilloma Q:

- Most common in children, where it arises from the **lateral ventricle** Q
- In adults, it arises from the **fourth ventricle** Q
- Presents with **hydrocephalus** (due to tumor obstructing the **ventricular system**)
- Rarer variant, **choroid plexus carcinoma** resemble **adenocarcinoma**

Ans. 18) D. All of the above (Ref: 8 ed. Robbins p.1335-36, 9 ed. 1311-12)

Gangliogliomas Q:

- **Most common neuronal tumors** of the **CNS**
- **Superficial lesions**, which presents with **seizures** Q

- **Most commonly** occur in the **temporal lobe** Q and have a **cystic component**
- 20% of these tumors have mutations of **BRAF** Q

Dysembryoblastic neuroepithelial tumor (DNET):

- Typically located in the **superficial temporal lobe** Q

Central Neurocytoma:

- **Low-grade** neuronal neoplasm found within the lateral or third ventricles

Ans. 19) D. All of the above (Ref: 8 ed. Robbins p.1336-37, 9 ed. 1312-13, f-28-52)

Medulloblastoma Q**:**

- Occurs **predominantly** in **children**
- Most common site – **cerebellum** Q

Microscopy Q**:**

- **Densely cellular** with sheets of anaplastic cells
- Tumor cells are small, with **scant cytoplasm** and **hyperchromatic nuclei** Q
- **Abundant** mitoses with increased Ki67 activity
- Tumor cells form **Homer-Wright rosettes** and express **GFAP** Q
- **Dissemination** through the **CSF and drop metastasis** are **common complications** Q
- On the basis of molecular alterations, it can be divided into **four groups** Q:
  a) **WNT type** b) **SHH type** c) Medulloblastoma with **MYC amplification** and **isochromosome 17 (i17q)** d) Medulloblastoma with **i17q cytogenetic alteration**

Note – Isochromosome 17 (i17q) indicates **worse prognosis** Q

Ans. 20) D. All of the above (Ref: 8 ed. Robbins p.1337, 9 ed. p. 1313)

Atypical Teratoid/Rhabdoid Tumor Q**:**

- **Highly aggressive tumor of children (< 5 years)** with **poor prognosis**
- Occurs in the **posterior fossa** and in **supra-tentorial compartments**

Molecular Genetics Q**:**

- Hallmark of **Rhabdoid tumor**: Genetic alterations in **chromosome 22** Q
- Gene involved in **Atypical Teratoid/Rhabdoid tumor** is **hSNF5/INI1** Q

Ans. 21) D. Desmin (Ref: 8 ed. Robbins p.1337, 9 ed. p. 1313)

- Cytoplasm of the **Rhabdoid cell** contains **intermediate filaments** Q
- **Rhabdoid cell** is **immunoreactive** for **epithelial membrane antigen, vimentin, smooth muscle actin and keratins** Q
- **Desmin** Q and **myoglobin** Q **positivity** is **absent**

Ans. 22) A. B cell type (Ref: 8 ed. Robbins p.1337, 9 ed. 1313-14)

- **Primary CNS lymphomas** are of **B-cell origin** Q
- **Diffuse large-cell B-cell lymphomas** Q are the **most common** histologic group
- Tumors express **B cell markers** such as **CD20** Q
- In **immunosuppressed individuals,** markers of **Epstein-Barr virus** Q are usually present within the tumor cells

Ans. 23) A. Diffuse large B-cell lymphoma (Ref: 8 ed. Robbins p.1337, 9 ed. 1313-14)

- **Diffuse large-cell B-cell lymphomas** Q are the most common **primary CNS lymphoma**
- **Intravascular lymphoma**, grows within the **small vessels** of the brain

Ans. 24) D. All of the above (Ref: 8 ed. Robbins p.1338, 9 ed. 1314)

Dural Based Tumors of CNS Q**:**

- **Meningiomas, metastases, solitary fibrous tumors** and **poorly differentiated sarcomas**

Ans. 25) C. Clear cell (Ref: 8 ed. Robbins p.1338-39, 9 ed. 1315, f-28-53)

- **Meningiomas** are graded according to **WHO grade I to IV** Q:

Grade I/IV meningiomas Q **includes:**

- **Syncytial ("meningothelial") – Whorled clusters** of cells in **tight groups**
- **Fibroblastic** – Elongated cells and abundant collagen deposition between them
- **Transitional** shows the features of **syncytial** and **fibroblastic** types
- **Psammomatous** with **psammoma bodies**, due to the calcification of syncytial nests of meningothelial cells
- **Secretory** with **PAS-positive intracytoplasmic droplets**
- **Microcystic** with a **loose, spongy appearance**

Atypical meningiomas (WHO grade II/IV) Q includes:

- **Clear cell** and **chordoid types**

Anaplastic (malignant) meningioma (WHO grade III/IV) Q **includes:**

- **Papillary meningioma** (with pleomorphic cells arranged around **fibrovascular cores)**
- **Rhabdoid meningioma** (sheets of tumor cells with **hyaline eosinophilic cytoplasm)**

Ans. 26) D. Psammomatous meningioma is considered Grade II meningioma (Ref: 8 ed. Robbins p.1338-39, 9 ed. 1314-15)

Features of Atypical Meningiomas (WHO grade II/IV) Q:

- Presence of **4/>4 mitoses** per 10 high power fields
- Presence of **three atypical features** (increased cellularity, small cells with a high N:C ratio, prominent nucleoli, pattern less growth or necrosis)
- **Higher rate of recurrence** and require radiation therapy in addition to surgery
- Includes **clear cell** Q and **chordoid types**

Ans. 27) C. Chordoid (Ref: 8 ed. Robbins p.1338-39, 9 ed. 1314-15)

Anaplastic (malignant) meningioma (WHO grade III/IV) Q:

- Mitotic rates are **>20 mitoses per 10 high power fields**
- Includes **Papillary meningioma** and **Rhabdoid meningioma**

Ans. 28) A. 22 q deletion (Ref: 8 ed. Robbins p.1338-39, 9 ed. 1314-15)

- **Most common cytogenetic abnormality** in **meningioma** is **loss of chromosome 22** especially the **long arm (22q)** Q
- **22q12 region** also harbors **NF-2 gene**

Ans. 29) D. Prostatic cancer (Ref: 8 ed. Robbins p.1339, 9 ed. 1315-16)

Most common primary sites Q which show **metastasis to brain** includes:

- Lung, breast, skin (melanoma), kidney and gastrointestinal tract, choriocarcinoma (rarely)
- **Prostatic adenocarcinoma** never shows **CNS metastasis**

Ans. 30) D. All of the above (Ref: 8 ed. Robbins p.1339-40, 9 ed. 1316)

Paraneoplastic Syndromes associated with **CNS tumors** Q:

- Sub-acute cerebellar degeneration (SACD)
- Limbic encephalitis
- Eye movement disorders (opsoclonus)
- Sub-acute sensory neuropathy
- Lambert-Eaton myasthenic syndrome

Ans. 31) D. All of the above (Ref: 8 ed. Robbins p.1342, 9 ed. 1316-17)

Familial Tumor Syndromes associated with **CNS Tumors:**

- **Cowden syndrome** [Q] associated with dysplastic **gangliogliocytoma** of the cerebellum, due to mutations in **PTEN gene**
- **Li-Fraumeni syndrome** [Q] associated with **Medulloblastoma,** due to mutations in **TP53**
- **Turcot syndrome** [Q] associated with **Medulloblastoma** or Glioblastoma, due to mutations in **APC gene**
- **Gorlin syndrome** [Q] associated with **Medulloblastoma**, due to mutations in the **PTCH gene**

Ans. 32) D. Lewy body (Ref: 9 ed. Robbin's p. 1294-95)

- Lewy body: Diagnostic hallmark of Parkinson disease
- Autosomal Dominant Parkinsonism Disease encodes α-synuclein protein
- α-synuclein protein forms a major component of Lewy body

Ans. 33) C. Mc Callum Plaques (Ref. 9 ed. Robbins p. 1316-1317)

Ans. 34) A. Autosomal recessive (Ref: 9 ed. Robbins p.298, 1156, 1317)

Ans. 35) D. Alzheimer's disease (Ref: 9 ed. Robbins p. 1288)

Ans. 36) D. X-linked recessive (Ref: 9 ed. Robbins p. 1303)

Adrenoleukodystrophy:

- X-linked recessive disease
- Associated with mutations in ATP-binding cassette transporter family of proteins (ABCD1)
- Results in accumulation of very-long chain fatty acid in the serum

Ans. 37) A. Alzheimer's disease (Ref: 9 ed. Robbins p. 1292) Refer Q 7 for details

Ans. 38) B. CD-133

CD-133 role in astrocytic gliomas is a matter of debate

Ans. 39) C. Primary CNS lymphoma (Ref: 9 ed. Robbins p. 1313-14) Refer Q 22 and 23 for details

Ans. 40) A. Misfolding of protein (Ref: 9 ed. Robbins p. 1281) Refer Q 4 for details

Ans. 41) A. Creutzfeldt-Jakob disease (Ref: 9 ed. Robbins p. 1281-82) Refer Q 4 for details

In CJD: Pathognomonic finding is a spongiform transformation of the cerebral cortex

Ans. 42) B. Frontal lobe (Ref: 9 ed. Robbins p. 1307-08) Refer Q 10 and 11 for details

- Most common site of Glioblastoma multiforme is temporal and frontal lobe and basal ganglia

Ans. 43) A. Astrocytoma (Ref: 9 ed. Robbins p. 1309) Refer Q 12 for details

Ans. 44) A. Pilocytic astrocytoma (Ref: 9 ed. Robbins p. 1309) Refer Q 12 for details

Ans. 45) B. Spongiform change in brain (9 ed. Robbins p. 1281)

- Classic histologic appearance in Creutzfeldt-Jakob disease is spongiform change in the gray matter

Ans. 46) B. CNS (Ref: 9ed. Robbins p. 1312-13) Refer Q 19 for details

Ans. 47) A. Haemangioblastoma (Ref: 9ed. Robbins p. 1317)

- Hemangioblastoma: Highly vascular neoplasms, seen in Von Hippel-Lindau Disease

Ans. 48) B. HIV encephalitis (Ref: 8 ed. Robbins p. 1375)

HIV encephalitis (Microscopy):

- Chronic inflammatory infiltrate forming microglial nodules, with associated tissue necrosis and reactive gliosis

Macrophage-derived multinucleated giant cell forms a component of microglial nodule

Ans. 49) D. Ependymoma (Ref: 9 ed. Robbins p. 1310) Refer Q 15 for details

Ans. 50) D. Neurocysticercosis (Ref: 9 ed. Robbins and Cotran, p. 259)

Retinoblastoma:

- Most common primary intraocular malignancy of children

- Tumor is composed of small, round cells with large hyperchromatic nuclei and scant cytoplasm, resembling undifferentiated retinoblasts
- Flexner-Wintersteiner rosettes: Consist of clusters of cuboidal or short columnar cells arranged around a central lumen

Ewing Sarcoma and Primitive Neuroectodermal Tumor:

- Primary malignant small round cell tumors of bone and soft tissue
- Composed of sheets of uniform small, round cells, larger than lymphocytes; with few mitotic figures and little intervening stroma

Ependymoma:

- Arises from next to the ependymal lined ventricular system
- Tumors are composed of cells with regular, round to oval nuclei and abundant granular chromatin
- Tumor cells form rosettes, with long, delicate processes extending into a lumen
- Tumor cells may form perivascular pseudo rosettes in which tumor cells are arranged around vessels

Medulloblastoma:

- Homer Wright or neuroblastic rosette is seen

27 Diseases of White Blood Cells, Lymph Nodes, Spleen and Thymus

How to go about this chapter?

- **One should be thorough with the following repeatedly asked topics:**
  - **Hemophagocytic Lymphohistiocytosis (HLH)**
  - **WHO classification of lymphoid neoplasms**
  - **Acute lymphoblastic leukemia**
  - **Chronic lymphocytic leukemia**
  - **Follicular lymphoma**
  - **Diffuse large B-cell lymphoma**
  - **Burkitt lymphoma**
  - **Plasma cell neoplasms**
  - **Mantle cell lymphoma**
  - **Lymphoplasmacytic lymphoma**
  - **Hairy cell leukemia**
  - **Anaplastic large cell lymphoma**
  - **Mycosis fungoides**
  - **Hodgkin disease**
  - **Non-Hodgkin disease**
  - **Acute myeloid leukemia**
  - **Myeloproliferative disorders**
  - **Langerhans cell histiocytosis (LCH)**
  - **Mediastinal lesions and thymoma**

INTRODUCTION

1) All are the components of myeloid lineage EXCEPT:
a) Red cells b) Platelets
c) Granulocytes d) Thymus

2) Following is/are true regarding the development of hematopoietic tissues:
a) Development starts in yolk sac during 3rd week of embryo development
b) During 3rd month, Hematopoietic stem cells (HSCs) migrate to liver
c) During 4th month, Hematopoietic stem cells (HSCs) migrate to bone marrow
d) All of the above

3) In normal adults, ratio of fat cells to hematopoietic cells in bone marrow is:
a) 1:1 b) 1:2
c) 2:1 d) 2:2

4) Lymphopenia is observed in:
a) HIV infection
b) Autoimmune disorders
c) Malnutrition
d) All of the above

5) Neutropenia is seen in:
a) Aplastic anemia
b) Megaloblastic anemias
c) SLE
d) Any of the above

6) Serious infections occur when neutrophil count falls below:
a) $1400/mm^3$ b) $1000/mm^3$
c) $500/mm^3$ d) None of the above

7) Causes of Neutrophilic leukocytosis include all EXCEPT:
a) Acute bacterial infections
b) Myocardial infarction

c) Burns
d) Tuberculosis

8) Döhle bodies are seen in:
a) Neutrophils
b) Lymphocytes
c) Monocytes
d) Any of the above

9) Tingible-body macrophages are seen in:
a) Follicular hyperplasia
b) Follicular lymphoma
c) Both of the above
d) None of the above

10) Follicular hyperplasia can be differentiated from Follicular lymphoma by following feature(s):
a) Preservation of lymph node architecture
b) Marked variation in size and shape of follicles
c) Presence of tingible body macrophages
d) All of the above

11) Follicular hyperplasia can be seen in:
a) Rheumatoid arthritis
b) Toxoplasmosis
c) HIV infection
d) All of the above

12) Sinus histiocytosis is/are seen in:
a) Langerhans cell histiocytosis
b) Whipple's disease
c) Rosai-Dorfmann disease
d) Any of the above

13) Monocytoid B cells in lymph node is/are seen in:
a) Toxoplasmosis
b) Infectious Mononucleosis
c) AIDS
d) Any of the above

14) Hemophagocytic Lymphohistiocytosis is due to activation of:
a) CD8 T cells b) Macrophages
c) CD4 T cells d) Both a and b

15) All are the features of Hemophagocytic Lymphohistiocytosis EXCEPT:
a) Anemia
b) Hepatosplenomegaly
c) Fever
d) Low levels of serum ferritin

16) Following is/are responsible for WBC malignancies:
a) Tyrosine kinase mutations
b) MYC translocation
c) BCL-2 translocation
d) Any of the above

17) Following etiological factors are associated with WBC neoplasia:
a) Bloom syndrome
b) Epstein-Barr Virus
c) Gluten sensitive enteropathy
d) All of the above

18) TRUE about leukemia and lymphoma:
a) Leukemia presents with widespread involvement of bone marrow
b) Lymphoma arises as discrete tissue masses
c) Lymphoma occasionally can have leukemic presentation
d) All of the above

19) All are B-cell neoplasms EXCEPT:
a) Plasma cell myeloma
b) Follicular lymphoma
c) Hairy cell leukemia
d) Mycosis fungoides

20) Lymphoid neoplasms which arises from germinal center of lymph node include(s):
a) Diffuse large B-cell lymphoma
b) Hodgkin lymphoma
c) Burkitt lymphoma
d) All of the above

21) T-cell associated markers include(s):
a) CD 1 b) CD3
c) CD5 d) Any of the above

22) Following is a NK-cell associated marker:
a) CD13 b) CD14
c) CD15 d) CD16

23) Which of the following is/are stem cell marker:
a) CD34 b) CD30
c) CD45 d) Any of the above

24) Langerhans cell show positivity of:
a) CD1a b) CD3
c) CD4 d) CD5

ACUTE LYMPHOBLASTIC LYMPHOMA

25) TRUE about Acute lymphoblastic lymphoma (ALL):
a) Most common cancer in children
b) B-cell ALL presents as childhood acute leukemia
c) T-cell ALL present in adolescents
d) All of the above

26) TRUE about the pathogenesis of ALL:
a) T-ALLs have gain-of-function mutations in NOTCH1
b) B-ALLs have loss-of-function mutations in PAX5
c) Hyperploidy is the most common structural chromosomal change
d) All of the above

27) All are the features differentiate lymphoblast from myeloblasts morphologically:
a) Lymphoblasts have more condensed chromatin
b) Lymphoblasts have small amount of cytoplasm

c) Lymphoblasts show MPO positivity
d) Lymphoblasts cytoplasm shows absence of granules

28) A young child presented with complaints of weakness, loss of appetite, weight loss, lymphadenopathy and hepatosplenomegaly of 15 days duration. Peripheral smear reveals blast > 20% and was labeled as acute leukemia. Bone marrow and flow cytometry studies were performed, the latter showed CD19, CD20 and PAX-5 positivity and CD1, CD2, CD5, CD7 and CD 10 negativity. The following should be the interpretation based on flow cytometry report:
a) T-cell ALL b) B-cell ALL
c) AML d) NHL

29) Favorable prognosis in ALL patients include all EXCEPT:
a) Age between 2 and 10 years
b) Low white cell count
c) Hyperdiploidy
d) t(9;22)

30) In B-ALL, BCR-ABL fusion protein is of following size:
a) 190 kDa b) 210 kDa
c) 250 kDa d) 300 kDa

CHRONIC LYMPHOCYTIC LEUKEMIA

31) Chronic Lymphocytic Leukemia diagnosis requires an absolute lymphocyte count of:
a) >2000/mm^3 b) >3000/mm^3
c) >4000/mm^3 d) >5000/mm^3

32) Following genetic mutation is/are seen in CLL/ SLL:
a) 13q14 deletion b) 11q deletion
c) Trisomy 12q d) All of the above

33) CLL cells are dependent on following signal transduction pathway(s):
a) Tyrosine kinase
b) Bruton tyrosine kinase
c) NF-KB
d) Any of the above

34) Proliferation centers are pathognomic of:
a) ALL b) CML
c) CLL d) NHL

35) CLL/ SLL cells express:
a) CD19 b) CD23
c) CD5 d) All of the above

36) 60-year-old male, presents with generalized lymphadenopathy and hepatosplenomegaly since 1 month. Peripheral smear shows spherocytes, schistocytes, nucleated red blood cell and atypical lymphoid cells. Most probable diagnosis with the history mentioned is:
a) CLL b) ALL
c) CML d) NHL

FOLLICULAR LYMPHOMA

37) TRUE about pathogenesis of Follicular Lymphoma:
a) Arises from germinal center B cells
b) t(14;18) is seen in 90% of patients
c) BCL-2 overexpression plays an important role
d) All of the above

38) Main cell population seen in Follicular lymphoma:
a) Centrocytes b) Centroblasts
c) Immunoblasts d) Both A and B

39) All of the following immunophenotype favors Follicular lymphoma EXCEPT:
a) CD19 b) CD20
c) CD5 d) BCL-2

DIFFUSE LARGE B-CELL LYMPHOMA

40) Most common form of NHL:
a) Diffuse large B-cell lymphoma (DLBCL)
b) Burkitt lymphoma
c) Follicular lymphoma
d) Marginal zone lymphoma

41) TRUE about the pathogenesis of Diffuse large B-cell lymphomas:
a) Overexpression of BCL-6
b) t(14;18)
c) *MYC* translocation
d) Any of the above

42) Following organ/s can be involved in DLBCL:
a) Waldeyer ring
b) Liver
c) GIT
d) All of the above

BURKITT LYMPHOMA

43) Following is/are seen in Burkitt lymphoma:
a) t(8;14) b) t(2;8)
c) t(8;22) d) Any of the above

44) All of the following are TRUE about Burkitt lymphoma EXCEPT:
a) Arises from germinal center
b) Endemic Burkitt lymphomas are infected with EBV
c) Expresses CD19, CD20
d) Expresses BCL-2

45) All are TRUE about Burkitt lymphoma EXCEPT:
a) Endemic form presents as mass in mandible
b) Sporadic form most often appears as mass involving peritoneum

c) Aggressive NHL
d) Does not respond to intensive chemotherapy

PLASMA CELL DYSCRASIA

46) Plasma cell neoplasms include(s):
a) Monoclonal gammopathy of unknown significance
b) Smoldering myeloma
c) Plasmacytoma
d) All of the above

47) TRUE about the molecular pathogenesis of Multiple Myeloma:
a) IgH-Cyclin D1 translocation
b) IgH-Cyclin D3 translocation
c) Chromosome 17p deletion
d) All of the above

48) Following is an important growth factor for plasma cells:
a) IL-1 b) IL-3
c) IL-4 d) IL-6

49) Cell of origin of Multiple Myeloma:
a) Pre-B-cell
b) Post-germinal center B-cell
c) T-cell
d) Pre T-cell

50) Bone most commonly involved in Multiple myeloma:
a) Vertebral column b) Ribs
c) Skull d) Pelvis

51) Most important diagnostic criteria for diagnosis of Multiple Myeloma:
a) Bone marrow plasma cells >30%
b) Bone marrow plasma cell >10%
c) M protein in serum or urine
d) Related organ or tissue impairment

52) Criteria for diagnosis of smoldering myeloma include(s):
a) M-protein in serum > 30 gm/l
b) 10% or more clonal plasma cells in bone marrow
c) No related organ or tissue impairment
d) All of the above

53) Diagnostic criteria for Monoclonal gammopathy of undetermined significance include(s):
a) M-protein in serum < 30 g/l
b) Bone marrow clonal plasma cells <10%
c) No lytic lesions or tissue impairment
d) All of the above

54) Following cell/s is/are seen in multiple myeloma:
a) Plasmablasts
b) Flame cells
c) Mott cells
d) All of the above

55) Plasma cell tumors shows positivity of:
a) CD138 b) Syndecan-1
c) CD56 d) All of the above

56) Rouleaux formation in peripheral smear can be seen in:
a) Multiple myeloma
b) SLE
c) Early HIV infection
d) Any of the above

57) Most common cause of death in multiple myeloma patients:
a) Recurrent infections
b) Renal failure
c) Pathological fractures
d) Hypercalcemia

58) Most common 'M-protein' in Multiple Myeloma:
a) IgM b) IgG
c) IgA d) IgD

59) Most common site for Extraosseous Plasmacytoma:
a) Lymph nodes b) Bladder
c) GIT d) Upper respiratory tract

LYMPHOPLASMACYTIC LYMPHOMA

60) All are TRUE regarding lymphoplasmacytic lymphoma EXCEPT:
a) B-cell neoplasm presenting in older individuals
b) Resembles CLL/SLL
c) Plasma cell component secretes IgG
d) Waldenstorm macroglobulinemia is a frequent presentation

61) An elderly male, presenting with complaints of weakness, weight loss and fatigue for 2 months. On examination, lymphadenopathy and hepatosplenomegaly were noted. Peripheral smear showed features of hemolysis. Bone marrow biopsy was done, which showed lymphoid cells, few of which shows plasmacytoid differentiation. What is the most likely diagnosis?
a) Multiple myeloma
b) Lymphoplasmacytic leukemia
c) CLL
d) ALL

MANTLE CELL LYMPHOMA

62) Translocation noted in mantle cell lymphoma:
a) t(4;14) b) t(14;18)
c) t(8;22) d) t(2;8)

63) Following are morphological features of Mantle cell lymphoma EXCEPT:
a) Lymphomatoid polyposis
b) Lymphadenopathy
c) Small cleaved lymphocytes
d) Proliferation centers

64) **Mantle cell lymphoma shows positivity of all EXCEPT:**
a) CD20 b) CD19
c) CD5 d) CD23

MARGINAL ZONE LYMPHOMA

65) **Features of Extranodal Marginal zone lymphoma include(s):**
a) Arises in tissues with chronic inflammatory disorders
b) Remain localized for prolonged periods
c) May regress if the inciting agent is eradicated
d) All of the above

66) **Which of the following is seen in Marginal zone lymphoma?**
a) t(11;18) b) t(14;18)
c) t(1;14) d) All of the above

HAIRY CELL LEUKEMIA

67) **TRUE about Hairy cell leukemia:**
a) Male: Female predilection ratio – 5:1
b) Activating point mutations of BRAF
c) Follows an indolent course
d) All of the above

68) **TRUE about morphology of Hairy cell leukemia:**
a) Leukemic cells with fine hairy like projections
b) Hairy cells have round, oblong, or reniform nuclei
c) Dry bone marrow aspirate tap
d) All of the above

69) **Markers of Hairy cell leukemia include(s):**
a) CD11c
b) CD25
c) CD103
d) Any of the above

PERIPHERAL NK/T-CELL LYMPHOMAS AND LEUKEMIAS

70) **TRUE about Anaplastic large cell lymphoma:**
a) ALK gene is expressed in lymphocytes
b) Occurs in elderly
c) Has poor prognosis
d) CD 30 positivity

71) **Adult T-cell leukemia is due to following infection:**
a) HIV b) HBV
c) EBV d) HTLV

72) **All of the following are TRUE about Mycosis Fungoides EXCEPT:**
a) Tumor of CD8+ T helper cells
b) Cutaneous lesions have three phases
c) Tumor cells have cerebriform appearance
d) Disease progression occurs to lymph nodes and spleen

73) **TRUE about Sezary syndrome:**
a) Generalized exfoliative erythema
b) Associated leukemia
c) Tumor cells express CCR4 and CCR10
d) All of the above

74) **TRUE about large granular lymphocytic leukemia:**
a) Acquired mutation in STAT3
b) Neutropenia and anemia is seen
c) T cell variant shows positivity of CD3
d) All of the above

75) **Most common site of Extranodal NK/T-cell lymphoma:**
a) Nasopharynx b) GIT
c) Skin d) Lymph nodes

HODGKIN LYMPHOMA

76) **TRUE about Hodgkin Lymphoma:**
a) Localized to a single axial group of lymph nodes
b) Spreads by contiguity
c) Mesenteric lymph nodes are rarely involved
d) All of the above

77) **Classical forms of Hodgkin Lymphoma include all EXCEPT:**
a) Nodular sclerosis
b) Mixed cellularity
c) Lymphocyte depletion
d) Lymphocyte predominance

78) **Activation of NF-κB in classical HL occurs due to:**
a) EBV infection
b) LMP-1
c) Loss-of-function mutations in TNF alpha-induced protein 3
d) All of the above

79) **Cells resembling Reed-Sternberg cells can be seen in:**
a) Infectious mononucleosis
b) Solid cancers
c) NHL
d) Any of the above

80) **Feature(s) of diagnostic RS cells:**
a) Large cells with multiple nuclei
b) Inclusion like nucleolus
c) Abundant cytoplasm
d) All of the above

81) **Peculiar form of cell death in Hodgkin disease:**
a) Apoptosis b) Mummification
c) Necroptosis d) Necrosis

82) **TRUE about Nodular sclerosis Hodgkin lymphoma:**
a) Lacunar variant of RS cell is seen
b) Deposition of collagen in bands
c) Association with EBV is not seen

d) All of the above

83) TRUE about Mixed cellularity Hodgkin lymphoma:
a) Frequent mononuclear and diagnostic RS cells
b) RS cells shows CD15+, CD30+; 70% EBV+
c) Males are affected more than females
d) All of the above

84) Pop-corn cells are a characteristic feature of:
a) Mixed cellularity Hodgkin lymphoma
b) Nodular sclerosis Hodgkin lymphoma
c) Lymphocyte predominant Hodgkin lymphoma
d) Lymphocyte rich Hodgkin lymphoma

85) Spread of Hodgkin lymphoma occurs in following manner:
a) Nodal disease, splenic disease, hepatic disease, bone marrow
b) Nodal disease, hepatic disease, bone marrow, splenic disease
c) Nodal disease, bone marrow, hepatic disease, splenic disease
d) Nodal disease, splenic disease, bone marrow, hepatic disease

86) Hodgkin disease patients are treated with radiotherapy has increased incidence of:
a) Lung cancer
b) Melanoma
c) Breast cancer
d) Any of the above

87) Patients treated with chemotherapy have highest incidence of:
a) Acute myeloid leukemia
b) Acute lymphoblastic lymphoma
c) Chronic lymphocytic lymphoma
d) Chronic myeloid leukemia

MYELOID NEOPLASMS

88) Which of the following has poor prognosis?
a) AML with t(8;21)
b) AML with t(15;17)
c) AML with t(11q23)
d) AML with inv16

89) All-trans retinoic acid is useful in the following genetic aberration:
a) RARα/PML fusion gene
b) CBFB/MYH11 fusion gene
c) RUNX1/ETO fusion gene
d) Any of the above

90) Most common AML in Down syndrome:
a) AML without maturation
b) AML with myelocytic maturation
c) AML with myelomonocytic maturation
d) AML with megakaryocytic maturation

91) Following blast percentage in bone marrow is required to diagnose AML:
a) 5% b) 10%
c) 15% d) 20%

92) Leukemia cutis is associated with:
a) AML without maturation
b) AML with myelomonocytic maturation
c) AML with monocytic maturation
d) Any of the above

93) Which of the following has best prognosis?
a) AML with t(15;17)
b) AML with t(8;21)
c) AML with inv16
d) AML following MDS

94) AML associated with DIC:
a) AML with t(15;17)
b) AML with t(8;21)
c) AML with inv 16
d) AML with t(11q23;v)

MYELODYSPLASTIC SYNDROMES (MDS)

95) Following chromosomal aberration(s) is/are seen in MDS:
a) 5q- b) 7q-
c) Trisomy 8 d) Any of the above

96) Following can be seen in Bone marrow biopsy of MDS EXCEPT:
a) Ring sideroblasts
b) Megaloblastoid maturation
c) Pseudo-Pelger-Huet cells
d) Myeloid blasts >20%

MYELOPROLIFERATIVE DISORDERS

97) TRUE about Myeloproliferative disorders:
a) Increased proliferative drive in bone marrow
b) Extra medullary hematopoiesis
c) Transformation to marrow fibrosis and leukemia
d) All of the above

98) TRUE about the mutation(s) seen in Myeloproliferative Disorders include(s):
a) Chronic myelogenous leukemia – BCR-ABL fusion gene
b) Polycythemia vera – JAK2 point mutations
c) Systemic mastocytosis – KIT point mutations
d) Any of the above

99) Philadelphia chromosome:
a) t(9;22) b) t(12;22)
c) t(14;11) d) t(14;22)

100) TRUE regarding marrow findings of CML includes all EXCEPT:
a) Hypercellular marrow
b) Maturing granulocyte precursors

c) Elevated eosinophils and basophils
d) Large megakaryocytes

101) Blood smear findings of CML includes all EXCEPT:
a) Leucocyte count > 100,000/mm^3
b) Precursors of myeloid lineage are seen
c) Blasts <10%
d) Reduced platelets

102) All are the features of accelerated phase of CML EXCEPT:
a) Persistent or increasing WBC count
b) Persistent thrombocytosis
c) Persistent thrombocytopenia
d) > 20% blasts

103) In blast crisis of CML, the following lineage blasts can be seen:
a) Myeloid lineage blasts
b) Lymphoid lineage blasts
c) Both of the above
d) Megakaryoblasts

104) CML can present clinically as:
a) Anemia, fatigability
b) Dragging sensation in lower abdomen
c) Acute pain abdomen
d) Any of the above

105) All are TRUE regarding the criteria for diagnosis of Polycythemia Vera EXCEPT:
a) Hb >18.5 gm% in males, Hb >16.5 gm% in females
b) Presence of JAK2 mutation
c) Panmyelosis
d) Normal erythropoietin levels

106) Following can be seen in Polycythemia Vera EXCEPT:
a) Primary myelofibrosis
b) AML
c) ALL
d) None of the above

107) Essential thrombocytosis is characterized by following mutation:
a) JAK2
b) MPL
c) Calreticulin
d) Any of the above

PRIMARY MYELOFIBOSIS:

108) TRUE regarding myelofibrosis:
a) Hallmark is to develop obliterative marrow fibrosis
b) Activating JAK 2 mutations are seen
c) PDGF and TGF-β are responsible for fibrosis
d) All of the above

109) Major criteria for diagnosing Primary Myelofibrosis includes all EXCEPT:
a) Megakaryocyte proliferation and atypia
b) Not meeting WHO criteria of other myeloproliferative neoplasms
c) Demonstration of JAK2V617F mutation
d) Leucoerythroblastosis

110) Peripheral blood findings of myelofibrosis include(s):
a) Leucoerythroblastosis
b) Dacrocytes
c) Basophilia
d) All of the above

111) Dacrocytes can be seen in:
a) Infiltrative diseases of marrow
b) Metastatic tumors
c) Granulomatous disorders
d) All of the above

LANGERHANS CELL HISTIOCYTOSIS

112) TRUE about Langerhans cell histiocytosis:
a) Shows BRAF mutation
b) Presence of Birbeck granules
c) Tumor cells express S 100
d) All of the above

113) All are TRUE regarding Langerhans cell histiocytosis (LCH), EXCEPT:
a) Letterer-Siwe disease affects predominantly adults
b) Eosinophilic granuloma most commonly involves the calvarium
c) Diabetes insipidus forms a part of Hand-Schuller Christian disease
d) Pulmonary LCH predominantly affects adult smokers

SPLEEN

114) Function of the spleen include(s):
a) Phagocytosis of blood cells
b) Antibody formation
c) Hematopoiesis
d) All of the above

115) Increased susceptibility to the following infection(s) occur following splenectomy:
a) Pneumococci
b) Meningococci
c) Haemophilus influenzae
d) All of the above

116) Splenic rupture in absence of physical blow is seen in:
a) Infectious mononucleosis
b) Malaria
c) Lymphoid neoplasms
d) All of the above

THYMUS

117) Thymic follicular hyperplasia most commonly occurs in:
a) Myasthenia gravis
b) Graves' disease
c) SLE
d) Scleroderma

118) Following neoplasm(s) can arise in thymus:
a) Germ cell tumors
b) Lymphomas
c) Carcinoid
d) All of the above

119) Most common site of thymoma:
a) Anterior superior mediastinum
b) Thyroid
c) Pulmonary hilus
d) Posterior mediastinum

120) Thymoma is associated with following autoimmune disorders EXCEPT:
a) Dermatomyositis
b) Cushing syndrome
c) Graves' disease
d) Hypergammaglobulinemia

121) Differential diagnosis of anterior mediastinal mass include(s):
a) Large cell lymphoma
b) Lymphoblastic lymphoma
c) Thymic seminoma
d) All of the above

122) Lacunar type of Reed Sternberg cell is seen in: (NEET 2014)
a) Nodular sclerosis
b) Lymphocyte predominance
c) Mixed cellularity
d) Lymphocyte depletion

123) Macrophage activation syndrome is characterized by all EXCEPT: (NEET 2014)
a) Activation of CD 8 + T cells
b) Presence of cytokine storm
c) Other name for Hemophagocytic Lymphohistiocytosis
d) Low levels of plasma ferritin

124) Birbeck granules in cytoplasm is seen in: (NEET 2014)
a) Langerhans cell histiocytosis
b) Hodgkin's lymphoma
c) Non-Hodgkin disease
d) Gastrointestinal stromal tumor

125) Most common type of Hodgkin Lymphoma: (NEET 2014)
a) Lymphocyte predominant
b) Lymphocyte depletion
c) Nodular sclerosis
d) Mixed cellularity

126) Most common site for eosinophilic granuloma is: (NEET 2014)
a) Radius b) Skull
c) Lumbar vertebra d) Femur

127) Translocation (8; 14) is characteristic of: (NEET 2014)
a) Burkitt's lymphoma
b) Ataxia telangieactasia
c) ALL
d) CML

128) Popcorn cells are seen in which variety of Hodgkin disease? (NEET 2014)
a) Nodular sclerosis
b) Mixed cellularity
c) Lymphocyte predominant
d) Lymphocyte depletion

129) Shape of Birbeck granules is: (NEET 2013, 2014)
a) Tennis racket
b) Hockey stick
c) Bat
d) Ball

130) EBV receptor mimics: (NEET 2014)
a) CD 20 b) CD 21
c) CD 22 d) CD 23

131) Poor prognosis in AML is indicated by: (NEET 2014)
a) Age < 2 years
b) t (15;17)
c) Blast cell with aeur rods
d) Leukemia without preceeding MDS

132) In multiple myeloma there is proliferation of: (NEET 2014)
a) Plasma cells b) Basophils
c) Eosinophils d) Neutrophils

133) Most important prognostic factor in ALL: (AIIMS Nov 2015)
a) Hyperploidy
b) Organomegaly
c) WBC more than 75000/mm^3
d) Response to steroids

134) Good prognosis of ALL: (NEET 2013)
a) Hyperdiploidy
b) Hypodiploidy
c) T cell line
d) Philadelphia chromosome

135) Progenitor hematopoietic stem cells originate in: (NEET 2013)
a) Bone Marrow b) Thymus
c) Lymph node d) Spleen

136) Starry sky appearance is seen in: (NEET 2013)
a) Burkitt's lymphoma
b) Hodgkin lymphoma
c) Diffuse large B cell lymphoma
d) ALCL

137) Mantle cell cancer shows: (NEET 2013)
a) CD5+, CD25- b) CD 5+, CD 10+
c) CD 5+, CD23+ d) CD 5+, CD 23-

138) B ALL is due to: (NEET 2013)
a) T cells b) Immature B cells
c) Immature T cells d) Both T & B cells

139) Features of type I histiocytosis: (NEET 2013)
a) Antigen processing cells
b) CD 1a marker present
c) CD 127 marker
d) More common in males

140) In thymoma, all are seen EXCEPT: (NEET 2013)
a) Hypogammaglobulinemia
b) Hyperalbuminemia
c) Red cell aplasia
d) Myasthenia Gravis

141) What is the chromosomal translocation in AML M3? (NEET 2013)
a) T (18,21) b) T (15,17)
c) T (8, 21) d) T (9,11)

142) Reed Sternberg cells are found in: (NEET 2013)
a) Hodkin's disease
b) Sickle cell anaemia
c) Thalassemia
d) CML

143) D.I.C. is seen in: (NEET 2013)
a) Acute promyelocytic leukemia
b) Acute myelomonocytic leukemia
c) CML
d) Autoimmune hemolytic anemia

144) Marginal lymphoma is type of: (NEET 2013)
a) B cell lymphoma
b) T cell lymphoma
c) NK cell lymphoma
d) Hodgkin's lymphoma

145) Specific stain for Myeloblasts is: (NEET 2013)
a) Sudan black
b) PAS
c) Myeloperoxidase
d) LAP

146) Mantle cell lymphomas are positive for all EXCEPT: (NEET 2013)
a) CD23 b) CD20
c) CD5 d) CD43

147) Russell bodies are found in: (NEET 2013)
a) Multiple myeloma
b) Gonadal tumor
c) Parkinsonism
d) Intracranial neoplasms

148) Leucocyte alkaline phosphatase (LAP) is raised in A/E: (NEET 2013)
a) Myelofibrosis
b) Essential thrombocythemia
c) Polycythemia
d) Chronic myeloid leukemia

149) Dohle bodies: (NEET 2013)
a) Dilated endoplasmic reticulum in Neutrophils
b) Mitochondria
c) Golgi apparatus
d) Lysosomes

150) Burkitt Lymphoma is associated with: (AIPGMEE 2010)
a) t (8:14) b) t (11:14)
c) t (15:17) d) t (14:18)

151) Translocation t (2:8) (p12:q24) is associated with: (AIPGMEE 2010)
a) Chronic Myeloid Leukemia (CML)
b) Acute Myeloid Leukemia (LML)
c) T cell - ALL
d) Burkitt Lymphoma

152) Necrotizing Lymphadenitis is seen in: (AIPGMEE 2012)
a) Kimura disease
b) Kikuchi disease
c) Hodgkin disease
d) Castelman disease

153) Poor prognostic factor in ALL is: (AIPGMEE 2012)
a) Hyperploidy
b) t (9;22) t(4;11)
c) 2-8 years of age
d) TLC < 50,000

154) Which of the following statements is true? (AIIMS May 2012)
a) Chronic myeloid leukemia occurs beyond 50 years of age
b) Hairy cell leukemia in less than 50 years has good prognosis
c) Acute lymphoid leukemia in less than 1 year has a poor prognosis
d) Chronic lymphocytic leukemia occurs in less than 50 years of age

155) Hematopoietic stem cell differ from progenitor stem cell in that they can: (AIIMS May 2012)
a) Form terminally differentiated cells
b) Long term reconstitution of bone marrow
c) Produce growth factors
d) Have receptors for anchoring proteins

156) In an ablated animal, myeloid series cells are injected. Which of following is seen after incubation period? (AIIMS May 2012)

a) RBC
b) Fibroblast
c) T-lymphocyte
d) Hematopoietic stem cell

157) A 23-year-old female presented with jaundice and pallor for 2 months. Her peripheral blood smear shows the presence of spherocytes. The most relevant investigation to arrive at a diagnosis is: (AIIMS May 2012)
a) Reticulocyte count
b) Osmotic fragility test
c) Coombs test
d) Tests for PNH

158) A 10-year-old boy with mass in the abdomen. On imaging the para-aortic LN is enlarged. On biopsy starry sky appearance is seen. What is the underlying abnormality? (AIIMS May 2015)
a) P53 gene mutation
b) RB gene mutation
c) Translocation involving BCR-ABL genes
d) Translocation involving MYC-gene

159) A 35-year-old male presents with history of bleeding. Peripheral smear shows leukocytosis, platelet count 50,000/mm3, increased neutrophils, normal lymphocyte, blast 20% and band form, myelocyte and metamyelocyte seen. Translocation (8; 21) is positive. What is diagnosis? (AIIMS May 2014)
a) CLL b) CML
c) AML d) MDS

160) Which of the following immunohistochemical stains is used for the diagnosis of lymphomas? (AIIMS Nov. 2015)
a) S-100
b) HMB-45
c) Leukocyte common antigen
d) Cytokeratin

161) Myelofibrosis leading to a dry tap on bone marrow aspiration is seen with which of the following condition? (AIIMS Nov 2015)
a) Burkitt's lymphoma
b) Acute erythroleukemia
c) Acute megakaryocytic leukemia
d) Acute myelomonocytic leukemia

162) A patient of more than 70 years, presented with generalized lymphadenopathy. WBC count was 20,000/mm^3 and blood film showed > 70% mature looking lymphocytes. Next investigation that should be done: (AIIMS Nov 2015)
a) Lymph node biopsy
b) Peripheral immunophenotyping
c) Bone marrow aspiration
d) Peripheral blood cytogenetics

163) A 45-year-old female patient presented with painless supraclavicular lymphadenopathy. Biopsy revealed bi-nucleated acidophilic owl eye appearance with floating lymphocytes in empty space which was CD15, CD30 positive. What is the most probable diagnosis? (AIIMS Nov 2013)
a. Lymphocytic predominant Hodgkin lymphoma
b. Nodular sclerosis Hodgkin lymphoma
c. Mixed cellularity Hodgkin lymphoma
d. Lymphocytic depleted lymphoma

164) 12-year-old boy presents with enlargement of bilateral cervical lymph nodes for 2 years. A biopsy from the lymph node reveals the following picture. Which of the following is the correct set of diagnosis, etiology and the cell described? (AIIMS Nov 2015)

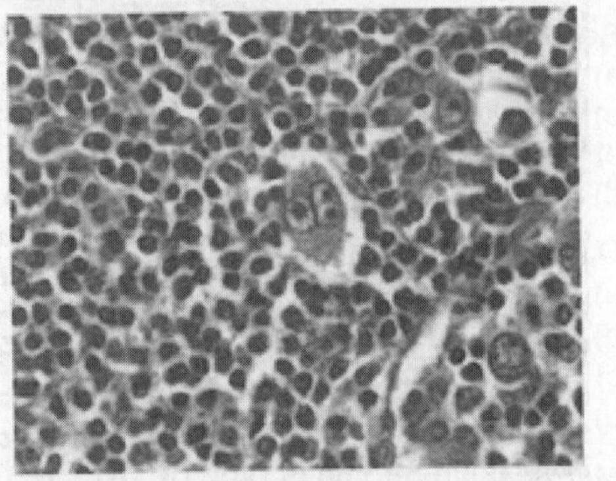

a) Hodgkin's lymphoma; Epstein Barr Virus and Reed Sternberg cells
b) Hodgkin's lymphoma; Epstein Barr Virus and Embryo cell
c) Non-Hodgkin's lymphoma; HIV and Giant B cell
d) Tuberculosis, Mycobacterium and Tiny granuloma

CHAPTER 27: DISEASES OF WHITE BLOOD CELLS, LYMPH NODES, SPLEEN AND THYMUS

Ans. 1) **D. Thymus (Ref: 8 ed. Robbins p.589-90, 9 ed. p. 579)**

Components of **hematopoietic system** Q:

- **Myeloid tissues** – which include bone marrow and the cells derived from it (i.e. red cells, platelets, granulocytes and monocytes)
- **Lymphoid tissues**, consisting of thymus, lymph nodes and spleen

Ans. 2) **D. All of the above (Ref: 8 ed. Robbins p.590, 9 ed. p.579-580)**

Development of Hematopoietic Tissues Q:

- **During third week** of embryonic development – Blood cell progenitors appears in the yolk sac
- During the **third month** of embryogenesis – **hematopoietic stem cells (HSC)**, migrate to the **liver** Q
- During the **fourth month**, **HSCs** reside in the bone marrow
- By **birth till puberty**, hematopoietically active marrow is found throughout the **skeleton** Q
- **After puberty**, hematopoietically active marrow is restricted to the **axial skeleton** Q

Two essential properties of HSCs: **Pluripotency** Q and capacity for **self-renewal** Q

Ans. 3) **A. 1:1 (Ref: 8 ed. Robbins p.592, 9 ed. p.582)**

- In normal adults, the ratio of **fat cells to hematopoietic elements** is **1 : 1** Q
- In **aplastic anemia**, the proportion of fat cells is **increased** Q
- **Hematopoietic fat cells** often **disappears**, when the marrow is involved by tumors, hemolytic anemias and leukemias Q

Ans. 4) **D. All of the above (Ref: 8 ed. Robbins p.592, 9 ed. p.582)**

Causes of **Lymphopenia** Q:

- Human immunodeficiency virus (HIV) infection
- Following glucocorticoids or cytotoxic drugs therapy
- Autoimmune disorders
- Malnutrition
- Acute viral disorders

Ans. 5) **D. Any of the above (Ref: 8 ed. Robbins p.592-93, 9 ed. p.582)**

Causes of Neutropenia Q:

Inadequate or ineffective granulopoiesis Q:

- Suppression of hematopoietic stem cells: **Aplastic anemia**, tumors, granulomatous disease
- Suppression of granulocytic precursors by **drugs**
- **Ineffective hematopoiesis** – As in **megaloblastic anemias** and **myelodysplastic syndromes**

Accelerated destruction or sequestration of neutrophils Q:

- Immunologically mediated injury – systemic lupus erythematosus
- Splenomegaly
- Increased peripheral utilization – bacterial, fungal, or rickettsial infections

Ans. 6) **C. 500/mm^3 (Ref: 8 ed. Robbins p.593, 9 ed. p.582)**

- **Serious infections** occurs when the **neutrophil count falls** below **500 per mm^3** Q

Ans. 7) **D. Tuberculosis (Ref: 8 ed. Robbins p.593-95, 9 ed. p.583-84, t-13-3)**

Causes of **Neutrophilic leukocytosis** Q:

- **Acute bacterial infections**
- Tissue necrosis (**myocardial infarction, burns**)

Causes of **Eosinophilic leukocytosis (eosinophilia)** Q:

- **Allergic disorders** such as asthma, hay fever, parasitic infestations
- Drug reactions
- Malignancies (e.g. Hodgkin and some non-Hodgkin lymphomas)
- Autoimmune disorders (e.g., pemphigus, dermatitis herpetiformis)
- Vasculitis; atheroembolic disease (transient)

Causes of **Monocytosis** Q:

- **Tuberculosis**, bacterial endocarditis, rickettsiosis and malaria
- Autoimmune disorders
- Inflammatory bowel disease

Causes of **Lymphocytosis** Q:

- **Tuberculosis**, Brucellosis
- **Viral infections** (e.g., hepatitis A, cytomegalovirus, Epstein-Barr virus); Bordetella pertussis infection

Ans. 8) **A. Neutrophils (Ref: 8 ed. Robbins p.594, 9 ed. p.583-84, f-13-2)**

Döhle Bodies: Q

- **Dilated endoplasmic reticulum** Q **patches** in cytoplasm of neutrophils
- Seen in patients with **bacterial sepsis** Q

Ans. 9) **A. Follicular hyperplasia (Ref: 8 ed. Robbins p.595-96, 9 ed. p.585, f-13-3)**

Tingible-body macrophages Q

- Seen in the **germinal center cells** of lymph nodes, **reactive lymphoid hyperplasia** Q and **follicular hyperplasia** Q

Ans. 10) **D. All of the above (Ref: 8 ed. Robbins p.595-96, 9 ed. p.585, f-13-3)**

Microscopic features favoring **Follicular hyperplasia** Q:

- Preservation of **lymph node architecture** Q
- **Marked variation** in shape and size of the follicles
- Presence of frequent **mitotic figures, phagocytic macrophages (tingible-body macrophages)** Q

All the above mentioned features are **absent** in **Follicular lymphoma**

Ans. 11) **D. All of the above (Ref: 8 ed. Robbins p.595-96, 9 ed. p.585, f-13-3)**

Causes of **follicular hyperplasia** Q include (Ref: Robbins):

- **Rheumatoid arthritis, Toxoplasmosis** and early stages of infection with **HIV**

Follicular hyperplasia Q can be seen in (Ref: Ackerman):

- **Hodgkin disease** (Nodular sclerosis, Nodular lymphocyte predominant), Castleman disease, Follicular lymphoma, Mantle cell lymphoma, Marginal zone lymphoma

Ans. 12) **D. Any of the above (Ref: 10 ed. Ackerman p. 1781, t-21.4)**

Sinus histiocytosis Q in a lymph node is seen in:

- Rosai-Dorfman disease
- Whipple disease
- Langerhans cell histiocytosis
- Hemophagocytic syndrome

Ans. 13) **D. Any of the above (Ref: 10 ed. Ackerman p. 1783-84, f-21.8)**

Monocytoid B cells Q in **lymph node** are seen in:

- Toxoplasmosis
- AIDS

- Infectious diseases
- Cat-scratch disease
- Autoimmune disorders
- Malignant lymphomas

Ans. 14) D. Both A & B (Ref: 9 ed. Robbins p.585-86)

Hemophagocytic Lymphohistiocytosis (HLH) Q:

- Characterized by **decreased cell lines**
- Signs and symptoms of **systemic inflammation** are present
- Due to the activation of macrophages, it is called as **macrophage activation syndrome** Q

Pathogenesis:

- Occurs due to **systemic activation of macrophages** and **CD8+ cytotoxic T cells** Q
- High levels of **inflammatory mediators – Interferon-γ, TNFα, IL-6, IL-12**, soluble **IL-2 receptor** are seen

Ans. 15) D. Low levels of serum ferritin (Ref: 9 ed. Robbins p.585-86)

Clinical Features of HLH Q:

- **Acute febrile illness** Q, Hepatosplenomegaly
- **Hemophagocytosis** seen on **bone marrow examination (not required** Q to make the diagnosis)
- **Anemia, thrombocytopenia, high levels** of **plasma ferritin** Q and **IL-2 receptor**
- Elevated liver function tests and triglyceride levels
- Coagulation studies show evidence of **disseminated intravascular coagulation** Q

Ans. 16) D. Any of the above (Ref: 8 ed. Robbins p.595-96, 9 ed. p.586-87, f-13-4)

Pathogenesis of **white blood cell** malignancies Q:

- **Pro-growth mutations** (mutations which effect **maturation** Q): e.g. **tyrosine kinase** mutations, **MYC translocation**
- Mutations leading to **increased self-renewal** Q: e.g. **MLL translocation, PML-RARA** fusion gene
- Mutations that prevent **apoptosis** Q: e.g. **BCL2 translocation**

Ans. 17) D. All of the above (Ref: 8 ed. Robbins p.597-98, 9 ed. p.587)

Etiological factors which play a role in **WBC malignancies**:

Inherited Genetic Factors Q:

- Bloom syndrome, Fanconi anemia and ataxia telangiectasia – increased incidence of **leukemia**
- **Down syndrome (Trisomy 21)** and **Type I neurofibromatosis** – increased incidence of **childhood leukemia**

Viruses Q:

- **Human T-cell leukemia virus-1 (HTLV-1)** – associated with adult T-cell leukemia/lymphoma
- **Epstein-Barr virus (EBV)** found in Burkitt lymphoma, Hodgkin lymphoma (HL), B-cell lymphomas
- Kaposi sarcoma herpes virus/human herpesvirus-8 **(KSHV/HHV-8)** – May lead to malignant pleural effusion

Chronic Inflammation Q:

- ***H. pylori*** infection – Gastric B-cell lymphomas
- **Gluten sensitive enteropathy** – Intestinal T-cell lymphomas
- **Breast implants** – T cell lymphoma
- **HIV infection** – B-cell lymphomas

Ans. 18) D. All of the above (Ref: 8 ed. Robbins p.598, 9 ed. p.588)

- **Leukemia** Q – Patient presents with widespread involvement of the **bone marrow** and **peripheral blood**
- **Lymphoma** – Proliferations that arise as **discrete tissue masses** Q
- Lymphoma occasionally have **leukemic presentations**

- Evolution to **leukemia** is not unusual in patients with lymphomas

Ans. 19) D. Mycosis fungoides (Ref: 8 ed. Robbins p.598, 9 ed. p.588, t-13-4)

WHO Classification of Lymphoid Neoplasms [Q]:

Precursor B-Cell Neoplasms

- B-cell acute lymphoblastic leukemia/lymphoma (B-ALL)

Peripheral B-Cell Neoplasms

- Chronic lymphocytic leukemia/small lymphocytic lymphoma
- B-cell prolymphocytic leukemia
- Lymphoplasmacytic lymphoma
- Splenic and nodal marginal zone lymphomas
- Extranodal marginal zone lymphoma
- Mantle cell lymphoma
- Follicular lymphoma
- Marginal zone lymphoma
- Hairy cell leukemia
- Plasmacytoma/plasma cell myeloma
- Diffuse large B-cell lymphoma
- Burkitt lymphoma

Precursor T-Cell Neoplasms

- T-cell acute lymphoblastic leukemia/lymphoma (T-ALL)

Peripheral T-Cell and NK-Cell Neoplasms

- T-cell prolymphocytic leukemia
- Large granular lymphocytic leukemia
- Mycosis fungoides/Sezary syndrome
- Peripheral T-cell lymphoma, unspecified
- Anaplastic large-cell lymphoma
- Angioimmunoblastic T-cell lymphoma
- Enteropathy-associated T-cell lymphoma
- Panniculitis-like T-cell lymphoma
- Hepatosplenic $\gamma\delta$T-cell lymphoma
- Adult T-cell leukemia/lymphoma
- Extranodal NK/T-cell lymphoma
- NK-cell leukemia

Hodgkin Lymphoma

Classical subtypes

- Nodular sclerosis
- Mixed cellularity
- Lymphocyte-rich
- Lymphocyte depletion
- Lymphocyte predominance

Note: Majority (85% to 90%) of lymphoid neoplasms are of **B-cell origin** [Q]

Ans. 20) D. All of the above (Ref: 8 ed. Robbins p.599, 9 ed. p.589, f-13-5)

Lymphoid neoplasms arising from **germinal center** Q of the lymph node:

- Follicular lymphoma
- Burkitt lymphoma
- Diffuse large B cell lymphoma
- Hodgkin disease

Lymphoid neoplasms arising from the **marginal zone** Q of lymph node:

- Diffuse large B cell lymphoma
- Marginal zone lymphoma
- Small lymphocytic lymphoma
- Chronic lymphocytic leukemia

Lymphoid neoplasms arising from the **mantle zone** Q of lymph node:

- Mantle zone lymphoma

Note: Plasma cells Q in bone marrow give rise to **Multiple myeloma**

Ans. 21) D. Any of the above (Ref: 8 ed. Robbins p.600, 9 ed. p.590, t-13-5)

Primarily **T-Cell associated markers** Q include:

- CD1, CD3, CD4, CD5, CD8

Primarily **B-Cell associated markers** Q include:

- CD10 (CALLA), CD19, CD20, CD21, CD23, CD79a

Ans. 22) D. CD16 (Ref: 8 ed. Robbins p.600, 9 ed. p.590, t-13-5)

Primarily **Monocyte or Macrophage** Q associated markers include:

- CD11c, CD13, CD14, CD15, CD33, CD64

Primarily **NK-Cell associated markers** Q include:

- CD16, CD56

Ans. 23) A. CD34 (Ref: 8 ed. Robbins p.600, 9 ed. p.590, t-13-5)

- **Stem Cell** marker – **CD34** Q
- **Activation Markers** (Activated B cells, T cells and monocytes; Reed-Sternberg cells) – **CD30** Q
- Pan-**leukocyte marker – CD45 (Leucocyte common antigen)** Q

Ans. 24) A. CD1 (Ref: 8 ed. Robbins p.600, 9 ed. p.590, t-13-5)

- **Langerhans cells** show positivity of **CD1** Q

Ans. 25) D. All of the above (Ref: 8 ed. Robbins p.600-02, 9 ed. p.590)

Acute Lymphoblastic Leukemia/Lymphoma (ALLs) Q:

- **Most common cancer** of children
- Neoplasms composed of immature **B (pre-B)** or **T (pre-T) cells**
- **B-ALLs (85%)** Q – Manifest as childhood **acute "leukemia"**
- **Peak incidence** at the age of **3 years**
- **T-ALLs** presents in adolescent males as **thymic "lymphomas"** Q

Ans. 26) D. All of the above (Ref: 8 ed. Robbins p.602-03, 9 ed. p.591-92)

Pathogenesis of ALL Q:

- **Most common** numerical or structural chromosomal change seen in **ALLs** is **hyperploidy** Q (>50 chromosomes)
- **70% of T-ALLs** have gain-of-function mutations in **NOTCH1** Q
- **B-ALLs** show loss-of-function mutations in **PAX5** Q, E2A and EBF genes

- **B-ALLs** shows balanced **t(12;21)** [Q] involving the genes **ETV6** and **RUNX1**

Ans. 27) C. Lymphoblasts show MPO positivity (Ref: 8 ed. Robbins p.602, 9 ed. p.591-92, f-13-6)

Morphological Features of **Lymphoblasts** [Q]:

- Shows condensed chromatin, less conspicuous nucleoli
- Smaller amounts of cytoplasm, which lacks granules

Histochemical Stains [Q]:

- Lymphoblast shows **periodic acid-Schiff (PAS) positivity**
- Lymphoblast are **myeloperoxidase (MPO) negative**

Ans. 28) B. B-cell ALL (Ref: 8 ed. Robbins p.602, 9 ed. p.591-92, f-13-6)

Immunophenotyping of ALL:

- **Pre-B** and **Pre-T lymphoblasts** show **terminal deoxynucleotidyl transferase (TdT)** positivity

B-ALLs immunophenotype [Q]:

- **Pan B-cell marker - CD 19, CD10** and transcription factor **PAX5**
- **CD20** and cytoplasmic IgM heavy chain
- However, in very immature B-ALLs, CD10 is negative

T-ALLs immunophenotype [Q]:

- **Shows** positivity for **CD1, CD2**, **CD5** and **CD7**

Ans. 29) D. t(9;22) (Ref: 8 ed. Robbins p.603, 9 ed. p.592-93)

Worse prognostic factors in **ALL** [Q]:

- Age younger than 2 years
- Presentation in adolescence or adulthood
- Peripheral blood blast counts greater than 100,000
- t(9;22) **(8 ed. Robbins)**

Favorable prognostic factors in ALL [Q]:

- Age between 2 and 10 years
- Low white cell count
- Hyperdiploidy
- Trisomy of chromosomes 4, 7 and 10
- Presence of t(12;21)

Ans. 30) A. 190kDa (Ref: 8 ed. Robbins p.603, 9 ed. p.592-93)

- **t(9;22)** creates a fusion gene that encodes **BCR-ABL tyrosine kinase** [Q]
- In **B-ALL, BCR-ABL protein** is **190 kDa** [Q] in size and has a **stronger** tyrosine kinase activity as found in **Chronic Myelogenous Leukemia (CML)**
- In **CML, BCR-ABL protein** is **210 kDa** [Q] in size and has a **weaker** tyrosine kinase activity

Ans. 31) D. >5000/mm³ (Ref: 8 ed. Robbins p.603, 9 ed. p.593)

Chronic Lymphocytic Leukemia (CLL):

- **Absolute lymphocyte count > 5000 per mm³** [Q] is the diagnostic requirement criteria
- **Absolute lymphocyte count >4000/mm³** is the diagnostic requirement of CLL **(8 ed. Robbins)**

Ans. 32) D. All of the above (Ref: 8 ed. Robbins p.604, 9 ed. p.593)

Genetic Anomalies in CLL/SLL:

- **Most common** genetic anomalies are **deletions of 13q14.3, 11q** and **17p** and **trisomy 12q**
- **Gain-of-function mutations** involving the **NOTCH1 receptor** [Q] are **also seen**

Ans. 33) B. Bruton tyrosine kinase (Ref: 9 ed. Robbins p. 593)

- Growth and survival of tumor cells (in CLL) depends on signals generated by the **B-cell receptor**
- Signals are transduced by **Bruton tyrosine kinase (BTK)** Q
- Hence, CLL cells are dependent on **BTK kinase** for its proliferation
- Most promising new therapy for the treatment of CLL patients is **BTK inhibitors** Q

Ans. 34) C. CLL (Ref: 8 ed. Robbins p.603-04, 9 ed. p.593-94, f-13-7,8)

Morphology of CLL Q**:**

- **Diffuse effacement** of lymph node architecture, which contains predominantly **small lymphocytes**
- Lymphocytes have round to slightly irregular nuclei, condensed chromatin and scant cytoplasm
- **Proliferation centers –** Larger activated lymphocytes are admixed in between small lymphocytes and form loose aggregates
- **Proliferation centers** Q are pathognomonic for **CLL/SLL**
- **Smudge cells** Q – Small round lymphocytes which are disrupted while making **peripheral smears**
- **Tumor cell infiltrates** are always seen in **white and red pulp** of spleen and **hepatic portal tracts**

Ans. 35) D. All of the above (Ref: 8 ed. Robbins p.604, 9 ed. p.594)

Immunophenotype of CLL/SLL Cells Q**:**

- Tumor cells express **pan B-cell markers CD19** and **CD20**
- Also expresses **CD23** and **CD5**
- Low-level expression of **surface Ig** (usually IgM or IgM and IgD) is also typical

Ans. 36) A. CLL (Ref: 8 ed. Robbins p.604-05, 9 ed. p.594-95, f-13-8)

Clinical Features of **Chronic Lymphocytic Leukemia** Q**:**

- **Easy fatigability, weight loss, anorexia, generalized lymphadenopathy** and **hepatosplenomegaly** Q
- **Hypogammaglobulinemia** Q is **common** and leads to increased susceptibility to infections
- 10% to 15% of patients develop **hemolytic anemia** Q
- **CLL/SLL** can transform to **diffuse large B-cell lymphoma**, so-called **Richter syndrome** Q

Note: Presence of **spherocytes** and **nucleated erythroid cell** suggests coexistent **autoimmune hemolytic anemia** Q, which can be seen in CLL

Ans. 37) D. All of the above (Ref: 8 ed. Robbins p.605, 9 ed. p.594-95, f-13-10)

Pathogenesis of **Follicular Lymphoma** Q**:**

- Arises from the **germinal center B cells** Q
- Associated with **chromosomal translocations** involving **BCL2** Q
- Hallmark is **t(14;18)** Q in which **IGH locus** on **chromosome 14** juxtaposes to the **BCL2 locus** on **chromosome 18**
- **t(14;18)** leads to overexpression of **BCL2** Q, which is an **anti-apoptotic gene**, thus inhibiting the **apoptosis**
- **MLL2 gene** Q mutations are also seen

Note: Follicular lymphomas patients can show histologic transformation to **diffuse large B-cell lymphoma** Q

Ans. 38) D. Both A and B (Ref: 8 ed. Robbins p.605, 9 ed. p.594-95, f-13-10)

Morphology of Follicular Lymphoma:

- **Lymph node** shows **nodular** or **diffuse** growth pattern of tumor cells
- Two principal cell types are : Centrocytes and centroblasts
- **Centrocytes** Q (small cleaved cells) – Small cells with irregular or cleaved nuclear contours and scant cytoplasm
- **Centroblasts** Q – Larger cells with moderate amount of cytoplasm, open nuclear chromatin and several nucleoli

Ans. 39) C. CD5 (Ref: 8 ed. Robbins p.605-06, 9 ed. p.594-96, f-13-12)

Immunophenotype of Follicular Lymphoma [Q]:

- Tumor cells express **CD19, CD20, CD10, surface Ig** and **BCL6**
- **CD5** [Q] **(positive in CLL/SLL** and **mantle cell lymphoma)** is **negative**
- **BCL2** is **expressed** in more than **90%** of cases

Ans. 40) A. DLBCL (Ref: 8 ed. Robbins p.606, 9 ed. p.595)

- **Diffuse Large B-Cell Lymphoma (DLBCL)** [Q] is the **most common** form of **NHL**

Ans. 41) D. Any of the above (Ref: 8 ed. Robbins p.607, 9 ed. p.596)

Pathogenesis of DLBCL [Q]:

- **BCL6 overexpression**: Inhibits germinal center **B-cell differentiation**, growth arrest and apoptosis
- **t(14;18):** Leads to the overexpression of **BCL2**
- ***MYC* translocation (worse prognosis)**

Ans. 42) D. All of the above (Ref: 8 ed. Robbins p.607, 9 ed. p.596-97, f-13-14)

DLBCL [Q] can affect:

- Waldeyer ring, tonsils and adenoids
- Liver and spleen
- Extra-nodal sites include gastrointestinal tract, skin, bone, brain

Subtypes of DLBCL [Q]:

A) **Immunodeficiency-associated large B-cell lymphoma:**
   - Predisposing factors – **HIV, allogeneic bone marrow transplantation**
   - B cells are infected with **EBV** [Q]

B) **Primary effusion lymphoma (PEL):**
   - Presents as **malignant pleural** or **ascitic effusion**
   - Tumor cells are infected with **KSHV/HHV-8** [Q]

Ans. 43) D. Any of the above (Ref: 8 ed. Robbins p.607-08, 9 ed. p.597)

Pathogenesis of Burkitt Lymphoma [Q]:

- Associated with **MYC gene** translocation on **chromosome 8**, leading to increased **MYC protein** [Q] levels

MYC [Q] **translocation** can be seen with:

- IgH locus [t(8;14)]
- Ig κl [t(2;8)]
- λ light chain loci [t(8;22)]

Ans. 44) D. Expresses BCL-2 (Ref: 8 ed. Robbins p.607-08, 9 ed. p.597, f-13-15)

Types of Burkitt Lymphoma [Q]:

- African **(endemic)** Burkitt lymphoma
- Sporadic **(non-endemic)** Burkitt lymphoma
- **Aggressive lymphomas** occurring in HIV patients

Morphology:

- **Diffuse infiltrate** of **intermediate sized** lymphoid cells
- Tumor cells have **high mitotic index**
- Tumor cells contain numerous **apoptotic cells**, which are phagocytosed by **macrophages**
- **"Starry sky" pattern** [Q]: Due to abundant clear cytoplasm of these macrophages

Immunophenotype [Q]:

- Tumor cells express **surface IgM, CD19, CD20, CD10 and BCL6**
- **Does not express anti-apoptotic protein BCL2** [Q] (unlike other tumors of germinal center origin)

Note: Latent infection with **EBV**, is noted in all three types of Burkitt lymphoma

Ans. 45) D. Does not respond to intensive chemotherapy (Ref: 8 ed. Robbins p.608, 9 ed. p.597)

Clinical Features of Burkitt Lymphoma [Q]:

- **Endemic** and **sporadic Burkitt lymphomas** are found in children or young adults
- **Endemic form** presents as a mass involving the **mandible** [Q]
- **Sporadic form** presents as a mass involving the **ileocecum** and **peritoneum** [Q]
- Though, being an **aggressive tumor**, it responds well to **intensive chemotherapy** [Q]

Ans. 46) D. All of the above (Ref: 4 ed. WHO Classification of Tumours of the Hematopoietic and Lymphoid Tissues p. 200, t-10.03)

Plasma cell neoplasms [Q] **include:**

a) **Monoclonal gammopathy of unknown significance**

b) **Plasma cell myeloma**
- Smoldering myeloma
- Plasma cell leukemia

c) **Plasmacytoma**
- Solitary Plasmacytoma of bone
- Extra osseous (Extra medullary Plasmacytoma)

d) **Immunoglobulin deposition diseases**
- Primary amyloidosis
- Systemic light and heavy chain deposition diseases

e) **Osteosclerotic myeloma (POEMS Syndrome)**

Ans. 47) D. All of the above (Ref: 8 ed. Robbins p.609, 9 ed. p.599)

Molecular Pathogenesis of **Multiple Myeloma** [Q]:

a) Translocations of **Ig heavy-chain gene (IgH)** on chromosome **14q32** with
- **Cyclin D1** on chromosome 11q13
- **Cyclin D3** on chromosome 6p21

b) Deletions of **chromosome 17p**

c) Mutations involving **NF-κB pathway** and rearrangements involving ***MYC***

Ans. 48) D. IL-6 (Ref: 8 ed. Robbins p.609, 9 ed. p.598-99)

IL-6:

- **Proliferation** and **survival of myeloma cells** depends on **IL-6** [Q]
- High serum levels of **IL-6** are associated with a **poor prognosis**

Note:

Pathogenesis of **bone destruction** in **Multiple Myeloma**:

- **MIP1α** increases **RANKL** [Q] expression, which in turn activates **osteoclasts** leading to **bone destruction**

Ans. 49) B. Post-germinal center B-cell (Ref: 8 ed. Robbins p.609)

- **Cell of origin** of Multiple myeloma is **post germinal center B-cell** [Q]

Ans. 50) A. Vertebral column (Ref: 8 ed. Robbins p.609-10, 9 ed. p.598-99, f-13-16)

- Bones **most commonly affected** (in descending order): **Vertebral column** [Q], ribs, skull, pelvis, femur, clavicle and scapula

- **Pathologic fractures** [Q] are most common in **vertebral column**
- **Bone lesions** appear as **punched-out defects** [Q] **(1 to 4 cm** in diameter) radiographically

Ans. 51) D. Related organ or tissue impairment (Ref: 4 ed. WHO Classification of Tumours of the Hematopoietic and Lymphoid Tissues, p. 202, t-10.05)

Diagnostic Criteria of **Symptomatic Plasma Cell Myeloma** [Q]:

a) M-protein in serum or urine
   - **No levels** of serum proteins are included. However, most cases have IgG >30g/l, IgA >25g/l or >1 gm/24 hr. of urine light chain

b) Bone marrow clonal plasma cells or plasmacytoma
   - **No minimal level** is designated, however monoclonal plasma cells exceed 10% of nucleated cells

c) Related organ or tissue impairment **(CRAB: hypercalcemia, renal insufficiency, anemia, bone lesions)** [Q]
   - **Most important criteria** [Q] of symptomatic myeloma are manifestations of **end organ damage** [Q]

Ans. 52) D. All of the above (Ref: 4th ed. WHO Classification of Tumours of the Hematopoietic and Lymphoid Tissues, p. 202, t-10.05)

Asymptomatic or smoldering myeloma [Q]:

- M-protein in serum >30 g/l AND/OR
- 10% or more clonal plasma cells in bone marrow
- **No related organ or tissue impairment** (i.e. CRAB)

Hence, the difference between symptomatic plasma cell myeloma and smoldering myeloma is **absence of symptoms related to organ damage (i.e. CRAB)** [Q] in the latter

Ans. 53) D. All of the above (Ref: 4th ed. WHO Classification of Tumours of the Hematopoietic and Lymphoid Tissues, p. 201, t-10.04)

- **MGUS** [Q] is the **most common plasma cell dyscrasia** [Q]

Diagnostic criteria for **Monoclonal Gammopathy of unknown significance (MGUS)** [Q]:

- **M-protein** in serum **< 30 g/l**
- Bone marrow clonal plasma cells **<10%**
- No lytic bone lesions
- No evidence of **CRAB**
- No evidence of B-cell proliferative disorder

Note: Risk of progression of **MGUS** to **plasma cell myeloma** is **1% per year** [Q]

Ans. 54) D. All of the above (Ref: 8 ed. Robbins p.610, 9 ed. p.599, f-13-17)

Morphology of cells in **Multiple myeloma** [Q]:

- **Plasma cells** [Q]: Show perinuclear clearing and an **eccentrically placed nucleus**
- **Plasmablasts**: Show **vesicular nuclear chromatin** and a prominent single nucleolus

Following cells are seen due to **dysregulated synthesis** and **secretion of Ig:**

- **Flame cells** [Q] with **fiery red cytoplasm**
- **Mott cells** [Q] with multiple **grape-like cytoplasmic droplets**
- **Russell bodies** [Q] – Cytoplasmic globular inclusions
- **Dutcher bodies** [Q] – Nuclear globular inclusions

Ans. 55) D. All of the above (Ref: 9 ed. Robbins p.599)

Plasma Cell Tumors:

- Express **CD138** [Q]/syndecan-1 (adhesion molecule) and **CD56** [Q]

Ans. 56) D. Any of the above (Ref: 8 ed. Robbins p.610, 9 ed. p.599)

Rouleaux formation in **peripheral smear** can be seen:
- **Multiple myeloma** [Q] (increased **M proteins** causes red cells to stick to one another in linear arrays)
- Also seen in **SLE** [Q] **and early HIV infection** [Q] with elevated Ig levels

Ans. 57) A. Recurrent infections (Ref: 8 ed. Robbins p.610-11, 9 ed. p. 600)

Clinical Features of **Multiple Myeloma** [Q]:
- **Recurrent bacterial infections** [Q]: Due to **immunoglobulin deficiency**, most common cause of death
- **Renal insufficiency**, after **infections** [Q] are a common cause of death
- Bone resorption leads to **pathological fractures** and chronic pain
- **Hypercalcemia** leads to confusion, weakness, lethargy, constipation and polyuria

Ans. 58) B. IgG (Ref: 8 ed. Robbins p.610-11, 9 ed. p. 600, f-13-18)
- Most common **monoclonal Ig ("M protein")** is **IgG** [Q], followed by **IgA** [Q]
- Myelomas expressing IgM, IgD or IgE are rare

Techniques to detect monoclonal Igs:
- **Serum or urine electrophoresis** [Q]: shows **abnormal protein "spikes"**
- **Immunofixation** [Q] **– Confirmation and characterization** of monoclonal Ig

Ans. 59) D. Upper respiratory tract (Ref: 4th ed. WHO Classification of Tumours of the Hematopoietic and Lymphoid Tissues, p. 208)

Extraosseous Plasmacytoma:
- 80% occurs in the **upper respiratory tract** (oropharynx, nasopharynx, sinuses and larynx)
- **Other sites** include – Gastrointestinal tract, lymph nodes, bladder, CNS, breast, thyroid, testis, parotid and skin

Ans. 60) C. Plasma cell component secretes IgG (Ref: 8 ed. Robbins p.612, 9 ed. p. 601, f-13-19)

Lymphoplasmacytic Lymphoma [Q]:
- **B-cell neoplasm**, presents in sixth or seventh decade and resembles **CLL/SLL**
- **Plasma cell** component of tumor cells secretes **monoclonal IgM** [Q]
- **Waldenstorm macroglobulinemia** [Q]: Due to **monoclonal IgM secretion** which predisposes to **hyperviscosity syndrome**
- **Bone destruction** does not occur

Ans. 61) B. Lymphoplasmacytic leukemia (Ref: 8 ed. Robbins p.612, 9 ed. p. 601-02, f-13-19)

Clinical Features of **Lymphoplasmacytic Lymphoma** [Q]:
- **Weakness, fatigue and weight loss**
- **On examination** – Lymphadenopathy, hepatomegaly and splenomegaly
- **Autoimmune hemolysis** [Q] occurs when the **cold agglutinins (IgM antibodies)** bind to red cells at temperatures **less than 37°C**

Hyperviscosity syndrome:
- Occurs due to increased IgM levels, which leads to **increased viscosity** of blood
- Presents with **visual impairment**, **neurological problems**, bleeding, **cryoglobulinemia** (precipitation of macroglobulins at low temperatures)

Ans. 62) A. t(11;14) (Ref: 8 ed. Robbins p.612-13, 9 ed. p. 601-02)

Pathogenesis of **Mantle Cell Lymphoma** [Q]:
- **t(11;14)** involving the **IgH** locus on **chromosome 14** and the **cyclin D1** locus on **chromosome 11** is **characteristic**
- Translocation leads to increased expression of **cyclin D1** [Q]
- **Cyclin D1** promotes **G1- to S-phase** [Q] progression

Ans. 63) D. Proliferation centers (Ref: 8 ed. Robbins p.612-13, 9 ed. p. 602-03, f-13-20)

Morphology of **Lymphoplasmacytic Lymphoma** Q:

- Presents with **generalized lymphadenopathy**, with or without peripheral blood involvement
- **Extra nodal** sites include: Bone marrow, spleen, liver and gut
- **Lymphomatoid polyposis** Q: **polyp-like lesions** in the **small bowel** or **colon**
- Composed of **small lymphocytes** with clefted (cleaved) nuclear contours
- **Centroblasts** (seen in **follicular lymphoma**) and **proliferation centers** Q (seen in **CLL/SLL**) are **absent**

Ans. 64) D. CD23 (Ref: 8 ed. Robbins p.612-13, 9 ed. p. 602-03)

Immunophenotype of **Mantle Cell Lymphoma** Q:

- Expresses increased levels of **cyclin D1**
- Shows positivity of **CD19, CD20** and surface **Ig**
- **CD5+** and **CD23** helps to distinguish it from **CLL/SLL** Q **(CD5 – and CD23+)**

Ans. 65) D. All of the above (Ref: 8 ed. Robbins p.613, 9 ed. p. 603)

Characteristic Features of Extra nodal marginal zone lymphomas Q:

- Arises in the tissues involved by **chronic inflammatory disorders** of **autoimmune** or **infectious** etiology
- **Examples:** Salivary gland in **Sjögren disease** Q, thyroid gland in **Hashimoto thyroiditis** Q and the stomach in ***Helicobacter gastritis*** Q
- Remains localized for **prolonged periods** and **spread systemically** late in their course
- **Can regress** Q if the inciting agent (e.g., *Helicobacter pylori*) is eradicated

Ans. 66) D. All of the above (Ref: 8 ed. Robbins p.613-14, 9 ed. p. 603)

- Chromosomal translocations, specific for **Extranodal marginal zone lymphomas: t(11;18)**, **t(14;18)**, or **t(1;14)** Q
- Translocations up-regulates the expression of **BCL10** or **MALT1**, that activates **NF-κB** Q and promotes the growth and survival of **B cells** Q

Ans. 67) D. All of the above (Ref: 8 ed. Robbins p.614, 9 ed. p. 603-04)

Hairy Cell Leukemia Q:

- **B-cell neoplasm** with **male-to-female ratio** of **5 : 1**
- Associated with **point mutation** in **BRAF**

Clinical Features:

- Tumor cells can infiltrate **bone marrow, liver** and **spleen**
- **Massive Splenomegaly** Q – Most common physical finding
- **Pancytopenia**
- **Infections** – Atypical mycobacterial infections
- Follows an **indolent course** Q and is highly sensitive to **"gentle" chemotherapeutic regimen** Q
- **BRAF inhibitors** produce excellent responses
- **Excellent** Q prognosis

Ans. 68) D. All of the above (Ref: 8 ed. Robbins p.614, 9 ed. p. 604, f-13-21)

Morphology of Hairy cell leukemia:

- **Phase contrast microscope** Q shows leukemic cells with **fine hair like projections**
- **Peripheral smear** Q – Hairy cells with **round, oblong**, or **reniform nuclei** with **pale blue cytoplasm** and **thread like or bleb like extensions**
- **Bone marrow biopsy** Q – Diffuse interstitial infiltrate of cells with oblong or reniform nuclei, condensed chromatin and pale cytoplasm
- **Bone marrow aspirate** shows **"dry tap"** Q – Tumor cells are enmeshed within the **reticulin fibrils**, hence cannot be aspirated

Ans. 69) D. Any of the above (Ref: 8 ed. Robbins p.614, 9 ed. p. 604)

Immunophenotyping of Hairy Cell Leukemia Q:

- Expresses **pan-B-cell markers CD19** and **CD20**, surface Ig (usually **IgG**) Q
- **CD11c, CD25, CD103** and **annexin A1** Q positive

Ans. 70) D. CD 30 positivity (Ref: 8 ed. Robbins p.615, 9 ed. p. 604-05, f-13-23)

Anaplastic Large-Cell Lymphoma (ALK Positive) Q:

- Shows rearrangements in **ALK gene** on **chromosome 2p23**
- **Hallmark cells** Q – Large anaplastic cells, having horseshoe-shaped nuclei and abundant cytoplasm
- **ALK** is **not expressed** in **normal lymphocytes** Q
- Presence of **ALK protein** in tumor cells indicates ALK gene rearrangement
- **Most common** in children or young adults and has **good prognosis** Q
- Both **ALK+** and **ALK - tumors** express **CD30** Q

Ans. 71) D. HTLV (Ref: 8 ed. Robbins p.615-16, 9 ed. p. 605)

Adult T-Cell Leukemia/Lymphoma:

- Neoplasm of CD4+ T cells
- Seen in the adults infected with **human T-cell leukemia retrovirus type 1 (HTLV-1)** Q
- **Clinical Features** – Skin lesions, generalized lymphadenopathy, hepatosplenomegaly, peripheral blood lymphocytosis and hypercalcemia
- **Cloverleaf or flower cells** Q – Tumor cells with **multilobated nuclei**
- **HTLV-1** encodes a protein called **Tax**, which is a potent activator of **NF-κB**

Note – **HTLV-1 infection** can lead to **progressive demyelinating disease** of the **central nervous system** and **spinal cord** Q

Ans. 72) A. Tumor of CD8+ T helper cells (Ref: 8 ed. Robbins p.616, 9 ed. p. 605-06)

Mycosis Fungoides Q:

- Tumor composed of **CD4+ helper T cells** Q, most commonly seen in skin
- Cutaneous lesions progresses through **three phases: Inflammatory premycotic phase, plaque phase** and **tumor phase** Q
- **Microscopically**: Epidermis and upper dermis are infiltrated by **neoplastic T cells**, which have **cerebriform appearance** Q
- **Extra-cutaneous spread** to **lymph nodes** Q and **bone marrow** Q can be seen

Ans. 73) D. All of the above (Ref: 8 ed. Robbins p.616, 9 ed. p. 606)

Sezary Syndrome Q:

- Manifests as **generalized exfoliative erythroderma** Q
- **Peripheral Blood smear** shows **"Sézary" cells** having characteristic **cerebriform nuclei** Q
- Tumor cells express the adhesion molecule **cutaneous leukocyte antigen (CLA)** Q and **chemokine receptors CCR4** and **CCR10** Q

Ans. 74) D. All of the above (Ref: 8 ed. Robbins p.616, 9 ed. p. 606)

Large Granular Lymphocytic Leukemia Q:

- Includes **T-cell** and **NK-cell** types
- Acquired mutations in transcription factor **STAT3** are seen
- Tumor cells are **large lymphocytes** with abundant blue cytoplasm and coarse azurophilic granules
- **T-cell** large granular lymphocytic leukemias are **CD3+**
- **NK-cell** large granular lymphocytic leukemias are **CD3–, CD56+**

- **Neutropenia** and **anemia** dominate the clinical picture
- Associated with **pure red cell aplasia** and **Felty syndrome** Q (rheumatoid arthritis, splenomegaly and neutropenia)

Ans. 75) A. Nasopharynx (Ref: 8 ed. Robbins p.616, 9 ed. p. 606)

Extranodal NK/T-cell Lymphoma Q:

- Most commonly presents as a **nasopharyngeal mass**
- Other sites includes **testis** and **skin**
- Highly associated with **EBV**

Ans. 76) D. All of the above (Ref: 8 ed. Robbins p.616-17, 9 ed. p. 606-07)

Differences between Hodgkin and Non-Hodgkin Lymphomas Q:

Hodgkin Lymphoma (HL)	Non-Hodgkin Lymphoma
Localized to a single axial group of nodes (cervical, mediastinal, para-aortic)	Multiple peripheral nodes can be involved
Contiguous spread	Noncontiguous spread
Mesenteric nodes and Waldeyer ring are rarely involved	Waldeyer ring and mesenteric nodes are commonly involved
Extranodal presentation is rare	Extranodal presentation is common

Reed-Sternberg Cell (R-S cell) Q

- HL is characterized by the presence of RS cells i.e. **neoplastic giant cells**
- Derived from **germinal center** or **post-germinal center** B cells

Ans. 77) D. Lymphocyte predominance (Ref: 8 ed. Robbins p.616-17, 9 ed. p. 606-07)

WHO classification recognizes **five subtypes** Q of HL:

1. Nodular sclerosis
2. Mixed cellularity
3. Lymphocyte-rich
4. Lymphocyte depletion
5. Lymphocyte predominance
   - In the **first four subtypes** — Reed-Sternberg cells have a similar immunophenotype and are called as **classical forms** Q of HL
   - In **lymphocyte predominance** Q subtype, Reed-Sternberg cells have distinctive B-cell immunophenotype

Ans. 78) D. All of the above (Ref: 8 ed. Robbins p.620, 9 ed. p. 607)

Pathogenesis of Hodgkin disease:

Activation of the transcription factor NF-κB Q in HL, occurs by:

- **EBV infection**
- **EBV+ tumor cells** which express **latent membrane protein-1 (LMP-1)**
- **Loss-of-function** mutation in **TNF alpha-induced protein 3**
- **REL proto-oncogene mutation** on chromosome 2p

Ans. 79) D. Any of the above (Ref: 8 ed. Robbins p.618, 9 ed. p. 608)

- **Reed-Sternberg like cells** can be seen in **infectious mononucleosis** Q, **solid tissue cancers** Q and **large-cell NHLs** Q

Ans. 80) D. All of the above (Ref: 8 ed. Robbins p.617-18, 9 ed. p. 607-08, f-13-24)

Reed-Sternberg Cells Q:

- Large cells with **multiple nuclei** or a **single nucleus** with multiple nuclear lobes

- **Large inclusion-like nucleolus**, same as a size of small lymphocyte
- Abundant cytoplasm

Variants of **Reed-Sternberg Cell** Q:

- **Mononuclear variant** Q containing a **single nucleus** with a **large inclusion-like nucleolus**
- **Lacunar cells** Q
- **Lymphohistiocytic variants** Q (L&H cells)

Ans. 81) B. Mummification (Ref: 8 ed. Robbins p.618, 9 ed. p. 608)

- In **Classical forms** of **Hodgkin Lymphoma**, **Reed-Sternberg cell** undergo **mummification** Q (cell death in which the cells **shrink** and become **pyknotic**)

Ans. 82) D. All of the above (Ref: 8 ed. Robbins p.618-19, 9 ed. p. 608, f-13-24, 25)

Nodular Sclerosis Hodgkin Lymphoma Q:

- **Most common form** of HL
- Characteristic histological feature is presence of **Lacunar cells** Q
- Lacunar cells have delicate, folded or multilobated nuclei and abundant pale cytoplasm, with the nucleus sitting in an empty hole
- **Collagen in bands** divide the involved lymph nodes into **circumscribed nodules**
- Background shows T cells, eosinophils, plasma cells and macrophages
- **RS cells** are positive for **PAX5** Q (a B-cell transcription factor), **CD15** Q and **CD30** Q
- **Not commonly** associated with **EBV**
- Equal frequency in males and females
- **Excellent** Q prognosis

Ans. 83) D. All of the above (Ref: 8 ed. Robbins p.619, 9 ed. p. 608-09, f-13-24,26)

Mixed cellularity Hodgkin Disease Q:

- **More common** in **males**
- Lymph node shows **heterogeneous cellular infiltrate** (T-cells, eosinophils, plasma cells, macrophages)
- **Diagnostic Reed-Sternberg cells** and **mononuclear variant** Q are seen
- **Reed-Sternberg cells** are infected with **EBV** Q **(70% of cases)**
- **Good prognosis**

Ans. 84) C. Lymphocyte predominant Hodgkin lymphoma (Ref: 8 ed. Robbins p.619-20, 9 ed. p. 609-10, f-13-27)

Lymphocyte Predominance Hodgkin Lymphoma Q:

- Lymph node architecture is effaced by a **nodular infiltrate** of **small lymphocytes** admixed with **macrophages**
- **Popcorn cells – L&H** Q **(lymphocytic and histiocytic)** variant are **characteristic**
- Expresses **B-cell markers** Q – **CD20** and **BCL6**
- **Negative for CD15** and **CD30** Q
- **EBV** is **not associated** with this subtype and it has **excellent prognosis** Q

Ans. 85) A. Nodal disease, splenic disease, hepatic disease, bone marrow (Ref: 8 ed. Robbins p.620, 9 ed. p. 610-11, t-13-9)

Spread of Hodgkin disease Q occurs in following manner:

- **Nodal disease** first, followed by **splenic disease, hepatic disease** and finally the involvement of the **marrow**

Ann Arbor Classification of HD and NHL

Stage	Distribution of disease
I	Involvement of a single lymph node region (I) or a single Extra-lymphatic organ or site (IE)
II	Involvement of two or more lymph node regions on the same side of the diaphragm alone (II) or localized involvement of an extralymphatic organ or site (IIE)
III	Involvement of lymph node regions on both sides of the diaphragm without (III) or with (IIIE) localized involvement of an extralymphatic organ or site
IV	Diffuse involvement of one or more extralymphatic organs or sites with or without lymphatic involvement

Ans. 86) D. Any of the above (Ref: 8 ed. Robbins p.620, 9 ed. p. 610)

- **Hodgkin lymphoma** patients treated with **radiotherapy** [Q] have higher incidence of **lung cancer, melanoma** and **breast cancer** [Q]

Ans. 87) A. Acute myeloid leukemia (Ref: 8 ed. Robbins p.620, 9 ed. p. 610-11)

- Patients treated with early **chemotherapy regimens** have high incidence of **acute myeloid leukemia** [Q]

Ans. 88) C. AML with t(11q23) (Ref: 8 ed. Robbins p.622, 9 ed. p. 612, t-13-10)

WHO Classification of Acute myeloid Leukemia:

- AML with Genetic Aberrations
- AML with MDS-like Features
- AML, therapy-related
- AML, Not Otherwise Specified

AML with genetic aberrations [Q]**:**

Class	Prognosis
AML with t(8;21)	Favorable
AML with inv(16)	Favorable
AML with t(15;17)	Intermediate
AML with t(11q23)	Poor
AML with normal cytogenetics and mutated NPM	Favorable

Ans. 89) A. RARA/PML fusion gene (Ref: 8 ed. Robbins p.622-24, 9 ed. p. 612, t-13-10)

AML with **t (15; 17) (acute promyelocytic leukemia)** [Q]**:**

- **t(15;17)** leads to fusion of **retinoic acid receptor-α (RARα)** with protein **PML** leading to formation of **RARA/PML fusion gene product** [Q]
- This **fusion protein** interferes with the maturation of granulocytes
- **All-trans retinoic acid** or **arsenic trioxide** [Q] is used in treatment as this inhibits the fusion protein effect
- **AMLs** with **t(15;17)** have frequent activating mutations in **FLT3**

Ans. 90) D. AML with megakaryocytic maturation (Ref: 8 ed. Robbins p.622, 9 ed. p. 612, t-13-10)

AML with **megakaryocytic maturation** [Q]:

- Composed of **blasts** of **megakaryocytic lineage** [Q]
- Shows antibodies against **megakaryocyte-specific markers (GPIIb/IIIa or vWF)** [Q]
- Associated with **marrow fibrosis**
- **Most common AML** in **Down syndrome** [Q]

Ans. 91) D. 20% (Ref: 8 ed. Robbins p.622, 9 ed. p. 613, f-13-29, 30)

Morphology of AML [Q]**:**

- **Diagnosis** is based on the presence of at least **20% myeloid blasts** in the **bone marrow**

Myeloblasts [Q]:

- Has moderate amount of cytoplasm, delicate nuclear chromatin, **two to four** nucleoli
- Cytoplasm contains **fine, peroxidase positive** azurophilic granules
- **Auer rods** [Q]**:** Distinctive **needle-like azurophilic granules**, present in patients with **AML** with **t(15;17) (acute promyelocytic leukemia)** [Q]

Monoblasts [Q]**:**

- Shows **folded** or **lobulated** nuclei, **lack Auer rods** and are **nonspecific esterase (NSE) positive** [Q]

Aleukemic Leukemia:

- Occasionally, **blasts are absent** from the blood, hence **bone marrow examination** is essential to exclude acute leukemia

Ans. 92) C. AML with monocytic maturation (Ref: 8 ed. Robbins p.624, 9 ed. p. 614)

Clinical Features of AML [Q]:

- **AML with monocytic differentiation** often infiltrate the **skin (leukemia cutis)** and **gingiva**
- **Central nervous system** spread is less common than **ALL**
- Can also present as a localized soft-tissue mass (**myeloblastoma, granulocytic sarcoma** or **chloroma**)

Ans. 93) A. AML with t(15;17) (Ref: 8 ed. Robbins p.624, 9 ed. p. 614)

Prognosis of AML:

- Due to treatment using **all-trans retinoic acid** and **arsenic salts**, AMLs with **t(15;17)** has **best prognosis** [Q]
- AMLs with **t(8;21)** or **inv(16)** has **good prognosis** with **chemotherapy**
- Bad prognosis is in **AML that follow MDS** or genotoxic therapy, or in older adults

Ans. 94) A. AML with t(15;17) (Ref: 8 ed. Robbins p.622, 9 ed. p. 612-14, t-13-10)

Clinical Features of AML with t (15; 17) [Q]**:**

- **Procoagulants** and **fibrinolytic factors** released by leukemic cells exacerbate the bleeding tendency
- Increased incidence of **DIC (disseminated intravascular coagulation)** [Q]

Ans. 95) D. Any of the above (Ref: 8 ed. Robbins p.625, 9 ed. p. 614-15)

Chromosomal abnormalities [Q] seen in **MDS** include:

- Monosomy 5 and 7
- Deletions of 5q, 7q and 20q
- Trisomy 8

Ans. 96) D. Myeloid blasts >20% (Ref: 8 ed. Robbins p.625, 9 ed. p. 615, f-13-31)

Morphology of MDS [Q]**:**

Bone Marrow Examination:

- **Cellularity**: Hypercellular marrow or can be normocellular or hypocellular
- **Most characteristic finding** is **dysplastic differentiation** [Q] affecting the erythroid, granulocytic, monocytic and megakaryocytic lineages

Erythroid series [Q]:

- **Ring sideroblasts** (erythroblasts with iron-laden perinuclear granules seen on Prussian blue-stain)
- **Megaloblastoid maturation** and **nuclear budding** abnormalities
- **Neutrophils** with reduced numbers of secondary granules, toxic granulations and/or Döhle bodies
- **Pseudo-Pelger-Hüet cells** i.e. neutrophils with only two nuclear lobes

Megakaryocytes Q:

- Shows **single nuclear lobe** or **multiple, separate nuclei (pawn ball megakaryocytes)**

Myeloid Series Q:

- Blasts may be increased but are **less than 20%** of the marrow cellularity

Peripheral Smear Q:

- **RBC**: macrocytes and poikilocytes
- **WBC**: Pseudo-Pelger-Hüet cells, monocytosis
- **Platelets**: Giant platelets
- **Myeloid blasts** are **less than 10%** of total leukocyte count

Ans. 97) D. All of the above (Ref: 8 ed. Robbins p.626, 9 ed. p. 616)

Common features among **myeloproliferative disorders** Q:

- **Increased proliferative drive** in the bone marrow
- Extramedullary hematopoiesis
- Can undergo transformation to **spent phase** characterized by **marrow fibrosis** and peripheral **blood cytopenias**
- Transformation to **acute leukemia** Q

Ans. 98) D. Any of the above (Ref: 8 ed. Robbins p.626, 9 ed. p. 616, t-13-11)

Tyrosine Kinase Mutations in **Myeloproliferative Disorders** Q:

Disorder	Mutation
Chronic myelogenous leukemia	BCR-ABL fusion gene
Polycythemia vera	JAK2 point mutations
Essential thrombocythemia	JAK2 point mutations
Primary myelofibrosis	JAK2 point mutations, MPL point mutations
Systemic mastocytosis	KIT point mutations
Chronic eosinophilic leukemia	FIP1L1-PDGFRA fusion gene
Stem cell leukemia	FGFR1 fusion genes (various)

Ans. 99) A. t(9;22) (Ref: 8 ed. Robbins p.627, 9 ed. p. 616-17, f-13-32)

Pathogenesis of **Chronic Myelogenous Leukemia** Q:

- **Characterized** by presence of **BCR-ABL gene translocation**, with **BCR gene** on **chromosome 22** and **ABL gene** on **chromosome 9**
- **BCR-ABL** leads to synthesis of **BCR-ABL tyrosine kinase**, which is **210 kDa** Q in size
- **BCR-ABL** increases proliferation of **granulocytic** and **megakaryocytic precursors**
- **BCR-ABL** leads to abnormal release of **immature granulocytic forms** Q from the marrow into the **blood**

Ans. 100) D. Large megakaryocytes (Ref: 8 ed. Robbins p.627, 9 ed. p. 617, f-13-33)

Morphology of Bone Marrow in CML Q:

- **Hypercellular marrow**
- **Marked increased numbers** of **maturing granulocytic precursors** Q
- Increased **eosinophils** and **basophils**
- **Megakaryocytes: Increased** in number and appear **"dwarf"** Q
- **Sea-blue histiocytes** Q: Scattered macrophages with abundant wrinkled, green-blue cytoplasm

Ans. 101) D. Reduced platelets (Ref: 8 ed. Robbins p.627, 9 ed. p. 617, f-13-33,34)

Blood Smear Findings in CML Q:

- **Leukocytosis > 100,000 cells/mm^3**

- **Predominant cell population** includes **neutrophils, band forms**, metamyelocytes, **myelocytes**, eosinophils and basophils
- **< 10%** [Q] **blasts**
- **Increased Platelet count**

Note: Massive splenomegaly [Q] is seen due to extensive **extramedullary hematopoiesis**

Ans. 102) D. > 20 % blasts (Ref: 4th ed. WHO Classification of Tumours of the Hematopoietic and Lymphoid Tissues, p. 32-35)

3 Phases of CML: Chronic phase, Accelerated phase and Blast crisis

Criteria for diagnosing **Accelerated phase (AP)** of **CML** [Q]:

a) **Persistent or increasing WBC count** and/or **persistent or increasing splenomegaly** unresponsive to therapy
b) **Persistent thrombocytosis** uncontrolled by therapy
c) **Persistent thrombocytopenia** unrelated to therapy
d) 20% or more **basophils** in the peripheral blood
e) **10-19% Myeloblasts** in the blood

Ans. 103) C. Both of the above (Ref: 8 ed. Robbins p.627-28, 9 ed. p. 618)

Blast crisis phase of CML [Q]:

- Blasts are of **myeloid origin (myeloid blast crisis)** or of **B cell origin (lymphoid blast crisis)**

Note: In patients with **lymphoid blast crisis**, additional mutations in ***"Ikaros"*** [Q] are seen

Ans. 104) D. Any of the above (Ref: 8 ed. Robbins p.627-28, 9 ed. p. 618)

Clinical Features of CML [Q]:

- Mild-to-moderate **anemia, fatigability, weakness, weight loss** and **anorexia**
- **Massive splenomegaly** leading to **dragging sensation** [Q] in the abdomen – first symptom
- **Left upper quadrant** abdominal pain due to **splenic infarction** [Q]

Ans. 105) D. Normal erythropoietin levels (Ref: 4th ed. WHO Classification of Tumours of the Hematopoietic and Lymphoid Tissues, p.40-41)

Diagnostic Criteria of Polycythemia Vera (PV) [Q]:

Major criteria [Q]

1. Hemoglobin >18.5 g/dL in men, 16.5 g/dl in women or other evidence of increased red cell volume
2. Presence of ***JAK2 V617F*** mutation

Minor criteria [Q]

1. **Panmyelosis – Erythroid**, **granulocytic** and **megakaryocytic** proliferation
2. **Serum erythropoietin** levels are below normal levels [Q]
3. Endogenous erythroid colony formation

Diagnosis requires **both major criteria** and **one minor** criterion **or first major** criterion with **two minor** criteria

Ans. 106) D. None of the above (Ref: 8 ed. Robbins p.629, 9 ed. p. 619)

Polycythemia Vera can **evolve into** [Q]:

- **"Spent phase"**, during which clinical features of **primary myelofibrosis** [Q] develop
- In **2%** of patients, **PCV transforms** to **AML** [Q]

Ans. 107) D. Any of the above (Ref: 8 ed. Robbins p.629-30, 9 ed. p. 619-20)

Essential Thrombocytosis (ET): [Q]

- Associated with point mutations in ***JAK2*** or ***MPL*** [Q]
- Mutations in **calreticulin** [Q] are also seen

- **Peripheral smears** reveal **abnormally large platelets** Q
- **Megakaryocytes** in **bone marrow** are **markedly increased** in number and shows **abnormally large forms** Q

Note: Causes of reactive thrombocytosis: **inflammatory disorders** Q and **iron deficiency** Q

WHO criteria for diagnosis of ET:

1. Sustained **platelet count > 450x 10^9/L**
2. **Bone marrow biopsy** specimen shows proliferation of **megakaryocytic lineage**
3. Not meeting WHO criteria of Polycythemia Vera, Primary myelofibrosis, BCR-ABL positive CML or myelodysplaslic syndrome
4. Demonstration of ***JAK2V617F*** mutation

Ans. 108) D. All of the above (Ref: 8 ed. Robbins p.630, 9 ed. p. 620)

Primary Myelofibrosis Q**:**

- **Hallmark** is the development of **marrow fibrosis**
- Activating ***JAK2***, ***MPL*** and ***calreticulin*** Q mutations are seen
- **Chief pathologic feature** – Extensive deposition of **collagen** in the marrow by non-neoplastic fibroblasts
- Fibrogenic factors includes **Platelet-derived growth factor** and **TGF-β** Q

Ans. 109) D. Leucoerythroblastosis (Ref: 4th ed. WHO Classification of Tumours of the Hematopoietic and Lymphoid Tissues, p.40-41)

WHO Criteria for Diagnosis of Primary myelofibrosis

Major criteria Q**:**

1. Presence of megakaryocyte proliferation (**cloud like appearance**) and **atypia** accompanied by collagen and reticulin fibrosis
2. Not meeting WHO criteria of polycythemia, BCR-ABL+ve chronic myelogenous leukemia, myelodysplastic syndrome
3. Demonstration of ***JAK2 V617F*** mutation

Minor criteria Q**:**

1. Leucoerythroblastosis
2. Increase in serum lactate dehydrogenase level
3. Anemia
4. Splenomegaly

Diagnosis requires **3 major** and **2 minor** criteria

Note: Extensive **extra medullary hematopoiesis** is seen in **spleen**

Ans. 110) D. All of the above (Ref: 8 ed. Robbins p.630-31, 9 ed. p. 620-21, f-13-37)

Peripheral smear findings in **Myelofibrosis** Q**:**

- **Leucoerythroblastosis** Q: Due to premature release of nucleated erythroid and early granulocyte progenitors
- **Teardrop-shaped** Q red cells (dacryocytes)
- Abnormally large platelets and
- Basophilia

Bone marrow aspirate: Shows **clusters of atypical megakaryocytes ("cloud-like")** Q and **hematopoietic elements** within the **dilated sinusoids** Q

Ans. 111) D. All of the above (Ref: 8 ed. Robbins p.630-31, 9 ed. p. 620-21, f-13-37)

Causes of **Leucoerythroblastosis** and **dacryocytes** Q:

- **Primary myelofibrosis**

- Infiltrative disorders of the marrow, including **granulomatous diseases** and **metastatic tumors**

Ans. 112) D. All of the above (Ref: 8 ed. Robbins p.631-32, 9 ed. p. 621-22, f-13-38)

Langerhans Cell Histiocytosis (LCH) Q:

- **Most common** activating **mutation** seen is **BRAF** Q mutation followed by mutations in **TP53, RAS** and the tyrosine kinase **MET**
- **Langerhans cells** have **abundant, vacuolated cytoplasm** and **vesicular nuclei** containing **linear grooves** or **folds** Q
- **Birbeck granules** Q in the cytoplasm is characteristic and **dilated terminal end** produces a **tennis racket-like appearance** Q
- Tumor cells **express HLA-DR, S-100** and **CD1a** Q

Ans. 113) A. Letterer-Siwe disease affects predominantly adults(Ref: 8 ed. Robbins p.631-32, 9 ed. p. 622)

Multifocal Multisystem LCH (Letterer-Siwe disease) Q:

- **Most commonly** seen in **children younger than 2 years** of age Q
- Presents as a **seborrheic eruption**, over the trunk and on **scalp**
- **Hepatosplenomegaly, lymphadenopathy, pulmonary lesions** and **osteolytic bone lesions** are seen
- Extensive infiltration of the marrow leads to **anemia, thrombocytopenia**
- Predisposition to **recurrent infections**, such as **otitis media** and **mastoiditis** Q
- Rapidly fatal diseases

Eosinophilic Granuloma Q:

- Characterized by **proliferation of Langerhans cells** with **eosinophils (predominant population)**, lymphocytes, plasma cells and neutrophils
- Most commonly affects the **calvarium, ribs and femur** Q
- **Bone lesions – Asymptomatic** or cause pain, tenderness, pathologic fractures
- **Diabetes insipidus** Q (due to involvement of **posterior pituitary stalk** of hypothalamus)
- **Hand-Schüller-Christian triad** Q: Includes **calvarial bone defects, diabetes insipidus** and **exophthalmos**

Pulmonary Langerhans Cell Histiocytosis:

- Seen in **adult smokers** and may **regress** after cessation of smoking

Ans. 114) D. All of the above (Ref: 8 ed. Robbins p.632-33, 9 ed. p. 623-24)

Major Functions of Spleen Q:

1. Phagocytosis of blood cells
   - **Heinz bodies** and **Howell-Jolly bodies** are formed due to **"pitting"** of **red cells** by **splenic macrophages**
2. Antibody production
3. Hematopoiesis
   - **In severe anemia**, spleen becomes a major site of **extra medullary hematopoiesis**
4. Sequestration of formed blood elements
   - **Enlarged spleen** can trap platelets and **leucocytes**
   - **Hypersplenism** Q is characterized by **anemia, leukopenia** and **thrombocytopenia**

Ans. 115) D. All of the above (Ref: 8 ed. Robbins p.632-33, 9 ed. p. 623-24)

- **Splenectomy** or **auto-infarction (sickle-cell disease)** leads to increased susceptibility to **sepsis**
- Sepsis occurs due to encapsulated bacteria – **Pneumococci, meningococci** and ***Haemophilus influenzae*** Q
- **Asplenic individuals** should be vaccinated against these **encapsulated bacteria** Q

Ans. 116) D. All of the above (Ref: 8 ed. Robbins p.635, 9 ed. p. 625)

- Splenic rupture is precipitated by **blunt trauma** Q

- **Splenic rupture** can also be seen in – **Infectious mononucleosis, malaria, typhoid fever** and **lymphoid neoplasms** Q

Ans. 117) A. Myasthenia gravis (Ref: 8 ed. Robbins p.635, 9 ed. p. 626)

Thymic Follicular Hyperplasia Q:

- Appearance of **B-cell germinal centers** within the thymus
- **Most frequently** occurs in **myasthenia gravis** Q
- Also seen in **Graves' disease, Systemic lupus erythematosus, Scleroderma, Rheumatoid arthritis** Q

Ans. 118) D. All of the above (Ref: 8 ed. Robbins p.636, 9 ed. p. 626)

- **Neoplasms** that can arise in **thymus** include **thymoma, germ cell tumors, lymphomas, carcinoids** Q

Ans. 119) A. Anterior superior mediastinum (Ref: 8 ed. Robbins p.636, 9 ed. p. 626)

- **Most common site** Q of **thymoma** is **anterior superior mediastinum** Q
- Thymoma can be seen in **neck, thyroid and pulmonary hilus** and rarely in the **posterior mediastinum** Q

Ans. 120) D. Hypergammaglobulinemia (Ref: 8 ed. Robbins p.637, 9 ed. p. 627)

Autoimmune disorders associated with **Thymoma** Q:

- **Myasthenia gravis**
- **Hypogammaglobulinemia**
- **Pure red cell aplasia**
- Graves' disease, pernicious anemia
- Dermatomyositis-polymyositis
- Cushing syndrome

Ans. 121) D. All of the above (Ref: Ackerman 10 ed. p. 445)

Differential diagnosis of tumors of the **anterior mediastinum** Q:

- Thymoma, Large cell lymphoma, Lymphoblastic lymphoma, Thymic Hodgkin lymphoma, Thymic seminoma, Thymic carcinoid

Ans. 122) A. Nodular sclerosis (Ref: Robbins 9 ed. p. 607-610) Refer Q 82 for details

Ans. 123) D. Low levels of plasma ferritin (Ref 9 ed. Robbins p. 585) Refer Q 15 for details

Ans. 124) A. Langerhans cell histiocytosis (Ref: 9 ed. Robbins p. 621-622) Refer Q 112 for details

Ans. 125) C. Nodular sclerosis (Ref: 9 ed. Robbins p. 607) Refer Q 82 for details

Ans. 126) B. Skull (Ref: ed. Robbins p. 622) Refer Q 113 for details

Ans. 127) A. Burkitt lymphoma (Ref: 9 ed. Robbins p. 597) Refer Q 44 for details

Ans. 128) C. Lymphocyte predominant (Ref: Robbins 9 ed. p. 609) Refer Q 84 for details

Ans. 129) A. Tennis racket (Ref: 9 ed. Robbins p.621-22) Refer Q 122 for details

Ans. 130) B. CD 21 (Ref: 9 ed. Robbins p. 590) CD 21 – EBV receptor, present on mature B-cells and Follicular dendritic cells

Ans. 131) A. Age <2 years (Ref: 9 ed. Robbins p. 611-14) Refer Q 88-94 form details

Ans. 132) A. Plasma cells (Ref: 9 ed. Robbins p. 598-599) Refer Q 54 for details

Ans. 133) D. Response to steroids (Ref: 9 ed. Robbins p.592-93) Refer Q 29 for details

Ans. 134) A. Hyperploidy (Ref: 9 ed. Robbins p. 592) Refer Q 29 for details

Ans. 135) A. Bone marrow (Ref: 9 ed. Robbins p. 580)

Ans. 136) A. Burkitt's lymphoma (Ref: 9 ed. Robbins p.597) Refer Q 14 for details

Ans. 137) D. CD 5+, CD 23- (Ref: 9 ed. Robbins p. 602-03) Refer Q 64 for details

Ans. 138) B. Immature B cells (Ref: 9 ed. Robbins p. 590) Refer Q 2 for details

Ans. 139) B. CD1a marker present (Ref: 9 ed. Robbins p. 621-22) Refer Q 112 for details

Ans. 140) B. Hyperalbuminemia (Ref: 9 ed. Robbins p. 627)

Ans. 141) B. t (15,17) (Ref: 9 ed. Robbins p. 612) Refer Q 89 for details

Ans. 142) A. Hodgkin disease (Ref: 9 ed. Robbins p. 606) Refer Q 75 for details

Ans. 143) A. Acute promyelocytic leukemia (Ref: 9 ed. Robbins p. 612-14) Refer Q 94 for details

Ans. 144) A. B cell lymphoma (Ref: 9 ed. Robbins p.588, 603) Refer Q 65 for details

Ans. 145) C. Myeloperoxidase

- Myeloperoxidase stain distinguishes between the immature cells in acute myeloblastic leukemia (cells stain positive) from those in acute lymphoblastic leukemia (cells stain negative)

Ans. 146) A. CD 23 (Ref: 9 ed. Robbins p. 602-03) Refer Q 64 for details

Ans. 147) A. Multiple Myeloma (Ref: 9 ed. Robbins p.599) Refer Q 54 for details

Ans. 148) D. Chronic myeloid leukemia

- Low LAP score is seen in CML, Paroxysmal nocturnal hemoglobinuria, Hematological neoplasm, Myelodysplastic syndrome

Ans. 149) A. Dilated endoplasmic reticulum in neutrophils (Ref: 9 ed. Robbins p.583-84) Refer Q8 for details

Ans. 150) A. t (8:14) (Ref: 9 ed. Robbins p.597) Refer Q 43 for details

Ans. 151) D. Burkitt lymphoma (Ref: 9ed. Robbins p. 597) Refer Q 43 for details

Ans. 152) B. Kikuchi disease (Ref: Ch. 21, 10 ed. Ackerman)

- In, Kikuchi disease, the affected nodes show focal, well-circumscribed, paracortical necrotizing lesions

Ans. 153) B. t (9; 22) t (4;11) (Ref: 9 ed. Robbins p. 592-93) Refer Q 29 for details

Ans. 154) C. Acute lymphoid leukemia in less than 1 year has a poor prognosis (Ref: 9 ed. Robbins p.592-93) Refer Q 29 for details

Ans. 155) B. Long term reconstitution of bone marrow (Ref: 8 ed. Robbins p 590-593)

- **Hematopoietic stem cells are pluripotent or totipotent undifferentiated cells capable of self-renewal through numerous cycles of cell division**

Ans. 156) A. R.B.C. (Ref: 8 ed. Robbins p 590-593)

- **Hematopoietic stem cells are able to generate every lineage found in the hematopoietic system including red blood cells, platelets and lymphoid cells**
- **If myeloid progenitor cells are injected in an ablated animal it would differentiate into cells of myeloid series i.e. red cells, platelets, granulocytes (WBC) and monocytes**
- **But, in an ablated animal, hematopoietic stem cells are not present and thus, bone marrow cannot be reconstituted i.e., mature blood cells of other lineage are not generated**

Hence, the answer here is RBC's only

Ans. 157) C. Coombs test (Ref: 9 ed. Robbins p. 631-32)

- Coombs test is used to differentiate between autoimmune hemolytic anemia (positive) from hereditary spherocytosis (negative)

Ans. 158) D. Translocation involving MYC-gene (Ref: 9 ed. Robbins p.597) Refer Q 43 & 44 for details

Ans. 159) C. AML (Ref: 9ed. Robbins p. 428-29)

- t (8;21)is seen in AML

Acute Leukemias has the following characteristics:

- Fatigue (due to anemia), fever (reflecting infections resulting from neutropenia) and bleeding (petechiae, ecchymosis, epistaxis, gum bleeding) secondary to thrombocytopenia
- Bone pain and tenderness
- Generalized lymphadenopathy, splenomegaly and hepatomegaly due to dissemination of the leukemic cells
- Central nervous system manifestations, including headache, vomiting and nerve palsies resulting from meningeal spread

Laboratory Findings in Acute Leukemias:

- White cell count can be greater than 100,000 cells/µL or less than 10,000 cells/µL
- Anemia is almost always present and the platelet count usually is below 100,000/µL
- Neutropenia is another common finding

1) Acute Lymphoblastic Leukemia/Lymphoblastic Lymphoma

- Acute lymphoblastic leukemia (ALL) and lymphoblastic lymphoma are aggressive tumors, composed of immature lymphocytes (lymphoblast), occur predominantly in children and young adults
- Karyotypic abnormalities in childhood pre-B cell tumors are hyperdiploidy and presence of t (12; 21) involving the TEL1 and AML1 genes, 25% of adult pre-B cell tumors harbor t(9; 22), involving the BCR and ABL genes

2) Chronic Lymphocytic Leukemia/Small Lymphocytic Lymphoma

- **Neoplasm arising from Mature B cells**

Immunophenotypic and Genetic Features:

- Expresses pan-B cell markers: CD19, CD20 and CD23, surface immunoglobulin heavy and light chains and CD5
- Karyotypic abnormalities include Trisomy 12 and deletions of chromosomes 11, 13 and 17
- Notch 1 receptor mutation predicts worst outcome

3) Acute Myeloid Leukemia

- Affects older adults; the median age is 50 years
- AML with recurrent genetic abnormalities includes:

Favorable prognosis – t (8; 21), inv16, t (15; 17)

Poor prognosis – t (11q23)

Myelodysplastic Syndromes (MDS)

- Marrow usually is hypercellular or normocellular
- Peripheral blood shows one or more cytopenias
- Some common karyotypic abnormalities include Monosomy 5 or 7; 5q, 7q and 20q deletions and trisomy 8

Ans. 160) C. Leukocyte common antigen (Ref: 9 ed. p.590)

- CD45 (leucocyte common antigen) is exclusively expressed in hematolymphoid cells
- 90% of malignant lymphomas are CD45 positive

Important Tumor Markers:

Epithelial cell carcinoma – Cytokeratin

Lymphoid cell carcinoma – CD45

Melanocytes – S100, HMB45

Mesenchymal markers – Vimentin

Neuroendocrine markers – Chromogranin, Neuron specific enolase

Ans. 161) C. Acute megakaryocytic leukemia (Ref: 9 ed. Robbins p. 612) Refer Q 90 for details

Ans. 162) B. Peripheral Immunophenotyping (Ref: 9 ed. Robbins p.593-95) Refer Q 31-36 for details

Ans. 163) B. Nodular sclerosis Hodgkin lymphoma (Ref: Robbins 8th p. 617-619) Refer Q 8 for details

Reed Sternberg Cells:

- Large cells and are either multinucleated or have a bi-lobed nucleus (owl eye's appearance) with prominent eosinophilic inclusion like nucleoli
- Negative for CD20 and CD45 and positive for CD15 and CD30
- Presence of these cells is necessary in diagnosis of Hodgkin lymphoma

Ans. 164) A. Hodgkin's lymphoma; Epstein Barr Virus and Reed Sternberg cells (Ref: 9 ed. Robbins p. 606) Refer Q 75 for details

28 Red Blood Cell and Bleeding Disorders

How to go about this chapter?

- **One should be thorough with the following topics:**
  - **Red cell indices**
  - **Hemolytic anemia**
  - **Hereditary spherocytosis, G-6 PD deficiency**
  - **Sickle cell anemia**
  - **Thalassemia**
  - **Paroxysmal Nocturnal Hemoglobinemia**
  - **Megaloblastic/Folic acid deficiency anemia**
  - **Iron deficiency anemia**
  - **Anemia of chronic disease**
  - **Hepcidin protein**
  - **Aplastic anemia**
  - **Polycythemia Vera**
  - **Thrombotic thrombocytopenic purpura (TTP) and Hemolytic uremic syndrome (HUS)**
  - **Disseminated blood transfusion**
  - **Complications of blood transfusion**

INTRODUCTION

1) **TRUE about red cell indices:**
   a) Mean cell volume is expressed in femtoliters
   b) Mean cell hemoglobin is expressed in picograms
   c) Mean cell hemoglobin concentration is expressed in gram/dl
   d) All of the above

2) **Significant bleeding in patient can lead to following changes:**
   a) Increased WBC count
   b) Increased reticulocyte count
   c) Increased platelet count
   d) All of the above

3) **All are TRUE about Intravascular hemolysis EXCEPT:**
   a) Caused by mechanical injury to the RBC's
   b) Hemoglobinuria is seen
   c) Normal haptoglobin levels
   d) Anemia and jaundice are seen

4) **Morphological changes of hemolytic anemia include(s):**
   a) Normoblasts
   b) Increased reticulocyte count
   c) Hemosiderosis
   d) All of the above

HEREDITARY SPHEROCYTOSIS

5) **Following protein defects can cause hereditary spherocytosis EXCEPT:**
   a) Ankyrin
   b) Paladin
   c) Glycophorin C
   d) Band 3

6) **Aplastic anemia in hereditary spherocytosis precipitated by:**
   a) Parvo virus
   b) HIV
   c) Adenovirus
   d) Influenza virus

7) **Osmotic fragility is increased in:**
   a) Sickle cell anemia
   b) Thalassemia
   c) Hereditary spherocytosis
   d) Chronic lead poisoning

GLUCOSE 6 PHOSPHATE DEHYDROGENASE DEFICIENCY

8) **TRUE about G6PD deficiency:**
a) X-linked recessive trait
b) G6PD deficient patients are resistant to plasmodium falciparum
c) Hemolysis is precipitated by oxidant stress
d) All of the above

9) **Trigger(s) that lead to hemolysis in G-6PD deficient patients:**
a) Infections b) Food
c) Drugs d) Any of the above

10) **Feature(s) of G-6PD deficient patients include(s):**
a) Hemoglobinemia b) Heinz bodies
c) Bite cells d) All of the above

SICKLE CELL ANEMIA

11) **Sickle cell anemia occurs due to a point mutation in which there is:**
a) Replacement of glutamine with valine at sixth codon of β-globin
b) Replacement of valine with glutamine at sixth codon of β-globin
c) Replacement of glutamine with valine at sixth codon of α-globin
d) Replacement of valine with glutamine at sixth codon of α-globin

12) **Rate of sickling of RBC's is affected by:**
a) Interaction of HbS with other hemoglobin
b) Mean cell hemoglobin concentration
c) Transit time of RBC's through the microvascular beds
d) All of the above

13) **Following is/are features of sickle cell anemia on peripheral smear:**
a) Irreversibly sickle cells
b) Howell-Jolly bodies
c) Reticulocytosis
d) All of the above

14) **Most common acute presentation of sickle cell anemia is:**
a) Priapism
b) Bone pain
c) Fever
d) Splenomegaly

15) **Crew haircut appearance in X-rays skull and Gamna Gandy bodies are seen in:**
a) G-6PD deficiency
b) Hodgkin lymphoma
c) Hereditary spherocytosis
d) Sickle cell anemia

16) **Sickle cell trait is protective against which infection?**
a) Hepatitis B b) Salmonella
c) Staphylococcus d) Plasmodium

17) **Most commonly used agent for treatment of Sickle cell anemia:**
a) Hydroxyurea b) Decitabine
c) Cytarabine d) 5-azacytidine

18) **Autosplenectomy is seen in:**
a) Sickle cell anemia
b) G-6PD deficiency
c) Hereditary spherocytosis
d) Any of the above

THALASSEMIA

19) **TRUE about molecular pathogenesis of β-Thalassemia:**
a) β^0 mutations are associated with absent β-globin synthesis
b) Splicing mutations are the most common cause of β^+-thalassemia
c) Chain terminator mutations are the most common cause of β^0-thalassemia
d) All of the above

20) **Ineffective erythropoiesis lead(s) to:**
a) Erythroid hyperplasia
b) Extramedullary hematopoiesis
c) Secondary hemochromatosis
d) All of the above

21) **In Beta thalassemia, there is:**
a) Increase in beta chain, decrease in alpha chain
b) Decrease in beta chain, increase in alpha chain
c) Decrease in beta chain, decrease in alpha chain
d) Increase in beta chain, increase in alpha chain

22) **TRUE about Beta thalassemia major:**
a) Manifestation of anemia after 6 months of birth
b) Hemoglobin levels between 3-6 gm%
c) Elevated HbF
d) All of the above

23) **All are TRUE about peripheral smear findings of Beta thalassemia major EXCEPT:**
a) Microcytic hypochromic anemia
b) Target cells
c) Low reticulocyte count
d) Basophilic stippling

24) **Crew-cut appearance in X-rays skull is seen in:**
a) Thalassemia
b) Hydrocephalus
c) Chronic malaria
d) Sickle cell anemia

25) **NESTROFT test used as screening test in:**
a) Beta thalassemia
b) Sickle cell anemia

c) AIHA
d) G6PD deficiency

26) All are TRUE about Beta thalassemia trait EXCEPT:
a) Raised HbF
b) Raised HbA2
c) Microcytosis
d) Severe anemia

27) HbH is associated with:
a) Deletion of 3 alpha chains
b) Deletion of 4 alpha chains
c) Deletion of 3 beta chains
d) Deletion of 4 beta chains

28) TRUE about a-thalassemia trait:
a) Increased HbF
b) Increased HbA2
c) Microcytosis
d) Severe anemia

PNH

29) Stem cell disorder affecting all the three cell line i.e. platelets, RBCs and leucocytes is:
a) Hemolytic anemia
b) Paroxysmal cold hemoglobinuria
c) Paroxysmal nocturnal hemoglobinemia
d) Blackfan Diamond syndrome

30) PNH blood cells are deficient in:
a) CD55 b) CD59
c) C8 d) All of the above

31) Which of the following is NOT seen in PNH?
a) Thrombosis
b) Hemosiderinuria
c) Decreased LDH
d) Thrombocytopenia

32) All are TRUE regarding PNH, EXCEPT:
a) Hemosiderinuria
b) Pancytopenia
c) Increased leukocyte alkaline phosphatase
d) Cellular marrow

33) Features of PNH are all EXCEPT:
a) Thrombosis
b) Pancytopenia
c) Splenomegaly
d) Can progress to myeloid leukemia

34) Gold standard test to diagnose PNH:
a) HAMS test
b) Sucrose lysis test
c) Flow cytometry
d) Bone marrow

35) Most common cause of death in PNH:
a) Venous thrombosis
b) Infection
c) Bleeding
d) None of the above

36) Treatment of PNH is:
a) Eculizumab b) Infliximab
c) Rituximab d) Alemtuzimab

IMMUNOHEMOLYTIC ANEMIA

37) Warm autoimmune hemolytic anemia may be seen in all of the following conditions EXCEPT:
a) Systemic lupus erythematous
b) Alpha-Methyl dopa therapy
c) Non-Hodgkin's lymphoma
d) Mycoplasma pneumonia

38) All of the following are TRUE about warm antibody type hemolytic anemia EXCEPT:
a) Most common form of Immune hemolytic anemia
b) Hemolysis is extravascular
c) Most common antibodies are of IgA type
d) Splenomegaly is seen

39) Causes of warm antibody immune hemolytic anemia:
a) Idiopathic
b) α-methyl dopa therapy
c) SLE
d) All of the above

40) Cold agglutinin antibody appears after following infection(s):
a) Mycoplasma pneumonia
b) Epstein-Barr virus
c) Cytomegalovirus
d) All of the above

41) Paroxysmal cold hemoglobinuria is caused by following antibody:
a) IgG b) IgM
c) IgA d) IgD

42) Microangiopathic hemolytic anemia most commonly occurs in:
a) DIC
b) TTP
c) SLE
d) Malignant hypertension

43) Following cell(s) is/are seen in hemolytic anemia:
a) Schistocyte
b) Burr cells
c) Helmet cells
d) Any of the above

44) Donath Landsteiner antibody is seen in:
a) PNH
b) Waldenstorm's macroglobulinemia
c) Paroxysmal cold hemoglobinuria
d) Malaria

45) Cold agglutinin is:
a) IgG b) IgM
c) IgA d) IgD

46) **Cold hemagglutinin is associated with:**
a) Anti IgM
b) Anti IgG
c) Anti IgA
d) Donath Landsteiner antibody

47) **Coombs positive hemolytic anemia is seen in:**
a) TTP b) SLE
c) ITP d) PNH

48) **Autoimmune hemolytic anemia is associated with:**
a) ALL b) AML
c) CML d) CLL

MEGALOBLASTIC ANEMIA

49) **Cause(s) of Vitamin B12 deficiency include(s):**
a) Diffuse intestinal disease
b) Parasitic infestation of GI tract
c) Intrinsic factor deficiency
d) Any of the above

50) **Cause(s) of Folic acid deficiency include(s):**
a) Alcoholism
b) Anticonvulsants
c) Pregnancy
d) Any of the above

51) **Megaloblastic anemia changes occurs due to:**
a) Impairment of DNA synthesis
b) Impairment of RNA synthesis
c) Impairment of mi-RNA synthesis
d) Any of the above

52) **All are TRUE about the morphology of megaloblastic anemia EXCEPT:**
a) Macro-ovalocytes
b) Low reticulocyte count
c) Elevated MCHC
d) Hyper-segmented neutrophils

53) **Bone marrow aspirate of Megaloblastic anemia show(s):**
a) Megaloblasts
b) Giant metamyelocyte/Band form
c) Delayed nuclear maturation
d) All of the above

54) **Marrow hyperplasia in megaloblastic anemia occurs due to:**
a) Increased erythropoietin levels
b) Ineffective erythropoiesis
c) Both of the above
d) None of the above

55) **Daily requirement of Vitamin B12:**
a) 1-2 μg
b) 2-3 μg
c) 3-4 μg
d) 4-5 μg

56) **TRUE about absorption of Vitamin B12:**
a) In stomach, vitamin B12 bind to haptocorrin
b) In duodenum, vitamin B12 associates with Intrinsic factor
c) In ileum, vitamin B12 is associated with Transcobalamin II
d) All of the above

57) **Megaloblastic anemia should be treated with both folic acid vitamin B12 because:**
a) Folic acid alone causes improvement of hematologic symptoms but worsening of neurological symptoms
b) Acts as a Co factor
c) Acts as an enzyme
d) None of the above

58) **Most common type of autoantibody responsible for pernicious anemia:**
a) Type I b) Type II
c) Type III d) Type IV

59) **All are TRUE about morphology of pernicious anemia EXCEPT:**
a) Atrophy of fundic glands
b) Intestinal metaplasia
c) Atrophic glossitis
d) Gastric atrophy is corrected by Vitamin B12 administration

60) **CNS lesions in Pernicious anemia include(s):**
a) Spastic paraparesis
b) Sensory ataxia
c) Paresthesias
d) Any of the above

61) **Diagnosis of pernicious anemia requires all EXCEPT:**
a) Leucopenia with hyper segmented granulocytes
b) Low serum Vitamin B12
c) Increased homocystine and methylmalonic acid
d) Low reticulocyte count following parenteral administration of Vitamin B12

62) **Complications associated with pernicious anemia include(s):**
a) Gastric carcinoma
b) Atherosclerosis
c) Thrombosis
d) Any of the above

63) **Daily requirement of Folic acid:**
a) 10-50 μg b) 50-200 μg
c) 200-400 μg d) 40-1000 μg

64) **Folic acid deficiency can be encountered in:**
a) Pregnancy
b) Infancy
c) Hemolytic anemia
d) All of the above

IRON DEFICIENCY ANEMIA

65) **TRUE about iron metabolism:**
a) Transported in plasma by transferrin
b) Iron is in storage pool either as ferritin or hemosiderin
c) Serum iron levels average 120 μg/dl in men and 100 μg in women
d) All of the above

66) **Ferritin is found in highest levels in:**
a) Liver b) Spleen
c) Bone marrow d) All of the above

67) **Iron in hemosiderin is detected by:**
a) MPO b) Von Kossa
c) Prussian blue d) Sudan Black

68) **All are TRUE about regulation of absorption of iron EXCEPT:**
a) Luminal iron (Fe^{3+}) must be reduced to Ferrous state (Fe^{2+}) by cytochrome B
b) Fe^{2+} is transported across the apical membrane by DMT-1
c) Fe^{2+} is transported from cytoplasm across basolateral membrane by ferroproten
d) Fe^{2+} before combining transferrin is converted to Fe^{3+} by hepcidin

69) **All of the following are TRUE about Hepcidin EXCEPT:**
a) Hepcidin is synthesized and released from liver
b) Hepcidin inhibits iron transfer by binding ferroprotein
c) With high iron levels hepcidin synthesis decreases
d) Hepcidin suppresses iron release from macrophages

70) **Pathology of anemia of chronic disease:**
a) Reduced hepcidin levels
b) Increased hepcidin levels
c) Both of the above
d) None of the above

71) **Hemochromatosis is associated with:**
a) High hepcidin levels
b) Low hepcidin levels
c) Both of the above
d) None of the above

72) **Daily iron requirement for adult men:**
a) 7-10 mg b) 10-15 mg
c) 15-25 mg d) 25-30 mg

73) **Absorption of inorganic iron is enhanced by all EXCEPT:**
a) Ascorbic acid
b) Citric acid
c) Oxalates
d) Sugars

74) **Plummer-Vinson syndrome include(s):**
a) Microcytic hypochromic anemia
b) Atrophic glossitis
c) Esophageal webs
d) All of the above

75) **Which of the following findings is diagnostic of iron deficiency anemia?**
a) Increased TIBC, decreased serum ferritin
b) Decreased TIBC, decreased serum ferritin
c) Increased TIBC, increased serum ferritin
d) Decreased TIBC, increased serum ferritin

ANEMIA OF CHRONIC DISEASE

76) **Anemia of chronic disease is characterized by all EXCEPT:**
a) Low serum iron
b) Reduced TIBC
c) Reduced ferritin
d) Increased bone marrow iron

77) **Cause(s) of Anemia of chronic disease:**
a) Osteomyelitis
b) Rheumatoid arthritis
c) Carcinoma lung
d) All of the above

78) **Following Interleukin is implicated in pathogenesis of Anemia of chronic disease:**
a) IL-1 b) IL-2
c) IL-5 d) IL-6

APLASTIC ANEMIA

79) **Cause(s) of aplastic anemia include(s):**
a) Idiopathic
b) Alkylating agents
c) Fanconi anemia
d) All of the above

80) **Following drug(s) has been implicated in Aplastic anemia:**
a) Chloramphenicol
b) Alkylating agents
c) Benzene
d) All of the above

81) **TRUE about aplastic anemia are all EXCEPT:**
a) Splenomegaly
b) Reticulocytopenia
c) Thrombocytopenia
d) Neutropenia

82) **Vashishta, 25-year-old-girl, presents with complaints of fever and weakness. On examination there is splenomegaly of 8 cm below the costal margin. Hb is 6 gm/dL, TLC is 3,500/mm³, and platelet count is 40,000/mm³. Which of the following is the least likely diagnosis?**

a) Acute lymphocytic leukemia
b) Anemia of chronic disease
c) Aplastic anemia
d) Megaloblastic anemia

83) Aplastic anemia can transform into:
a) Myeloid neoplasms
b) Lymphoid neoplasms
c) Non-Hodgkin's disease
d) Any of the above

84) Diagnostic modality for aplastic anemia:
a) Bone marrow aspirate
b) Bone marrow biopsy
c) Flow-cytometry
d) Peripheral smear

85) Clinical features of aplastic anemia includes all EXCEPT:
a) Pancytopenia
b) Reticulocytopenia
c) Splenomegaly
d) Predisposition to infections

86) Treatment of choice for aplastic anemia:
a) Anti-thymocyte globulin
b) Cyclosporine
c) Methotrexate
d) Bone marrow transplantation

PURE RED CELL APLASIA

87) Pure red cell aplasia is associated with:
a) Thymoma
b) Large granular cell lymphoma
c) Parvovirus infection
d) All of the above

88) Cause(s) of Myelophthisic anemia include(s):
a) Metastatic cancer
b) Granulomatous disease
c) Both of the above
d) None of the above

89) Features of myelophthisic anemia(s):
a) Nucleated erythroid precursors in peripheral smear
b) Immature granulocytes in peripheral smear
c) Tear drop shape of RBC's
d) All of the above

90) Anemia in chronic renal failure occurs due to:
a) Decreased synthesis of erythropoietin
b) Increased synthesis of erythropoietin
c) Both of the above
d) None of the above

POLYCYTHEMIA

91) Relative polycythemia occurs in:
a) Dehydration
b) Gaisbock syndrome
c) Excessive use of diuretics
d) All of the above

92) Causes of secondary polycythemia includes all EXCEPT:
a) Renal cell carcinoma
b) Hepatocellular carcinoma
c) Polycythemia vera
d) Cerebellar hemangioblastoma

BLEEDING DISORDERS

93) Prolonged Prothrombin time is seen due to deficiency of following factors EXCEPT:
a) Factor V b) Factor VII
c) Factor VIII d) Factor X

94) Cause(s) of petechial and purpuric hemorrhage:
a) Infections b) Drugs
c) Scurvy d) All of the above

95) Perivascular amyloidosis is seen with:
a) AA b) AL
c) Both of the above d) None of the above

96) Spontaneous bleeding can occur when the platelet count is less than:
a) 150,000/μL b) 100,000/μL
c) 50,000/μL d) 20,000/μL

97) Following is/are cause(s) of thrombocytopenia:
a) Aplastic anemia
b) SLE
c) Splenic sequestration
d) Any of the above

98) In Immune thrombocytopenic purpura auto-antibodies are of:
a) IgA class b) IgG class
c) IgD class d) IgM class

99) All of the following can cause megakaryocytic thrombocytopenia, EXCEPT:
a) Idiopathic thrombocytopenic purpura
b) Systemic lupus erythematosus
c) Aplastic anemia
d) Disseminated intravascular coagulation

100) Idiopathic thrombocytopenic purpura is associated with all of the following EXCEPT:
a) Splenomegaly
b) Mucosal bleeding
c) Thrombocytopenia
d) Increased megakaryocytes in bone marrow

101) A 6-year-old boy presents with ecchymoses and petechiae all over the body 2 weeks after an upper respiratory tract infection. Abdominal examination is unremarkable with no hepatosplenomegaly. All of the following statements about the affecting condition are TRUE EXCEPT:

a) Bleeding into the joints is a common manifestation
b) Bone marrow will show increased megakaryocytes
c) Platelet count is decreased
d) Condition resolves spontaneously in 80% of patients in 2 to 6 weeks

102) Following features are TRUE about Idiopathic thrombocytopenia, EXCEPT:
a) Acute ITP is often proceeded by viral infections
b) Chronic ITP is common in females
c) Spontaneous remission is common in chronic ITP
d) Acute ITP is more common in children

103) Following laboratory determinants is abnormally prolonged in ITP:
a) APTT
b) Prothrombin time
c) Bleeding time
d) Clotting time

104) Treatment options of Chronic ITP include(s):
a) Glucocorticoids
b) Splenectomy
c) Rituximab
d) Any of the above

THROMBOTIC THROMBOCYTOPENIC PURPURA (TTP) AND HEMOLYTIC UREMIC SYNDROME (HUS)

105) TTP includes all EXCEPT:
a) Renal failure
b) Macrocytic anemia
c) Thrombocytopenia
d) Fever

106) TTP is associated with deficiency of:
a) vWF metalloprotease
b) vWF
c) High molecular weight vWF
d) Metalloproteases

107) HUS includes all EXCEPT:
a) Microangiopathic hemolytic anemia
b) Thrombocytopenia
c) Neurological deficits
d) Acute renal failure

108) Atypical HUS is associated with all EXCEPT:
a) E. Coli 0157:H7
b) Complement factor H
c) CD46
d) Factor I

109) Following is TRUE about coagulation tests in TTP/HUS:
a) Prolonged PT
b) Prolonged APTT
c) Prolonged PT and APTT
d) Normal PT and APTT

110) TRUE about glycoprotein Ib-IX:
a) Deficiency leads to Bernard-Soulier syndrome
b) Receptor for vWF
c) Essential for normal platelet adhesion to sub-endothelial extracellular matrix
d) All of the above

111) TRUE about Glanzmann thrombasthemia:
a) Transmitted as autosomal recessive trait
b) Platelets fail to aggregate in response to ADP
c) Deficiency of gpIIb-IIIa
d) All of the above

112) Vitamin K deficiency leads to impaired synthesis of following EXCEPT:
a) Factor II b) Factor VIII
c) Factor X d) Protein C

113) Hemophilia A occurs due to deficiency of:
a) Factor VIII b) Factor IX
c) Factor X d) Factor II

114) Hemophilia B occurs due to deficiency of:
a) Factor VIII b) Factor IX
c) Factor X d) Factor II

115) Vitamin K deficiency results in impaired synthesis of:
a) Factor II b) Factor VII
c) Factor IX d) All of the above

116) Factor VIII is produced in:
a) Sinusoidal endothelial cells in liver
b) Kupffer cells in liver
c) Tubular epithelial cells in kidney
d) Any of the above

117) vWF factor is produced by:
a) Endothelial cells
b) Megakaryocytes
c) α-granules of platelets
d) Any of the above

118) Factor VIII bound to vWF has half-life of:
a) 2 hours b) 5 hours
c) 10 hours d) 12 hours

119) Following is the most common inherited bleeding disorder of humans:
a) vWD
b) Factor VIII deficiency
c) Factor X deficiency
d) Factor V Leidin mutation

120) Ristocetin test is used for diagnosis of:
a) Factor VIII deficiency
b) vWF deficiency
c) Factor X deficiency
d) None of the above

121) vWF function is assessed by:
a) Ristocetin agglutination test
b) ADP aggregation test
c) Both of the above
d) None of the above

122) vWD is treated by:
a) Desmopressin
b) Transfusion of Factor VIII
c) Transfusion of vWF
d) All of the above

123) TRUE about vWD:
a) Patients have defects in platelet function despite normal platelet count
b) Active vWF is reduced
c) vWF deficiency gives rise to secondary decrease in Factor VIII levels
d) Any of the above

124) TRUE about Hemophilia A:
a) Transmitted as Autosomal recessive disorder
b) Can affect heterozygous females
c) 30% patients have no family history
d) Patients with 2%-5% of normal factor VIII levels have severe disease

125) Genetic lesion of Factor VIII leading to most severe Hemophilia A:
a) Deletion
b) Non sense mutation
c) Inversion of X chromosome
d) Point mutation

126) Following features characterize Hemophilia EXCEPT:
a) Easy bruising
b) Spontaneous hemorrhage
c) Hemarthoses
d) Petechiae

127) Following is seen in Hemophilia A:
a) Normal PT, Prolonged APTT
b) Normal APTT, Prolonged PT
c) Normal PT, Normal APTT
d) Prolonged PT, Prolonged APTT

128) Following treatment of Hemophilia A has least rate of transmission of HIV:
a) Recombinant factor VIII therapy
b) Plasma derived factor VIII concentrates
c) Cryoprecipitate
d) Any of the above

129) Christmas disease occurs due to deficiency of:
a) Factor VIII
b) Factor IX
c) Factor X
d) Factor XI

DISSEMINATED INTRAVASCULAR COAGULATION (DIC)

130) Condition(s) associated with DIC:
a) Abruption placenta
b) Massive trauma
c) Burns
d) All of the above

131) Following are seen in DIC EXCEPT:
a) Prolonged PT
b) Prolonged APTT
c) Normal platelet count
d) Decreased fibrinogen levels

132) Following cancers are associated with DIC, EXCEPT:
a) Acute promyelocytic leukemia
b) Lung carcinoma
c) Colon carcinoma
d) Breast carcinoma

133) In DIC, thrombi are seen most commonly in:
a) Brain b) Heart
c) Lungs d) Kidney

134) Waterhouse-Friderichsen syndrome occurs due to thrombus in:
a) Adrenal b) Pituitary
c) Thyroid d) Kidney

135) TRUE about DIC:
a) 50% of patients have obstetric complications
b) Acute DIC is dominated by bleeding diathesis
c) Chronic DIC presents with thrombotic complications
d) All of the above

COMPLICATIONS OF TRANSFUSION

136) Most common complication of transfusion reaction:
a) Febrile non hemolytic reaction
b) Allergic reactions
c) Hemolytic reactions
d) Transfusion Related Acute Lung Injury

137) Fatal allergic reactions may occur in patients with deficiency of:
a) IgG b) IgA
c) IgM d) IgD

138) Urticarial allergic reaction can be recognized by presence of following antibody in recipient:
a) IgE b) IgD
c) IgM d) IgG

139) Acute hemolytic reaction is caused by the following preformed antibodies against donor red cells:
a) IgM b) IgG
c) IgA d) IgE

140) Delayed hemolytic transfusion reactions occurs due to following antibody:
a) IgG b) IgM
c) IgD d) IgE

141) Transfusion Related Acute Lung Injury occurs due to activation of:
a) Neutrophils
b) Lymphocytes
c) Monocytes
d) Eosinophils

142) Transfusion Related Acute Lung Injury is associated with transfusion of:
a) Plasma containing blood products
b) Fresh frozen plasma
c) Platelets
d) Any of the above

143) Antibodies associated with Transfusion Related Acute Lung Injury binds to:
a) MHC I b) MHC II
c) MHC III d) MHC IV

144) Transfusion which leads to increased risk of bacterial infection:
a) Plasma b) Platelet
c) Red cell d) Whole blood

145) Rate of transmission of following infection is highest after transfusion:
a) HIV
b) Hepatitis B
c) Hepatitis C
d) West-Nile virus

146) Which of the following is not TRUE about idiopathic thrombocytopenic purpura? (NEET 2014)
a) Antibodies of IgM class
b) Autoantibodies to Gp IIb/ IIIa or IB IX
c) Increased megakaryocytes in bone marrow
d) Spleen is normal in size

147) Hemophilia A occurs due to deficiency of: (NEET 2014)
a) Factor VIII
b) Factor IX
c) Factor X
d) Factor XI

148) Blood is stored at what temperature in blood bank? (NEET 2014)
a) -2 to -4 degrees Celsius
b) -2 to 0 degrees Celsius
c) 1 to 6 degrees Celsius
d) 6 to 12 degrees Celsius

149) Reticulocytes are stained by: (NEET 2014)
a) Supravital stain
b) Purssian blue stain
c) H & E stain
d) Reticulin stain

150) Normal reticulocyte count in newborn is: (NEET 2014)
a) 0 - 1% b) 1 - 1.5%
c) 3 - 6% d) 6 - 9%

151) Giant platelets are seen in: (NEET 2014)
a) Bernard-Soulier syndrome
b) vWD
c) Polycythemia rubra vera
d) Leukemia

152) Pelger Huet anomaly shows presence of: (NEET 2014)
a) Hyposegmented neutrophil
b) Hypersegmented neutrophil
c) Unsegmented neutrophil
d) None of the above

153) DIC is seen in all EXCEPT: (NEET 2014)
a) Carcinoma pancreas
b) Carcinoma prostate
c) Carcinoma lung
d) Carcinoma kidney

154) PT is used to test: (NEET 2014)
a) Extrinsic and common pathway
b) Intrinsic and common pathway
c) Intrinsic pathway
d) Extrinsic pathway

155) Most common cause of aplastic anemia is: (NEET 2014)
a) Exposure to drugs
b) Viral hepatitis
c) Fanconi anemia
d) Fungal infection

156) FFP is stored at what temperature? (NEET 2014)
a) 2 - 4 degrees Celsius
b) 0- (-25) degrees Celsius
c) Below (-25) degrees Celsius
d) 2 - 10 degrees Celsius

157) TRUE about hereditary spherocytosis: (NEET 2014)
a) Autosomal dominant
b) Shows phenomenon of extravascular hemolysis
c) Defect of spectrin is most common
d) There is no defect in ankyrin protein in this condition

158) Defect in paroxysomal nocturnal hemoglobinuria lies in: (NEET 2014)
a) Alpha globulin gene
b) Beta globulin gene
c) Cell membrane
d) None of the above

159) Defect in Bernard-Soulier lies in: (NEET 2014)
a) GpIb-IX
b) GpIIIa-IIb
c) GpIIa-IIIb
d) GpIIIb-IIa

160) Ringed sideroblasts are seen in: (NEET 2014)
a) Iron deficiency anemia
b) Sideroblastic anemia
c) Thalassemia
d) Anemia of chronic disease

161) Test used for factor VIII deficiency identification is: (NEET 2014)
a) PT b) APTT
c) D dimer d) FDP

162) Most common defect in hereditary spherocytosis in: (NEET 2014)
a) Spectrin b) Ankyrin
c) Band 3 d) Band 4.2

163) Triad of PNH includes all EXCEPT: (NEET 2014)
a) Pancytopenia
b) Renal failure
c) Hemolysis
d) Venous thrombosis

164) Normal red cell distribution width is: (NEET 2014)
a) 8.5-11.5% b) 11.5-14.5%
c) 14.5-17.5% d) 17.5-20.5%

165) Hemophilia is associated with: (NEET 2013)
a) X Chromosome
b) Y Chromosome
c) Chromosome 3
d) Chromosome 16

166) Dohle bodies are seen in: (NEET 2013)
a) Multiple myeloma
b) May-Hegglin anomaly
c) Waldenstorm Macroglobulinemia
d) Lymphoma

167) In α thalassemia:
a) Excess α chain b) No α chain
b) Excess β chain d) No β chain

168) Glanzmann disease is: (NEET 2013)
a) Congenital defect of platelets
b) Congenital defect of RBCs
c) Defect of neutrophils
d) Clotting factor deficiency

169) Primary defect which leads to sickle cell anemia is: (NEET 2013)
a) An abnormality in porphyrin part of hemoglobin
b) Replacement of glutamate by valine in β chain of HbA
c) A non-sense mutation in the β chain of HbA
d) Substitution of valine by glutamate in the a-chain of HbA

170) In DIC, following are seen EXCEPT: (NEET 2013)
a) Fibrinogen decreased
b) Thrombocytopenia
c) Normal APTT
d) PT elevation

171) Not TRUE regarding fresh frozen plasma: (NEET 2013)
a) Supplies major coagulation factors
b) ABO match not required
c) Should be used in replacement of factors in DIC/ trauma
d) To be used within 30 minutes of having trauma

172) Intravascular hemolysis occurs in: (NEET 2013)
a) Hereditary spherocytosis
b) Autoimmune hemolytic anemia
c) PNH
d) Thalassemia

173) All of the following provide protection against malaria EXCEPT: (NEET 2013)
a) Duffy blood group
b) Sickle cell anemia
c) Hereditary spherocytosis
d) PNH

174) PNH occurs due to defect in:
a) CD 59 b) CD 15
c) CD 100 d) CD 20

175) Bite cells are seen in: (NEET 2013)
a) G6 PD deficiency
b) Sickle cell anemia
c) Hereditary spherocytosis
d) Trauma

176) Cold agglutinin is: (NEET 2013)
a) IgG
b) IgM
c) IgA
d) IgD

177) Sideroblastic anemia is caused by all EXCEPT: (NEET 2013)
a) Collagen vascular disease
b) Iron deficit
c) Lead poisoning
d) Cutaneous porphyria

178) Anemia associated with leukemia is: (NEET 2013)
a) Iron deficiency
b) Megaloblastic type
c) Myelophthisic type
d) All of the above

179) Helmet cells are characteristic of anemia of: (NEET 2013)
a) Hemolytic uremic syndrome
b) Polysplenia
c) Spherocytosis
d) Acanthocytosis

180) Schistocyte is/are found in: (NEET 2013)
a) TTP
b) DIC
c) Severe iron deficiency
d) March hemoglobinuria

181) Hypersegmented neutrophils are seen in: (NEET 2013)
- a) Microcytic hypochromic anemia
- b) Sideroblastic anemia
- c) Megaloblastic anemia
- d) Hemolytic anemia

182) All of the following are associated with Coombs positive hemolytic anemia EXCEPT: (NEET 2013)
- a) Thrombotic Thrombocytopenic purpura
- b) Scleroderma
- c) SLE
- d) PAN

183) Maximum spherocytes are seen in: (NEET 2013)
- a) Autoimmune hemolytic anemia
- b) Vit. B12 deficiency
- c) Aplastic anemia
- d) None of the above

184) HbA2 is raised in: (NEET 2013)
- a) Beta thal trait
- b) Sickle cell anemia
- c) Hereditary spherocytosis
- d) None of the above

185) PNH is associated with deficiency of: (AIPGMEE 2010)
- a) DAF (Decay accelerating factor)
- b) MIRL (Membrane inhibitor of reactive lysis)
- c) GPI Anchored Protein (Glycosyl phosphatidyl inosital anchored proteins)
- d) LFA (Lymphocyte function associated antigen)

186) Heterozygous sickle cell anemia gives protection against: (AIPGMEE 2010)
- a) G6PD
- b) Malaria
- c) Thalassemia
- d) Dengue fever

187) Which is not an autoimmune disease? (AIPGMEE 2011)
- a) SLE
- b) Graves' disease
- c) Myasthenia gravis
- d) Sickle cell disease

188) True **about platelet function defect: (AIPGMEE 2011)**
- a) Normal platelet count with prolonged bleeding time
- b) Thrombocytopenia with prolonged bleeding time
- c) Normal bleeding time with normal platelet number
- d) Normal platelet count with decreased bleeding time

189) Which is false about Bernard-Soulier syndrome? (AIPGMEE 2011)
- a) Ristocetin Aggregation is normal
- b) Aggregation with collagen and ADP is normal
- c) Large platelets
- d) Thrombocytopenia

190) HbH occurs due to: (AIPGMEE 2012)
- a) Deletion of Three alpha genes
- b) Deletion of all four alpha genes
- c) Deletion of three beta genes
- d) Deletion of all four beta genes

191) A newborn baby presented with profuse bleeding from the umbilical stump after birth. Rest of the examination and PT, APTT are within normal limits. Most of probable diagnosis is: (AIIMS May 2012)
- a) Factor X deficiency
- b) Glanzmann thrombasthenia
- c) von-Willebrand disease
- d) Bernard-Soulier disease

192) A 28-year-female presents with recurrent abortions and pain in the calves. She is most likely suffering from a deficiency of which of the following? (AIIMS May 2013)
- a) Protein C
- b) Thrombin
- c) Factor XIII
- d) Plasmin

193) The clot formed is not stable unless extensive cross linking occurs. This is done by: (AIIMS May 2015)
- a) Plasmin
- b) Thrombin
- c) Factor XIII
- d) HMWK

194) Platelet adhesion to vessel wall is due to: (AIIMS May 2015)
- a) Factor IX
- b) Fibrinogen
- c) vWF
- d) Fibronectin

195) HAM test is done for: (Nov 2011)
- a) G.P.I. anchor protein
- b) Complement defect
- c) Spectrin defect
- d) Mannose binding protein

196) NESTROFT test is used in: (Nov 2011)
- a) Thalassemia
- b) Autoimmune hemolytic anemia
- c) Spherocytosis
- d) Sickle cell disease

197) A child with fever shows CD 10 positive; CD 19 positive; MPO positive; CD 117 positive; CD 3 negative; CD 33 negative; TC= 6000; Hb.= 4.5;

Platelet count= 20,000. The most probable diagnosis is: (AIIMS Nov 2011)

a) ALL
b) AML
c) Bi-phenotypic
d) Undifferentiated

198) A 25-year-old lady on treatment for rheumatoid arthritis has the following lab findings. Hemoglobin – 6 g, MCV – 60 fl, RBC= 2.5 lakhs, Ferritin – 200ng/ml. Transferrin – 298 mg/dl. Iron -=30. What is the probable diagnosis? (AIIMS Nov 2011)

a) Thalassemia
b) Autoimmune hemolytic anemia
c) Anemia of chronic disease
d) Iron deficiency anemia

199) Person having heterozygous sickle cell trait is protected from infection of: (AIIMS Nov. 2013)

a) Plasmodium falciparum
b) P. vivax
c) Pneumococcus
d) Salmonella

200) Which of the following does not indicate megaloblastic anemia? (AIIMS Nov 2013)

a) Increased reticulocyte count
b) Raised bilirubin
c) Mild splenomegaly
d) Nucleated RBC

201) Platelet adhesion to collagen occurs via: (AIIMS Nov 2013)

a) Factor VIII
b) Factor IX
c) von Willebrand factor
d) Fibronectin

202) Not specific for iron metabolism: (AIIMS Nov 2015)

a) DMT-1
b) Hepcidin
c) Ferroprotein
d) Ferritin

203) Schilling test is used for: (NEET 2013)

a) Fat absorption
b) Vit K absorption
c) Vitamin B12 absorption
d) Vitamin D absorption

CHAPTER 28: RED BLOOD CELL AND BLEEDING DISORDERS

Ans. 1) **D. All of the above (Ref: 8 ed. Robbins p.640-41, 9 ed. p. 630-31)**

Red Cell Indices Q:

- **Mean cell volume (MCV)**: Average volume of red cell, expressed in **femtoliters (fL)** Q
- **Mean cell hemoglobin (MCH)**: Average content (mass) of hemoglobin per red cell, expressed in **picograms** Q
- **Mean cell hemoglobin concentration (MCHC):** Average concentration of hemoglobin in a given volume of packed red cells, expressed in **grams per deciliter** Q

Red cell distribution width: Coefficient of variation of **red cell volume** Q

Adult Reference Ranges for Red Cells Q

Measurement	Men	Women
Hemoglobin (gm/dL)	13.6-17.2	12-15
Hematocrit (%)	39-49	33-43
Red cell count (× 10^6/μL)	4.3-5.9	3.5-5.0
Reticulocyte count (%)	0.5-1.5	0.5-1.5
Mean cell volume (fL)	82-96	82-96
Mean cell hemoglobin (pg)	27-33	27-33
Mean cell hemoglobin concentration (gm/dL)	33-37	33-37
Red cell distribution width	11.5-14.5	11.5-14.5

Ans. 2) **D. All of the above (Ref: 8 ed. Robbins p.641, 9 ed. p. 631)**

Significant bleeding leads to **following changes** Q:

Leukocytosis (increased WBC count) Q:

- Due to the release of **adrenergic hormones**, which mobilizes **granulocytes** from the intravascular marginal pool

Reticulocytosis Q (increased reticulocyte count):

- Due to blood loss, marrow production of **RBC increases** and as a result of which **reticulocyte count increases** to **10% to 15%** after 7 days
- Reticulocytes are larger in size than normal RBC's and have blue-red polychromatophilic cytoplasm

Thrombocytosis Q:

- Early recovery from blood loss is associated with **increased platelet production**

Ans. 3) **C. Normal haptoglobin levels (Ref: 8 ed. Robbins p.641-42, 9 ed. p. 631-32)**

Intravascular Hemolysis Q:

- Red cell destruction occurs within circulation
- **Causes** – Transfusion reaction, G6PD deficiency, falciparum malaria, septicemia, autoimmune hemolytic anemia, Paroxysmal Nocturnal Hemoglobinuria
- **Laboratory features** – Anemia, hemoglobinemia, hemoglobinuria, hemosiderinuria and jaundice, **decreased or absent haptoglobin** Q
- **Splenomegaly** is **absent**

Extravascular Hemolysis Q:

- Occurs due to **alterations** that make **red blood cells less deformable** Q
- **Less deformable RBC's**, pass through the **splenic sinusoids** with great difficulty, leading to red cell **phagocytosis** by **macrophages** in splenic cords
- **Clinical features** – Anemia, splenomegaly, jaundice, mild decrease in haptoglobin

	Intravascular	Extravascular
Peripheral smear	Schistocytes	Spherocytes
Haptoglobin	Decrease/absent	Mild decrease
Urine hemosiderin	++	Negative
Urine hemoglobin	++	Negative
Direct Coombs test	Negative	++++

Ans. 4) D. All of the above (Ref: 8 ed. Robbins p.642, 9 ed. p. 632, f-14-1)

Morphological changes seen in **hemolytic anemia** Q:

- **Increased erythropoietin levels**, leading to increased production of erythroid precursors **(normoblasts)**
- **Increased reticulocyte count** Q – Due to compensatory increase in erythropoiesis
- **Hemosiderin accumulation (Hemosiderosis)** in spleen, liver and bone marrow
- **Extramedullary hematopoiesis** Q – Seen in liver, spleen and lymph nodes
- **Formation of pigment gallstones (cholelithiasis)** – Due to chronic hemolysis and elevated biliary excretion of bilirubin

Ans. 5) C. Glycophorin C (Ref: 8 ed. Robbins p.642-44, 9 ed. p. 632-33, f-14-2,3)

Hereditary spherocytosis:

- **Life span** of RBC's is reduced to **10 to 20 days** Q from the normal 120 days
- **Pathogenic mutations** most commonly affect **ankyrin, band 3, spectrin** or **band 4.2** Q
- Due to these mutations, RBC's assume a **spherical shape (smallest possible diameter** for a **given volume)** Q
- Spherocytes get **trapped in splenic cords** and are engulfed by **macrophages** Q
- **Splenectomy** produces **beneficial effects** in HS patients

Ans. 6) A. Parvo virus (Ref: 8 ed. Robbins p.644, 9 ed. p. 633-34)

Aplastic Crisis Q:

- Triggered by an acute **parvovirus infection** Q
- **Parvovirus** Q infects and kills red cell precursors
- Treatment includes blood transfusion

Note: In **Infectious mononucleosis** Q, hemolytic crises occur due to **increased splenic destruction** of **red cells**

Ans. 7) C. Hereditary spherocytosis (Ref: 8 ed. Robbins p.644, 9 ed. p. 633-34)

Causes of increased osmotic fragility Q:

- Hereditary spherocytosis
- Autoimmune hemolytic anemia
- Hemolytic disease of newborn

Causes of decreased osmotic fragility Q:

- Sickle cell disease
- Thalassemia

Note: Hereditary Spherocytosis is the only condition which is characterized by an **increased MCHC** Q

Ans. 8) D. All of the above (Ref: 8 ed. Robbins p.644-45, 9 ed. p. 634-35, f-14-5)

G6PD Deficiency Q

- **X-linked recessive** trait
- Patients have protective effect against **Plasmodium falciparum malaria** Q
- Older RBC's are more prone to **hemolysis** Q than younger ones

- **Most common trigger** of hemolysis: Infections, Drugs and Food

Ans. 9) D. Any of the above (Ref: 8 ed. Robbins p.644-45, 9 ed. p. 634-35)

Most common trigger of **hemolysis** Q **in G6PD deficient** patients:

- **Infections** (viral hepatitis, pneumonia and typhoid fever)
- **Drugs** (primaquine, chloroquine, sulfonamides, nitrofurantoins)
- **Food** (fava bean)

Ans. 10) D. All of the above (Ref: 8 ed. Robbins p.644-45, 9 ed. p. 634-35, f-14-6)

Features of G6PD Deficiency Q:

- Oxidants leads to **intravascular** and **extravascular** hemolysis
- Following exposure of G6PD-deficient individuals to oxidants, acute **intravascular hemolysis** Q (anemia, hemoglobinemia and hemoglobinuria) begins in 2-3 days
- **Heinz bodies** – Precipitates of **denatured globin**, seen as **dark inclusions** within red cells, can be visualized by **supravital staining** Q
- As the blood flows within the spleen, **splenic macrophages** pluck out **Heinz bodies**, resulting in appearance of a **bite** taken out of RBC's **(bite cell)** Q

Ans. 11) A. Replacement of glutamine with valine at sixth codon of β-globin (Ref: 8 ed. Robbins p.645, 9 ed. p. 635)

- Normal adult red cells contain mainly **HbA ($\alpha_2\beta_2$)**, along with small amounts of **HbA2 ($\alpha_2\beta_2$)** and **HbF ($\alpha_2\gamma_2$)** Q
- **Sickle cell disease** is caused by a **point mutation** in the **sixth codon of β-globin**
- Point mutation results in the replacement of **glutamate residue** with **valine residue** Q and thus formation of **HbS**
- **HbS** like **G6PD deficiency** and **thalassemia**, protects against **falciparum malaria** Q

Ans. 12) D. All of the above (Ref: 8 ed. Robbins p.645-46, 9 ed. p. 635-36, f-14-7)

Factors affecting the rate and degree of sickling Q:

a) Interaction of HbS with other types of hemoglobin in the cell Q:

- **HbF** Q and **HbA** Q inhibits sickling
- **HbC** Q (in which **lysine** is substituted for **glutamate** in sixth amino acid residue of **β-globin**) with HbS in heterozygous state promote sickling

b) Mean cell hemoglobin concentration (MCHC) Q:

- **Intracellular dehydration**, which **increases MCHC**, facilitates sickling
- **β-thalassemia**, which **reduces Hb synthesis** when coexist with HbS has a milder disease

c) Intracellular pH Q:

- **Decreased pH (acidosis)** reduces the **oxygen affinity** of **hemoglobin**, increasing the fraction of **deoxygenated HbS** and increases sickling

d) Transit time of red cells through microvascular beds Q:

- Transit time in **normal microvascular beds is short** and thus significant aggregation of **deoxygenated HbS** is not seen
- Movement of blood through **inflamed tissues** is slow, making them prone to sickling and occlusion
- **Blood flow** is **sluggish** in normal **spleen** and **bone marrow**, which are **prominently** affected in **sickle cell disease**

Ans. 13) D. All of the above (Ref: 8 ed. Robbins p.646-47, 9 ed. p. 636-37, f-14-8,9)

Peripheral smear findings in **Sickle cell anemia** Q:

- **Irreversibly sickled cells, reticulocytosis** and **target cells**
- **Howell-Jolly bodies** (small nuclear remnants) can also be seen

Ans. 14) B. **Bone pain (Ref: 8 ed. Robbins p.647-48, 9 ed. p. 637-38)**

Clinical Features of Sickle Cell Anemia Q:

Vaso-occlusive crises (pain crises) Q:

- Associated with **severe pain** in the affected region
- Most common affected sites are the **bones**, lungs, liver, brain, spleen and penis
- In children, **bone pains** resembles that of **acute osteomyelitis**
- **Acute chest syndrome**, due to vaso-occlusive crisis involving the lungs
- **Priapism, stroke, blindness** (due to retinopathy) can be seen

Sequestration crises Q:

- Occurs in **children** with **intact spleens**
- **Massive entrapment** of sickle red cells in spleen, leads to rapid splenic enlargement, hypovolemia and shock

Aplastic Crises:

- Due to infection of red cell progenitors by **parvovirus B19** Q

Infections:

- **Pneumococcus pneumoniae** Q, **Haemophilus influenzae** Q septicemia and **meningitis** are commonly seen

Note: Most common cause of death – **Sepsis** and **acute chest syndrome**

Ans. 15) D. **Sickle cell anemia (Ref: 8 ed. Robbins p.648, 9 ed. p. 638)**

Gamna Gandy Bodies

- Most characteristic features of **congestive splenomegaly, sickle cell anemia** Q
- Also seen in **Portal hypertension, hemolytic anemia, Hemochromatosis**

Bone Changes in Sickle Cell Anemia:

- **Crew haircut** Q appearance (Hair on end)
- Fish mouth vertebrae

Ans. 16) D. **Plasmodium (Ref: 8 ed. Robbins p.645, 9 ed. p. 635)**

- **HbS** protects against **falciparum malaria** Q

Ans. 17) A. **Hydroxyurea (Ref: 8 ed. Robbins p.648, 9 ed. p. 638)**

- Mainstay of treatment in **sickle cell anemia** is **Hydroxyurea (inhibitor of DNA synthesis)** Q
- Hydroxyurea leads to **increase in red cell HbF levels** and has an **anti-inflammatory effect** Q
- **Hematopoietic stem cell transplantation** Q can be curative

Ans. 18) A. **Sickle cell anemia (Ref: 8 ed. Robbins p.647, 9 ed. p. 637, f-14-9,10)**

- Early in **sickle cell anemia**, spleen is enlarged by **red pulp congestion** Q, due to trapping of sickled red cells in cords and sinuses
- **Autosplenectomy** Q: **Chronic erythrostasis**, leads to **splenic infarction** Q, **fibrosis** and progressive shrinkage

Ans. 19) D. **All of the above (Ref: 8 ed. Robbins p.648-49, 9 ed. p. 638-39, f-14-11,12)**

Molecular Pathogenesis of Thalassemia Q:

- **Two α chains** in HbA are encoded by **pair of α-globin genes** on **chromosome 16** Q
- **Two β chains** in HbA are encoded by **single β-globin gene** on **chromosome 11** Q
- **β-thalassemia** occurs due to **deficient β chain** synthesis, whereas **α-thalassemia** occurs due to deficient synthesis of **α chains** Q
- β^0 **mutation** is associated with **absent β-globin synthesis** Q
- β^+ **mutation** is characterized by **reduced β-globin synthesis** Q
- **Splicing mutations** are the **most common** cause of β^+**-thalassemia** Q
- **Chain terminator mutations** are the **most common** cause of β^0**-thalassemia** Q

Ans. 20) D. All of the above (Ref: 8 ed. Robbins p.649, 9 ed. p. 639)

Ineffective Erythropoiesis:

- **Imbalance in α- and β-globin synthesis,** leads to diminished survival of **red cells** and their precursors
- **α chains** precipitate within the **red cell precursors** and forms **inclusions** Q
- These inclusions leads to **RBC membrane damage**, resulting in apoptosis of RBC's in marrow and thus **ineffective erythropoiesis** Q

Consequences of **ineffective erythropoiesis** Q:

- **Massive erythroid hyperplasia** in the **marrow** Q
- **Extensive extramedullary hematopoiesis** Q, which involves the liver, spleen and lymph nodes
- Excessive absorption of **dietary iron** occurs due to **low hepcidin levels** Q (negative regulator of iron absorption)
- **Secondary hemochromatosis** Q **(Systemic iron overload)** – Excessive **iron deposition** most commonly damages the **liver** Q

Ans. 21) B. Decrease in beta chain, increase in alpha chain (Ref: 8 ed. Robbins p.648-49, 9 ed. p. 638-39)

- Refer answer 19 for details

Ans. 22) D. All of the above (Ref: 8 ed. Robbins p.649, 9 ed. p. 640)

β-Thalassemia Major Q:

- Anemia manifests **6 to 9 months** after birth
- At **6-9 months** of age, hemoglobin synthesis switches from **HbF to HbA** Q
- Hemoglobin levels are **3 to 6 gm/dL** Q
- Red cells may completely **lack HbA (β^0/β^0 genotype)** or contain small amounts of HbA (β^+/β^+ or β^0/β^+ genotypes)
- **Markedly elevated HbF** Q (major red cell hemoglobin)
- **HbA2 levels** can be **high** but more often are **normal or low** Q

Ans. 23) C. Low reticulocyte count (Ref: 8 ed. Robbins p.650-51, 9 ed. p. 640-41)

Morphology of **β-Thalassemia Major** Q:

RBC picture on **peripheral smear:**

- **Microcytic hypochromic anemia** with **anisocytosis** (marked variation in size) and **poikilocytosis** (variation in shape)
- **Target cells, basophilic stippling** and **fragmented red cells** are seen
- **Elevated** reticulocyte count Q

Ans. 24) A. Thalassemia (Ref: 8 ed. Robbins p.650-51, 9 ed. p. 640-41, f-14-12, 13)

- **Expansion** of **hematopoietically active marrow** occurs in **thalassemic** patients
- **Marrow expansion** of **facial** and **skull** bones leads to erosion of **existing cortical bone** and **induces new bone formation** – gives **"crew-cut" appearance** Q on X-ray

Ans. 25) A. Beta thalassemia (Hemoglobinopathies by Anupam Sachdev 1st ed. p.100)

- **NESTROFT (Naked Eye Single Tube Red cell Osmotic Fragility Test)** is used as a screening test for **beta thalassemia trait** Q
- Confirmation of **positive NESTROFT** is done by **Hemoglobin electrophoresis** Q

Positive NESTROFT test is seen with:

- Iron deficiency anemia
- Alpha thalassemia trait
- Homozygous and heterozygous HbE
- HbS and Hereditary persistence of Fetal Hemoglobin

Ans. 26) D. Severe anemia (Ref: 8 ed. Robbins p.651, 9 ed. p. 641)

Beta Thalassemia Trait [Q]:

- Majority of patients are **asymptomatic**, but it can present as **mild anemia**
- **Peripheral smear** reveals **microcytic hypochromic anemia, basophilic stippling** and **target cells** [Q]
- **Bone marrow** reveals **mild erythroid hyperplasia**
- **Hemoglobin electrophoresis** shows increase in **HbA2 (α2δ2)** to **4% to 8% (normal, 2.5%** ± 0.3%) and normal **HbF** levels

Ans. 27) A. Deletion of 3 alpha chains (Ref: 8 ed. Robbins p.651-52, 9 ed. p. 641-42, t-14-3)

α-Thalassemia [Q]:

Condition	Defect	Genotype	Clinical syndrome
Silent carrier	Deletion of 1 alpha chains	–/α α/α	Normal
α-Thalassemia trait	Deletion of 2 alpha genes	–/–α/α (homozygous)	Microcytic hypochromic anemia
		–/α–/α (heterozygous)	No/minimal anemia
HbH disease	Deletion of 3 alpha genes	–/– –/α	Hemolytic anemia
Hydrops fetalis	Deletion of 4 alpha genes	–/– –/–	Fatal in utero or birth

Ans. 28) C. Microcytosis (Ref: 8 ed. Robbins p.651-52, 9 ed. p. 641-42, t-14-3)

α-thalassemia Trait [Q]:

- Similar to **β-thalassemia minor**
- Shows **microcytosis** (small red cells) and minimal or no anemia
- Normal or low HbA_2 levels

Ans. 29) C. Paroxysmal nocturnal hemoglobinemia (Ref: 8 ed. Robbins p.652, 9 ed. p. 642)

Paroxysmal Nocturnal Hemoglobinemia:

- **Hemolytic anemia** caused by an **acquired genetic defect** [Q]
- Results due to **acquired mutations** in the **phosphatidylinositol glycan complementation group A gene (PIGA)** [Q]
- PIGA mutation leads to deficiency of **GPI linked proteins** [Q]
- **Increased susceptibility** of all **three cell lines** (RBC, WBC, Platelet) to **complement mediated lysis** [Q]

Ans. 30) D. All of the above (Ref: 8 ed. Robbins p.652, 9 ed. p. 642)

- **PNH** blood cells are **deficient** in three **GPI-linked proteins:** [Q]
  a) Decay accelerating factor, or **CD55**
  b) Membrane inhibitor of reactive lysis, or **CD59**; and
  c) C8 binding protein
- Most important protein is **CD59**, a potent inhibitor of **C3 convertase** [Q]
- **CD59** prevents the spontaneous activation of **alternate complement pathway**

Ans. 31) C. Decreased LDH (Ref: 8 ed. Robbins p.652-53, 9 ed. p. 642)

Intravascular Hemolysis [Q]:

- **Red cells** deficient in **GPI-linked factors** are susceptible to lysis by **C5b-C9 membrane attack complex**
- **Chronic hemolysis** occurs without hemoglobinuria
- **Hemosiderinuria** leads to **iron deficiency**

Thrombosis:

- **Most common cause of death** [Q] in individuals with **PNH**
- Involves hepatic, portal or cerebral veins

Hematological Complications [Q]**:**

- **Acute myeloid leukemia**
- **Myelodysplastic syndrome**
- **Aplastic anemia**

Ans. 32) C. Increased leukocyte alkaline phosphatase (Ref: 8 ed. Robbins p.652, 9 ed. p. 642)

- **Neutrophil alkaline phosphatase** is **decreased** [Q] in **P.N.H**

Ans. 33) C. Splenomegaly (Ref: 8 ed. Robbins p.652, 9 ed. p. 642-43)

Features of PNH:

- **Activation of the complement** leads to **intravascular hemolysis, leukopenia, thrombocytopenia** [Q] (Pancytopenia)
- **Splenomegaly is not seen** [Q]

Ans. 34) C. Flow cytometry (Ref: 8 ed. Robbins p.652, 9 ed. p. 642-43, f-14-14)

Diagnostic Tests for PNH [Q]**:**

- HAMS test
- Sucrose lysis test
- Flow cytometry

Flow cytometry (gold standard) in PNH shows **RBCs population** deficient in **CD55** [Q] and **CD59** [Q]

Ans. 35) A. Venous thrombosis (Ref: 8 ed. Robbins p.652, 9 ed. p. 642-43)

Causes of Death [Q] in PNH:

- Venous thrombosis
- Infection
- Bleeding

Note: Most common cause of death in PNH is cortical **vein thrombosis** [Q]

Ans. 36) A. Eculizumab (Ref: 8 ed. Robbins p.652, 9 ed. p. 643)

Eculizumab [Q]**:**

- **Monoclonal antibody** which binds to **complement protein C5** and prevents the conversion of **C5 to C5a**
- **Inhibits** complement mediated **intravascular hemolysis in PNH patients**

Ans. 37) D. Mycoplasma pneumonia (Ref: 8 ed. Robbins p.653-54, 9 ed. p. 643, t-14-4)

Causes of Warm antibody type hemolytic anemia [Q]**:**

Primary (idiopathic)

Secondary

- Autoimmune disorders (**systemic lupus erythematosus**)
- Drugs (penicillin, cephalosporins, **α-methyldopa**)
- Lymphoid neoplasms

Causes of Cold Agglutinin type hemolytic anemia [Q]**:**

Acute

- Mycoplasma infection
- Infectious mononucleosis

Chronic

- Idiopathic
- Lymphoid neoplasms

Ans. 38) C. Most common antibodies are of IgA type (Ref: 8 ed. Robbins p.653-54, 9 ed. p. 643-44)

Warm Antibody Type Hemolytic Anemia [Q]**:**

- **Most common** form of **immunohemolytic anemia**

- **Causative** antibodies are of **IgG class** [Q] followed by **IgA antibodies**
- Leads to **extravascular** red cell hemolysis
- Moderate splenomegaly is seen

Ans. 39) D. All of the above (Ref: 8 ed. Robbins p.653-54, 9 ed. p. 643-44, t-14-4)

- Refer to answer 40

Ans. 40) C. All of the above (Ref: 8 ed. Robbins p.653-54, 9 ed. p. 644)

Cold agglutinin type hemolytic anemia [Q]**:**

- Caused by **IgM antibodies** which bind red cells at **low temperatures (0°C to 4°C)**

Associated infections include:

- **Mycoplasma pneumoniae** [Q]
- Epstein-Barr virus
- Cytomegalovirus
- Influenza virus
- Human immunodeficiency virus (HIV)

Ans. 41) A. IgG (Ref: 8 ed. Robbins p.653-54, 9 ed. p. 644)

Paroxysmal cold hemoglobinuria [Q]**:**

- **IgG** [Q] **autoantibodies (Donath-Landsteiner antibody)** binds to **P-blood group antigen** on RBC
- **Antigen antibody** complexes on RBC's activates **complement**
- Complement activation leads to formation of **membrane attack complex**, which destroys RBC's, leading to **intravascular hemolysis** and **hemoglobinuria** [Q]

Ans. 42) A. DIC (Ref: 8 ed. Robbins p.654, 9 ed. p. 644, f-14-15)

Microangiopathic hemolytic anemia [Q]**:**

- Characterized by **fragmentation** of **red blood cells** due to obstruction of small blood vessels

Causes:

- Disseminated intravascular coagulation **(DIC)** [Q] – **most common**
- Thrombotic thrombocytopenic purpura **(TTP)**
- Hemolytic-uremic syndrome **(HUS)**
- **Malignant hypertension**
- **Systemic lupus erythematosus**
- **Disseminated cancer**

Ans. 43) D. Any of the above (Ref: 8 ed. Robbins p.654, 9 ed. p. 644, f-14-15)

- **Traumatic damage** to RBC's, leads to the appearance of **red cell fragments (schistocytes)**, **"burr cells"**, **"helmet cells"**, and **"triangle cells"** in **blood smears** [Q]

Ans. 44) C. Paroxysmal cold hemoglobinuria (Ref:7 ed. Robbins p.637)

Paroxysmal cold hemoglobinuria [Q]**:**

- Characterized by intermittent **massive intravascular hemolysis**, with **hemoglobinuria** at low temperature
- Due to **IgG** autoantibodies, also known as **Donath-Landsteiner antibody** [Q]

Ans. 45) B. IgM (Ref: 8 ed. Robbins p.654, 9 ed. p. 644)

Cold Agglutinin Hemolytic Anemia [Q]**:**

- Caused by cold agglutinin **IgM antibodies** [Q]
- Antibodies react with RBCs at **0°C to 4°C**
- Both **intravascular** and **extravascular** hemolysis may occur

Ans. 46) D. Donath Landsteiner antibody (Ref: 8 ed. Robbins p.654)

- Answer here is not "a" as option is anti-IgM and not IgM
- Cold agglutinins are IgM antibodies against RBC

Anti-erythrocyte antibodies Q:

a) Warm antibodies

b) **Cold antibodies – Cold agglutinin (IgM)** and **Donath Landsteiner (IgG)** Q

Ans. 47) B. SLE (Ref: 8 ed. Robbins p.653, 9 ed. p. 643)

Autoimmune Hemolytic Anemia Q:

- Diagnosis of **immune-hemolytic anemia** requires the detection of antibodies and/or complement on patient red cells
- Done by using Coomb's test; hence this anemia is also called as **Coomb's positive hemolytic anemia** Q
- **Autoimmune hemolytic anemia** can be divided (according to temperature at which this antibody reacts with RBC):
  - a) Warm antibody autoimmune hemolytic anemia
  - b) Cold antibody autoimmune hemolytic anemia
  - c) Paroxysmal cold hemoglobinuria

Causes of Warm antibody Autoimmune Hemolytic Anemia Q:

- **Autoimmune disorders**: **SLE** Q, RA, Ulcerative colitis, Scleroderma, Antiphospholipid antibodies
- **Chronic Lymphocytic leukemia** Q
- Hodgkin disease
- Non-Hodgkin Lymphoma
- Multiple myeloma
- Thymoma
- Drugs

Note: Also refer Q 40, 41

Ans. 48) D. CLL (Ref: 8 ed. Robbins p.653, 9 ed. p. 643) Refer to answer 50

Ans. 49) D. Any of the above (Ref: 8 ed. Robbins p.655, 9 ed. p. 645)

Causes of Vitamin B12 Deficiency Q:

a) Decreased Intake

- Inadequate diet, Vegetarianism

b) Impaired Absorption

- **Intrinsic factor deficiency** – Pernicious anemia, Gastrectomy
- Malabsorption states

c) Diffuse intestinal disease (e.g., **lymphoma**, systemic sclerosis)

d) **Ileal resection, ileitis** – Competitive parasitic uptake, Fish tapeworm infestation

e) Bacterial overgrowth in blind loops and diverticula of bowel

Ans. 50) D. Any of the above (Ref: 8 ed. Robbins p.655, 9 ed. p. 645)

Causes of Folic Acid Deficiency Q:

a) **Decreased Intake**

- Inadequate diet, **alcoholism**, infancy
- Impaired Absorption

- Malabsorption states
- Intrinsic intestinal disease
- **Anticonvulsants**, oral contraceptives
- Hemodialysis

b) **Increased Requirement**

- **Pregnancy** Q, infancy, disseminated cancer, markedly increased hematopoiesis

c) **Impaired Utilization**

- Folic acid antagonists

d) Unresponsive to Vitamin B12 or Folic Acid Therapy

- DNA Synthesis and/or Folate Metabolism inhibitors (e.g., Methotrexate)

Ans. 51) A. Impairment of DNA synthesis (Ref: 8 ed. Robbins p.654-55, 9 ed. p. 645)

Peripheral smear Q and **bone marrow** changes in Megaloblastic anemia occur due to:

- **Impairment of DNA synthesis** Q that leads to **ineffective hematopoiesis**

Ans. 52) C. Elevated MCHC (Ref: 8 ed. Robbins p.655, 9 ed. p. 645)

Peripheral smear findings in **Megaloblastic anemia** Q:

RBC Q:

- Predominantly **macrocytic** and **oval (macro-ovalocytes) red cells** Q
- Marked variation in size **(anisocytosis)** and shape **(poikilocytosis)** of red cells
- **Nucleated RBC** Q may appear in the circulating blood

WBC Q:

- Neutrophils are larger than normal (macropolymorphonuclear)
- Neutrophils show **nuclear hyper segmentation** Q, having **five or more nuclear lobules**

Platelets:

- Can be reduced or normal in number

Note:

- **Reticulocyte count is low** Q
- **MCHC is not elevated** Q

Ans. 53) D. All of the above (Ref: 8 ed. Robbins p.655, 9 ed. p. 645, f-14-16,17)

Bone Marrow Aspirate in **Megaloblastic Anemia** Q:

a) **Hyper-cellular marrow** for age

b) **Erythroid lineage:**

- **Megaloblasts** replaces all erythroid precursors
- **Megaloblasts** – Large cells, with **deeply basophilic cytoplasm**, prominent nucleoli and a **distinctive, fine nuclear chromatin pattern** Q
- **Nuclear maturation** is delayed than the cytoplasmic maturation, leading to **nuclear-to-cytoplasmic asynchrony** Q
- **Giant metamyelocytes** and **band forms** Q – Due to **impaired DNA synthesis** there occurs release of immature **granulocytic precursors**

c) **Megakaryocytes**:

- Abnormally large with bizarre, **multilobated nuclei** Q

Ans. 54) A. Increased erythropoietin levels (Ref: 8 ed. Robbins p.655, 9 ed. p. 645)

- **Bone marrow hyperplasia** occurs due to **increased levels** of growth factors, such as **erythropoietin** Q

- **Pancytopenia** [Q] occurs due to **derangement in DNA synthesis**, which leads to **apoptosis** of precursor forms in the marrow (an example of **ineffective hematopoiesis**)

Ans. 55) B. 2-3 μg (Ref: 8 ed. Robbins p.656, 9 ed. p. 646)

- **Daily requirement** of **Vitamin B_{12}** is **2 to 3 μg** [Q]

Ans. 56) D. All of the above (Ref: 8 ed. Robbins p.656, 9 ed. p. 646, f-14-18)

Vitamin B12 metabolism:

- **Vitamin B12** in the **stomach** binds to a salivary protein called **haptocorrin**
- In **duodenum**, vitamin B12 after being released from haptocorrin by pancreatic proteases, combines with **intrinsic factor** [Q]
- **Intrinsic factor-Vitamin B12 complex** is transported to the **ileum** [Q]
- In **ileum**, it is endocytosed by **ileal enterocytes** that express **cubilin** (receptor for intrinsic factor)
- Within the **ileal cells**, **Vitamin B12** combines with **transcobalamin II** [Q] (major carrier protein) and is **secreted into plasma**
- **Transcobalamin II** delivers **vitamin B12** to the **liver**, rapidly proliferating cells in **bone marrow** and **gastrointestinal tract** [Q]

Ans. 57) A. Folic acid alone causes improvement of hematologic symptoms but worsening of neurological symptoms (Ref: 8 ed. Robbins p.657, 9 ed. p. 647)

- **Neurological complications** associated with **vitamin B12 deficiency** are **not improved by folate administration** [Q]
- Hence, it becomes essential to exclude **vitamin B12 deficiency** in **megaloblastic anemia** before initiating therapy with **folate**

Ans. 58) A. Type I (Ref: 8 ed. Robbins p.657, 9 ed. p. 647-48)

Three types of **autoantibodies** seen in **Pernicious anemia** patients:

Type I antibody [Q]**:**

- **75%** [Q] of patients have antibody which blocks the binding of **Vitamin B12 to intrinsic factor**
- Found in both the plasma and gastric juice

Type II antibodies:

- Prevents the binding of **intrinsic factor-vitamin B12 complex** to **ileal receptor**

Type III antibodies:

- Recognize α **and** β **subunits** of **gastric proton pump**, localized to the **gastric parietal cell**

Ans. 59) D. Gastric atrophy is corrected by Vitamin B12 administration (Ref: 8 ed. Robbins p.658, 9 ed. p. 648)

Morphology of Pernicious Anemia [Q]

- **Bone marrow** and **blood findings** in pernicious anemia are similar to megaloblastic anemia
- Stomach shows **diffuse chronic gastritis** [Q]
- **Most characteristic finding** is **Fundic gland atrophy** [Q]
- **Intestinal metaplasia** [Q] – Glandular epithelium is replaced by **mucus-secreting goblet cells** that resemble those lining the **large intestine**
- **Atrophic glossitis** – Tongue may become shiny, glazed and "beefy"
- **Gastric atrophy** and **metaplastic changes** occurs due to **autoimmunity** and it persists even after parenteral administration of **vitamin B12**

Ans. 60) D. Any of the above (Ref: 8 ed. Robbins p.658, 9 ed. p. 648)

Dorsal and **lateral spinal tracts** undergo demyelination in **pernicious anemia** and leads to:

- **Spastic paraparesis** [Q]
- **Sensory ataxia** [Q]
- **Severe paresthesias** in lower limbs [Q]

Ans. 61) D. Low reticulocyte count following parenteral administration of Vitamin B12 (Ref: 8 ed. Robbins p.658, 9 ed. p. 648)

Clinical Features of Pernicious Anemia Q:

- **Moderate to severe** megaloblastic anemia
- **Leukopenia** with **hypersegmented granulocytes**
- Low serum **vitamin B12**
- **Elevated** serum levels of **homocysteine** and **methylmalonic acid**
- **Increased reticulocyte count** and hematocrit levels **after 5 days** Q of parenteral administration of **vitamin B12**

Ans. 62) D. Any of the above (Ref: 8 ed. Robbins p.658, 9 ed. p. 648)

Complications associated with **pernicious anemia** Q:

- **Gastric atrophy** and **metaplasia** are at increased risk for developing **gastric carcinoma** Q
- **Elevated homocysteine levels** are risk factors for **atherosclerosis** and **thrombosis** Q

Ans. 63) B. 50-200 µg (Ref: 8 ed. Robbins p.658, 9 ed. p. 649)

- Daily requirement for **folic acid** is **50 to 200 µg daily** Q
- **Richest sources** are **green vegetables** such as lettuce, spinach, asparagus and broccoli Q

Ans. 64) All of the above (Ref: 8 ed. Robbins p.658, 9 ed. p. 649)

Folic acid requirement is **increased in**:

- Pregnancy, infancy, hemolytic anemia and disseminated cancer

In **folic acid deficiency**:

- **Serum homocysteine levels** are **increased**, but methylmalonate concentrations are **normal** Q
- **Hematologic symptoms** of **vitamin B12 deficiency anemia** responds to **folate** Q
- **Folate** does not prevent the **neurologic deficits** seen in **vitamin B12 deficiency** Q

Ans. 65) D. All of the above (Ref: 8 ed. Robbins p.659, 9 ed. p. 649-50, f-14-21)

Iron Metabolism Q:

- **Free iron** is **highly toxic** and exists in storage pool as **ferritin** or **hemosiderin**
- **Storage pool** of iron is represented by **hemosiderin** and **ferritin** Q
- Iron is **transported** in plasma by an **iron-binding glycoprotein** called **transferrin** Q
- Serum iron levels average **120 µg/dL** in **men** and **100 µg/dL** in women Q

Ans. 66) D. All of the above (Ref: 8 ed. Robbins p.659, 9 ed. p. 650)

- **Ferritin** is found at highest levels in **liver, spleen, bone marrow and skeletal muscles** Q
- In **liver**, **ferritin** is stored within the **parenchymal cells** Q, in **spleen** and **bone marrow**, it is found mainly in **macrophages** Q

Ans. 67) C. Prussian blue (Ref: 8 ed. Robbins p.660, 9 ed. p. 650)

Prussian Blue Stain Q:

- Iron in hemosiderin gives a **blue-black** color, when exposed to **potassium ferrocyanide** in the stain

Ans. 68) D. $Fe2^{+}$ before combining transferrin is converted to Fe3+ by hepcidin (Ref: 8 ed. Robbins p.660-61, 9 ed. p. 650-51, f-14-22)

Regulation of Iron Absorption Q:

- Luminal **nonheme iron** is in the **Fe^{3+} (ferric)** state and is reduced to **Fe^{2+} (ferrous)** iron by **cytochrome B** Q
- **Fe^{2+} iron** is transported across the **apical membrane** of duodenum by **divalent metal transporter 1 (DMT1)** Q
- **Fe^{2+} iron** that enters into circulation is **transported from the cytoplasm** across the **basolateral enterocyte** membrane by **ferroprotein** Q
- **Hephaestin** and **ceruloplasmin** Q leads to **oxidation** of **Fe^{2+} iron to Fe^{3+} iron**
- **Fe^{3+}** iron binds with **transferrin** (which delivers iron to the red cell progenitors in marrow)

Hepcidin:

- Regulates iron absorption
- Synthesized and released from the liver
- Released in response to **increased hepatic iron** levels
- Inhibits **iron transfer** from **enterocyte** to plasma by binding to **ferroprotein**
- When there are sufficient iron stores, increased **hepcidin levels,** inhibits iron absorption into the **blood** [Q]
- With **low iron stores**, hepcidin levels **fall**, which facilitates **iron absorption** [Q]

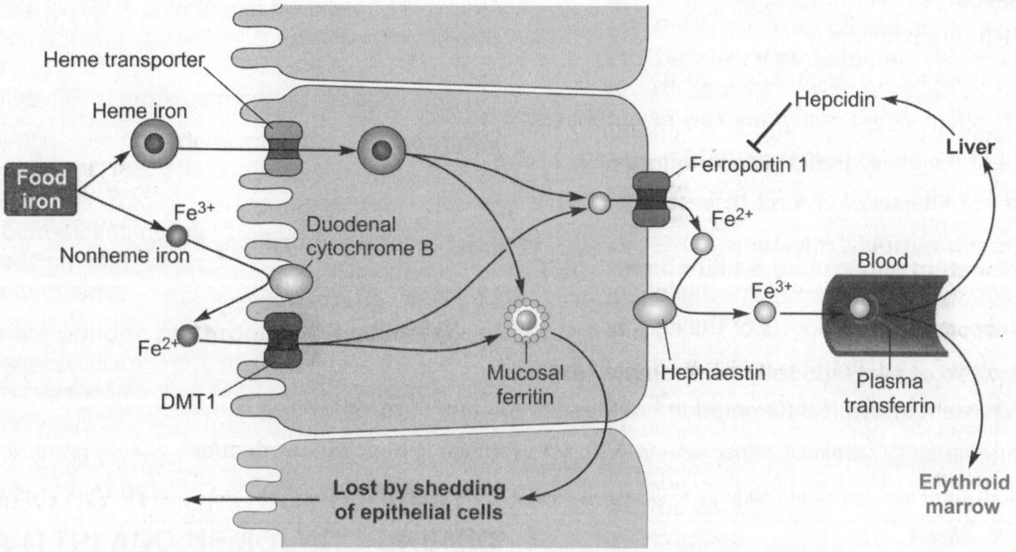

Regulation of iron absorption

Ans. 69) C. With high iron levels hepcidin synthesis decreases (Ref: 8 ed. Robbins p.660-61, 9 ed. p. 650-51, f-14-22)

- When iron stores are adequate, **hepcidin** [Q] synthesis increases and inhibits iron absorption into the blood
- With **low body iron stores, hepcidin synthesis falls** [Q], which **facilitates iron absorption**
- **Hepcidin**, inhibits **ferroprotein**, which reduces **iron uptake** from enterocytes and suppresses iron release from **macrophages** [Q]

Ans. 70) B. Increased hepcidin levels (Ref: 8 ed. Robbins p.660-61, 9 ed. p. 650-51)

- **Anemia of chronic disease** is caused by **inflammatory mediators** that **increases hepatic hepcidin** [Q]

Ans. 71) B. Low hepcidin levels (Ref: 8 ed. Robbins p.660, 9 ed. p. 651)

- **Hepcidin activity** is **low** [Q] in both **primary** and **secondary hemochromatosis** [Q] (a syndrome caused by systemic iron overload)

Ans. 72) A. 7-10 mg (Ref: 8 ed. Robbins p.661, 9 ed. p. 651)

- Daily iron requirement is **7 to 10 mg** for **adult men** [Q] and **7 to 20 mg** for **adult women** [Q]

Ans. 73) C. Oxalates (Ref: 8 ed. Robbins p.661, 9 ed. p. 651)

Absorption of **inorganic iron** is:

- Enhanced by **ascorbic acid, citric acid, amino acids** and **sugars** [Q] in the diet
- Inhibited by **tannates (found in tea), carbonates, oxalates** and **phosphates** [Q]

Ans. 74) D. All of the above (Ref: 8 ed. Robbins p.662, 9 ed. p. 652)

Plummer-Vinson Syndrome [Q]**:**

- **Triad** of **Esophageal webs, microcytic hypochromic anemia** and **atrophic glossitis**

Ans. 75) A. Increased TIBC, decreased serum ferritin (Ref: 8 ed. Robbins p.662, 9 ed. p. 652)

Laboratory Features of **Iron Deficiency Anemia** [Q]:

- **Low serum iron** and **ferritin**
- **High Total iron-binding capacity** (TIBC)
- **Transferrin saturation** is **reduced (<15%)**

Ans. 76) C. Reduced ferritin (Ref: 8 ed. Robbins p.662, 9 ed. p. 652)

Laboratory Features of Anemia of Chronic Disease [Q]:

- **Low** serum iron
- **High** serum ferritin level
- **Reduced** total iron-binding capacity
- Abundant stored iron in **marrow macrophages**

Ans. 77) D. All of the above (Ref: 8 ed. Robbins p.662, 9 ed. p. 652)

Causes of **Anemia of Chronic Disease** [Q]:

a) **Chronic microbial infections** – Osteomyelitis, bacterial endocarditis and lung abscess

b) **Chronic immune disorders** – Rheumatoid arthritis and regional enteritis

c) **Neoplasms** – Carcinomas of the lung, breast and Hodgkin lymphoma

Ans. 78) D. IL-6 (Ref: 8 ed. Robbins p.662, 9 ed. p. 652)

- **Persistent systemic inflammation** [Q] can lead to **Anemia of chronic disease**
- Inflammatory mediator – **Interleukin-6 (IL-6)** [Q], stimulates **hepcidin production**
- **High hepcidin** levels inhibits transfer of iron from **storage pools** to developing **erythroid precursors** in bone marrow [Q]

Ans. 79) D. All of the above (Ref: 8 ed. Robbins p.662-63, 9 ed. p. 653, t-14-7)

Major Causes of Aplastic Anemia [Q]:

Acquired

- Idiopathic
- Acquired stem cell defects
- Immune mediated

Chemical Agents

a) Dose related

- Alkylating agents
- Antimetabolites
- Benzene
- Chloramphenicol
- Inorganic arsenicals

b) Idiosyncratic

- Chloramphenicol
- Phenylbutazone
- Organic arsenicals
- Methylphenylethylhydantoin
- Carbamazepine
- Penicillamine
- Gold salts

Physical Agents

- Whole-body irradiation
- Viral Infections
- Hepatitis
- Cytomegalovirus infections
- Epstein-Barr virus infections
- Herpes zoster (varicella zoster)

Inherited

- Fanconi anemia, Telomerase defects

Ans. 80) D. All of the above (Ref: 8 ed. Robbins p.662-63, 9 ed. p. 653, t-14-7)

Aplastic Anemia:

- **Def.:** Syndrome of **chronic primary hematopoietic failure** resulting in **pancytopenia (anemia, neutropenia** and **thrombocytopenia)** Q
- Drugs implicated in aplastic anemia are mentioned in **Answer 79**

Ans. 81) A. Splenomegaly (Ref: 8 ed. Robbins p.664, 9 ed. p. 654)

Clinical Features of **Aplastic Anemia** Q:

- **Pancytopenia** Q i.e. neutropenia, anemia and thrombocytopenia
- **Splenomegaly** Q is characteristically **absent**
- **Reticulocytopenia** Q is the rule

Ans. 82) C. Aplastic anemia (Ref: 8 ed. Robbins p.664, 9 ed. p. 654-55)

- Presence of **splenomegaly** rules out **Aplastic anemia** Q

Ans. 83) A. Myeloid neoplasms (Ref: 8 ed. Robbins p.664, 9 ed. p. 654-55)

- **Aplastic anemia** can undergo transformation into **myeloid neoplasms**, typically **myelodysplasia** or **acute myeloid leukemia** Q

Ans. 84) B. Bone marrow biopsy (Ref: 8 ed. Robbins p.664, 9 ed. p. 654, f-14-25)

- **Diagnostic modality** of choice of **aplastic anemia** is **bone marrow biopsy** Q
- In **aplastic anemia, marrow** is **hypocellular**, whereas **myeloid neoplasms** are associated with **hypercellular marrow** Q

Ans. 85) C. Splenomegaly (Ref: 8 ed. Robbins p.664, 9 ed. p. 654-55)

- Refer to answer 84 and 85

Ans. 86) D. Bone marrow transplantation (Ref: 8 ed. Robbins p.664, 9 ed. p. 655)

- **Bone marrow transplantation** Q is the **treatment of choice** of **aplastic anemia**
- **Antithymocyte globulin** Q and other **immunosuppressive drugs** such as **cyclosporine** Q are effective in older patients or without suitable donors

Ans. 87) D. All of the above (Ref: 8 ed. Robbins p.664-65, 9 ed. p. 655)

Pure Red Cell Aplasia Q occurs in association with:

- **Thymoma** Q
- **Large granular lymphocytic leukemia** Q
- Drug exposures
- Autoimmune disorders
- **Parvovirus B 19** infection

Ans. 88) C. Both of the above (Ref: 8 ed. Robbins p.665, 9 ed. p. 655)

Myelophthisic Anemia [Q]:

- Form of **marrow failure** in which **space-occupying lesions** replace **normal marrow elements**

Causes:

- **Metastatic cancer** – Carcinomas of breast, lung and prostate
- **Infiltrative process (granulomatous disease)** [Q]
- **Spent phase** of **myeloproliferative disorders** [Q]

Ans. 89) D. All of the above (Ref: 8 ed. Robbins p.665, 9 ed. p. 655)

Marrow involvement in myelophthisic anemia leads to:

- **Leucoerythroblastosis** [Q] – Abnormal release of **nucleated erythroid precursors** and **immature granulocytic forms** into peripheral smears
- **Teardrop-shaped red cells** [Q] are seen

Ans. 90) A. Decreased synthesis of erythropoietin (Ref: 8 ed. Robbins p.665, 9 ed. p. 655)

Causes of Anemia in Chronic Renal Failure [Q]:

- **Decreased synthesis of erythropoietin** [Q] by **damaged kidneys (most common cause)**
- **Extra-corpuscular defect** that reduces **red cell life span**
- **Iron deficiency** due to **platelet dysfunction** and **increased bleeding**

Ans. 91) D. All of the above (Ref: 8 ed. Robbins p.665, 9 ed. p. 656)

Causes of Polycythemia Vera [Q]:

a) Relative Polycythemia [Q]:

- Occurs due to **hemoconcentration (decreased plasma volume)**

Causes:

- **Dehydration**, prolonged **vomiting or diarrhea**, or excessive use of **diuretics**
- Gaisbock syndrome

b) Absolute polycythemia [Q]:

- **Due to increased total red cell mass**

Causes can be Primary or **Secondary:**

Primary (Low Erythropoietin) [Q]:

- Polycythemia Vera
- Inherited erythropoietin receptor mutations (rare)

Secondary (High Erythropoietin) [Q]:

Compensatory

- Lung disease, High-altitude living, Cyanotic heart disease

Paraneoplastic

- Erythropoietin-secreting tumors (e.g., **renal cell carcinoma, hepatocellular carcinoma, cerebellar hemangioblastoma)**

Hemoglobin mutants with high O_2 affinity

Inherited defects that stabilize HIF-1α

Ans. 92) C. Polycythemia vera (Ref: 8 ed. Robbins p.665, 9 ed. p. 656, t-14-8)

Polycythemia Vera is an example of **primary polycythemia** [Q] and is associated with **low erythropoietin levels** [Q]

Ans. 93) C. Factor VIII (Ref: 8 ed. Robbins p.666, 9 ed. p. 656)

Prothrombin Time (PT) [Q]:

- Used to assess **extrinsic** and **common coagulation pathway**

- **Prolonged PT** results from deficiency or dysfunction of **factor V**, **factor VII**, **factor X**, **prothrombin**, or **fibrinogen** [Q]

Partial Thromboplastin Time (PTT) [Q]:

- Used to assess **intrinsic** and **common clotting pathways** [Q]
- **Prolonged PTT** can result due to deficiency or dysfunction of **factors V, VIII, IX, X, XI, XII, prothrombin, or fibrinogen** [Q]

Ans. 94) D. All of the above (Ref: 8 ed. Robbins p.666, 9 ed. p. 656-57)

Causes of **bleeding disorders** due to **vessel wall abnormalities** [Q]:

a) **Infections** [Q]:
   - Meningococcemia, infective endocarditis, rickettsioses
   - **Mechanism** – due to **vasculitis** and **disseminated intravascular coagulation**

b) **Drug reactions** – deposition of **drug-induced immune complexes** in vessel walls, which leads to **hypersensitivity (leukocytoclastic) vasculitis** [Q]

c) **Scurvy and Ehlers-Danlos syndrome**

d) **Henoch-Schönlein purpura**

e) **Hereditary hemorrhagic telangiectasia** (Weber-Osler-Rendu syndrome)

f) **Perivascular amyloidosis**

Ans. 95) B. AL (Ref: 8 ed. Robbins p.666, 9 ed. p. 657)

Perivascular Amyloidosis:

- Can weaken **blood vessel walls** and cause **bleeding**
- **Most common** with **amyloid light-chain (AL) amyloidosis** [Q]

Ans. 96) D. 20,000/μL (Ref: 8 ed. Robbins p.667, 9 ed. p. 657)

- **Thrombocytopenia** [Q] – When platelet count is **less than 100,000 platelets/μL**
- **Posttraumatic bleeding** [Q] – Can occur when platelet count occurs in range of **20,000 to 50,000 platelets/μL**
- **Spontaneous (non-traumatic) bleeding** [Q] – Can occur when platelet count is less than **20,000 platelets/μL**

Ans. 97) D. Any of the above (Ref: 8 ed. Robbins p.667, 9 ed. p. 657, t-14-9)

Causes of Thrombocytopenia [Q]

a) **Decreased platelet production**

Selective impairment of platelet production:

- Drug-induced: Alcohol, thiazides, cytotoxic drugs
- Infections: Measles, human immunodeficiency virus (HIV)

Nutritional deficiencies:

- B12, folate deficiency (megaloblastic leukemia) [Q]

Bone marrow failure:

- Aplastic anemia [Q]

Bone marrow replacement:

- Leukemia, disseminated cancer, granulomatous disease

Ineffective hematopoiesis:

- Myelodysplastic syndromes

b) **Decreased Platelet Survival**

Immunologic destruction [Q]:

Primary autoimmune

- Chronic immune thrombocytopenic purpura
- Acute immune thrombocytopenic purpura

Secondary autoimmune
- Systemic lupus erythematosus, B-cell lymphoid neoplasms
- Alloimmune: Post-transfusion and neonatal
- Drug-associated: Quinidine, heparin, sulfa compounds
- Infections: HIV, infectious mononucleosis (transient, mild), dengue fever

Non-immunologic destruction [Q]:
- Disseminated intravascular coagulation
- Thrombotic microangiopathies
- Giant hemangiomas

c) Sequestration
- Hypersplenism

d) Dilution
- Transfusions

Ans. 98) B. IgG class (Ref: 8 ed. Robbins p.667, 9 ed. p. 658)

Pathogenesis of **Immune thrombocytopenic purpura** [Q]:
- **Autoantibodies** are directed against **platelet membrane glycoproteins IIb-IIIa or Ib-IX** [Q]
- **Antiplatelet antibodies** are of **IgG class** [Q]

Ans. 99) C. Aplastic anemia (Ref: 8 ed. Robbins p.667-68, 9 ed. p. 657, t-14-9)
- Refer to answer 100 explanation

Ans. 100) A. Splenomegaly (Ref: 8 ed. Robbins p.668, 9 ed. p. 658)

Clinical Features of ITP [Q]:
- Characterized by **bleeding** into the skin and mucosal surfaces
- **Cutaneous bleeding** is seen in form of **pinpoint hemorrhages (petechiae)** [Q]
- **Ecchymosis** – i.e. confluent petechiae
- Easy bruising, nosebleeds, bleeding from gums and hemorrhage into soft tissues
- Disease may manifest with **melena, hematuria**, or excessive menstrual flow
- **Splenomegaly** and **lymphadenopathy** are not seen [Q]

Lab Findings [Q]:
- Low platelet count
- **Bone marrow**: Normal or increased megakaryocytes
- Peripheral blood show **large platelets**
- **Normal PT and PTT**

Ans. 101) A. Bleeding into the joints is a common manifestation (Ref: 8 ed. Robbins p.668, 9 ed. p. 658)

Diagnosis as given per history suggests Idiopathic Thrombocytopenic purpura

Bleeding in the joints is not a feature of **ITP**

Acute ITP [Q]:
- Commonly seen in childhood
- Seen in equal frequency in both sexes
- Symptoms appear **abruptly**, often 1 to 2 weeks after a self-limited **viral illness**
- Unlike chronic ITP, **acute ITP resolves spontaneously** [Q] within 6 months

Ans. 102) C. Spontaneous remission is common in Chronic ITP (Ref: 8 ed. Robbins p.668, 9 ed. p. 658)

Differences between Acute and Chronic ITP [Q]

	Acute ITP	Chronic ITP
Age	Children 2-6 years	Adults 20-40 years
Sex ratio	None	F:M::3:1 female
Antecedent infection	1-2 week prior	Unusual
Onset	Abrupt	Insidious
Bullae in mouth	Present	None
Platelet count	<20,000	50000-80000
Eosinophilia and lymphocytosis	Common	Rare
Duration	2-6 weeks	Months or years
Spontaneous remission	Present in 80%	Uncommon

Ans. 103) C. Bleeding time (Ref: 8 ed. Robbins p.668, 9 ed. p. 658)

- In **ITP, bleeding time is increased but clotting time is normal** Q

Ans. 104) D. Any of the above (Ref: 8 ed. Robbins p.668, 9 ed. p. 658)

Treatment of Chronic ITP Q**:**

- Excellent response to Glucocorticoids
- **Splenectomy** Q in patients with **severe thrombocytopenia**
- **Intravenous immunoglobulin** or **anti-CD20 antibody (rituximab)** are effective in patients who relapse after **splenectomy** Q
- **Thrombopoietin (TPO) mimetic** Q – Effective in stimulating platelet production and improving platelet counts

Ans. 105) B. Macrocytic anemia (Ref: 8 ed. Robbins p.669-70, 9 ed. p. 659-660)

Thrombotic Thrombocytopenic Purpura (TTP):

- Defined as **pentad** of **fever, thrombocytopenia, microangiopathic hemolytic anemia, transient neurologic deficits and renal failure** Q

Hemolytic-Uremic Syndrome (HUS) Q**:**

- Occurs frequently in **children**
- Associated with **microangiopathic hemolytic anemia** and **thrombocytopenia** Q
- **Acute renal failure** is a **prominent feature**
- **Absence** of **neurologic symptoms** Q

Ans. 106) A. vWF metalloprotease (Ref: 8 ed. Robbins p.669-70, 9 ed. p. 659-660)

- **TTP** is associated with **deficiency** in plasma enzyme called **ADAMTS 13**, also designated **"vWF metalloprotease".** Q
- **ADAMTS 13** degrades **very high-molecular-weight multimers** of **von Willebrand factor (vWF)** Q
- **Deficiency of ADAMTS 13** leads to accumulation of these multimers in plasma and tend to promote **platelet activation** and **aggregation** Q

Ans. 107) C. Neurological deficits (Ref: 8 ed. Robbins p.669-70, 9 ed. p. 659-660)

- **Neurological deficits** is a **characteristic feature** of **TTP** and **not HUS** Q

Ans. 108) A. E. Coli 0157:H7 (Ref: 8 ed. Robbins p.669-70, 9 ed. p. 659-660)

- **HUS** is associated with **normal levels of ADAMTS 13**

"Typical" HUS:

- Associated with **Escherichia coli strain 0157:H7** Q, which elaborates **Shiga-like toxin**

"Atypical" HUS:

- Associated with defects in **complement factor H, membrane cofactor protein (CD46)** or **factor I** Q

- Defects in these three proteins **prevents excessive activation** of **alternative complement pathway**

Ans. 109) D. Normal PT and APTT (Ref: 8 ed. Robbins p.669-70, 9 ed. p. 659-660)

- **Coagulation cascade** activation is **not seen** Q in TTP and HUS
- Coagulation tests, such as the **PT** and **PTT**, are usually **normal** Q

Ans. 110) D. All of the above (Ref: 8 ed. Robbins p.670, 9 ed. p. 660)

Bernard-Soulier Syndrome Q:

- Caused by **inherited deficiency** of platelet membrane **glycoprotein complex Ib-IX** Q
- **Glycoprotein complex Ib-IX** Q is a **receptor for vWF** Q and is essential for **normal platelet adhesion** to **sub-endothelial extracellular matrix** Q

Ans. 111) D. All of the above (Ref: 8 ed. Robbins p.670, 9 ed. p. 660)

Glanzmann Thrombasthenia Q:

- Transmitted as an **autosomal recessive** trait
- Occurs due to **deficiency of glycoprotein IIb-IIIa** Q
- Bleeding occurs due to **defective platelet aggregation** Q
- Platelets fail to aggregate in response to **adenosine diphosphate (ADP), collagen, epinephrine, or thrombin** Q

Ans. 112) B. Factor VIII (Ref: 8 ed. Robbins p.670, 9 ed. p. 660)

- **Vitamin K deficiency** Q results in the **impaired synthesis** of **factors II, VII, IX, X** and **protein C** Q

Ans. 113) A. Factor VIII (Ref: 8 ed. Robbins p.670, 9 ed. p. 661)

- Deficiency of **factor VIII** leads to **Hemophilia A** Q

Ans. 114) B. Factor IX (Ref: 8 ed. Robbins p.670, 9 ed. p. 661)

- Deficiency of **factor IX** leads to **Hemophilia B** Q

Ans. 115) D. All of the above (Ref: 8 ed. Robbins p.670, 9 ed. p. 661)

- **Vitamin K deficiency** Q results in the impaired synthesis of **factors II, VII, IX, X** and **protein C** Q

Ans. 116) D. Any of the above (Ref: 8 ed. Robbins p.670, 9 ed. p. 661)

- **Factor VIII** is produced in the **sinusoidal endothelial cells, Kupffer cells** in the **liver** and **tubular epithelial cells** in **kidney** Q

Ans. 117) D. Any of the above (Ref: 8 ed. Robbins p.670, 9 ed. p. 662)

vWF:

- Produced by **endothelial cells, megakaryocytes, α-granules** of **platelets** Q
- **Most important** function of **vWF** is to **promote the adhesion of platelets** to the **sub-endothelial matrix** Q

Ans. 118) D. 12 hours (Ref: 8 ed. Robbins p.670-71, 9 ed. p. 662)

- **vWF stabilizes factor VIII** Q
- **Factor VIII** has a **half-life** of about **2.4 hours** when it is **not bound** to **vWF** Q
- **Factor VIII** has a **half-life** of **12 hours** Q when bound to **vWF** in the circulation

Ans. 119) A. vWD (Ref: 8 ed. Robbins p.671, 9 ed. p. 662)

- **von Willebrand disease** Q is the **most common inherited bleeding disorder** Q of humans

Ans. 120) B. vWF deficiency (Ref: 8 ed. Robbins p.671-72, 9 ed. p. 662)

vWF Function:

- Assessed by **ristocetin agglutination test** Q

- Performed by mixing the **patient's plasma** with **formalin-fixed platelets** and **ristocetin** (which binds and "activates" vWF)
- **Ristocetin** induces **vWF multimers** to bind **platelet glycoprotein Ib-IX** Q and form interplatelet "bridges"
- Resulting **agglutination** of platelets is measured by a device called an **aggregometer** Q

Ans. 121) A. Ristocetin agglutination test (Ref: 8 ed. Robbins p.671-72, 9 ed. p. 662)

- Refer answer 123 for details

Ans. 122) D. All of the above (Ref: 8 ed. Robbins p.672, 9 ed. p. 662)

Treatment of patients having **von Willebrand disease** Q is done with:

- **Desmopressin** Q, which stimulates **vWF release** or
- **Infusions** of plasma concentrates containing **factor VIII** Q and **vWF** Q

Ans. 123) D. Any of the above (Ref: 8 ed. Robbins p.672, 9 ed. p. 662)

von Willebrand Disease:

- Patients have defects in **platelet function** despite a **normal platelet count** Q
- **Active vWF** (measured as **ristocetin cofactor activity) is reduced** Q
- **vWF stabilizes factor VIII**, thus it will lead to a **decrease in factor VIII levels** Q
- **Prolonged PTT**

Ans. 124) C. 30 % patients have no family history (Ref: 8 ed. Robbins p.672, 9 ed. p. 662)

Hemophilia A (Factor VIII Deficiency) Q:

- Caused by mutations in **factor VIII** Q
- Inherited as **an X-linked recessive trait**
- Affects mainly males and homozygous females
- **30%** of patients have **no family history** Q
- Patients with **less than 1% of factor VIII normal levels** have **severe disease** Q
- Patients with **2% to 5% of normal factor VIII levels** have **moderately severe disease** Q
- Patients with **6% to 50%** of **normal factor VIII levels** have **mild disease** Q

Ans. 125) C. Inversion of X chromosome (Ref: 8 ed. Robbins p.672, 9 ed. p. 662-63)

- **Severe hemophilia A** results from an **inversion** involving the **X chromosome** Q

Ans. 126) D. Petechiae (Ref: 8 ed. Robbins p.672, 9 ed. p. 663)

Clinical Features of **Hemophilia A** Q:

- **Easy bruising** Q and **massive hemorrhage** after **trauma** or **operative procedures**
- **Hemarthroses** Q **– Spontaneous hemorrhages** in the **joints**
- **Recurrent bleeding** into the joints leads to **progressive deformities** Q that can be crippling
- **Petechiae** are characteristically **absent** Q

Ans. 127) A. Normal PT, Prolonged APTT (Ref: 8 ed. Robbins p.672, 9 ed. p. 663)

- Patients with **hemophilia A** have **prolonged PTT** and **normal PT** Q, due to abnormality of the **intrinsic coagulation pathway**
- **Factor VIII-specific assays** are required for **diagnosis** Q

Ans. 128) A. Recombinant factor VIII therapy (Ref: 8 ed. Robbins p.672, 9 ed. p. 663)

Treatment of Hemophilia A:

- **Plasma derived factor VIII concentrates**[Q] can lead to transmission of **HIV infection**
- **Recombinant factor VIII therapy** is the **treatment of choice** for **Hemophilia A**[Q]

Ans. 129) B. Factor IX (Ref: 8 ed. Robbins p.672, 9 ed. p. 663)

- **Factor IX deficiency** produces a disorder known as **Christian disease (hemophilia B)**[Q]
- Hemophilia B is clinically indistinguishable from **Hemophilia A**

Ans. 130) D. All of the above (Ref: 8 ed. Robbins p.673-74, 9 ed. p. 663-664, f-14-27)

DIC:

- Characterized by **excessive activation** of **coagulation** pathways and **formation of thrombi**[Q] in microvasculature of the body
- Associated with **obstetric complications, malignant neoplasms, sepsis** and **major trauma**[Q]

Two major mechanisms that **trigger DIC**[Q]:

- Release of **procoagulant** i.e. **tissue factor**[Q] into the circulation
- Widespread injury to the **endothelial cells**[Q]

Tissue factor can be derived from **placenta**[Q] in **obstetric complications** or tissues injured by **trauma** or **burns**[Q]

Ans. 131) C. Normal platelet count (Ref: 8 ed. Robbins p.673-74, 9 ed. p. 663-664)

Laboratory Findings of DIC[Q]**:**

- Hypofibrinogenemia
- Elevated fibrin degradation products (**D-dimer** is the **most sensitive test**)[Q]
- Thrombocytopenia
- Prolonged prothrombin time

Ans. 132) D. Breast carcinoma (Ref: 8 ed. Robbins p.673, 9 ed. p. 664)

Cancers associated with **DIC**[Q]:

- **Acute promyelocytic leukemia**[Q]
- **Adenocarcinomas** of the **lung, pancreas, colon** and **stomach**[Q]

Ans. 133) A. Brain (Ref: 8 ed. Robbins p.674, 9 ed. p. 664)

- In **decreasing order** of frequency, **thrombus**[Q] in DIC are most often found in the **brain**[Q], **heart, lungs, kidneys, adrenals, spleen** and **liver**

Ans. 134) A. Adrenal (Ref: 8 ed. Robbins p.674, 9 ed. p. 664)

Waterhouse-Friderichsen Syndrome[Q]**:**

- In **meningococcemia**, **fibrin thrombi** in the microcirculation of **adrenal cortex** leads to **massive adrenal hemorrhages**

Kasabach-Merritt Syndrome[Q]**:**

- DIC occurring in association with **giant hemangiomas**

Ans. 135) D. All of the above (Ref: 8 ed. Robbins p.674, 9 ed. p. 664)

Clinical Features of DIC[Q]**:**

- 50% patients have **complications of pregnancy** as a **cause**[Q]
- **Acute DIC**[Q], associated with **obstetric complications** or **major trauma** presents with **bleeding diathesis**[Q]
- **Chronic DIC**[Q], as seen in **cancer** patients, present with **thrombotic complications**[Q]

Ans. 136) A. Febrile non hemolytic reaction (Ref: 9 ed. Robbins p. 665)

Febrile Nonhemolytic Reaction Q

- **Most common** complication of transfusion Q
- Presents with **fever** and **chills**, mild dyspnea, occurs within **6 hours** of **transfusion** of red cells or platelets Q

Ans. 137) B. IgA (Ref: 9 ed. Robbins p. 665)

- **Fatal allergic reactions** commonly occur in patients with **IgA deficiency** Q

Ans. 138) A. IgE (Ref: 9 ed. Robbins p. 665)

- **Urticarial allergic reactions** occurs due to the presence of **allergen** in the donated blood that is recognized by **IgE antibodies** Q in the recipient

Ans. 139) A. IgM (Ref: 9 ed. Robbins p. 666)

Acute Hemolytic Reaction:

- Caused by **preformed IgM antibodies** Q against **red cells** of the **donor**
- **Direct Coombs test** is **positive** Q
- Can progress to **DIC, shock, acute renal failure** and occasionally **death**

Ans. 140) A. IgG (Ref: 9 ed. Robbins p. 666)

- **Delayed hemolytic reactions** are caused by **IgG antibodies** Q that **recognize** previously sensitized **red cell antigens** in the recipient

Ans. 141) A. Neutrophils (Ref: 9 ed. Robbins p. 666)

Transfusion-Related Acute Lung Injury Q **(TRALI):**

- **Severe, fatal complication** of **transfused blood product**
- Triggers the activation of **neutrophils** Q in **lung microvasculature**

Ans. 142) D. Any of the above (Ref: 9 ed. Robbins p. 666)

TRALI has been **associated** with:

- **Plasma-containing blood products** Q
- Transfusion of **fresh frozen plasma** Q and **platelets** Q

Ans. 143) A. MHC I (Ref: 9 ed. Robbins p. 666)

- **Most common antibodies** associated with **TRALI** bind with **major histocompatibility complex (MHC) class I antigens (MHC I)** Q

Ans. 144) B. Platelet (Ref: 9 ed. Robbins p. 666)

- **Platelets** are stored at **room temperature**
- Also know that significant bacterial contamination is **more common** in **platelet preparations** Q than **red cell preparations**

Ans. 145) B. Hepatitis B (Ref: 9 ed. Robbins p. 666)

- **HIV, hepatitis C** and **hepatitis B** are **transfusion-related viruses** Q
- **Rates of transmission** of **HIV, hepatitis C** and **hepatitis B** are 1 in 2 million, 1 in 1 million and 1 in 500,000, respectively Q
- Thus, **hepatitis B** has highest transmission rate

Ans. 146) A. Antibodies of IgM class (Ref: 9 ed. Robbins p. 659) Refer: Ans 98 and 100 for details

Ans. 147) A. Factor VIII (Ref: 9 ed. Robbins p. 661) Refer Q 113 and Q 124-28 for details

Ans. 148) C. 1 to 6 degrees Celsius

- Recommend temperature for storage of blood is 1-6°C, which can be stored for 21 days)

Ans. 149) A. Supravital stain (Ref: 9ed Robbins p. 631)

- Supravital stains (Methylene blue and Brilliant cresyl blue) are used for staining reticulocytes

Ans. 150) C. 3 - 6% (Ref: 9 ed. Robbins p. 631)

Ans. 151) A. Bernard-Soulier syndrome (Ref: 9 ed. Robbins p. 660)

Ans. 152) A. Hyposegmented neutrophil

Ans. 153) D. Carcinoma kidney (Ref: 9 ed. Robbins p. 663-665) Refer Q 132 for details

Ans. 154) A. Extrinsic and common pathway (Ref: 9 ed. Robbins p. 656) Refer Q 93 for details

Ans. 155) A. Exposure to drugs (Ref: 9 ed. Robbins p. 653) Refer Q 79 and 89 for details

Ans. 156) C. Below (-25) degrees Celsius

Fresh frozen plasma must be stored in blood bank at or below -25 degrees Celsius

Ans. 157) A. Autosomal dominant (Ref: 9ed. Robbins p. 632 - 634) Refer Q 5 and 7 for details

Ans. 158) C. Cell membrane (Ref: 9ed. Robbins p. 642-643) Refer Q 29 and 30 for details

- Paroxysmal nocturnal hemoglobinuria occurs due to acquired defect in cell membrane

Ans. 159) A. GpIb-IX (Ref: 9 ed. Robbins p. 660) Refer Q 110 for details

Ans. 160) B. Sideroblastic anemia

Sideroblastic Anemia:

- Failure to completely form heme molecules
- Iron enters the mitochondria, but is not synthesized into heme
- Thus, iron, accumulates in mitochondria, giving a ringed appearance to Ringed sideroblasts
- Ringed sideroblasts are recognized on bone marrow by Prussian blue stain

Ans. 161) B. APTT (Ref: 9 ed. Robbins p. 663) Refer Q 123 for details

Ans. 162) B. Ankyrin (Ref: 9 ed. Robbins p. 632-34)

Ans. 163) B. Renal failure (Ref: 9 ed. Robbins p. 642-43)

Ans. 164) B. 11.5-14.5% (Ref: 9 ed. Robbins P.630-31) Refer Q 1 for details

Ans. 165) A. X chromosome (Ref: 9 ed. Robbins p. 662-63)

Hemophilia A:

- Characterized by deficient Factor VIII levels
- Most severe deficiencies occurs due to inversion involving the X chromosome, which leads to absence of factor VIII synthesis

Ans. 166) B. May-Hegglin anomaly (Ref: Clinical Hematology: Theory and practices volume 936 p. 213)

Döhle Bodies:

- Patches of dilated endoplasmic reticulum that appear as sky-blue cytoplasmic "puddles".
- Seen in : Burns, Infections, Physical trauma, Neoplastic diseases, Wissler's disease, May-Hegglin anomaly, Chediak-Higashi's syndrome

Ans. 167) B. No α chain (Ref: 9 ed. Robbins p. 641-42) Refer Q 27 for details

Ans. 168) A. Congenital defects of platelets (Ref: 9 ed. Robbins p. 660) Refer Q 111 for details

Ans. 169) B. Replacement of glutamate by valine in β chain of HbA (Ref: 9 ed. Robbins p. 635) Refer Q 11-15 for details

Ans. 170) C. Normal APTT (Ref: 9 ed. Robbins p. 663-664) Refer Q 130, 131 and 135 for details

Ans. 171) D. To be used within 30 minutes of having trauma

Fresh Frozen Plasma (FFP):

- Fluid portion of human blood that has been centrifuged, separated and frozen solid at -18°c within 6 hours
- FFP contains stable coagulation factors and plasma proteins: i) Fibrinogen ii) Antithrombin iii) Albumin and Immunoglobulin iv) Protein C, S v) Factor II, V, VII, IX, X, XI

Ans. 172) C. PNH (Ref: 9 ed. Robbins p. 642) Refer Q 29 to Q 32 for details

Ans. 173) D. PNH (Ref: 9ed. Robbins p. 635) Refer Q 8 and 16 for details

Ans. 174) A. CD 59 (Ref: 9 ed. Robbins p. 642) Refer Q 30 for details

Ans. 175) A. G6PD deficiency (Ref: 9 ed. Robbins 634-35) Refer Q 10 for details

Ans. 176) B. IgM (Ref: 9 ed. Robbins p. 644) Refer Q 40 for details

Ans. 177) B. Iron deficit (Ref: 6 ed. Postgraduate hematology p. 43-45)

- Sideroblastic anemia is characterized with an excess of iron in the bone marrow

Ans. 178) C. Myelophthisis type (Ref: 9 ed. Robbins p. 655) Refer Q 88 for details

Ans. 179) A. Hemolytic uremic syndrome (Ref: 9 ed. Robbins p. 644) Refer Q 43, 105, 107, 108 for details

Ans. 180) All of the above (Ref: 9 ed. p. 631-32) Refer Q 3 and 45 for details

March hemoglobinuria is an example of Microangiopathic hemolytic anemia

Ans. 181) C. Megaloblastic anemia (Ref: 9 ed. Robbins p. 645) Refer Q 52 for details

Ans. 182) A. Thrombotic thrombocytopenia purpura (TTP)

Ans. 183) A. Autoimmune hemolytic anemia (Ref: 9ed. Robbins p. 631-32) Refer Q 3 for details

Ans. 184) A. Beta thalassemia trait (Ref: 9 ed. Robbins p. 641) Refer Q26 for details

Ans. 185) C. GPI Anchored Protein (Glycosyl phosphatidyl inosital anchored proteins) (Ref: 9 ed. Robbins p. 642)

Refer Q 29 and 30 for details

Ans. 186) B. Malaria (Ref: 9 ed. Robbins p. 635) Refer Q 14 for details

Ans. 187) D. Sickle cell disease (Ref: 9 ed. Robbins p. 635) Refer Q 11 for details

Ans. 188) A. Normal platelet count with prolonged bleeding time

Ans. 189) A. Ristocetin Aggregation is normal (Ref: 9 ed. Robbins p. 662) Refer Q 120 and 123 for details

Ans. 190) A. Deletion of three alpha genes (Ref: 9 ed. Robbins p. 641-42) Refer Q 27 for details

Ans. 191) B. Glanzmann thrombasthemia (Ref: 9 ed. Robbins p. 660) Refer Q 110 and 111 for details

Glanzmann Thrombasthenia:

- **Can present as bleeding since birth (bleeding from the umbilical cord stump: as said in question)**

Ans. 192) A. Protein C

Inherited thrombophilia:

Predisposes to venous thromboembolism due to deficiency of any anticoagulant

Causes:

- Factor V Leiden, Prothrombin gene mutations are the most common causes
- Deficiencies in Protein S, Protein C and Antithrombin

Ans. 193) Factor XIII

Explanation:

- Cross-linking reaction is catalyzed by activated factor XIII

Ans. 194) C. vWF (Ref: 9 ed. Robbins p. 662) Refer Q 117 for details

Ans. 195) A. G.P.I. anchor protein (Ref: 9 ed. Robbins p. 642-45) Refer Q 29-35 for details

Ans. 196) A. Thalassemia (Hemoglobinopathies by Anupam Sachdev 1st ed. p.100)

- NESTROFT as a screening test for the detection of thalassemia and common hemoglobinopathies

Ans. 197) D. Mixed phenotypic acute leukemia

Immunophenotype pattern for B-cell lineage: CD10+ve and CD19 +ve

Immunophenotype pattern for myeloid lineage: MPO and CD117 +ve

Thus, it is bi-phenotypic leukemia as both B-cell and myeloid lineage tumor cells are there

Ans. 198) C. Anemia of chronic disease (Ref: 9 ed. Robbins p.652) Refer Q 70, 75-78 for details

Ans. 199) A. Plasmodium falciparum (Ref: 9 ed. Robbins p. 635) Refer Q 11 and 16 for details

Ans. 200) A. Increased reticulocyte count (Ref: Harrison 18th 865 - 866; Wintrobe's clinical hematology 12th 1151, Robbins 8 ed p. 655) Refer Q 52 for details

- **In megaloblastic anemia, reticulocyte count is decreased due to destruction of fragile and abnormal megaloblastic erythroid precursors**

Ans. 201) A. Von Willebrand factor (Ref: Robbins 8 ed p. 116-118)

- **Platelet adhesion to the endothelial surface is brought about by vWF-Gp Ib interactions**
- **Platelet aggregation is accomplished by fibrinogen bridging Gp IIb-IIIa receptors**
- **Factors promoting platelet aggregation:**
  1. **ADP**
  2. **Epinephrine**
  3. **Thromboxane A2**
  4. **Serotonin**
  5. **von-Willebrand Factor**
  6. **Fibrinogen**
  7. **Thrombospondin**
  8. **Collagen**
  9. **Immune complex**
  10. **Thrombin**

Ans. 202) A. DMT-1 (Ref: 9 ed. Robbins p. 650) Refer Q 68 for details

Ans. 203) C. Vitamin B 12 absorption

29

Miscellaneous

1) **Koenen tumor is seen in: (NEET 2014)**
   a) Neurofibromatosis
   b) Tuberous sclerosis
   c) Struge-Weber syndrome
   d) Tuberculosis

2) **Pearl's stain is used to demonstrate the following in tissues: (NEET 2014)**
   a) Hemosiderin b) Fat
   c) Reticulin d) Fibrin

3) **Most common fixative used in electron microscopy:**
   a) Glutaraldehyde b) Formalin
   c) Picric acid d) Absolute alcohol

4) **Flow cytometry is done on:**
   a) Polycythemia b) Thrombocytosis
   c) Basophil d) Lymphocytes

5) **Pendred syndrome occurs due to mutation of: (NEET 2014)**
   a) Bartillin b) Pendrin
   c) Fibrillin d) Reticulin

6) **Non-professional antigen presenting cell is A/E: (NEET 2014)**
   a) Endothelial cell b) Epidermal cell
   c) Fibroblasts d) Red blood cells

7) **Infra-clavicular lesion of tuberculosis is known as: (NEET 2014)**
   a) Assman's focus b) Puhl's focus
   c) Simmon's focus d) Ghon's focus

8) **RAST detects: (NEET 2014)**
   a) IgE b) Histamine
   c) IgG d) IgM

9) **Stain used for melanin: (NEET 2013)**
   a) Oil red
   b) Gomori methamine silver stain
   c) Masson fontana stain
   d) PAS stain

10) **Which of the following is a negative stain? (NEET 2013)**
   a) Nigrosin b) Fontana
   c) ZN stain d) Albert stain

11) **Slide fixing in pathology most commonly done by: (AIPGMEE 2011)**
   a) Formaldehyde b) Alcohol
   c) Picric acid d) Glutraldehyde

12) **The fixative used in histopathology: (AIIMS May 2012)**
   a) 10% buffered neutral formalin
   b) Bouins fixative
   c) Glutaraldehyde
   d) Ethyl alcohol

13) **About Bombay Blood Group, true is: (AIIMS May 2012)**
   a) Lack of A, B and H antigen on RBC
   b) Lack of A, B and H antigen in Saliva
   c) Lack of other Blood Group Antigens
   d) Presence of Anti-A, Anti-B and Anti-H antibody in blood

14) **Forward dispersion or scatter in flow cytometry signifies: (AIIMS May 2015)**
   a) Cell death b) Cell size
   c) Cell granularity d) Cell fluorescence

15) **Oil red O stain used for: (AIIMS May 2015)**
   a) Frozen specimen
   b) Glutaraldehyde specimen
   c) Alcohol specimen
   d) Formalin specimen

16) **What is the anticoagulant of choice for coagulation test? (AIPGMEE 2013)**
   a) 3.2% sodium citrate b) EDTA
   c) Heparin d) Sodium oxalate

17) **If you are in PHC, which anticoagulant is used to send the blood sample for blood glucose? (AIIMS Nov 2011)**
   a) EDTA
   b) Heparin
   c) Potassium Oxalate + sodium fluoride (NaF)
   d) Potassium Oxalate

18) **A patient presents with increase serum ferritin, decreased TIBC, increased serum iron, increased % saturation. Most probable diagnosis is: (AIIMS)**
   a) Anemia of Chronic disease
   b) Sideroblastic anemia
   c) Iron deficiency anemia
   d) Thalassemia minor

CHAPTER 29: MISCELLANEOUS

Ans. 1) B. Tuberous sclerosis (Ref: Neena Khanna 4 ed. p. 33)

Periungual Fibromas (Koenen's tumors):

- Present in 20% of patients of tuberous sclerosis and are seen in adult life
- Small, pink, sausage-shaped growths arising under the nail folds
- May lead to distortion of the nail plate

Ans: 2) A. Hemosiderin (Ref: Textbook of histopathology 4 ed. p. 662)

Perl's iron stain used for hemosiderin deposition in a tissue and imparts blue color to hemosiderin

Ans. 3) A. Glutaraldehyde (Ref: 7 ed. Bancroft Theory and practice of histological techniques p. 78)

- Preferred fixatives for electron microscopy – Glutaraldehyde and formaldehyde

Ans. 4) D. Lymphocytes

Ans. 5) B. Pendrin

- Occurs due to mutations in the PDS gene, which codes for the pendrin protein
- Gene is located on the long arm of chromosome 7 (7q31)

Ans. 6) D. Red blood cells (Ref: Internet)

- RBC's lack nucleus and are one of the cells in the body that cannot display antigens

Ans. 7) A. Assman's focus (Ref: 8 ed. Robbins p. 370)

Assman's focus: In secondary tuberculosis, the initial lesion is seen at the apex of lung (infra-clavicular) without involvement of any lymph node

Ans. 8) A. IgE (Ref: Patterson's allergic diseases p. 28)

RAST: Radioallergosorbent assay

- Method used to measure total as well as specific IgE against a particular allergen or a complex

Ans. 9) C. Masson Fontana (Ref: Bancroft's theory and practice of histological techniques. p. 248)

Most reliable methods for identification of melanin:

a) Masson-Fontana stain

b) Schmorl's ferric ferricyanide reduction test

c) DOPA reaction

Ans. 10) A. Nigrosin

Ans. 11) A. Formaldehyde

Ans. 12) A. 10% buffered neutral formalin

- Formaldehyde in its 10% neutral buffered form is the most common fixative used in diagnostic pathology
- Aqueous form of formaldehyde is formalin

Ans. 13) A. Lack of A, B and H antigen on RBC

Ans. 14) B. Cell size

Flow Cytometry

- Measurement of characteristics of single cells suspended in a flowing saline stream
- Properties measured include – particle relative size, granularity and fluorescence intensity

Forward Light Scatter:

Large objects (cell size) will refract more light than smaller objects (cell size) leading to high forward scatter signals

Ans. 15) A. Frozen specimen

Explanation:

Oil Red O is used to demonstrate the presence of fat or lipids in fresh, frozen tissue sections

Ans. 16) A. 3.2% sodium citrate (Ref: Dacie and Lewis)

Different types of Vacutainers and its uses:

Color of vacutainer cap	Anticoagulant used	Quantity of anticoagulant and blood	Use
Blue	3.2% Na_3 citrate	2.7 ml blood + 0.3 ml of anticoagulant (9:1)	Coagulation studies
Red	Not used	4 ml of blood	Serum studies
Green (contains Lithium Heparin)	-	4 ml of blood	Arterial blood gas analyses, Osmotic fragility test, Pyruvate kinase deficiency, G6PD deficiency
Lavender	K_2 EDTA	-	Routine hematological investigations
Grey	K_2 EDTA/oxalate and contains antimetabolite (NaF)	2 ml of blood	Blood glucose
Black	Na_3 citrate (3.8%)	1.6 ml of blood and 0.4 ml of citrate (4:1)	For ESR

Be thorough with the above table for answering such questions

Ans. 17) C. NaF + Potassium oxalate

- Potassium oxalate is used as a standard anticoagulant for glucose estimation
- But the RBC's in the sample continue utilizing glucose for glycolysis. This is inhibited by adding a glycolysis inhibitor i.e. sodium fluoride

Ans. 18) B, D (Ref: Clinical laboratory hematology by McKenzie)

- Total Iron Binding Capacity: total amount of iron in body, that can bind with transferrin present in plasma
- Transferrin saturation: Normally, transferrin binding sites are one-third saturated with iron (Serum iron/ TIBC X 100)

Please be thorough with the following table to deal with such questions:

Disease	Iron	TIBC/Transferrin	UIBC	% Transferrin Saturation	Ferritin
Iron Deficiency	Low	High	High	Low	Low
Hemochromatosis	High	Low	Low	High	High
Chronic Illness	Low	Low	Low/Normal	Low	Normal/High
Hemolytic Anemia	High	Normal/Low	Low/Normal	High	High
Sideroblastic Anemia	Normal/High	Normal/Low	Low/Normal	High	High
Iron Poisoning	High	Normal	Low	High	Normal